Older Adults: Physical, Mental and Social Aspects of Health and Well-being

Older Adults: Physical, Mental and Social Aspects of Health and Well-being

Editor: Freya Phillips

MURPHY & MOORE
www.murphy-moorepublishing.com

www.murphy-moorepublishing.com

MURPHY & MOORE

Cataloging-in-Publication Data

Older adults : physical, mental and social aspects of health and well-being / edited by Freya Phillips.
p. cm.
Includes bibliographical references and index.
ISBN 978-1-63987-407-1
1. Older people--Health and hygiene. 2. Older people--Physiology.
3. Older people--Health and hygiene--Psychological aspects.
4. Older people--Health and hygiene--Social aspects. 5. Aging. I. Phillips, Freya.
RA564.8 .O43 2022
362.198 97--dc23

Murphy & Moore Publishing,
1 Rockefeller Plaza,
New York City, NY 10020, USA

ISBN 978-1-63987-407-1 (Hardback)

Contents

Preface

This book was inspired by the evolution of our times; to answer the curiosity of inquisitive minds. Many developments have occurred across the globe in the recent past which has transformed the progress in the field.

A state of social, mental and physical well-being where infirmity and disease are absent is referred to as health. It can be promoted by encouraging various healthful activities such as physical exercise and by avoiding unhealthful activities like stress and smoking. Physical environment, social and economic environment, and the individual characteristics and behaviors of a person are the primary determinants of health. Other determinants of health are lifestyle, environmental and biomedical factors. All aspects of health of an individual are influenced by the genetic make-up of the individual. This book unravels the recent studies in the field of health and well-being of older adults. It presents researches and studies performed by experts across the globe. Scientists and students actively engaged in this field will find this book full of crucial and unexplored concepts.

This book was developed from a mere concept to drafts to chapters and finally compiled together as a complete text to benefit the readers across all nations. To ensure the quality of the content we instilled two significant steps in our procedure. The first was to appoint an editorial team that would verify the data and statistics provided in the book and also select the most appropriate and valuable contributions from the plentiful contributions we received from authors worldwide. The next step was to appoint an expert of the topic as the Editor-in-Chief, who would head the project and finally make the necessary amendments and modifications to make the text reader-friendly. I was then commissioned to examine all the material to present the topics in the most comprehensible and productive format.

I would like to take this opportunity to thank all the contributing authors who were supportive enough to contribute their time and knowledge to this project. I also wish to convey my regards to my family who have been extremely supportive during the entire project.

Editor

1

Chronic Disease Self-Management Education (CDSME) program delivery and attendance among urban-dwelling African Americans

Chivon A. Mingo[1]*, Matthew Lee Smith[2], SangNam Ahn[3,4], Luohua Jiang[5], Jinmyoung Cho[4,6], Samuel D. Towne Jr.[4] and Marcia G. Ory[4]

[1] *Gerontology Institute, College of Arts and Sciences, Georgia State University, Atlanta, GA, USA*
[2] *Department of Health Promotion and Behavior, College of Public Health, The University of Georgia, Athens, GA, USA*
[3] *Division of Health Systems Management and Policy, School of Public Health, The University of Memphis, Memphis, TN, USA*
[4] *Department of Health Promotion and Community Health Sciences, School of Public Health, Texas A&M Health Science Center, College Station, TX, USA*
[5] *Department of Epidemiology and Biostatistics, School of Public Health, Texas A&M Health Science Center, College Station, TX, USA*
[6] *Baylor Scott & White Health, Center for Applied Health Research, Temple, TX, USA*

Edited by:
Renae L. Smith-Ray, University of Illinois at Chicago, USA

Reviewed by:
Pankaja Desai, University of Illinois at Chicago, USA
Debra Evelyn Krotish, University of South Carolina School of Medicine, USA
Renae L. Smith-Ray, University of Illinois at Chicago, USA

***Correspondence:**
Chivon A. Mingo, Gerontology Institute, Georgia State University, P.O. Box 3984, Atlanta, GA 30302-3984, USA
e-mail: cmingo2@gsu.edu

Background: Older African Americans carry a disproportionate share of chronic diseases. The purpose of this study was to identify the characteristics of urban-dwelling African Americans with chronic disease participating in Chronic Disease Self-Management Education (CDSME) programs and to examine factors related to successful program completion (i.e., attending at least four of the six sessions).

Methods: Data were analyzed from 11,895 African Americans who attended a CDSME program at one of the five leading delivery sites (i.e., senior center, health care organization, residential facility, community location, faith-based organization). Logistic regression analyses were used to assess the associations of demographic, delivery site, and neighborhood characteristics with CDSME program successful completion.

Results: Approximately, half of the African American participants were aged 65–79 years, 83% were female, and 92% lived alone. Approximately, 44% of participants had three or more chronic conditions and 35% resided in an impoverished area (i.e., 200% below federal poverty level). Successful completion of the CDSME program was associated with being between the ages of 50–64 and 65–79 years, being female, living alone, living in an impoverished community, and attending a CDSME program at a residential facility or community center.

Conclusion: Findings highlight the unique patterns of attendance and delivery within the context of self-management interventions among this unique and traditionally underserved target population. Understanding such patterns can inform policy and practice efforts to engage more organizations in urban areas to increase CDSME program adoption. Particularly, employing strategies to implement CDSME programs across all delivery site types may increase reach to African American participants.

Keywords: African American, urban, chronic disease self-management, delivery site, evidence-based program

INTRODUCTION

Currently, over 43 million US residents are 65+ years of age with that number projected to increase to approximately 80 million by the year 2040 (1). Along with the overall growth of the aging population, a significant increase in the racial/ethnic diversity of this population is also occurring. Racial/ethnic minority populations are projected to increase to 20.2 million making up 28% of the aging population in 2030 (1). Specifically, between the years of 2012 and 2030, it is projected that the non-Hispanic African American population aged 65 years and above will increase 104% in comparison to the 54% projected increase for non-Hispanic Whites in the same age group (1).

The drastic increase in the number of older adults, particularly those from diverse racial/ethnic groups, is associated with burgeoning rates of chronic disease. Approximately, 50% of aging adults report two or more chronic conditions, and data show that the prevalence of having two or more comorbidities is higher among aging African Americans than other racial/ethnic groups (i.e., Whites, Hispanics) (2). Moreover, African Americans are more likely to be diagnosed with a chronic condition at a younger age and be more physically disabled than Whites (3). Although African Americans are at a greater risk for a chronic disease diagnosis and negative health outcomes associated with chronic conditions in comparison to Whites, African Americans are underrepresented in access to chronic disease self-management education programs as a result of a variety of biopsychosocial and sociocultural factors (e.g., racism, low socioeconomic status, discrimination, unequal access to goods and services, lack of trust in the health care system) (4–6). It is plausible that the context in which one experiences negative health outcomes may impact their perceptions about health, health behaviors, and disease management (7–9). However, very little attention has been given to cultural milieu and unique experiences for African Americans that may influence utilization, participation, and even completion of evidenced-based health prevention and management programs [e.g., Chronic Disease Self-Management Program (CDSMP)].

Considerable efforts have been made nationally to address issues surrounding the management of chronic illnesses among underserved and disadvantaged individuals (10–13). In fact, public health efforts have focused on reducing the burden of chronic disease for all and minimizing health disparities in chronic disease among racial/ethnic minorities by redirecting society's attention to the benefits of evidence-based health prevention and management programs. Notably, there has been a concerted effort by the US Administration on Aging, Centers for Disease Control and Prevention (CDC), and Centers for Medicare and Medicaid Services (CMS) to disseminate and implement Chronic Disease Self-Management Education (CDSME) programs nationally (14).

As a result, a national study of the CDSMP was conducted resulting in greater racial/ethnic diversity among participants than had been seen in previous research focused on self-management (10, 11, 13). Specifically, the national study included approximately 45% of participants who self-identified as African American, Latino, or other minority groups (11). Although substantial efforts to widely disseminate and implement the program have been made, there is still a great deal of information to be learned about how individuals living with multiple chronic conditions (MCC) successfully manage their conditions by participating in and completing evidenced-based self-management programs (e.g., CDSMP) and how this may vary by race/ethnicity.

While much has been written about national dissemination and implementation of the CDSME programs (10–12) as well as the benefits of completing a CDSME program (13), there is little empirical data that examine the effectiveness of the program or the unique predictors of participation and successful completion among African Americans with chronic conditions. Moreover, few studies have reported on completers (i.e., individuals who complete four out of six sessions) and non-completers (i.e., individuals who stop attending the program prior to completing four sessions) within this context. Thus, the fact that African Americans are already disproportionately affected by chronic conditions is made worse by the relative gap in what is known about the management of chronic diseases among this target population.

In addition to African Americans facing unique challenges (e.g., racism, discrimination, cultural mistrust) that may influence health behaviors, health status, and utilization of health care (4–6), African Americans living in urban areas may add another layer of complexity that is not well addressed or understood in the chronic disease self-management literature. African Americans who reside in urban areas often experience unique health-related vulnerabilities in comparison to Whites and other minority racial/groups. A significant proportion of African Americans reside in urban areas overwhelmed with violence, dilapidated housing, limited options for fresh fruits and vegetables, and in close proximity to toxic waste sites (15–17). Further, research has shown that specifically urban-dwelling aging African Americans have greater levels of disability as a result of chronic conditions in comparison to not only Whites but also aging African Americans living outside of urban areas (18, 19).

The aforementioned findings suggest the importance of extending CDSME research in an effort to understand the patterns of chronic disease management among urban-dwelling aging African Americans. Studying African Americans specifically in this context is a unique contribution to the literature in that African Americans embody cultural similarities but also intragroup differences. It is important for researchers, health care providers, and policy makers to recognize the vast array of characteristics that may be represented in aging African Americans in order to provide services that are appealing, feasible, and that lead to successful completion of effective behavioral health programs.

Therefore, the objective of this study is to (1) determine the characteristics of urban-dwelling African Americans with at least one chronic condition who participated in a CDSME program, and (2) determine factors associated with successfully completing the program.

MATERIALS AND METHODS

DATA SOURCE AND STUDY POPULATION

Cross-sectional data for this study was obtained from a nationwide delivery of CDSME programs as part of the American Recovery and Reinvestment Act of 2009 (i.e., Recovery Act) *Communities Putting Prevention to Work: Chronic Disease Self-Management Program* initiative (20). The US Administration on Aging led this initiative in collaboration with CDC and CMS to support the translation of CDSME programs in 45 states, Puerto Rico, and the District of Columbia (14). This initiative was originally designed to have 50,000 Americans complete CDSME program sessions between 2010 and 2012 and to embed CDSME program delivery structures into statewide systems (20). Based on the aforementioned unique challenges facing the target population, the focus of this study is on the 11,895 urban-dwelling African Americans who attended the program at one of the five leading delivery sites (i.e., senior center, health care organization, residential facility, community location, faith-based organization) and reported having at least one chronic condition. Specifically, 2,170 unique workshops were delivered to African American participants in this study. Of these workshops, 754 were delivered in senior centers/AAA, 518 in healthcare organizations, 479 in residential facilities, 242 in community/multi-purpose facilities, and 177 in faith-based organizations. Participants attending other sites were small in sample size and omitted from the analyses in this study. Institutional Review Board approval for this study was given by Texas A&M University.

PROGRAM DESCRIPTION

The CDSMP, a program included within a larger suite of Stanford's CDSME programs, has been introduced and widely disseminated in the US as a method to empower patients with self-management skills to deal with their chronic conditions (21). Drawing upon Social Learning Theory (22), CDSME programs are evidence-based, peer-led interventions consisting of six highly participative classes held for 2.5 hours each, once a week, for six consecutive weeks (21). During the tenure of these programs, participants receive a copy of the book, *Living a Healthy Life with Chronic Conditions, Fourth Edition* (23) as well as an audio relaxation CD titled *Relaxation for Mind and Body* (24). In addition, content for the workshops focus on teaching individuals ways to deal with frustration, isolation, pain, and fatigue. Furthermore, participants are taught how to develop an action plan to meet intended goals; how to develop an individualized exercise program; how to appropriately use medications; how to solve chronic disease-related problems; and how to communicate with family, friends, and health care providers. In particular, the CDSMP has resulted in improved health care (e.g., exercise, communication with physician) and health (e.g., pain, self-reported health, fatigue, disability, depression) (11–13), while potentially saving health care costs (25).

MEASURES

Independent variables

In an effort to identify characteristics associated with participating and successfully completing the CDSME program that are specific to urban-dwelling African Americans with chronic conditions, various measures (i.e., demographics, health status, delivery site types) were included.

Demographics. Participants were asked to self-report age (i.e., in years), sex (i.e., male or female), and living arrangement (i.e., living alone, living with others). In addition, residential ZIP Codes provided by participants were used to determine percentage of residents within the ZIP Code that fell below a 200% federal poverty level, and the percent of African American residents residing within the participants' ZIP Code.

Health status. Health status was determined using the participants' self-reported chronic conditions. Participants were presented with a list of chronic conditions (i.e., arthritis, cancer, depression, diabetes, heart disease, hypertension, lung disease, stroke, osteoporosis, other) and asked to indicate whether or not they had been diagnosed with each condition by a health care provider. The number of self-reported chronic conditions were summed to create one count variable, and the prevalence of each individual disease was calculated based on participants' self-report.

Delivery site type. Delivery site information was collected through administrative procedures. For the purposes of this study, analyses focused on the five leading delivery sites (i.e., senior center, health care organization, residential facility, community location, faith-based organization). Participants attending CDSME programs at any other delivery site types (e.g., workplaces, educational institutions, tribal centers) were omitted because of inadequate case sizes. Reports of participants attending the CDSME program at any delivery sites or delivery sites labeled as "other" were omitted from analyses due to the complexities of interpretation.

Dependent variable

Successful completion. Completion of the CDSME program was the dependent variable of interest in this study. Attending at least four of the six classes was considered successful completion of the program. This criterion is consistent with criterion used in previous work focused on the CDSMP (11, 12, 20).

STATISTICAL ANALYSIS

First, frequencies were examined to assess demographics, health status, and utilization by delivery site type among the total sample of urban-dwelling African Americans with chronic disease. Next, independent samples *t*-test, one-way ANOVA, and chi-square analyses were conducted to examine differences in sample characteristics by number of chronic conditions (i.e., one, two, or three or more chronic conditions) and by CDSME programs completion status (i.e., non-successful completion, successful completion). Specifically, independent samples *t*-test analyses and one-way ANOVA were used for continuous variables and chi-square analyses were used for categorical variables. Subsequently, a multiple logistic regression model was employed to determine the association between the independent variables (i.e., age, sex, living situation, number of chronic conditions, delivery site, poverty level) and successful completion of CDSME programs.

RESULTS

Descriptive statistics for the sample of urban-dwelling African Americans ($N = 11{,}895$) are displayed in **Table 1**. Descriptive statistics are presented for the total sample and stratified by the number of self-reported chronic conditions and CDSME program completion status. On average, participants were 68 (±12.06) years of age. The majority of the participants were female (83%) and lived with someone (92%). On average, participants reported having 2.5 (±1.41) chronic conditions with approximately 44% reporting 3 or more. Arthritis (50%), diabetes (48%), and hypertension (64%) were the three most commonly reported chronic conditions among the total sample. The largest percentage of participants attended the CDSME program at a senior center (37%) or residential facility (24%). Thirty-five percent of our sample resided in an impoverished area (i.e., 200% below federal poverty level).

When examining differences in characteristics across number of chronic conditions (i.e., one chronic condition, two chronic conditions, three or more chronic conditions), a statistically significant difference was found among the three groups on age, sex, living situation, disease prevalence, poverty level, and delivery site type. Notably, larger proportions of participants reporting three or more chronic conditions were ages 65–79 years (53%), female (86%), and living with someone (98%). As expected, larger proportions of participants who reported having any of the chronic conditions ultimately had more comorbidities. A larger proportion of participants who attended workshops at senior centers and faith-based organizations (40%, 16%; respectively) reported only one chronic condition. Conversely, a larger proportion of participants who attended a workshop at a health care organization or community center (17%, 13%; respectively) reported two chronic conditions. Lastly, a larger proportion of participants

Table 1 | Sample characteristics by number of chronic conditions and CDSME program completion.

	Total ($n = 11,895$)	1 Chronic condition ($n = 3,331$)	2 Chronic conditions ($n = 3,294$)	3+ Chronic conditions ($n = 5,270$)	X^2 or f	p	Non-successful completion ($n = 2,445$)	Successful completion ($n = 9,450$)	X^2 or t	p
Age (years)	68.46 (±12.06)	66.95 (±13.70)	68.46 (±12.21)	69.41 (±10.69)	42.57	<0.001	67.21 (±12.69)	68.78 (11.87)	−5.53	<0.001
Under 50	6.6%	10.8%	6.9%	3.7%	180.53	<0.001	8.4%	6.1%	35.89	<0.001
50–64	26.5%	25.5%	27.2%	26.8%			29.4%	25.8%		
65–79	49.7%	46.6%	47.8%	53.0%			46.0%	50.7%		
80+	17.1%	17.2%	18.1%	16.5%			16.2%	17.4%		
Sex										
Male	16.8%	22.1%	16.0%	13.9%	100.52	<0.001	19.6%	16.1%	16.69	<0.001
Female	83.2%	77.9%	84.0%	86.1%			80.4%	83.9%		
Lives alone										
No	92.3%	79.3%	97.3%	97.5%	1115.18	<0.001	96.4%	91.3%	70.28	<0.001
Yes	7.7%	20.7%	2.7%	2.5%			3.6%	8.7%		
Number of chronic conditions	2.53 (±1.41)	–	–	–	–	–	2.64 (±1.47)	2.51 (±1.40)	3.93	<0.001
1	28.0%	–	–	–	–	–	25.8%	28.6%	8.42	0.015
2	27.7%	–	–	–			27.8%	27.7%		
3+	44.3%	–	–	–			46.4%	43.8%		
Disease prevalence										
Arthritis	50.3%	14.9%	44.7%	76.3%	3139.78	<0.001	52.1%	49.9%	3.98	0.046
Cancer	7.4%	2.0%	4.9%	12.4%	369.93	<0.001	7.9%	7.3%	1.21	0.271
Depression	14.4%	3.1%	8.2%	25.3%	960.76	<0.001	18.1%	13.4%	35.38	<0.001
Diabetes	47.9%	34.8%	38.4%	62.1%	777.04	<0.001	44.2%	48.9%	16.87	<0.001
Heart disease	17.5%	2.3%	9.5%	32.2%	1465.08	<0.001	18.5%	17.3%	2.05	0.152
Hypertension	64.1%	26.3%	66.2%	86.6%	3234.57	<0.001	65.1%	63.8%	1.37	0.242
Lung disease	18.9%	3.9%	8.1%	35.2%	1651.38	<0.001	21.7%	18.2%	15.30	<0.001
Stroke	7.7%	1.3%	4.3%	13.9%	530.15	<0.001	8.6%	7.5%	3.67	0.055
Osteoporosis	10.0%	1.6%	5.3%	18.1%	729.44	<0.001	10.4%	9.8%	0.78	0.378
Other	15.0%	9.9%	10.4%	21.1%	276.60	<0.001	16.8%	14.6%	7.27	0.007
Percent of ZIP Code under 200% poverty level	34.59 (±8.22)	35.14 (±8.02)	34.33 (±8.21)	34.40 (±8.34)	10.73	<0.001	34.72 (±8.15)	34.55 (±8.24)	0.89	0.375
Percent of African American residents in ZIP Code	47.48 (±29.20)	47.80 (±29.49)	47.81 (±29.22)	47.06 (±29.01)	0.96	0.381	48.67 (±27.70)	47.17 (±29.07)	2.24	0.025
Delivery site type										
Senior Center/AAA	36.5%	40.0%	34.5%	35.6%	178.72	<0.001	31.2%	37.9%	82.70%	<0.001
Healthcare organization	15.5%	13.7%	16.6%	15.8%			18.0%	14.8%		
Residential facility	24.1%	18.6%	22.7%	28.4%			29.4%	22.7%		
Community/multipurpose-facility/library	11.2%	11.6%	12.5%	10.0%			10.6%	11.3%		
Faith-based organization	12.8%	16.0%	13.7%	10.2%			10.8%	13.3%		

who attended the CDSME program at a residential facility (28%) reported three or more chronic conditions.

Table 1 also reports differences in completion status across all independent variables. Significant differences in non-successful completion/successful completion were found across age, sex, living situation, number of chronic conditions, prevalence of disease by disease type, and type of delivery site. A larger proportion of participants who successfully completed the CDSME program were older ($p < 0.001$), female ($p < 0.001$), report living alone ($p < 0.001$), and report fewer chronic conditions ($p < 0.001$). A significantly smaller proportion of successful completers reported arthritis ($p = 0.05$), depression ($p < 0.001$), lung disease ($p < 0.001$), whereas a larger proportion of successful completers reported having diabetes ($p < 0.001$). There were no significant differences found in cancer, heart disease, hypertension, stroke, and osteoporosis disease prevalence between successful and non-successful completers. Lastly, significant differences were found across delivery sites between those who successfully completed CDSME programs and those who did not. A larger proportion of participants who successfully completed CDSME programs attended senior centers, whereas a smaller proportion of successful completers attended CDSME programs at other delivery sites (i.e., health care organization, residential facility, community center, faith-based organization) ($p < 0.001$).

Table 2 provides results of the logistic regression analyses. Compared to participants below the age of 50 years, being between the ages of 50–64 and 65–79 years decreased the odds of successfully completing the CDSME program [odds ratio (OR) = 0.71, $p = 0.001$ and OR = 0.85, $p = 0.025$; respectively). However, the odds of successfully completing the program increased for females (OR = 1.24, $p < 0.001$) and those that live alone (OR = 2.38, $p < 0.001$). Number of chronic conditions was not significantly associated with successful completion. Compared to senior centers, attending the CDSME program at a residential facility or a community center decreased the odds of successfully completing the program (OR = 0.70, $p < 0.001$; OR = 0.61, $p < 0.001$). In addition, living in an impoverished neighborhood reduced the odds of successfully completing the CDSME program (OR = 0.99, $p < 0.024$).

DISCUSSION

IDENTIFICATION OF SIMILARITIES AND DIFFERENCES

An initial research objective was to identify the characteristics of African American participants and the program delivery infrastructure that served them. In many regards, the urban-dwelling African American participants with chronic disease had profiles similar to participants seen in earlier CDSMP studies (11, 20, 26, 27). For example, participants were older, predominantly female, reported their most prevalent chronic conditions as hypertension, arthritis, and diabetes, and were more likely to participate in the program at senior centers, residential facilities and health care organizations. Notably, in our sample participating in CDSME programs at a residential facility was more prevalent than participating at a health care organization; the order of prevalence was reverse in the overall national level sample (20, 27).

Although the participants in our study were demographically similar in many ways to those in previous research describing populations and delivery characteristics, this study clearly demonstrates unique characteristics that are worthy of highlighting, and important to consider in policy, practice, and future research.

Table 2 | Factors associated with successful completion.

	OR	P	95% CI Lower	95% CI Upper
Age: under 50 years	1.00	–	–	–
Age: 50–64 years	0.71	0.001	0.578	0.863
Age: 65–79 years	0.85	0.025	0.738	0.980
Age 80+ years	1.02	0.763	0.897	1.160
Male	1.00	–	–	–
Female	1.24	<0.001	1.106	1.397
Live alone: no	1.00	–	–	–
Live alone yes	2.38	<0.001	1.892	3.007
Number of chronic conditions: 1	1.00	–	–	–
Number of chronic conditions: 2	1.04	0.454	0.932	1.172
Number of chronic conditions: 3+	1.05	0.365	0.944	1.171
Senior Center/AAA	1.00	–	–	–
Healthcare organization	0.92	0.280	0.785	1.073
Residential facility	0.70	<0.001	0.590	0.833
Community/multipurpose facility/library	0.61	<0.001	0.523	0.720
Faith-based organization	0.87	0.155	0.719	1.054
Percent of ZIP Code under 200% poverty level	0.99	0.024	0.988	0.999

OR, odds ratio; 95% CI, 95% confidence interval; attending fewer than four workshop sessions, referent.

Particularly, the burden of chronic disease among urban-dwelling African Americans cannot be ignored. While the ranking of chronic condition prevalence rates for specific disease type was similar to CDSME program participants in other studies (20), the actual prevalence rates for the individual chronic conditions were substantially higher. National prevalence rates indicate that irrespective of racial/ethnic group 21% of US community-dwelling adults report having three chronic conditions and approximately 5% report four or more (28). Overall, 44% of our sample reported having three or more chronic conditions. Moreover, our research findings indicated that participants with different comorbidity levels (i.e., one, two, three or more) participated in the CDSME program at different delivery site types. Specifically, larger proportions of participants who attended the CDSME at senior centers and faith-based organizations reported only having one chronic condition, whereas a larger proportion of those participating at a residential facility reported three or more chronic conditions. This is not overwhelmingly surprising in that residential facilities may be servicing individuals living within their community. Oftentimes, decisions to move into residential facilities particularly for aging individuals is predicated on disabilities and health challenges associated with common chronic conditions (29).

ASSOCIATIONS WITH PROGRAM COMPLETENESS

In addition to examining differences across chronic conditions, our study also closely examined differences in characteristics for successful completers and non-completers of the program as well as identified factors that were associated with successful completion. Results indicated that successful completers of the program were older than those who did not complete the program. However, the regression analyses showed that compared to participants below the age of 50 years, being between the ages of 50–64 and 65–69 years decreased the odds of successfully completing CDSME programs.

Considering that African Americans are diagnosed with chronic conditions much earlier in life in comparison to other groups (6), it may be that those between the age of 50–64 and 65–79 years have been dealing with the condition(s) for a longer period of time and either feel that they have learned how to successfully manage their health or have a perception that nothing can really be done for their condition. For example, in a study examining perceptions of arthritis, the authors found that individuals were less likely to believe a person diagnosed with arthritis could improve their condition with better health care (30). Perceptions of this type would make one more vulnerable to not completing the program. Studies have shown that the perception of chronic conditions and symptoms associated with chronic conditions influences health care decisions among African Americans (30, 31). In addition to age, a larger proportion of females and those living alone were successful completers. Moreover, being female and living alone increased the odds of successfully completing the CDSME program. Our findings on gender differences are consistent with findings in previous research (26, 32).

IMPLICATIONS FOR REACHING MALES

Due to the limited number of African American male participants and the findings highlighting gender differences in completion status, it is important to note the implications for the health of African American males. Unfortunately, the health of African American males has been likened to that of individuals living in developing countries (33). African American males fare worse than other segments of the population (e.g., African American females, Whites, and other racial/ethnic minority groups) on almost every chronic condition (33). While there is a dismal focus on African American men in chronic disease self-management research (13), our findings suggest that it is paramount that emphasis is put on empowering urban-dwelling African American men to engage in health promotion that would ultimately lead to positive health outcomes and providing other health-related benefits (e.g., symptom management, reduction of health care cost, reduction in emergency room visits, reduction in work disability) at both the individual and societal level.

ASSOCIATIONS WITH CHRONIC CONDITIONS

When examining health status in this study, individuals who completed the CDSME program had fewer total number of chronic conditions and reported lower prevalence rates of arthritis, depression, and lung disease. Interestingly, successful completers in comparison to non-completers reported higher rates of diabetes and no significant differences for the other conditions. Moreover, the total number of chronic conditions was not associated with successful completion. Erdem and Korda (26) reported similar findings in a study that examined characteristics of participants with diabetes who completed both the CDSMP and Diabetes Self-Management Program (DSMP). Future research is warranted to further examine the impact of MCC on participation and completion of behavioral health interventions.

ASSOCIATIONS WITH ENVIRONMENTAL CHARACTERISTICS

While there were no significant differences in successful completers and non-completers based on neighborhood level poverty, living in an impoverished community was associated with a lower likelihood of successfully completing the program. Research has consistently documented the association between socioeconomic factors and health, particularly highlighting the vulnerabilities of living in poverty (34). It is plausible that living in areas of concentrated poverty introduces additional barriers that may interfere with not only participating but completing health programs that are beneficial. As previously stated, a significant proportion of urban-dwelling African Americans live in impoverished areas that are associated with violence, poor housing, and limited access and availability to options that promote health (15–17).

To our knowledge, no research has closely examined the association of living in an impoverished community with completing the CDSME program among urban-dwelling African Americans. Findings not only suggest the need for future research in this area but also provide preliminary results that should be considered when implementing and disseminating the CDSME program in certain communities. Providing additional support that would foster increased completion rates of the CDSME program to residents of this community could lead to positive health outcomes for a population that is at risk for continued health and health care disparities.

ASSOCIATIONS WITH DELIVERY SITE

Finally, our analyses indicated that delivery site type is an important factor for urban-dwelling African Americans when considering program completion. Senior centers had the largest proportion of completers whereas faith-based organizations and community centers had the smallest proportion of completers. However, it is important to note among African Americans only that faith-based organizations and community centers had the smallest proportion of program participants. When examining the association between delivery sites and successful completion, findings indicated that the odds of successfully completing the program were significantly decreased if one attended the CDSME program at a residential facility or community center compared to attending the program at a senior center. Interestingly, there was no significant relationship between successful completion and faith-based organizations or health care organizations. This is in contrast to another study including participants from multiple racial/ethnic groups that found that completion rates for the CDSME program are lowest at residential facilities but highest at faith-based organizations (26). Other studies focused on delivery preferences of a self-management program among aging individuals who lived in an urban area have found that, in comparison to Whites, African Americans were more likely to prefer a self-management program that would be delivered at a local church or a health care organization (35). Notably, implementing programs within faith-based organizations have shown to be effective in increasing utilization of health promotion programs for African Americans (36–41). Therefore, the finding that faith-based and health care organizations have no association with successful completion may be more about reach and less about preference for participating or completing at that site type.

Therefore, one promising strategy for increasing the reach of CDSME programs may be to work more closely with faith-based organizations and health care organizations in urban African American communities. Embedding the program in existing infrastructures (e.g., church health ministry, senior ministry) may yield greater participation and completion of the program. Findings indicating that the odds of successfully completing the program are lowered for those participating at a residential facility or at a community center may be a result of a number of barriers. For example, residential facility participants may have a number of health complications resulting in the inability to successfully complete the program. Individuals participating in CDSME programs at a local community center may have other family responsibilities or transportation issues that could serve as a barrier to participating in a program for six consecutive weeks.

STUDY LIMITATIONS

Given that many of the measures were collected using self-reports, it is possible that participants may over- or underreport health status variables. However, self-report of chronic conditions is used as a valid measure in studies examining health in aging individuals (42). In addition, the cross-sectional nature of the data does not allow for us to determine a causal relationship between the independent variables and outcome variables. Although the delivery site type is available, lack of information concerning how participants were recruited to participate in the program is unavailable. It may not just be the differences in the types of delivery sites that result in significant differences in successful completion of the CDSME program, but also the methods that delivery sites use to initially recruit participants in the program. While lay leaders are trained to offer the program in a standardized manner, another limitation to consider would be unaccounted variance in program implementation that may or may not impact participants to remain in the program. Lastly, limited information is available about the lay leaders who served as instructors for the workshops. Therefore, an additional limitation of the study is the inability to examine the impact of instructor-level factors on completion rates (e.g., race, gender, age, health status).

CONCLUSION

The *American Recovery and Reinvestment Act Communities Putting Prevention to Work: Chronic Disease Self-Management Program* (14) has made a large public impact on the ongoing national dissemination and implementation of CDSME programs. The present study yields findings that can contribute to the ongoing research, practice, and policy efforts associated with this initiative. Particularly, our findings indicate that for vulnerable populations such as urban-dwelling African Americans, the influence of the individual, social, and environmental context in which one may experience CDSME programs must be considered. Strategies to encourage employment of CDSME programs across all available delivery site types can foster participation and completion. Working closely with health care providers and community gatekeepers to inform individuals about the availability and benefits of completing CDSME programs is one method for moving forward. In addition, considerations for program modifications that would still yield similar outcomes, but foster greater levels of completion should be discussed. Also, it is likely that putting policies in place that allow for allocation of resources that would provide support to individuals in impoverished communities may also yield positive outcomes. In summary, our study indicates that in order to increase reach and positively impact, a diverse population, practice, policy, and research strategies must consider the cultural milieu for African Americans that ultimately influence chronic disease self-management.

ACKNOWLEDGMENTS

Funding: The American Recovery and Reinvestment Act of 2009 (i.e., Recovery Act) Communities Putting Prevention to Work: Chronic Disease Self-Management Program initiative, led by the U.S. Administration on Aging in collaboration with the Centers for Disease Control and Prevention and the Centers for Medicare and Medicaid Services, allotted $32.5 million to support the translation of the Stanford program in 45 States, Puerto Rico, and the District of Columbia. The National Council on Aging served as the Technical Assistance Resource Center for this initiative and collected de-identified data on program participation. This study was supported by a grant from the National Institutes of Health, 5P30 AG015281, and the Michigan Center for Urban African American Aging Research.

REFERENCES

1. Administration on Aging. *A Profile of Older Americans.* (2013). p. 1–15. Available from: http://www.aoa.gov/Aging_Statistics/Profile/2013/docs/2013_Profile.pdf
2. Fried VM, Bernstein AB, Bush MA. *Multiple Chronic Conditions among Adults Aged 45 and over: Trends over the Past 10 Years.* (2013). Available from: http://www.cdc.gov/nchs/data/databriefs/db100.htm
3. Centers for Disease Control and Prevention. *Minority Health: Black or African American Populations.* (2013). Available from: http://www.cdc.gov/minorityhealth/populations/REMP/black.html
4. Becker G, Gates RJ, Newsom E. Self-care among chronically ill African Americans: culture, health disparities, and health insurance status. *Am J Public Health.* (2004) **94**(12):2066–73.
5. Dell JL, Whitman S. A history of the movement to address health disparities. In: Whitman S, Shah AM, Benjamins MR, editors. *Urban Health: Combating Disparities with Local Data.* New York: Oxford University Press (2011). p. 8–30.
6. Rooks RN, Whitfield KE. Health disparities among older African Americans: past, present, and future perspectives. In: Whitfield KE, editor. *Closing the Gap: Improving the Health of Minority Elders in the New Millennium.* Washington, DC: Gerontological Society of America (2004). p. 45–54.
7. McLeroy KR, Bibeau D, Steckler A, Glanz K. An ecological perspective on health promotion programs. *Health Educ Q* (1988) **15**(4):351–77. doi:10.1177/109019818801500401
8. Solar O, Irwin A. A conceptual framework for action on the social determinants of health. *Social Determinants of Health Discussion. Paper 2.* (2010). Available from: http://www.who.int/sdhconference/resources/ConceptualframeworkforactiononSDH_eng.pdf
9. Probst JC, Moore CG, Glover SH, Samuels ME. Person and place: the compounding effects of race/ethnicity and rurality on health. *Am J Public Health.* (2004) **94**(10):1695–703.
10. Smith ML, Belza B, Altpeter M, Ahn S, Dickerson JB, Ory M. Disseminating an evidence-based disease self-management program for older Americans: implications for diversifying participant reach through delivery site adoption. In: Maddock J, editor. *Public Health: Social and behavioral health.* Rijeka: InTech (2012). p. 385–404.
11. Ory MG, Ahn S, Jiang L, Lorig K, Ritter P, Laurent DD, et al. National study of chronic disease self-management six-month outcome findings. *J Aging Health* (2013) **25**(7):1258–74. doi:10.1177/0898264313502531
12. Ory MG, Ahn S, Jiang L, Smith ML, Ritter PL, Whitelaw N, et al. Successes of a national study of the chronic disease self-management program: meeting the triple aim of health care reform. *Med Care* (2013) **51**(11):992–8. doi:10.1097/MLR.0b013e3182a95dd1
13. Brady TJ, Murphy L, O'Colmain BJ, Beauchesne D, Daniels B, Greenberg M. A meta-analysis of health status, health behaviors, and health care utilization outcomes of the chronic disease self-management program. *Prev Chronic Dis* (2013) **10**:E07. doi:10.5888/pcd10.120112
14. US Department of Health and Human Services. *American Recovery and Reinvestment Act Communities Putting Prevention to Work: Chronic Disease Self-Management Program.* (2012). Available from: http://www.aoa.gov/AoA_programs/HPW/ARRA/index.aspx
15. Cooper RS. Health and the social status of blacks in the United States. *Ann Epidemiol* (1993) **3**(2):137–44. doi:10.1016/1047-2797(93)90126-O
16. Johnson BL, Coulberson SL. Environmental epidemiologic issues and minority health. *Ann Epidemiol* (1993) **3**(2):175–80. doi:10.1016/1047-2797(93)90133-O
17. Zenk SN, Schulz AJ, Hollis-Neely T, Campbell RT, Holmes N, Watkins G, et al. Fruit and vegetable intake in African Americans income and store characteristics. *Am J Prev Med* (2005) **29**(1):1–9. doi:10.1016/j.amepre.2005.03.002
18. Miller DK, Carter ME, Miller JP, Fornoff JE, Bentley JA, Boyd SD, et al. Inner-city older blacks have high levels of functional disability. *J Am Geriatr Soc* (1996) **44**(10):1166–73.
19. Miller DK, Wolinsky FD, Malmstrom TK, Andresen EM, Miller JP. Inner city, middle-aged African Americans have excess frank and subclinical disability. *J Gerontol A Biol Sci Med Sci* (2005) **60**(2):207–12. doi:10.1093/gerona/60.2.207
20. Ory MG, Smith ML, Patton K, Lorig K, Zenker W, Whitelaw N. Self-management at the tipping point: reaching 100,000 Americans with evidence-based programs. *J Am Geriatr Soc* (2013) **61**(5):821–3. doi:10.1111/jgs.12239
21. Lorig K, Holman H, Sobel D, Laurent D. *Living a Healthy Life with Chronic Conditions: Self Management of Heart Disease, Arthritis, Diabetes, Asthma, Bronchitis, Emphysema, and Others.* 3rd ed. Boulder, CO: Bull Publishing Company (2006).
22. Bandura A. Social cognitive theory of self-regulation. *Organ Behav Hum Decis Process* (1991) **50**(2):248–87. doi:10.1016/0749-5978(91)90022-L
23. Lorig K, Holman H, Sobel D, Laurent D, Gonzalez V, Minor M. *Living a Healthy Life with Chronic Conditions: Self-Management of Heart Disease, Arthritis, Diabetes, Depression, Asthma, Bronchitis, Emphysema and Other Physical and Mental Health Conditions.* Boulder, CO: Bull Publishing Company (2012).
24. Regan C, Seidel R. *Relaxation for Mind and Body: Pathways to Healing [CD].* Boulder, CO: Bull Publishing Company (2012).
25. Ahn S, Basu R, Smith ML, Jiang L, Lorig K, Whitelaw N, et al. The impact of chronic disease self-management programs: healthcare savings through a community-based intervention. *BMC Public Health* (2013) **13**(1):1141. doi:10.1186/1471-2458-13-1141
26. Erdem E, Korda H. Self-management program participation by older adults with diabetes: chronic disease self-management program and diabetes self-management program. *Fam Community Health* (2014) **37**(2):134–46. doi:10.1097/FCH.0000000000000025
27. Korda H, Erdem E, Woodcock C, Kloc M, Pedersen S, Jenkins S. Racial and ethnic minority participants in chronic disease self-management programs: findings from the communities putting prevention to work initiative. *Ethn Dis* (2013) **23**(4):508–17.
28. Ward BW, Schiller JS. Prevalence of multiple chronic conditions among US adults: estimates from the national health interview survey, 2010. *Prev Chronic Dis* (2013) **10**:1–15. doi:10.5888/pcd10.120203
29. Ball MM, Perkins MM, Hollingsworth C, Whittington FJ, King SV. Pathways to assisted living: the influence of race and class. *J Appl Gerontol* (2009) **28**(1):81–108. doi:10.1177/0733464808323451
30. Mingo CA, McIlvane JM, Haley WE. Impact of the diagnostic label of osteoarthritis on perceptions of disability and willingness to help a parent in African Americans and whites. *Arthritis Care Res* (2006) **55**(6):913–9. doi:10.1002/art.22352
31. Mingo CA, McIlvane JM, Haley WE, Luong M-LN. Impact of race and diagnostic label on older adults' emotions, illness beliefs, and willingness to help a family member with osteoarthritis. *J Appl Gerontol* (2013). doi:10.1177/0733464812471893
32. Hawkins J, Kieffer EC, Sinco B, Spencer M, Anderson M, Rosland A-M. Does gender influence participation? Predictors of participation in a community health worker diabetes management intervention with African American and Latino adults. *Diabetes Educ* (2013) **39**(5):647–54. doi:10.1177/0145721713492569
33. Gadson SL. The third world health status of black American males. *J Natl Med Assoc* (2006) **98**(4):488–91.
34. World Health Organization. *Social Determinants of Health: The Solid Facts.* (2003). Available from: http://www.euro.who.int/__data/assets/pdf_file/0005/98438/e81384.pdf
35. Mingo CA, McIlvane JM, Jefferson M, Edwards LJ, Haley WE. Preferences for arthritis interventions: identifying similarities and differences among African Americans and whites with osteoarthritis. *Arthritis Care Res* (2013) **65**(2):203–11.
36. Campbell MK, Demark-Wahnefried W, Symons M, Kalsbeek WD, Dodds J, Cowan A, et al. Fruit and vegetable consumption and prevention of cancer: the black churches united for better health project. *Am J Public Health* (1999) **89**(9):1390–6. doi:10.2105/AJPH.89.9.1390
37. Campbell MK, Hudson MA, Resnicow K, Blakeney N, Paxton A, Baskin M. Church-based health promotion interventions: evidence and lessons learned. *Annu Rev Public Health* (2007) **28**:213–34. doi:10.1146/annurev.publhealth.28.021406.144016
38. Irvin TM, Sutherland MS, Harris GJ. A faith-based arthritis self-help program for rural African Americans. *Am J Health Stud* (2006) **21**(2):107–14.
39. Darnell JS, Chang C-H, Calhoun EA. Knowledge about breast cancer and participation in a faith-based breast cancer program and other predictors of mammography screening among African American women and Latinas. *Health Promot Pract* (2006) **7**(3 Suppl):201S–12S. doi:10.1177/1524839906288693
40. Kerner JF, Dusenbury L, Mandelblatt JS. Poverty and cultural diversity: challenges for health promotion among the medically underserved. *Annu Rev Public Health* (1993) **14**:355–77. doi:10.1146/annurev.pu.14.050193.002035
41. Kotecki CN. Developing a health promotion program for faith-based communities. *Holist Nurs Pract* (2002) **16**(3):61–9. doi:10.1097/00004650-200204000-00011

2

The role of Session Zero in successful completion of Chronic Disease Self-Management Program workshops

Luohua Jiang[1]*, Matthew Lee Smith[2], Shuai Chen[3], SangNam Ahn[4,5], Kristie P. Kulinski[6], Kate Lorig[7] and Marcia G. Ory[5]

[1] *Department of Epidemiology and Biostatistics, School of Public Health, Texas A&M Health Science Center, College Station, TX, USA*
[2] *Department of Health Promotion and Behavior, College of Public Health, The University of Georgia, Athens, GA, USA*
[3] *Department of Statistics, Texas A&M University, College Station, TX, USA*
[4] *Division of Health Systems Management and Policy, School of Public Health, The University of Memphis, Memphis, TN, USA*
[5] *Department of Health Promotion and Community Health Sciences, School of Public Health, Texas A&M Health Science Center, College Station, TX, USA*
[6] *National Council on Aging, Washington, DC, USA*
[7] *Stanford Patient Education Research Center, Department of Medicine, Stanford School of Medicine, Palo Alto, CA, USA*

Edited by:
Sue Ellen Levkoff, University of South Carolina, USA

Reviewed by:
Xiaoguang Ma, University of South Carolina, USA
Nilesh Chandrakant Gawde, Tata Institute of Social Sciences, India

Correspondence:
Luohua Jiang, Department of Epidemiology and Biostatistics, Texas A&M Health Science Center, 219 SRPH Administration Building, TAMU 1266, College Station, TX 77843-1266, USA
e-mail: ljiang@sph.tamhsc.edu

Background: The Chronic Disease Self-Management Program (CDSMP) has been widely disseminated among various racial and ethnic populations. In addition to the six required CDSMP workshop sessions, the delivery sites have the option to offer a Session Zero (or zero class), an information session offered prior to Session One as a marketing tool. Despite assumptions that a zero class is helpful, little is known about the prevalence of these additional sessions or their impact on retaining participants in CDSMP workshops. This study aims to describe the proportion of CDSMP workshops that offered Session Zero and examine the association between Session Zero and workshop completion rates.

Methods: Data were analyzed from 80,987 middle-aged and older adults collected during a two-year national dissemination of CDSMP. Generalized estimating equation regression analyses were conducted to assess the association between Session Zero and successful workshop completion (attending four or more of the six workshop sessions).

Results: On average, 21.04% of the participants attended workshops that offered Session Zero, and 75.33% successfully completed the CDSMP workshop. The participants of the workshops that offered Session Zero had significantly higher odds of completing CDSMP workshops than those who were not offered Session Zero ($OR = 1.099$, $P = <0.001$) after controlling for participants' demographic characteristics, race, ethnicity, living status, household income, number of chronic conditions, and workshop delivery type.

Conclusion: As one of the first studies reporting the importance of an orientation session for participant retention in chronic disease management intervention projects, our findings suggest offering an orientation session may increase participant retention in similar translational efforts.

Keywords: attrition, retention, orientation session, evidence-based programs, chronic disease self-management program

INTRODUCTION

In recent years, an increasing number of interventions have been deemed highly efficacious in the prevention and management of chronic diseases in randomized clinical trials (1). To disseminate the findings of those clinical trials, the critical next step is to examine whether the research-based studies can be translated into effective community-based programs that can recruit and retain large numbers of participants with various chronic diseases. Program retention is often a challenge in controlled clinical studies (2), but it can be even more pronounced in large-scale implementation efforts of community-based interventions (3–5). Participant attrition not only threatens the internal validity and statistical power of a project, but also compromises the intervention benefits received by participants because of the lack of adequate intervention dose (6, 7). Less rigorously controlled than clinical trials, translational efforts pose special challenges for participant engagement. For example, grand-scale translational intervention efforts typically allocate fewer resources to intensively track and follow-up with participants over time, which may impact retention success.

To address problems associated with participant attrition, a wide range of studies have investigated factors related to retaining participants in clinical trials and observational studies (8–15). A previous meta-analysis identified 12 basic themes for successful retention in longitudinal studies, which include community involvement, contact and scheduling methods, and financial incentives (16). To date, however, the strategies for successful retention in translational initiatives remain underexplored (17, 18).

The Chronic Disease Self-Management Program (CDSMP) has been introduced and widely disseminated into US communities as a method to empower patients to deal with their chronic conditions by enhancing their self-management skills (19). Drawing upon Social Learning Theory (20), CDSMP is an evidence-based, peer-led intervention consisting of six highly participative classes held for 2.5 h each, once a week, for six consecutive weeks (19). In addition to the six workshop sessions, some delivery sites are offering a Session Zero (or zero class), an information session offered prior to Session One as a marketing tool (21). The primary purpose of Session Zero is to provide an overview of the workshop, explain expectations for workshop participation, and confirm commitment of those who are interested in or have already registered for a workshop. This additional session also serves as an opportunity to collect baseline data from participants to alleviate administrative burden on workshop instructors and ensure time is not taken away from Session One of the workshop. Although designed as a recruitment tool, we believe that incorporating a Session Zero to CDSMP workshops may boost participant retention rates because those who were not firmly committed to the workshop might decide to opt out of the program at this time. The goals of the current study are to (1) describe the proportion of CDSMP workshops that offered Session Zero and (2) examine the association between Session Zero and workshop completion rates.

MATERIALS AND METHODS

DATA SOURCE AND STUDY POPULATION

Data for this study were obtained from a two-year nationwide delivery of CDSMP as part of the American Recovery and Reinvestment Act of 2009 (i.e., Recovery Act) Communities Putting Prevention to Work: Chronic Disease Self-Management Program Initiative (22). The U.S. Administration on Aging led this initiative in collaboration with the Centers for Disease Control and Prevention (CDC) and the Centers for Medicare and Medicaid Services (CMS) to support the translation of CDSMP in 45 states, Puerto Rico, and the District of Columbia (23). This initiative was executed between 2010 and 2012 to embed CDSMP delivery structures into statewide systems (22). Within the first two years of this initiative, more than 100,000 adults participated in 9305 workshops in 1234 U.S. counties (22). For this study, administrative records were utilized to determine whether or not a Session Zero was held. Data were analyzed from 80,987 participants aged 50 years or older whose programmatic records contained data about Session Zero attendance.

MEASURES

DEPENDENT VARIABLE

CDSMP workshop attendance was the dependent variable for this study. As defined by the program developers and used in a variety of studies (24, 25), successful completion was defined as when CDSMP participants attended four or more of the six workshop sessions (22, 26), excluding Session Zero.

INDEPENDENT VARIABLES

Whether or not a workshop offered a Session Zero was recorded administratively and included in the database along with workshop attendance. Participants' actual attendance of a Session Zero was not recorded. If offered, the Session Zero was usually offered 1–4 weeks prior to the workshop and targeted those who had already registered or who might have shown an interest in the workshop. This orientation session was also used to recruit acquaintances and/or family members of those who already registered for the workshop. The specific content of Session Zero varied by site; however, all of them should have provided an overview of the CDSMP workshop and its expectations for participation. Session Zero may also be used to collect baseline data to reduce interference with Session One of the workshop.

Workshop delivery sites included area agencies on aging (AAAs), healthcare organizations, residential facilities, community or multipurpose centers, faith-based organizations, educational institution, county health department, tribal center, workplace, and other (e.g., recreational center).

Socio-demographic factors included age (in years), sex (male vs. female), median household income (in $10,000 units), and living arrangement (living with others vs. living alone). Participants' health status was measured by their number of self-reported chronic conditions (i.e., arthritis, cancer, depression, diabetes, heart disease, hypertension, lung disease, stroke, osteoporosis, and other chronic conditions).

STATISTICAL ANALYSIS

To compare the characteristics of the participants who attended workshops with a Session Zero and those who attended workshops without a Session Zero, we used χ^2 tests for categorical variables and two-sample t-tests for continuous variables. Because the participants were nested in workshops, generalized estimating equation (GEE) regression models were employed to investigate the association between successful workshop completion and Session Zero attendance. Specifically, the dependent variable of these regression models was successful workshop completion, while the independent variables were participant-level demographic and health characteristics. Furthermore, delivery site type was also included as an independent variable in the second GEE regression model. All the models included an exchangeable working covariance to account for the intraclass correlation among participants from the same workshop. Because the dependent variable is a binary variable; GEE analyses were conducted using SAS GENMOD procedure with a logit link function (SAS 9.3, SAS Institute, Inc., Cary, NC, USA).

RESULTS

Table 1 shows the proportions of participants who attended Session Zero and the workshop completion rates among the 10 types of delivery sites. Overall, 21.04% of the participants attended workshops with a Session Zero and 75.33% of participants successfully completed the CDSMP workshop. Among the 10 different types of delivery sites, the largest proportion of participants attending workshops with a Session Zero were at residential facilities (26.27%), while the smallest proportion of participants attending workshops with a Session Zero were at tribal centers (9.76%).

Table 1 | Session Zero attendance and CDSMP workshop completion rates by delivery site type.

Workshop delivery site	Total, *N* (%)	Attended workshops with a Session Zero (%)	CDSMP completion (%)
Senior Center/AAA	24,653 (30.44)	25.81	77.27
Health care organization	15,026 (18.55)	10.71	72.53
Residential facility	14,439 (17.83)	26.27	70.03
Community/multipurpose	8303 (10.25)	21.63	75.74
Faith-based organization	7127 (8.80)	22.25	78.88
Educational institution	1844 (2.28)	17.35	77.77
County health department	1013 (1.25)	19.64	69.89
Tribal center	205 (0.25)	9.76	69.76
Workplace	410 (0.51)	18.05	82.44
Other	7967 (9.84)	16.08	80.48
Total	80,987 (100.00)	21.04	75.33

CDSMP, chronic disease self-management program; AAA, area agency on aging.

With respect to workshop completion rates, workplaces had the highest completion rate (82.44%) and tribal center had the lowest completion rate (69.76%).

As presented in **Table 2**, CDSMP participants who attended workshops with a Session Zero had significantly higher workshop completion rate than those who attended workshops without a Session Zero (77.85% vs. 74.66%, $P < 0.001$). Participants who attended workshops with a Session Zero were more likely to be female, African American or other race group, Hispanic, and live alone. In terms of chronic conditions, they were more likely to have diabetes and hypertension, but less likely to have arthritis, cancer, depression, and lung disease. The average numbers of chronic conditions were not significantly different based on Session Zero status. Finally, the participants who attended workshops with a Session Zero were significantly older and had lower household incomes.

Table 3 illustrates the results of GEE regressions for workshop completion. As seen in Model 1, the participants of the workshops that offered Session Zero had significantly higher odds of completing CDSMP workshops than those who participated the workshops that did not offer a Session Zero (odds ratio [OR] = 1.087, $P = 0.003$). In addition, the likelihood of completing CDSMP

Table 2 | Baseline characteristics of CDSMP participants by Session Zero status.

	Total ($n = 80{,}987$)	Attended workshops without a Session Zero ($n = 63{,}946$)	Attended workshops with a Session Zero ($n = 17{,}041$)	*P*
Workshop completion	61,007 (75.33%)	47,740 (74.66%)	13,267 (77.85%)	<0.001
Female	59,669 (78.17%)	46,571 (77.47%)	13,098 (80.77%)	<0.001
Race				<0.001
White	45,673 (65.10%)	37,430 (67.63%)	8243 (55.64%)	
African American	15,929 (22.70%)	11,438 (20.67%)	4491 (30.32%)	
Asian/Pacific Islander	3057 (4.36%)	2511 (4.54%)	546 (3.69%)	
American Indian/Alaskan Native	1156 (1.65%)	969 (1.75%)	187 (1.26%)	
Other	4344 (6.19%)	2997 (5.42%)	1347 (9.09%)	
Hispanic	10,771 (15.78%)	7328 (13.49%)	3443 (24.74%)	<0.001
Living alone	10,968 (13.55%)	7868 (12.32%)	3100 (18.19%)	<0.001
Chronic conditions				
Arthritis	34,769 (42.93%)	27,672 (43.27%)	7097 (41.65%)	<0.001
Cancer	7585 (9.37%)	6135 (9.59%)	1450 (8.51%)	<0.001
Depression	16,729 (20.66%)	13,819 (21.61%)	2910 (17.08%)	<0.001
Diabetes	26,033 (32.14%)	19,453 (30.42%)	6580 (38.61%)	<0.001
Heart disease	13,480 (16.64%)	10,630 (16.62%)	2850 (16.72%)	0.753
Hypertension	36,531 (45.11%)	28,647 (44.80%)	7884 (46.26%)	<0.001
Lung disease	14,045 (17.34%)	11,231 (17.56%)	2814 (16.51%)	0.001
Stroke	4220 (5.21%)	3316 (5.19%)	904 (5.30%)	0.534
	Mean (±SD)	Mean (±SD)	Mean (±SD)	
Age	67.03 (±14.60)	66.58 (±14.79)	69.87 (±13.03)	<0.001
Median income	5.07 (±1.30)	5.02 (±1.27)	4.87 (±1.40)	<0.001
Number of chronic conditions	2.20 (±1.71)	2.29 (±1.71)	2.26 (±1.70)	0.060

CDSMP, Chronic Disease Self-Management Program.

Table 3 | Generalized estimating equation regression models for successful workshop completion.

	Model 1		Model 2	
	OR (95% CI)	*P*	OR (95% CI)	*P*
Session Zero offered	1.087 (1.030, 1.147)	0.003	1.099 (1.041, 1.161)	<0.001
Age	1.002 (1.001, 1.004)	0.003	1.004 (1.002, 1.005)	<0.001
Female	1.089 (1.039, 1.141)	<0.001	1.105 (1.054, 1.158)	<0.001
Race				<0.001[a]
White	0.989 (0.904, 1.082)	0.805	0.986 (0.900, 1.079)	0.751
African American	1.147 (0.904, 1.082)	0.007	1.133 (1.025, 1.251)	0.014
Asian/Pacific Islander	1.354 (1.179, 1.554)	<0.001	1.293 (1.126, 1.485)	< 0.001
American Indian/Alaska Native	0.916 (0.771, 1.088)	0.318	0.908 (0.760, 1.084)	0.284
Other	Ref	NA	Ref	NA
Hispanic	1.171 (1.087,1.263)	<0.001	1.145 (1.063,1.236)	<0.001
Living Alone	1.084 (0.977, 1.202)	0.127	0.930 (0.838, 1.031)	0.168
Median Income	0.979 (0.963, 0.994)	0.008	0.988 (0.972, 1.004)	0.128
Number of chronic conditions	1.005 (0.993, 1.017)	0.455	1.010 (0.998, 1.023)	0.093
Workshop delivery site				<0.001[a]
Senior Center/AAA			Ref	NA
Health Care Organization			0.837 (0.785, 0.893)	<0.001
Residential Facility			0.696 (0.655, 0.738)	<0.001
Community/Multipurpose			0.901 (0.835, 0.971)	0.007
Faith-based organization			1.150 (1.057, 1.251)	0.001
Educational institution			1.003 (0.871, 1.155)	0.968
County health department			0.797 (0.666, 0.954)	0.013
Tribal center			0.815 (0.559, 1.187)	0.286
Workplace			1.627 (1.166, 2.271)	0.004
Other			1.260 (1.158, 1.370)	<0.001

[a] *Overall Type 3 P value.*
AAA, area agency on aging.

workshops was higher among older participants (OR = 1.002, $P = 0.003$), females (OR = 1.089, $P < 0.001$), African Americans (OR = 1.147, $P = 0.007$), Asians and Pacific Islanders (OR = 1.354, $P < 0.001$), and Hispanics (OR = 1.171, $P < 0.001$). Conversely, the likelihood of completing the workshop was lower among those with higher household incomes (OR = 0.979, $P = 0.008$).

After adding types of delivery site into the GEE regression model (Model 2), we found participants of the workshops that offered Session Zero still had significantly higher odds of completing CDSMP workshops (OR = 1.099, $P < 0.001$). Furthermore, the average workshop completion rates were significantly different among different delivery site types ($P < 0.001$), with residential facility had the lowest likelihood of completing the workshop (OR = 0.696, $P < 0.001$) while workplace had the highest likelihood (OR = 1.627, $P = 0.004$).

DISCUSSION

The results of the current study show about one in five CDSMP workshops in this national initiative offered a Session Zero. Among the 10 delivery site types, senior centers/AAAs and residential facilities had the highest rates of offering a Session Zero, while tribal centers and healthcare organizations had the lowest rates. These differences might be related to variation in population subgroups served by each delivery site type (27, 28), as well as site staff availability and facility constraints (e.g., space, time, competing commitments).

As suggested in a review of lessons learned from the National Institute of Aging's Behavior Change Consortia (21), this study also demonstrates that participants who were offered orientation sessoins were more likely to complete intervention protocols. This finding indicates offering a Session Zero may not only facilitate participant recruitment, but also increase participant retention in grand scale community-based program dissemination efforts. Participants attending workshops with a Session Zero before the formal start of the workshop might have developed more support for and positive views of the program because they were given an opportunity to better understand the purpose, content, and expectations of the workshop. Meanwhile, attending a Session Zero may have given individuals who were not fully committed to the program a chance to re-evaluate their intention and opt out of the program if they felt they were not completely ready for it or thought it might not be beneficial for their preferences/needs. Therefore, the functions of a Session Zero with respect to retention might be twofold: (1) to strengthen the commitment of the participants by providing relevant information in advance and (2) to serve as a screening tool to identify those who are truly interested in the program and ready to participate. Future studies are warranted to study the details of these two potential functions of Session Zero.

Our results regarding the relationships between participants' demographic characteristics and retention are consistent with the existing literature (11–13, 29–32). Specifically, we found that older participants and females had higher workshop completion rates. The relationship between race/ethnicity and participant retention in previous studies are mixed, although most report minority populations were harder to retain (33), some have reported relatively lower attrition rates among Hispanic participants (8, 10, 34). Here, we found that African American, Asian Pacific Islanders, and Hispanic participants had higher likelihood of completing the workshop successfully. Differences in CDSMP workshop attendance rates by participant demographics may have been reflective of the type of delivery site at which workshops were attended. Other studies have shown that certain delivery sites attract and serve different community subgroups (22, 27, 28). For example, better workshop attendance among older participants may reflect that larger proportions of older participants attend CDSMP workshops at residential facilities (also with higher attendance rates).

The strengths of this study include a large sample size and diverse race and ethnicity representation included in the analysis. The large sample not only allowed us to have high power to detect relatively small differences and associations, but also implies potential good generalizability of our findings. Furthermore, the study sample included 16% Hispanics, 23% African Americans, 4% Asian and Pacific Islanders, and 2% American Indian and Alaskan Natives. The substantial diversity of the sample composition further supports the generalizability of these study results.

Despite the study's evident strengths, our findings need to be carefully interpreted in light of a few limitations. First, while data were collected that indicated whether or not workshops offered a Session Zero, participant attendance in these zero class sessions was not recorded. This means that participant attendance in a Session Zero could not be directly linked to their workshop attendance data. Second, these results were based on observational data, which limit our ability to determine a causal relationship between Session Zero attendance and CDSMP completion. Third, the number of variables collected at baseline was relatively small; therefore, although we were able to control for several important participant characteristics in the regression analyses, the identified associations in this study may be confounded by other unmeasured variables. Last, we were not able to investigate the relationship between Session Zero attendance and changes in health- and healthcare-related outcomes among these CDSMP participants because outcome measures were not available in this data collection effort.

In summary, including a Session Zero when delivering CDSMP workshops may be an important strategy for participant retention. Our findings suggest hosting a Session Zero may have implications for workshop attendance in similar translational efforts involving evidence-based programs for older adults. Given potential challenges associated with retaining participants in grand scale community-based interventions, offering a Session Zero before the formal start of the intervention might represent a feasible and efficient two-prong approach to help with participant retention in future translational projects.

ACKNOWLEDGMENTS

This work was supported by the Administration on Aging [90OP0001/03] and the National Institute of Child Health and Human Development [R01HD047143].

REFERENCES

1. Brady TJ, Murphy L, O'Colmain BJ, Beauchesne D, Daniels B, Greenberg M, et al. A meta-analysis of health status, health behaviors, and healthcare utilization outcomes of the chronic disease self-management program. *Prev Chronic Dis* (2013) **10**:120112. doi:10.5888/pcd10.120112
2. Warner ET, Glasgow RE, Emmons KM, Bennett GG, Askew S, Rosner B, et al. Recruitment and retention of participants in a pragmatic randomized intervention trial at three community health clinics: results and lessons learned. *BMC Public Health* (2013) **13**:192. doi:10.1186/1471-2458-13-192
3. Escobar-Chaves SL, Tortolero SR, Masse LC, Watson KB, Fulton JE. Recruiting and retaining minority women: findings from the women on the move study. *Ethn Dis* (2002) **12**(2):242–51.
4. Coday M, Boutin-Foster C, Goldman Sher T, Tennant J, Greaney ML, Saunders SD, et al. Strategies for retaining study participants in behavioral intervention trials: retention experiences of the NIH behavior change consortium. *Ann Behav Med* (2005) **29**(Suppl):55–65. doi:10.1207/s15324796abm2902s_9
5. Glasgow RE, Nelson CC, Kearney KA, Reid R, Ritzwoller DP, Strecher VJ, et al. Reach, engagement, and retention in an Internet-based weight loss program in a multi-site randomized controlled trial. *J Med Internet Res* (2007) **9**(2):e11. doi:10.2196/jmir.9.2.e11
6. Mody L, Miller DK, McGloin JM, Freeman M, Marcantonio ER, Magaziner J, et al. Recruitment and retention of older adults in aging research. *J Am Geriatr Soc* (2008) **56**(12):2340–8. doi:10.1111/j.1532-5415.2008.02015.x
7. King AC, Rejeski WJ, Buchner DM. Physical activity interventions targeting older adults. A critical review and recommendations. *Am J Prev Med* (1998) **15**(4):316–33. doi:10.1016/S0749-3797(98)00085-3
8. Hessol NA, Schneider M, Greenblatt RM, Bacon M, Barranday Y, Holman S, et al. Retention of women enrolled in a prospective study of human immunodeficiency virus infection: impact of race, unstable housing, and use of human immunodeficiency virus therapy. *Am J Epidemiol* (2001) **154**(6):563–73. doi:10.1093/aje/154.6.563
9. Williams PL, Van Dyke R, Eagle M, Smith D, Vincent C, Ciupak G, et al. Association of site-specific and participant-specific factors with retention of children in a long-term pediatric HIV cohort study. *Am J Epidemiol* (2008) **167**(11):1375–86. doi:10.1093/aje/kwn072
10. McGuigan WM, Katzev AR, Pratt CC. Multi-level determinants of retention in a home-visiting child abuse prevention program. *Child Abuse Negl* (2003) **27**(4):363–80. doi:10.1016/S0145-2134(03)00024-3
11. O'Brien RA, Moritz P, Luckey DW, McClatchey MW, Ingoldsby EM, Olds DL. Mixed methods analysis of participant attrition in the nurse-family partnership. *Prev Sci* (2012) **13**(3):219–28. doi:10.1007/s11121-012-0287-0
12. Anderson RT, Ory M, Cohen S, McBride JS. Issues of aging and adherence to health interventions. *Control Clin Trials* (2000) **21**(5 Suppl):171S–83S. doi:10.1016/S0197-2456(00)00075-1
13. Brown DR, Fouad MN, Basen-Engquist K, Tortolero-Luna G. Recruitment and retention of minority women in cancer screening, prevention, and treatment trials. *Ann Epidemiol* (2000) **10**(8 Suppl):S13–21. doi:10.1016/S1047-2797(00)00197-6
14. Manson SM, Jiang L, Zhang L, Beals J, Acton KJ, Roubideaux Y. Special diabetes program for Indians: retention in cardiovascular risk reduction. *Gerontologist* (2011) **51**(Suppl 1):S21–32. doi:10.1093/geront/gnq083
15. Jiang L, Manson SM, Dill EJ, Beals J, Johnson A, Huang H, et al. Participant and site characteristics related to participant retention in a diabetes prevention translational project. *Prev Sci* (2014). doi:10.1007/s11121-013-0451-1
16. Robinson KA, Dennison CR, Wayman DM, Pronovost PJ, Needham DM. Systematic review identifies number of strategies important for retaining study participants. *J Clin Epidemiol* (2007) **60**(8):757–65. doi:10.1016/j.jclinepi.2006.11.023

17. Rosal MC, White MJ, Borg A, Scavron J, Candib L, Ockene I, et al. Translational research at community health centers: challenges and successes in recruiting and retaining low-income Latino patients with type 2 diabetes into a randomized clinical trial. *Diabetes Educ* (2010) **36**(5):733–49. doi:10.1177/0145721710380146
18. Davis RM, Hitch AD, Nichols M, Rizvi A, Salaam M, Mayer-Davis EJ. A collaborative approach to the recruitment and retention of minority patients with diabetes in rural community health centers. *Contemp Clin Trials* (2009) **30**(1):63–70. doi:10.1016/j.cct.2008.09.007
19. Lorig K, Holman H, Sobel D, Laurent D. *Living a Healthy Life with Chronic Conditions: Self Management of Heart Disease, Arthritis, Diabetes, Asthma, Bronchitis, Emphysema and Others.* 3rd ed. Boulder, CO: Bull Publishing Company (2006).
20. Bandura A. Social cognitive theory of self-regulation. *Organ Behav Hum Decis Process* (1991) **50**(2):248–87. doi:10.1016/0749-5978(91)90022-L
21. Frank JC, Coviak CP, Healy TC, Belza B, Casado BL. Addressing fidelity in evidence-based health promotion programs for older adults. *J Appl Geron* (2008) **27**(1):14–33. doi:10.1177/1090198114543007
22. Ory MG, Smith ML, Patton K, Lorig K, Zenker W, Whitelaw N. Self-management at the tipping point: reaching 100,000 Americans with evidence-based programs. *J Am Geriatr Soc* (2013) **61**(5):821–3. doi:10.1111/jgs.12239
23. U.S. Department of Health and Human Services Administration on Aging. *ARRA – Communities Putting Prevention to Work: Chronic Disease Self-Management Program 2012 April 15* (2014). Available from: www.cfda.gov/?s=program&mode=form&tab=step1&id=5469a61f2c5f25cf3984fc3b94051b5f
24. Ory MG, Ahn S, Jiang L, Smith ML, Ritter PL, Whitelaw N, et al. Successes of a national study of the chronic disease self-management program: meeting the triple aim of health care reform. *Med Care* (2013) **51**(11):992–8. doi:10.1097/MLR.0b013e3182a95dd1
25. Standford University, Patient Education in the Department of Medicine. Available from: http://patienteducation.stanford.edu/programs/cdsmp.html
26. Ahn S, Basu R, Smith ML, Jiang L, Lorig K, Whitelaw N, et al. The impact of chronic disease self-management programs: healthcare savings through a community-based intervention. *BMC Public Health* (2013) **13**(1):1141. doi:10.1186/1471-2458-13-1141
27. Smith ML, Belza B, Altpeter M, Ahn S, Dickerson JB, Ory MG. Disseminating an evidence-based disease self-management program for older Americans: implications for diversifying participant reach through delivery site adoption. In: Maddock J, editor. *Public Health: Social and Behavioral Health.* Rijeka, Croatia: InTech (2012). p. 385–404.
28. Smith ML, Ory MG, Ahn S, Belza B, Mingo CA, Towne Jr. SD, et al. Reaching diverse participants utilizing a diverse delivery infrastructure: a replication study. *Front Public Health* (2015) **3**:77. doi:10.3389/fpubh.2015.00077
29. Bailey JM, Bieniasz ME, Kmak D, Brenner DE, Ruffin MT. Recruitment and retention of economically underserved women to a cervical cancer prevention trial. *Appl Nurs Res* (2004) **17**(1):55–60. doi:10.1016/j.apnr.2003.12.002
30. Warren-Findlow J, Prohaska TR, Freedman D. Challenges and opportunities in recruiting and retaining underrepresented populations into health promotion research. *Gerontologist* (2003) **43**(Spec No 1):37–46. doi:10.1093/geront/43.suppl_1.37
31. Chang MW, Brown R, Nitzke S. Participant recruitment and retention in a pilot program to prevent weight gain in low-income overweight and obese mothers. *BMC Public Health* (2009) **9**:424. doi:10.1186/1471-2458-9-424
32. Gappoo S, Montgomery ET, Gerdts C, Naidoo S, Chidanyika A, Nkala B, et al. Novel strategies implemented to ensure high participant retention rates in a community based HIV prevention effectiveness trial in South Africa and Zimbabwe. *Contemp Clin Trials* (2009) **30**(5):411–8. doi:10.1016/j.cct.2009.05.002
33. Probstfield JL, Frye RL. Strategies for recruitment and retention of participants in clinical trials. *JAMA* (2011) **306**(16):1798–9. doi:10.1001/jama.2011.1544
34. Smith ML, Ahn S, Jiang L, Kulinski KP, Ory MG. Factors associated with Hispanic adults attending Spanish-language disease self-management program workshops and workshop completion. *Front Public Health* (2015) **2**:155. doi:10.3389/fpubh.2014.00155

3

The reach of chronic-disease self-management education programs to rural populations

Samuel D. Towne Jr.[1]*, Matthew Lee Smith[2], SangNam Ahn[1,3] and Marcia G. Ory[1]

[1] Department of Health Promotion and Community Health Sciences, Texas A&M Health Science Center, School of Public Health, College Station, TX, USA
[2] Department of Health Promotion and Behavior, College of Public Health, University of Georgia, Athens, GA, USA
[3] Division of Health Systems Management and Policy, School of Public Health, The University of Memphis, Memphis, TN, USA

Edited by:
Renae L. Smith-Ray, University of Illinois at Chicago, USA

Reviewed by:
Jim P. Stimpson, University of Nebraska Medical Center, USA
Pankaja Desai, University of Illinois at Chicago, USA
Jo Ann Shoup, Kaiser Permanente Colorado, USA
Renae L. Smith-Ray, University of Illinois at Chicago, USA

***Correspondence:**
Samuel D. Towne Jr., Department of Health Promotion and Community Health Sciences, Texas A&M Health Science Center, School of Public Health, 1266 TAMU, College Station, TX 77843/1266, USA
e-mail: towne@sph.tamhsc.edu

This study assessed the sociodemographic characteristics of rural residents who participated in chronic-disease self-management education (CDSME) program workshops and the extent to which CDSME programs were utilized by those with limited access to health care services. We analyzed data from the first 100,000 adults who attended CDSME program workshops during a national dissemination spanning 45 states, the District of Columbia, and Puerto Rico. Approximately 24% of participants lived in rural areas. Overall, 42% of all participants were minorities; urban areas reached more minority participants (48%) than rural areas (25%). The average age of participants was high in rural (age, $\mu = 66.1$) and urban (age, $\mu = 67.3$) areas. In addition, the average number of chronic conditions was higher ($p < 0.01$) in rural ($\mu = 2.6$ conditions) versus urban ($\mu = 2.4$ conditions) areas. Successful completion of CDSME programs (i.e., attending four or more of the six workshop sessions) was higher ($p < 0.01$) in rural versus urban areas (78% versus 77%). Factors associated with higher likelihood of successful completion of CDSME programs included being Black (OR = 1.25) versus White and living in rural (versus urban) areas (OR = 1.09). Factors associated with lower likelihood of successful completion included being male (OR = 0.92) and residing in a primary care Health Professional Shortage Area or HPSA (versus a non-HPSA) (OR = 0.93). Findings highlight the capability of CDSME programs to reach rural residents, yet dissemination efforts can be further enhanced to ensure minorities and individuals in a HPSA utilize this program. Tailored strategies are needed to increase participant recruitment and retention in rural areas to overcome traditional barriers to health service access.

Keywords: chronic-disease self-management, evidence-based program, rural, intervention dose, older adults

INTRODUCTION

While it is known that individuals with chronic diseases are more likely to utilize health care services (1–3), we are still learning about their use of health promotion resources available in community settings. Further, less is known about the unique community characteristics and infrastructures that influence the delivery and adoption of evidence-based chronic-disease self-management education (CDSME) programs in traditionally underserved areas and populations.

Compared to metropolitan or urban areas, there is limited research about aging in rural areas. And, studies about rural populations are primarily demographic or epidemiological in focus. Disproportionately, more older adults live in rural areas (15% in rural, 12% in urban) (4), and rural areas have less health care service availability and fewer health care providers compared to urban areas (5–7). Relative to those living in urban areas, rural area residents are disproportionately affected by poor health outcomes and health care access barriers, which contributes to them having higher disease rates, disability rates, and risk factors for poor health outcomes (8–10).

Studies have shown that rural areas traditionally encounter geographic barriers limiting access to health care resources, as exemplified by areas designed as rural highly overlapping with health professional shortage area (HPSA) and medically underserved area designations (11, 12). Using geographic information systems (GIS), researchers have identified geospatial barriers hindering rural area residents, especially minority older adults, from accessing resources (e.g., longer distances, lower availability of health care providers) (13).

Prior research has documented the benefits of delivering evidence-based programs (EBP) in rural communities [e.g., improving health-related outcomes (14), falls efficacy (15)]. However, the extent to which CDSME programs are delivered in rural areas remains unknown. Because of the known effectiveness of CDSME programs (e.g., improved health outcomes, lower hospitalization, better chronic-disease management) (16–19), it is important to identify whether residents of rural areas have access to these EBP, especially in vulnerable rural areas with fewer health-related resources and services. Additionally, even when EBP are available in rural areas, it is important to assess whether or not participants in these areas attend enough sessions to receive adequate intervention dose. This is especially important considering individuals in rural areas may have greater distances to resources (e.g., health care resources), which may act as a barrier to program participation (8, 13).

As such, the objectives of this study were to: (1) assess the extent to which CDSME programs were utilized by rural residents and identify characteristics of these rural residents as compared to their urban counterparts; (2) investigate the geographic distribution of CDSME program participation based on the rurality of participants' residence; and (3) examine factors associated with successful workshop completion.

MATERIALS AND METHODS

PROGRAM DESCRIPTION

With the goal of improving self-management skills among adults with chronic conditions, CDSME programs have been widely delivered across the US (20). The CDSME program suite of evidence-based self-management programs, developed at Stanford University Patient Education Research Center, uses the Social Learning Theory (21) to deliver these peer-led interventions (i.e., six sessions, once a week at 2.5 h each for six consecutive weeks) (20). The results of participation in this program include improved health, health care utilization (e.g., lower rate of hospitalizations) (19, 22), and health care cost savings (23).

DATA SOURCE AND STUDY POPULATION

We conducted a cross-sectional analysis using data collected via the national delivery (45 states, Puerto Rico, and the District of Columbia) (24) of the CDSME programs. As part of the American Recovery and Reinvestment Act of 2009, CDSME programs were delivered via the *Communities Putting Prevention to Work: Chronic-Disease Self-Management Program* initiative led by the US Administration on Aging in partnership with the Centers for Disease Control and Prevention (CDC) and the Centers for Medicare and Medicaid Services (CMS) (25). Analyses were conducted using data on the first 100,000 participants targeted in this initiative (25). Institutional Review Board approval for this study was given by Texas A&M University.

MEASURES

Geospatial variables

Geospatial analyses were those examining differences across rurality. We were interested in characterizing participants and delivery sites by rural and urban categories. To accomplish this, the 2013 Area Health Resource File (AHRF) was used to identify geographic characteristics (i.e., rural residency, health professional resources) (26). We defined rurality based on county and separately ZCTA (ZIP Code Tabulation Areas)/ZIP Codes. For counties, urban influence codes (UIC) were merged with data from the National Council on Aging (NCOA) using Federal Information Processing Standards (FIPS) Codes. We compare results using both county and ZIP Code levels of rurality. We used county-level rurality in fully adjusted analyses. We dichotomized UIC into Metropolitan (UIC = 1–2) and Non-Metropolitan (UIC = 3–12) (27). For ZCTA/ZIP Codes, we merged Rural-Urban Commuting Area Codes (RUCA) into urban and non-urban (large rural cities, small rural towns, isolated small rural towns) areas (28). We also coded rurality into more than a two-way split (i.e., rural and urban). We coded rurality into a 4-way split including *Urban, Large Rural City/Town, Small Rural Town,* and *Isolated Small Rural Town.* These multiple rurality measurements allowed us to identify differences within rural areas with a greater degree of specificity in selected analysis.

Primary Care HPSA are defined based on geographic area, population groups, and facilities, with more detailed definitions available from the Health Resources Services Administration (HRSA) (http://www.hrsa.gov/shortage/) (29). Primary Care HPSAs were defined as either full, partial, or non-HPSA at the county level. A full-HPSA is defined as an entire county designated as a HPSA versus partial-HPSA. A non-HPSA is a county not designated as a HPSA.

Areas served by CDSME were defined as unique ZCTA/ZIP codes where at least one participant was located. These were spread nationwide throughout 9,599 unique ZCTA/ZIP Codes.

Dependent variable

Our primary dependent variable was successful workshop completion. Participant's attendance was recorded to determine if adequate intervention dose was received. As defined by the program developers, a participant has "successfully" completed the program if they attended four or more of the six offered workshop sessions (19, 22, 25, 30).

Sociodemographics

Personal characteristics of the participants included age, sex, and race/ethnicity. We used one variable for race and ethnicity with categories of non-Hispanic White, non-Hispanic Black or African American, non-Hispanic Native American or Alaskan Native, non-Hispanic Asian American, and "other" race/ethnicity category (including non-Hispanic Native Hawaiian or other Pacific Islander, those identified as "other," and those identified as belonging to multiple race/ethnic groups), and Hispanic. We also included living arrangement to specify whether participants lived alone or lived with others.

The number of chronic conditions among participants was identified as having any one or more of the following chronic diseases: diabetes, heart disease, hypertension, lung disease, arthritis, cancer, or "other" (another chronic disease). We summed the number of chronic diseases into one variable and grouped it into the following categories: one condition, two conditions, three conditions, four conditions, and five or more conditions (due to small sample sizes with six chronic conditions).

Statistical analyses

We conducted analyses on the first 100,000 participants reached in this initiative who had observations with complete data on all variables of interest. Those with missing data for age ($n = 12,447$), sex ($n = 8,826$), race/ethnicity ($n = 12,124$), living arrangement ($n = 1,605$), number of chronic conditions ($n = 1,539$), and geographic identifiers ($n = 12,314$) were omitted. Some participants had more than one of these exclusionary characteristics. Therefore our final sample size was 82,044. Analyses on observations with missing information (e.g., missing rurality) were not conducted because our primary goal was to measure outcomes across study characteristics (e.g., rurality). We did not attempt to measure program success independent of study characteristics.

We used independent sample t-tests and Chi Square for bivariate comparisons. Logistic regression analyses were used to investigate factors associated with successful workshop completion. We used logistic regression to predict the dichotomous outcome of successful completion (versus not attending at least four of the six workshop sessions). Fully adjusted analyses (logistic regression) includes participant race/ethnicity, rurality (county-level), HPSA status, participant sex, living arrangement (living alone or not), participant age, and the number of chronic conditions. SAS version 9.4 was used for all analysis (31). ArcGIS version 10.2 was used for mapping (32).

RESULTS

Overall, 1,721 counties throughout the US had a CDSME program available to residents, while 1,421 counties did not offer a CDSME workshop. There were 922 rural counties and 799 urban counties offering CDSME workshops. Rural counties without a CDSME workshop totaled 1,130 versus 291 for urban counties. Here, 74.3% of areas lacking a CDSME workshop were rural. Some states had more workshop clustering, and others had wider coverage throughout the states (e.g., South Carolina and North Carolina). The distribution of rural CDSME program participants varied across the US (see **Figure 1**). Analysis across rurality indicated that approximately 22.1% (using county-level rurality) to 24.4% (using ZCTA/ZIP Code-level rurality) of CDSME program participants resided in rural areas.

Characteristics of participants across rurality are provided in **Table 1**. Age ranged from 18 to over a 100 across all observations. The bulk of participants were female (approximately 78.0%). Approximately 48.9% of participants lived alone. In general, participants had at least two chronic conditions, where the average number of chronic conditions was 2.5.

When compared by the geography of residence, participants residing in rural areas were younger ($p < 0.01$) on average compared to those in urban areas (approximately 66.1 years versus 67.3 years). The percent of individuals living alone was higher ($p < 0.01$) in rural areas (i.e., ranging from 52.1 to 52.6% in rural areas versus 47.9 to 47.8% in urban areas by ZCTA/ZIP Code and county, respectively). Participants residing in rural areas had more ($p < 0.01$) chronic conditions on average compared to those in urban areas (approximately 2.6 conditions versus 2.4 conditions).

Table 2 presents the successful completion rates by rurality. Successful completion of the CDSME program was uniformly high at 77.3% overall; however, it was slightly higher in rural areas (77.9%) than in urban areas (77.1%). When we specified a 4-level categorization for rurality, we found participants residing in large rural towns (78.4%) and isolated small rural towns (78.3%) had higher successful completion rates than those participants residing in small rural towns (76.6%).

Table 3 presents the distribution of areas with a CDSME program presence (i.e., having one or more CDSME workshops available in the county) by rurality. The majority of areas with CDSME workshops were urban (70.0%). Approximately 9.3% of all CDSMP workshops were located in isolated small rural towns, and approximately 8.2% were located in small rural towns. The average number of participants in areas with a CDSME workshop

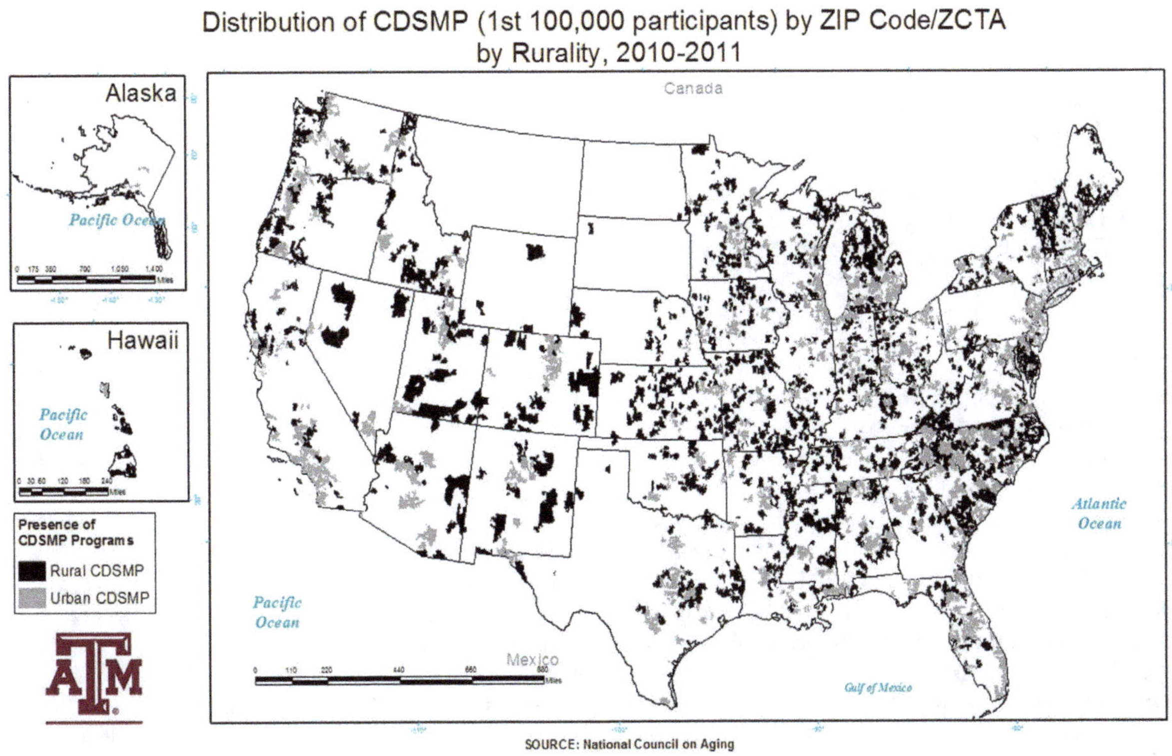

FIGURE 1 | Distribution of the chronic-disease self-management program by ZIP Code/ZCTA and rurality.

Table 1 | Distribution of key characteristics across rurality.

	Rural		Urban		Total
	ZIP Code/ZCTA	County	ZIP Code/ZCTA	County	
Sample size	(n = 19,982) 24.38%*	(n = 18,111) 22.09%*	(n = 61,991) 75.62%*	(n = 63,862) 77.91%*	(n = 81,973) 100%
Number of chronic conditions	2.59*	2.59*	2.42	2.43	2.46
Sex (% Female)	77.70%	78.00%	78.06%	77.96%	77.97%
Age	66.06*	66.13*	67.32	67.27	67.01
Living alone	52.12%*	52.75%*	47.88%	47.83%	48.92%
Race/ethnicity					
White	74.52%	75.48%	52.19%	52.57%	57.63%
Black	13.20%	13.21%	22.33%	22.06%	20.11%
AIAN	2.56%	2.48%	0.92%	0.99%	1.32%
Asian	1.07%	1.17%	3.99%	3.88%	3.28%
Other	6.77%	6.36%	13.11%	13.04%	11.56%
Hispanic	1.87%	1.29%	7.46%	7.46%	6.10%
HPSA					
Full HPSA	8.48%	7.59%	34.12%	35.01%	42.60%
Partial HPSA	11.36%	10.26%	33.58%	34.68%	44.94%
Non-HPSA	4.52%	4.23%	7.94%	8.23%	12.46%

**Indicates significantly different (p < 0.01) from urban areas using independent group t-test for continuous variables (number of chronic conditions, percent female, age, and percent living alone). The overall sample size is different (p < 0.01) by rurality (Chi Square).*

Table 2 | Successful completion rates by rurality.

	Successful completion	Standard deviation	Total (n = 82,044)
Rurality			
Urban	77.1%	0.42	62,051
Large rural city/town	78.4%	0.41	10,054
Small rural town	76.6%	0.42	5,900
Isolated small rural town	78.3%	0.41	4,039

Operational definition of rurality (4-way) includes Urban: RUCA 1.0, 1.1, 2.0, 2.1, 4.1, 5.1, 7.1, 8.1, and 10.1; Large Rural City/Town: 3.0, 4.0, 4.2, 5.0, 5.2, 6.0, 6.1, 7.2, 8.2, and 10.2; Small Rural Town: 7.0, 7.3, 7.4, 8.0, 8.3, 8.4, 9.0, 9.1, 9.2, and 10.3; Isolated Small Rural Town: 10.0, 10.4, 10.5, and 10.6.

Table 3 | Distribution of CDSMP sites (unique ZCTA/ZIP codes with a participant) by rurality.

	Average number of participants	Standard deviation	Range		Total (n = 9,599)
Rurality					
Urban	9.23	13.67	1	208	6,725 (70.01%)
Large rural city/town	8.46	28.11	1	884	1,192 (12.42%)
Small rural town	7.40	9.37	1	62	791 (8.24%)
Isolated small rural town	4.54	5.50	1	45	891 (9.28%)

Operational definition of rurality (4-way) includes Urban: RUCA 1.0, 1.1, 2.0, 2.1, 4.1, 5.1, 7.1, 8.1, and 10.1; large rural city/town: 3.0, 4.0, 4.2, 5.0, 5.2, 6.0, 6.1, 7.2, 8.2, and 10.2; Small Rural Town: 7.0, 7.3, 7.4, 8.0, 8.3, 8.4, 9.0, 9.1, 9.2, and 10.3; isolated small rural town: 10.0, 10.4, 10.5, and 10.6.

by rurality (calculated at the ZCTA/ZIP Code) was 9.2 participants in urban areas, which was almost twice the amount of participants in isolated small rural towns. Among areas with a CDSME workshop present, the range of the average number of participants in urban areas was much higher than small rural towns or isolated small rural towns (1–208 participants versus 1–62 participants and 1–45 participants, respectively). However, the highest range in the number of participants in a ZCTA/ZIP Code was measured in areas identified as a large rural city/town (1–884 participants).

Table 4 presents factors associated with successful completion of the CDSME program. A greater likelihood of successful completion was associated with being Black (OR = 1.25), or another race/ethnicity (OR = 1.32) versus being non-Hispanic White. A greater likelihood of successful completion was also associated with living in a rural county (OR = 1.10). Factors associated with lower likelihood of successful completion of the CDSME program included being male (OR = 0.92) and residing in a full-HPSA (OR = 0.93) versus a non-HPSA.

DISCUSSION

Our findings support earlier work about rural–urban differences in access to health-related resources (33). As expected, CDSME programs were less prevalent in rural versus urban areas. However, this study highlights that CDSME workshops are reaching rural areas in the US, although this reach is less than 25% of all rural areas. This is critical because CDSME programs have been shown to facilitate improvements in health status and other health-related outcomes among adults. CDSME programs assist participants to set goals, problem solve and do action planning

Table 4 | Likelihood of successful completion of the CDSMP.

	Odds ratio	*p*-Value	Confidence intervals (95%)	
Race				
White (referent)				
Black	1.249*	<0.0001	1.194	1.305
AIAN	0.923	0.0023	0.804	1.060
Asian	1.209**	0.0342	1.098	1.331
Other	1.318*	<0.0001	1.246	1.395
Hispanic	0.994	0.0008	0.927	1.067
Rurality				
Rural county	1.095*	<0.0001	1.051	1.140
HPSA				
Non-HPSA (referent)				
Partial HPSA	0.988	0.1588	0.936	1.042
Full HPSA	0.926*	0.0002	0.877	0.977
Sex				
Female (referent)				
Male	0.924*	<0.0001	0.888	0.961
Household status				
Lives with others (referent)				
Lives alone	1.017	0.3376	0.983	1.052

**Indicates significant differences ($p < 0.01$) using logistic regression.*

***Indicates significant differences ($p < 0.05$) using logistic regression.*

that can help in medical, emotional, and social role management of chronic conditions (16–18).

Rural residents face several issues related to health care and disease prevention program access (5–7). Identifying efficient ways to bridge access issues in rural areas is critically important for those who are older and have one or more chronic conditions. Improving the rural reach of EBP is one example of bridging this gap and linking rural residents to appropriate health care services intended to improve-health outcomes (34). Thus, examining strategies that bolster participation rates in rural and urban areas is warranted. More research is needed to identify why rural residents had somewhat higher completions rates when compared to urban residents. Overall, rural adults may be harder to reach and have other barriers related to social support, as exemplified by rural participants reporting higher rates of living alone (35, 36). In addition, the somewhat higher rates in the number of chronic conditions among rural residents may make this population potentially more vulnerable to self-care issues and in need of CDSME programs.

In the current study, the smaller number of participants in rural versus urban ZCTA/ZIP Codes may be related to the smaller number of eligible participants in these areas (i.e., population density and geographic isolation) (37) and the difficulty of some potential participants getting to centralized locations (e.g., longer distance, limited transportation) (38–41). To adequately serve rural populations, efforts are needed to ensure these programs are delivered in areas closer to potential/existing participants' homes. Offering these programs in closer proximity to rural participants' residences has potential to increase attendance rates because it can reduce the time and distance traveled to get to workshop sessions. Strategies make CDSME programs available rural residents' homes include embedding programs into existing local community infrastructures such as health care clinics or agricultural extension health services. Engaging multiple delivery sites in these communities (through the aging services network and public health system) is encouraged. For example, offering programs in faith-based organizations have been shown to improve participant reach (34). Embedding these programs in as regular offerings in organizations where rural residents frequently attend may increase their participation and foster long-term program sustainability.

Another strategy to better serve rural communities with CDSME programs includes cross-training workshop facilitators to be certified to an array of EBP (e.g., disease self-management, fall prevention). Cross-training these facilitators can increase the capacity of rural areas to deliver a collection of diverse EBP, each of which differ in purpose to meet the needs of rural residents and their caregivers. While increasing the availability of EBP in rural communities is essential, increasing access (and repeated access) to workshops is of equal importance. Once recruited into the program, additional efforts are needed to ensure participants remain in the program long enough to receive sufficient intervention dose for desired effects. Possible strategies to improve participants' access to and retention within workshops may include the creation of participant "buddy systems," exploring options for free or low-cost transportation services (e.g., shared rides or volunteer drivers), including technologically driven approaches, or holding meetings in community settings where older adults are already congregating.

More research should be conducted to identify differences in how programs are delivered in rural versus urban areas (e.g., strategies for recruitment and retention of different community partners; targeting different delivery settings; and determining ideal but feasible class size). Further investigation is also needed to assess the health-related impact of programs in rural versus urban areas, with special attention to cost-benefit issues. Future efforts should also examine whether differences by region or US territory exist (e.g., comparisons between continental US and Hawaii/Puerto Rico).

LIMITATIONS

The measure of rurality used in health services research is an important consideration in studies about rurality because the designated selection has potential to change areas of comparison and influence study findings (42). Our definition of rurality varied across the level of analysis. We used both a county-level measure (UIC) and the ZCTA/ZIP Code-level measure (RUCA), which assessed rurality in both larger areas (i.e., counties) and on a more micro-level (i.e., ZCTA/ZIP Codes). Thus, our use of different levels of rurality in this study provides a more complete picture of geospatial differences. While CDSME workshops were delivered in Puerto Rico, the measure of rurality used (i.e., 2006 RUCA Codes) was not available for Puerto Rico (43). As such, we were unable to provide accurate estimates of delivery by rurality for this area in the current study.

Data presented in the current study is based on the level of rural residents reached by the CDSME programs only among those who participated in this initiative. We do however, provide the rural reach by geographic distribution (i.e., reach within areas). Further, distances traveled by participants to attend workshops were not measured, thus we could not determine if time or distance traveled influenced workshop attendance. Additionally, the level of missing data is not uncommon to community-based interventions (44–46). While there was substantial missing data, this may have been attributed more to the sites' administrative ability to collect field data than from individual data refusal (47). Because the analyses performed in this study were not longitudinal, we could not measure changes in the rural reach of the CDSME programs over time. Designing such longitudinal analyses is highly recommended as a next step in identifying whether progress is being made in reaching rural residents. We acknowledge that because of our large sample size seemingly small comparative differences were statistically significant. To be more conservative and protect against Type I error, we used a p-value of 0.01 in all study analyses.

CONCLUSION

The current study helps lessen the gap in what is known about the rural reach of CDSME programs and factors affecting successful completion. Findings highlight the capability of CDSME programs to reach rural residents, yet dissemination efforts can be enhanced to ensure minorities and individuals in HPSAs utilize this program. Tailored strategies are needed to increase participant recruitment and retention in rural areas to overcome traditional barriers to health service access. Assessing the infrastructure in rural areas may be helpful for identifying viable partners for those seeking to deliver EBP to residents of rural areas, creating greater uptake, reach, and sustainability.

ACKNOWLEDGMENTS

The American Recovery and Reinvestment Act of 2009 (i.e., Recovery Act) Communities Putting Prevention to Work: Chronic-Disease Self-Management Program initiative, led by the U.S. Administration on Aging in collaboration with the Centers for Disease Control and Prevention and the Centers for Medicare and Medicaid Services, allotted $32.5 million to support the translation of the Stanford program in 45 States, Puerto Rico, and the District of Columbia. The National Council on Aging served as the Technical Assistance Resource Center for this initiative and collected de-identified data on program participation.

REFERENCES

1. Anderson G, Horvath J. The growing burden of chronic disease in America. *Public Health Rep* (2004) **119**(3):263–70. doi:10.1016/j.phr.2004.04.005
2. Broemeling AM, Watson DE, Prebtani F. Population patterns of chronic health conditions, co-morbidity and healthcare use in Canada: implications for policy and practice. *Healthc Q* (2007) **11**(3):70–6. doi:10.12927/hcq.2008.19859
3. Nolte E, McKee M. *Caring For People with Chronic Conditions: A Health System Perspective.* Berkshire: McGraw-Hill International (2008).
4. Glasgow N, Berry EH. *Rural Aging in 21st Century America.* Heidelberg: Springer (2013). doi:10.1007/978-94-007-5567-3
5. Council on Graduate Medical Education. *Physician Distribution and Health Care Challenges in Rural and Inner City Areas: Tenth Report to Congress and the Department of Health and Human Services Secretary.* Rockville, MD: Health Resources and Services Administration, US Dept of Health and Human Services (1998).
6. Knapp KK, Paavola FG, Maine LL, Sorofman B, Politzer RM. Availability of primary care providers and pharmacists in the United States. *J Am Pharm Assoc* (1999) **39**(2):127–35.
7. MacDowell M, Glasser M, Fitts M, Nielsen K, Hunsaker M. A national view of rural health workforce issues in the USA. *Rural Remote Health* (2010) **10**(3):1531.
8. Gamm L, Hutchison L, Dabney BJ, et al. *Rural Healthy People 2010: A companion document to Healthy People 2010.* College Station, TX: The Texas A&M University System Health Science Center, School of Rural Public Health, Southwest Rural Health Research Center (2003).
9. Norton CH, McManus MA. Background tables on demographic characteristics, health status, and health services utilization. *Health Serv Res* (1989) **23**(6):725–56.
10. Jones CA, Parker TS, Ahearn M, Mishra AK, Variyam JN. Health Status and Health Care Access of Farm and Rural Populations., EIB-57. Washington, DC: U.S. Department of Agriculture, Economic Research Service (2009). p. 1–64.
11. Bennett KJ, Olatosi B, Probst JC. *Health Disparities: A Rural – Urban Chartbook.* South Carolina: Rural Health Research Center (2008).
12. Lengerich EJ, Wyatt SW, Rubio A, Beaulieu JE, Coyne CA, Fleisher L, et al. The Appalachia cancer network: cancer control research among a rural, medically underserved population. *J Rural Health* (2004) **20**(2):181–7. doi:10.1111/j.1748-0361.2004.tb00026.x
13. Towne SD, Smith ML, Ory MG. Geographic variations in access and utilization of cancer screening services: examining disparities among American Indian and Alaska Native Elders. *Int J Health Geogr* (2014) **13**:18. doi:10.1186/1476-072X-13-18
14. Smith ML, Quinn C, Gipson R, Wilson AD, Ory MO. Serving rural communities for falls prevention: the dissemination of a matter of balance in the Brazos Valley Region of Texas. *Tex Pub Health J* (2011) **63**(1):54–8.
15. Smith ML, Ahn SN, Sharkey JR, Horel S, Mier N, Ory MG. Successful falls prevention programming for older adults in Texas Rural–Urban Variations. *J Appl Gerontol* (2012) **31**(1):3–27. doi:10.1177/0733464810378407
16. Lorig KR, Sobel DS, Stewart AL, Brown BW, Bandura A, Ritter P, et al. Evidence suggesting that a chronic disease self-management program can improve health status while reducing hospitalization: a randomized trial. *Med Care* (1999) **37**(1):5–14. doi:10.1097/00005650-199901000-00003
17. Lorig KR, Sobel DS, Ritter PL, Laurent D, Hobbs M. Effect of a self-management program on patients with chronic disease. *Eff Clin Practi* (2001) **4**(6):256–62.
18. Lorig KR, Ritter P, Stewart AL, Sobel DS, Brown BW Jr, Bandura A, et al. Chronic disease self-management program: 2-year health status and health care utilization outcomes. *Med Care* (2001) **39**(11):1217–23. doi:10.1097/00005650-200111000-00008
19. Ory MG, Ahn S, Jiang L, Smith ML, Ritter PL, Whitelaw N, et al. Successes of a national study of the chronic disease self-management program: meeting the triple aim of health care reform. *Med Care* (2013) **51**(11):992–8. doi:10.1097/MLR.0b013e3182a95dd1
20. Lorig K, Holman H, Sobel D, Laurent D. *Living a Healthy Life with Chronic Conditions: Self Management of Heart Disease, Arthritis, Diabetes, Asthma, Bronchitis, Emphysema and others.* 3rd ed. Boulder, CO: Bull Publishing Company (2006).
21. Bandura A. Social cognitive theory of self-regulation. *Organ Behav Hum Decis Process* (1991) **50**(2):248–87. doi:10.1016/0749-5978(91)90022-L
22. Ory MG, Ahn S, Jiang L, Lorig K, Ritter P, Laurent DD, et al. National study of chronic disease self-management six-month outcome findings. *J Aging Health* (2013) **25**(7):1258–74. doi:10.1177/0898264313502531
23. Ahn S, Basu R, Smith ML, Jiang L, Lorig K, Whitelaw N, et al. The impact of chronic disease self-management programs: healthcare savings through a community-based intervention. *BMC Public Health* (2013) **13**(1):1141. doi:10.1186/1471-2458-13-1141
24. U.S. Department of Health and Human Services Administration on Aging. *ARRA – Communities Putting Prevention to Work: Chronic Disease Self-Management Program.* Washington, DC. (2012).
25. Ory MG, Smith ML, Patton K, Lorig K, Zenker W, Whitelaw N. Self-management at the tipping point: reaching 100,000 Americans with evidence-based programs. *J Am Geriatr Soc* (2013) **61**(5):821–3. doi:10.1111/jgs.12239
26. Area Health Resources Files (ARF). *US Department of Health and Human Services, Health Resources and Services Administration.* Rockville, MD: Bureau of Health Professions (2013).
27. United States Department of Agriculture Economic Research Service. Available from: http://www.ers.usda.gov/data-products/urban-influence-codes.aspx#.UwahVfldV8E
28. WWAMI Rural Health Research Center. *RUCA Data: Using RUCA Data.* Available from: http://depts.washington.edu/uwruca/ruca-uses.php

29. Health Resources and services Administration (HRSA). *Primary Medical Care HPSA Designation Overview.* Available from: http://bhpr.hrsa.gov/shortage/hpsas/designationcriteria/primarycarehpsaoverview.html
30. Stanford School of Medicine. *Chronic Disease Self-Management Program (Better Choices, Better Health®Workshop)* (2014). Available at: http://patienteducation.stanford.edu/programs/cdsmp.html
31. SAS Institute Inc. Sas 9.4 by SAS Institute Inc. Cary, NC: SAS Institute Inc. Copyright © 2002–2013.
32. ESRI Inc. ArcGIS: Release 10.2 by ESRI Inc. Redlands, CA: Environmental Systems Research Institute. Copyright ©1999–2013.
33. Towne SD, Lee C, Smith ML, Pulczinski J, Swierc SM, Coughlin R, et al. Health-related quality of life & well-being. In: Bolin J, editor. *Rural Health People 2020: A Companion Document to Healthy People 2020,* Vol. 2, Chapter 14. Southwest Rural Health Research Center, School of Public Health, Texas A&M University System Health Science Center (2014).
34. Smith ML, Belza B, Altpeter M, Ahn S, Dickerson JB, Ory MG. Disseminating an evidence-based disease self-management program for older Americans: implications for diversifying participant reach through delivery site adoption. In: Maddock J, editor. *Public Health: Social and Behavioral Health.* Rijeka: InTech (2012). p. 385–404.
35. Eshbaugh EM. Perceptions of living alone among older adult women. *J Commun Health Nurs* (2008) **25**(3):125–37. doi:10.1080/07370010802221685
36. Culo S. Risk assessment and intervention for vulnerable older adults. *B C Med J* (2011) **53**(8):421–5.
37. United States Department of Agriculture. *Economic Research Service. What is Rural* (2014). Available from: http://www.ers.usda.gov/topics/rural-economy-population/rural-classifications/what-is-rural.aspx#.UyCRHPldV8E
38. Freeman VA, Patterson D, Slifkin RT. *Issues in Staffing Emergency Medical Services: Results from a National Survey of Local Rural and Urban EMS Directors. Report no. 93.* Chapel Hill: University of North Carolina at Chapel Hill, US Department of Health and Human Services (2008).
39. Genovesi AL, Hastings B, Edgerton EA, Olson LM. Pediatric emergency care capabilities of Indian Health Service emergency medical service agencies serving American Indians/Alaska Natives in rural and frontier areas. *Rural Remote Health* (2014) **14**(2):2688.
40. Peck J, Alexander K. *Maternal, Infant, and Child Health in Rural Areas: A Literature Review. Rural Healthy People 2010: A Companion Document to Healthy People 2010* (Vol. 2) (2010).
41. Velaga NR, Beecroft M, Nelson JD, Corsar D, Edwards P. Transport poverty meets the digital divide: accessibility and connectivity in rural communities. *J Transp Geography* (2012) **21**:102–12. doi:10.1016/j.jtrangeo.2011.12.005
42. Smith ML, Dickerson JB, Wendel ML, Ahn S, Pulczinski JC, Drake KN, et al. The utility of rural and underserved designations in geospatial assessments of distance traveled to healthcare services: implications for public health research and practice. *J Environ Public Health* (2013) **2013**:960157. doi:10.1155/2013/960157
43. WWAMI Rural Health Research Center. Available from: http://depts.washington.edu/uwruca/ruca-projects.php (2014).
44. Edwards KE, Gibson N, Martin J, Mitchell S, Andersson N. Impact of community-based interventions on condom use in the Tłicho region of Northwest Territories Canada. *BMC Health Serv Res* (2011) **11**(Suppl 2):S9. doi:10.1186/1472-6963-11-S2-S9
45. Mayworm AM, Sharkey JD. Gender-specific mental health outcomes of a community-based delinquency intervention. *J Juv Just* (2013) **3**(1).
46. Temel S, van Voorst SF, Jack BW, Denktas S, Steegers EA. Evidence-based preconceptional lifestyle interventions. *Epidemiol Rev* (2014) **36**(1):19–30. doi:10.1093/epirev/mxt003
47. Kulinski K, Boughtaugh M, Smith ML, Ory MG, Lorig K. Setting the stage: measure selection, coordination, and data collection for a national self-management initiative. *Front Public Health* (2015) **2**:206. doi:10.3389/fpubh.2014.00206

Factors associated with Hispanic adults attending Spanish-language disease self-management program workshops and workshop completion

Matthew Lee Smith[1]*, SangNam Ahn[2,3], Luohua Jiang[4], Kristie P. Kulinski[5] and Marcia G. Ory[3]

[1] Department of Health Promotion and Behavior, College of Public Health, The University of Georgia, Athens, GA, USA
[2] Division of Health Systems Management and Policy, School of Public Health, The University of Memphis, Memphis, TN, USA
[3] Department of Health Promotion and Community Health Sciences, Texas A&M Health Science Center, School of Public Health, College Station, TX, USA
[4] Department of Epidemiology and Biostatistics, Texas A&M Health Science Center, School of Public Health, College Station, TX, USA
[5] National Council on Aging, Washington, DC, USA

Edited by:
Sue Ellen Levkoff, University of South Carolina, USA

Reviewed by:
Marta Enid Pagan-Ortiz, Environment and Health Group, USA
Dharma E. Cortes, Northeastern University, USA

***Correspondence:**
Matthew Lee Smith, Department of Health Promotion and Behavior, College of Public Health, The University of Georgia, 330 River Road, 315 Ramsey Center, Athens, GA 30602, USA
e-mail: health@uga.edu

Many factors influence ways in which middle-aged and older Hispanic adults prefer to receive health-related information. While Spanish-language disease management programs are increasingly offered in community and healthcare settings, less is known about their utilization among the Hispanic population. This study aimed to identify participant and workshop factors associated with middle-aged and older Hispanic adults attending Spanish-language disease self-management program workshops and receiving the recommended intervention dose (i.e., successful workshop completion is defined as attending four or more of the six workshop sessions). Data were analyzed from 12,208 Hispanic adults collected during a national dissemination of the Stanford suite of Chronic Disease Self-Management Education (CDSME) programs spanning 45 states, the District of Columbia, and Puerto Rico. Two logistic regression analyses were performed. Over 65% of participants attended Spanish-language workshops, and 78.3% of participants successfully completed workshops. Relative to participants in English-language workshops, participants who attended Spanish-language CDSME workshops were more likely to successfully complete workshops, as were those aged 80 years and older, females, and those who lived alone. Participants who were aged 50–79 years and female were significantly more likely to attend Spanish-language workshops than their counterparts under age 50. Conversely, those with more chronic conditions were less likely to attend Spanish-language workshops. Those who attended workshops with more participants and where the Hispanic population was less affluent were more likely to attend Spanish-language workshops. This study provides insight into Spanish-language CDSME program recruitment and utilization with implications for program adoption in underserved Hispanic community settings.

Keywords: chronic disease self-management, evidence-based program, Hispanic adults, intervention dose, Spanish language

INTRODUCTION

The United States is becoming increasingly more racially and ethnically diverse (1). The Hispanic population is the largest and fastest growing minority group in the United States (2). This population is expected to represent nearly one-third of the American population and one-fifth of the older adult population by 2050 (3). Growth rates are anticipated to be even higher in some parts of America such as the Texas–Mexico border (4).

The pattern of chronic disease differs among minority groups, and Hispanic individuals often acquire chronic conditions at younger ages than their non-Hispanic white counterparts (5). Additionally, as a group, Hispanic individuals are disproportionately burdened by chronic conditions including obesity, diabetes, and heart disease (6–9). They are also less likely to have access to health care (10, 11) or evidence-based health promotion programs (12). Despite the growing availability of evidence-based disease prevention programs for seniors (13, 14), language and/or cultural barriers may prevent Hispanic individuals from accessing these services (10).

English or Spanish-language preferences for receiving health information and materials among Hispanic individuals vary by a multitude of factors (15–17), but less is known about language-based preferences for evidence-based programs among this population. As such, this study draws from national data to examine participant and workshop characteristics associated with Hispanic individuals' attending Spanish-language disease self-management program workshops. Further, this study examines if this participant subgroup received the recommended intervention dose (i.e., successfully completed the workshop by attending four or more of the six workshop sessions).

MATERIALS AND METHODS

PROGRAM DESCRIPTION

The Chronic Disease Self-Management Program (CDSMP) is one intervention in a suite of Chronic Disease Self-Management Education (CDSME) programs licensed through the Stanford Patient Education Research Center. CDSMP has been introduced and widely disseminated in the U.S. as a method to empower patients with self-management skills to deal with their chronic conditions (18). CDSMP is an evidence-based, peer-led intervention consisting of six highly participative classes held for 2.5 h each, once a week, for consecutive 6 weeks. (18) CDSMP has resulted in improved health care and health (19, 20), while potentially saving healthcare costs (21). While some of the CDSME programs are general (e.g., CDSMP), others are disease specific (e.g., diabetes, arthritis, chronic pain). While the chronic condition may vary, all CDSME programs are based upon social learning theory (22), highly interactive, and apply the principles of goal setting, problem solving, and action planning (22).

DATA SOURCE AND STUDY POPULATION

Cross-sectional data for this study were obtained from a nationwide delivery of CDSME programs as part of the American Recovery and Reinvestment Act of 2009 (i.e., ARRA) *Communities Putting Prevention to Work: Chronic Disease Self-Management Program* initiative (13, 23). The U.S. Administration on Aging led this initiative in collaboration with the Centers for Disease Control and Prevention and the Centers for Medicare and Medicaid Services to support the translation of CDSME programs in 45 states, Puerto Rico, and the District of Columbia (24). For this study, cases were only drawn from Hispanic participants within the first 100,000 participants enrolled in CDSME program workshops and who had complete data on variables of interest. Based on these inclusion criteria, the final analytic sample was 12,208 middle-aged and older Hispanic adults who attended a CDSMP workshop.

MEASURES

Dependent variables

Two dependent variables were used for this study. Participants' attendance was recorded to determine if the recommended intervention dose was received. As defined by the program developers, a participant has "successfully" completed the program if they attended four or more of the six offered workshop sessions (13, 19, 20, 25). Therefore, successful program completion was used as the first dependent variable in this study (i.e., non-successful completion served as the referent group). The second dependent variable was the workshop language in which attended. Workshops are offered in approximately 20 languages worldwide (25). Although CDSME program workshops are available in a variety of languages other than English (e.g., Mandarin Chinese, Korean, Farsi, Tagalog), the most predominant non-English workshop language is Spanish. Therefore, participants' enrollment in Spanish-language workshops was used as the second dependent variable in this study (i.e., enrollment in English-language workshops served as the referent group). Spanish-language CDSME programs offered in this nationwide rollout included *Tomando Control de su Salud* (i.e., Spanish version of CDSMP), *Programa de Manejo Personal de la Diabetes* (i.e., Spanish version of the diabetes self-management program), and *Curso de Manejo Personal de la Artritis* (i.e., Spanish version of the arthritis self-management program).

Personal characteristics

Personal characteristics of the participants included age group (i.e., under 50 years, 50–64 years, 65–79 years, 80+ years), sex (i.e., male, female), living situation (i.e., lives alone, lives with others), and self-reported number of chronic conditions (i.e., ranging from 0 to 10). Chronic condition types included arthritis, cancer, depression, diabetes, heart disease, hypertension, lung disease, stroke, osteoporosis, and other chronic conditions.

Delivery site types

Data pertaining to CDSME program delivery site types were gathered administratively, as described previously. Delivery site types included healthcare organizations, senior centers or area agencies on aging (AAAs), residential facilities, community or multipurpose centers (including libraries), faith-based organizations, educational institutions, and site types classified as "other" (e.g., correctional facilities malls, RV parks, fire departments, county administration buildings, private residences, casinos, career centers).

Neighborhood characteristics

Using participants' residential ZIP Codes, geographic information system (GIS) software was used to generate neighborhood-level variables for each participant. Neighborhood characteristics included residential rurality (i.e., metro residence or non-metro residence based on the rural–urban commuting area codes (RUCA) (26)) and the percent of Hispanic families below the federal poverty line residing in the participants' ZIP Code (27). Using organizational ZIP Codes, GIS software was used to generate neighborhood-level variables for each delivery site (i.e., site rurality, percent of Hispanic families below the federal poverty line).

ANALYSES

All statistical analyses were performed using SPSS (version 21). Of the first 100,000 participants reached in this initiative, all non-Hispanic cases ($n = 86,191$) were immediately omitted from analyses based on specified study aims, which left 13,809 Hispanic participants. Of these Hispanic participants, those with missing data for age ($n = 661$), sex ($n = 291$), living situation ($n = 8$), residential rurality ($n = 973$), delivery site rurality ($n = 11$), and class size ($n = 85$) were omitted. Some participants had more than one of these exclusionary characteristics, thus the final sample was 12,208 middle-aged and older Hispanic adults who attended a CDSMP workshop. When comparing characteristics between Hispanic participants in the analytic sample with Hispanic participants omitted from analyses, participants in the analytic sample were significantly younger, lived with others, and had more chronic conditions. No significant differences were observed based on participants' sex or the rurality of their residence.

For participants meeting study inclusion criteria, frequencies were calculated for all major study variables, which were initially examined in relationship to participants' successful workshop completion and the workshop language in which participants attended. Pearson's chi-square tests were performed to assess differences between categorical independent variables. Independent sample t-tests were used to examine mean differences for continuous variables. Two logistic regression analyses were performed to identify factors associated with attending Spanish-language workshops (i.e., attending English-language workshops served as the referent group) and successful workshop attendance (i.e., non-successful attendance served as the referent group). Odds ratios and 95% confidence intervals are reported.

RESULTS

SAMPLE CHARACTERISTICS

Sample characteristics of study participants are presented in **Table 1**. Of the 12,208 study participants, 65.1% attended Spanish-language workshops and 78.3% successfully completed the program (i.e., attended four or more of the six offered workshop sessions). Over 55% of participants were aged 64 years or younger and 78.4% was female. On average, participants self-reported 1.96 (±1.54) chronic conditions. The majority of participants lived with others (92.2%) and resided in metro areas (93.2%). The largest proportion of these Hispanic participants attended workshops at healthcare organizations (32.1%), followed by senior centers or AAAs (22.3%), residential facilities (11.1%), and community or multi-purpose centers (10.1%). On average, workshops had 13.14 (±4.08) participants, and participants attended 4.49 (±1.64) of the six workshop sessions.

ATTENDING SPANISH-LANGUAGE WORKSHOPS

Significant differences were observed when comparing sample characteristics by workshop language in bivariate analyses (see **Table 1**). A significantly larger proportion of participants who enrolled in Spanish-language workshops also received the recommended intervention dose (i.e., attended four or more of the six workshop sessions) ($\chi^2 = 58.52$, $P < 0.001$). Significantly larger proportions of younger participants ($\chi^2 = 149.44$, $P < 0.001$) and female participants ($\chi^2 = 59.47$, $P < 0.001$) attended Spanish-language workshops. On average, participants who attended Spanish-language workshops had fewer chronic conditions ($t = 14.36$, $P < 0.001$). Significantly larger proportions of participants who lived alone ($\chi^2 = 14.09$, $P < 0.001$) and lived in metro areas ($\chi^2 = 374.95$, $P < 0.001$) attended Spanish-language workshops. On average, those attending Spanish-language workshops resided ($t = -40.79$, $P < 0.001$) and attended delivery sites ($t = -41.30$, $P < 0.001$) in areas with higher percentages of Hispanic families below the federal poverty line. Larger proportions of participants who attended Spanish-language workshops did so at healthcare organizations and educational institutions, whereas smaller proportions of participants who attended Spanish-language workshops did so at senior centers or AAAs and residential facilities ($\chi^2 = 464.88$, $P < 0.001$). On average, participants who attended Spanish-language workshops had larger class sizes ($t = -10.61$, $P < 0.001$) and attended more workshop sessions ($t = -7.56$, $P < 0.001$).

Table 2 presents the logistic regression modeling factors associated with Hispanic participants' enrollment in Spanish-language workshops (i.e., attending English-language workshops served as the referent group). Compared to participants under age 50 years, those who were aged 50–64 years (OR = 1.68, $P < 0.001$) and 65–79 years (OR = 1.29, $P = 0.002$) were significantly more likely to attend Spanish-language workshops. Female participants were also more likely to attend Spanish-language workshops (OR = 1.26, $P < 0.001$), whereas, those with fewer chronic conditions (OR = 0.85, $P < 0.001$) and who resided in non-metro areas (OR = 0.28, $P < 0.001$) were less likely to attend Spanish-language workshops. Relative to those who attended workshops in healthcare organizations, participants who attended workshops at all other delivery site types, except residential facilities, were significantly more likely to attend Spanish-language workshops ($P < 0.001$). Participants in workshops with more participants (OR = 1.03, $P < 0.001$) and those attending workshops at delivery sites in areas with higher percentages of Hispanic families below the federal poverty line (OR = 1.15, $P < 0.001$) were significantly more likely to attend Spanish-language workshops.

SUCCESSFUL WORKSHOP COMPLETION

Significant differences were observed when comparing sample characteristics by workshop completion in bivariate analyses (see **Table 1**). A significantly larger proportion of participants aged 65–79 years ($\chi^2 = 26.16$, $P < 0.001$) and female participants ($\chi^2 = 22.42$, $P < 0.001$) successfully completed workshops. Significantly larger proportions of participants who lived alone ($\chi^2 = 20.41$, $P < 0.001$) and lived in metro areas ($\chi^2 = 4.72$, $P = 0.030$) successfully completed workshops. On average, those who successfully completed workshops resided in ($t = -5.10$, $P < 0.001$) and attended delivery sites in ($t = -4.34$, $P < 0.001$) areas with higher percentages of Hispanic families below the federal poverty line. Larger proportions of participants who successfully completed workshops did so at senior centers or AAAs and other delivery sites, whereas smaller proportions of participants who successfully completed workshops did so at healthcare facilities and residential facilities ($\chi^2 = 86.17$, $P < 0.001$). On average, participants who successfully completed workshops were in workshops with fewer participants ($t = 3.09$, $P = 0.002$).

Table 3 presents the logistic regression modeling factors associated with successful workshop completion (i.e., attending fewer than four workshops served as the referent group). Compared to participants under age 50 years, those who were aged 85 years and older were significantly more likely to be successful completers (OR = 1.36, $P < 0.001$). Female participants (OR = 1.22, $P < 0.001$), those who lived alone (OR = 1.34, $P = 0.002$), and those who resided in areas with higher percentages of Hispanic families below the federal poverty line (OR = 1.05, $P = 0.002$) were more likely to successfully complete workshops. Relative to those who attended workshops in healthcare organizations, participants who attended workshops at all other delivery site types, except educational institutions, were significantly less likely to successfully complete workshops ($P < 0.05$). Participants enrolled in Spanish-language workshops were significantly more likely to successfully complete workshops (OR = 1.50, $P < 0.001$), whereas, those in workshops with larger class sizes (OR = 0.98, $P < 0.001$) were significantly less likely to successfully complete workshops. Those attending workshops at delivery sites in areas with higher percentages of Hispanic families below the federal

Table 1 | Sample characteristics by workshop language and completion.

	Total (*n* = 12,208)	Workshop language				Workshop completion			
		English (*n* = 4,262)	Spanish (*n* = 7,946)	χ^2 or *t*	*P*	Not successful (*n* = 2,652)	Successful (*n* = 9,556)	χ^2 or *t*	*P*
Work shop completion				58.52	<0.001				
Not successful	21.7%	25.6%	19.6%			–	–	–	–
Successful	78.3%	74.4%	80.4%			–	–	–	–
Work shop language								58.52	<0.001
English	34.9%	–	–	–	–	41.2%	33.2%		
Spanish	65.1%	–	–	–	–	58.8%	66.8%		
Age				149.44	<0.001			26.16	<0.001
Under 50	25.6%	19.5%	28.9%			26.9%	25.2%		
50–64	29.8%	30.0%	29.7%			31.3%	29.4%		
65–79	34.8%	39.6%	32.2%			30.8%	35.9%		
80+	9.8%	11.0%	9.1%			11.0%	9.4%		
Sex				59.47	<0.001			22.42	<0.001
Male	21.6%	25.6%	19.5%			25.0%	20.7%		
Female	78.4%	74.4%	80.5%			75.0%	79.3%		
Living situation				14.09	<0.001			20.41	<0.001
Lives with others	92.2%	93.4%	91.5%			94.3%	91.6%		
Lives alone	7.8%	6.6%	8.5%			5.7%	8.4%		
Rurality (participant residence)				374.95	<0.001			4.72	0.030
Metro	93.2%	87.2%	96.4%			92.3%	93.5%		
Non-metro	6.8%	12.8%	3.6%			7.7%	6.5%		
Number of chronic conditions	1.96 (±1.54)	2.24 (±1.62)	1.81 (±1.47)	14.36	<0.001	1.96 (±1.57)	1.96 (±1.53)	−0.22	0.825
Percent of Hispanics below poverty (participant residence)	10.41 (±10.26)	6.30 (±5.66)	12.61 (±11.43)	−40.79	<0.001	9.59 (±8.96)	10.63 (±10.58)	−5.10	<0.001
Delivery site type				464.88	<0.001			86.17	<0.001
Healthcare Organization	32.1%	24.7%	36.0%			38.2%	30.4%		
Senior center/AAA	22.3%	29.5%	18.4%			20.1%	22.9%		
Residential facility	11.1%	13.2%	10.0%			12.1%	10.9%		
Community/Multi-Purpose Center	10.1%	10.1%	10.2%			10.2%	10.1%		
Faith-based Organization	6.6%	5.1%	7.5%			5.6%	6.9%		
Educational Institution	4.1%	1.3%	5.6%			3.5%	4.2%		
Other	13.6%	16.0%	12.3%			10.3%	14.5%		
Rurality (delivery site location)				390.99	<0.001			0.38	0.537
Metro	93.7%	87.7%	96.9%			93.4%	93.7%		
Non-metro	6.3%	12.3%	3.1%			6.6%	6.3%		
Class size	13.14 (±4.08)	12.60 (±4.16)	13.43 (±4.00)	−10.61	<0.001	13.35 (±4.06)	13.08 (±4.08)	3.09	0.002
Number of sessions attended	4.49 (±1.64)	4.33 (±1.70)	4.57 (±1.61)	−7.56	<0.001	1.76 (±0.82)	5.25 (±0.79)	−195.38	<0.001
Percent of Hispanics below poverty (delivery site location)	10.51 (±10.25)	6.35 (±5.64)	12.73 (±11.42)	−41.30	<0.001	9.80 (±9.20)	10.70 (±10.52)	−4.34	<0.001

Table 2 | Factors associated with enrollment in Spanish-language workshops.

	OR	*P*	95% CI	
			Lower	Upper
Age: under 50	1.00	–	–	–
Age: 50–64	1.68	<0.001	1.41	1.99
Age: 65–79	1.29	0.002	1.10	1.51
Age: 80+	0.97	0.681	0.83	1.13
Male	1.00	–	–	–
Female	1.26	<0.001	1.15	1.40
Lives with others	1.00	–	–	–
lives alone	1.12	0.179	0.95	1.33
Metro (participant-level)	1.00	–	–	–
Non-metro (participant-level)	0.28	<0.001	0.21	0.39
Number of chronic conditions	0.85	<0.001	0.82	0.87
Percent of Hispanics below poverty (participant-level)	0.98	0.287	0.95	1.02
Delivery site: Healthcare Organization	1.00	–	–	–
Delivery site: senior center/AAA	2.27	<0.001	1.98	2.60
Delivery site: residential facility	1.07	0.400	0.92	1.24
Delivery site: Community/Multi-Purpose Center	1.60	<0.001	1.35	1.90
Delivery site: Faith-Based Organization	1.96	<0.001	1.64	2.34
Delivery site: Educational Institution	3.46	<0.001	2.82	4.24
Delivery site: other	5.14	<0.001	3.72	7.11
Metro (delivery site-level)	1.00	–	–	–
Non-metro (delivery site-level)	0.74	0.072	0.53	1.03
Class size	1.03	<0.001	1.02	1.04
Percent of Hispanics below poverty (delivery site-level)	1.15	<0.001	1.11	1.19

Table 3 | Factors associated with successful workshop completion.

	OR	*P*	95% CI	
			Lower	Upper
Age: under 50	1.00	–	–	–
Age: 50–64	1.09	0.320	0.92	1.30
Age: 65–79	1.14	0.103	0.97	1.34
Age: 80+	1.36	<0.001	1.17	1.59
Male	1.00	–	–	–
Female	1.22	<0.001	1.10	1.35
Lives with others	1.00	–	–	–
Lives alone	1.34	0.002	1.11	1.61
Metro (participant-level)	1.00	–	–	–
Non-metro (participant-level)	0.81	0.210	0.57	1.13
Number of chronic conditions	1.01	0.530	0.98	1.04
Percent of Hispanics below poverty (participant-level)	1.05	0.002	1.02	1.08
Workshop: English	1.00	–	–	–
Workshop: Spanish	1.50	<0.001	1.36	1.66
Delivery site: Healthcare Organization	1.00	–	–	–
Delivery site: senior center/AAA	0.52	<0.001	0.45	0.61
Delivery site: residential facility	0.74	0.001	0.63	0.88
Delivery site: Community/Multi-Purpose Center	0.60	<0.001	0.50	0.73
Delivery site: Faith-based Organization	0.64	<0.001	0.53	0.78
Delivery site: Educational Institution	0.81	0.060	0.64	1.01
Delivery site: other	0.71	0.013	0.55	0.93
Metro (delivery site-level)	1.00	–	–	–
Non-metro (delivery site-level)	1.19	0.341	0.83	1.69
Class size	0.98	<0.001	0.97	0.99
Percent of Hispanics below poverty (delivery site-level)	0.96	0.004	0.93	0.99

poverty line ($OR = 0.96$, $P = 0.004$) were also significantly less likely to successfully complete workshops.

DISCUSSION

Hispanic participants represented 17.4% of the first 100,000 participants reached through this ARRA implementation effort (28), a percentage that is representative of the overall Hispanic population in the United States (29). However, relative to the larger population reached in this initiative, participants in our sample are younger (25.6% under age 50 compared to 12.0% in the larger group) (28). This finding is important because it reinforces that Hispanics in the United States are acquiring chronic conditions at younger ages and living with those conditions for longer periods of time (5), thus highlighting the necessity for self-management programs. With approximately two-thirds of sample participants ($n = 7,946$) attending Spanish-language CDSME program workshops, this study supports previous studies' assumptions about preferences among Hispanic individuals for receiving health-related information delivered in Spanish (15–17). While the proportion of Hispanic participants electing to attend Spanish-language workshops is substantial, further inspection of the larger initiative (28) reveals that the majority of workshops delivered to the first 100,000 participants were English-language CDSMP (78.4%) and the Diabetes Self-Management Program (10.3%), whereas only about 10% were specialized Spanish versions of the CDSME (i.e., Tomando Control de su Salud, Programa de Manejo Personal de la Diabetes, and Curso de Manejo Personal de la Artritis). Therefore, it remains to be determined if the number of Hispanic participants would have been larger if more Spanish-language workshops were available across the country, or if older Hispanics are becoming increasingly assimilated and comfortable with English for health-related information.

The overall completion rates among Hispanic participants were higher than for the total population of CDSME program participants (28) (i.e., 74.9% completion among all participants, 78.3% completion among Hispanic participants, and 80.4% completion among Spanish-language workshop participants), and can be attributed, in part, to the availability of Spanish-language workshops. This study identified participant and workshop characteristics associated with attendance at Spanish speaking versus English-language workshops. Relative to English-language workshops, Spanish-language workshops attracted a different population base (e.g., younger, female, fewer chronic conditions) and were held in different settings (e.g., more urban, less affluent settings). These differences may be attributed to other characteristics associated with successful Spanish-language workshop completion such as attending more workshops in healthcare facilities and senior centers/AAAs or attending workshops with larger class sizes.

Several research and practice implications emerge from this study. First, in future research, it will be important to stratify Hispanic participants by ethnic origin to identify characteristics contributing to their program enrollment, attendance, and benefits. As indicated in new census designations (30), there is growing awareness of the importance of differentiating among different Hispanic populations (e.g., Mexican, Mexican American, Chicano, Puerto Rican, or Cuban), as well as the degree of acculturation (e.g., native or recent immigrant) and available social support (31). Including these types of measures is also important to address inherent biases associated with the current study, in that they are likely attributed to Spanish-language workshop preferences.

Second, additional efforts are needed to understand differences between surface and deeper intervention approaches, which identify language as a defining characteristic as opposed to other intervention strategies that resonate with cultural preferences (32, 33). These elements are especially important for tailoring participant recruitment and delivery efforts, which may be more or less feasible based on the delivery site type and socio-economics of the residents and service area. Further investigations are warranted to better understand program preferences among this population within the context of existing delivery systems and referral patterns. Healthcare settings are already primed to reach diverse populations because of their capacity to use bilingual patient navigators and community health workers (34). This study's findings suggest that healthcare systems had more capacity to deliver Spanish-language workshops, in contrast to faith-based organizations. Given the traditional importance of religion and church involvement within the Hispanic population (35–38), it may be necessary to increase delivery capacity at faith-based organizations to reach and enroll more Spanish-speaking CDSME program participants.

Third, it will be important to understand how the geography of service delivery affects program utilization. Prior research has revealed a service gap in predominantly Hispanic residential areas, which was combined with a tendency for Hispanic participants to travel further distances to attend CDSMP classes (9). Strategies and partnerships may be needed in certain areas and settings to coordinate transportation for participants without means of travel, which can increase participant retention rates.

Fourth, in future research and practice efforts, it will be important to examine whether Spanish- versus English-language workshops are more effective in terms of achieving positive health and quality of life outcomes among participants. Further investigations should also identify the participant and delivery characteristics associated with greater health benefits received. Some evidence suggests that Hispanic participants in evidence-based programs have greater benefits than White non-Hispanic participants (12, 39), but it is not clear whether these advantages are due to baseline disadvantages of Hispanic participants, or the way the classes are structured or made available in community settings.

CONCLUSION

The American Recovery and Reinvestment Act of 2009 (i.e., ARRA) *Communities Putting Prevention to Work: Chronic Disease Self-Management Program* initiative shows the potential for reaching Hispanic participants in a variety of delivery sites. This study provides insight into Spanish-language CDSME program recruitment and utilization with implications for program adoption in underserved Hispanic community settings. To grow the numbers of Hispanic participants reached, it may be important to increase the capacity of communities and organizations to deliver Spanish-language programs and utilize culturally tailored and appropriate recruitment materials and channels.

ACKNOWLEDGMENTS

The American Recovery and Reinvestment Act of 2009 *Communities Putting Prevention to Work: Chronic Disease Self-Management Program* initiative, led by the U.S. Administration on Aging in collaboration with the Centers for Disease Control and Prevention and the Centers for Medicare and Medicaid Services, allotted $32.5 million to support the translation of the Stanford program in 45 States, Puerto Rico, and the District of Columbia. The National Council on Aging served as the Technical Assistance Resource Center for this initiative and collected de-identified data on program participation.

REFERENCES

1. U.S. Census Bureau. *The Next Four Decades: The Older Population in the United States: 2010 to 2050.* Washington, DC: U.S. Census Bureau (2010). 138 p.
2. Humes K, Jones N, Ramirez R. *Overview of Race and Hispanic Origin: 2010.* Washington, DC: U.S. Department of Commerce Economics and Statistics Administration (2011).
3. Passel JS, Cohn DV. *US Population Projections: 2005-2050.* Washington, DC: Pew Research Center (2008).
4. United States-México Border Health Commission. *Health Disparities and the US-México Border: Challenges and Opportunities.* El Paso, TX: United States-México Border Health Commission (2010).
5. Angel JL, Whitfield KE. *The Health of Aging Hispanics: The Mexican-Origin Population.* New York, NY: Springer (2007). 294 p.
6. Agency for Healthcare Research and Quality. *2013 National Healthcare Disparities Report.* Rockville, MD: U.S. Department of Health and Human Services (2014).
7. Federal Interagency Forum on Aging-Related Statistics. *Population: Indicator 1. Number of Older Americans* (2012) [cited 2014 July 8]. Available from: http://www.agingstats.gov/Main_Site/Data/2012_Documents/Population.aspx
8. Administration on Aging. *A Statistical Profile of Hispanic Older Americans Aged 65+* (2014) [updated 2010; cited 2014 July 9]. Available from: http://www.aoa.gov/Aging_Statistics/minority_aging/Facts-on-Hispanic-Elderly.aspx
9. Salazar C, Smith ML, Perez A, Ahn S, Ory MG. Geospatial characteristics of the chronic disease self-management program: reaching diverse ethnic population in San Antonio, Texas. *Tex Public Health Assoc J* (2011) **63**:16–20.
10. Livingston G, Minushkin S, Cohn DV, Center PH. *Hispanics and Health Care in the United States: Access, Information and Knowledge.* Washington, DC: Pew Hispanic Center (2008).

11. Escarce J, Kapur K. Access to and quality of health care. In: Tienda M, Mitchell F, editors. *Hispanics and the Future of America.* (Chap. 10), Washington, DC: National Academies Press (2006). p. 410–46.
12. Smith ML, Ahn S, Mier N, Jiang L, Ory MG. An evidence-based program to reduce fall-related risk among older adults: a comparison of program efficacy by ethnicity. *Calif J Health Promot* (2012) **10**(1):28–44.
13. Ory MG, Smith ML, Kulinski KP, Lorig K, Zenker W, Whitelaw N. Self-management at the tipping point: reaching 100,000 Americans with evidence-based programs. *J Am Geriatr Soc* (2013) **61**(5):821–3. doi:10.1111/jgs.12239
14. National Council on Aging. *Evidence-Based Health Promotion Programs for Older Adults: Key Factors and Strategies Contributing to Program Sustainability.* Washington, DC: National Council on Aging (2012).
15. DuBard CA, Gizlice Z. Language spoken and differences in health status, access to care, and receipt of preventive services among US Hispanics. *Am J Public Health* (2008) **98**(11):2021–8. doi:10.2105/AJPH.2007.119008
16. Pearson WS, Ahluwalia IB, Ford ES, Mokdad AH. Language preference as a predictor of access to and use of healthcare services among Hispanics in the United States. *Ethn Dis* (2008) **18**(1):93–7.
17. Cheng EM, Chen A, Cunningham W. Primary language and receipt of recommended health care among Hispanics in the United States. *J Gen Intern Med* (2007) **22**(Suppl 2):283–8. doi:10.1007/s11606-007-0346-6
18. Lorig K. *Living a Healthy Life with Chronic Conditions: Self-Management of Heart Disease, Arthritis, Diabetes, Asthma, Bronchitis, Emphysema & Others.* 3rd ed. Boulder, CO: Bull Publishing Company (2006). 8, 382 p.
19. Ory MG, Ahn S, Jiang L, Lorig K, Ritter P, Laurent DD, et al. National study of chronic disease self-management six-month outcome findings. *J Aging Health* (2013) **25**(7):1258–74. doi:10.1177/0898264313502531
20. Ory MG, Ahn S, Jiang L, Smith ML, Ritter PL, Whitelaw N, et al. Successes of a national study of the chronic disease self-management program: meeting the triple aim of health care reform. *Med Care* (2013) **51**(11):992–8. doi:10.1097/MLR.0b013e3182a95dd1
21. Ahn S, Basu R, Smith ML, Jiang L, Lorig K, Whitelaw N, et al. The impact of chronic disease self-management programs: healthcare savings through a community-based intervention. *BMC Public Health* (2013) **13**(1):1141. doi:10.1186/1471-2458-13-1141
22. Bandura A. Social cognitive theory of self-regulation. *Organ Behav Hum Decis Process* (1991) **50**(2):248–87. doi:10.1016/0749-5978(91)90022-L
23. Kulinski KP, Boughtaugh M, Smith ML, Ory MG, Lorig K. Setting the stage: measure seletion, coordination, and data collection for a national self-management initiative. *Front Public Health* (2015) **2**:206. doi:10.3389/fpubh.2014.00206
24. U.S. Department of Health and Human Services, Administration on Aging. *ARRA – Communities Putting Prevention to Work: Chronic Disease Self-Management Program* (2012) [cited 2014 June 14]. Available from: www.cfda.gov/index?s=program&mode=form&tab=step1&id=5469a61f2c5f25cf3984fc3b94051b5f
25. Stanford School of Medicine. *Chronic Disease Self-Management Program (Better Choices, Better Health® Workshop)* (2014) [updated 2014; cited 2014 July 12]. Available from: http://patienteducation.stanford.edu/programs/cdsmp.html
26. United States Department of Agriculture Economic Research Service. *Rural-Urban Commuting Area Codes: Overview* (2014) [updated 2014; cited 2014 August 7]. Available from: http://www.ers.usda.gov/data-products/rural-urban-commuting-area-codes.aspx#.U-ObPmPqlZU
27. U.S. Census Bureau. Census 2000, Summary File 1, Table S1702; generated by Scott Horel; using American FactFinder (2012). Available from: http://factfinder2.census.gov
28. Smith ML, Ory MG, Ahn S, Kulinski KP, Jiang L, Horel S, et al. National dissemination of chronic disease self-management education programs: an incremental examination of delivery characteristics. *Front Public Health* (2015) **2**:227. doi:10.3389/fpubh.2014.00227
29. U.S. Census Bureau. *State & County QuickFacts: USA* (2014) [updated 2014; cited 2014 August 3]. Available from: http://quickfacts.census.gov/qfd/states/00000.html
30. U.S. Census Bureau. *Hispanic Origin* (2012) [cited 2014 August 5]. Available from: http://www.census.gov/population/hispanic/
31. Gonzalez-Barrera A, Lopez MH. *A Demographic Portrait of Mexican-Origin Hispanics in the United States. Pew Research Hispanic Trends Project [Internet]* (2013). Available from: http://www.pewhispanic.org/2013/05/01/a-demographic-portrait-of-mexican-origin-hispanics-in-the-united-states/
32. Mier N, Ory MG, Medina A. Anatomy of culturally sensitive interventions promoting nutrition and exercise in Hispanics: a critical examination of existing literature. *Health Promot Pract* (2010) **11**(4):541–54. doi:10.1177/1524839908328991
33. Mier N, Ory MG, Toobert DJ, Smith ML, Osuna D, McKay JR, et al. A qualitative case study examining intervention tailoring for minorities. *Am J Health Behav* (2010) **34**(6):822–32.
34. Riddick S. Improving access for limited English-speaking consumers: a review of strategies in health care settings. *J Health Care Poor Underserved* (1998) **9**(5):S40–61. doi:10.1353/hpu.2010.0672
35. Koenig H, King D, Carson VB. *Handbook of Religion and Health.* 2nd ed. New York, NY: Oxford University Press (2012). 1192 p.
36. Koenig HG, Pargament KI, Nielsen J. Religious coping and health status in medically ill hospitalized older adults. *J Nerv Ment Dis* (1998) **186**(9):513–21. doi:10.1097/00005053-199809000-00001
37. Musgrave CF, Allen CE, Allen GJ. Spirituality and health for women of color. *Am J Public Health* (2002) **92**(4):557–60. doi:10.2105/AJPH.92.4.557
38. Ahn S, Hochhalter AK, Moudouni DK, Smith ML, Ory MG. Self-reported physical and mental health of older adults: the roles of caregiving and resources. *Maturitas* (2012) **71**(1):62–9. doi:10.1016/j.maturitas.2011.10.011
39. Smith ML, Cho J, Salazar CI, Ory MG. Changes in quality of life indicators among chronic disease self-management program participants: an examination by race and ethnicity. *Ethn Dis* (2013) **23**(2):182–8.

5

Setting the stage: Measure selection, coordination, and data collection for a national self-management initiative

Kristie P. Kulinski[1]*, Michele Boutaugh[2], Matthew Lee Smith[3], Marcia G. Ory[4] and Kate Lorig[5]

[1] *National Council on Aging, Washington, DC, USA*
[2] *Administration on Aging, Administration for Community Living, Atlanta, GA, USA*
[3] *Department of Health Promotion and Behavior, College of Public Health, The University of Georgia, Athens, GA, USA*
[4] *Department of Health Promotion and Community Health Sciences, School of Public Health, Texas A&M Health Science Center, College Station, TX, USA*
[5] *Stanford Patient Education Research Center, Department of Medicine, Stanford School of Medicine, Palo Alto, CA, USA*

Edited by:
Will R. Ross, Washington University School of Medicine, USA

Reviewed by:
Lalit Raghunath Sankhe, Grant Government Medical College, India
Lynda Anderson, Centers for Disease Control and Prevention, USA

****Correspondence:***
Kristie P. Kulinski, National Council on Aging, 1901 L Street NW, 4th Floor, Washington, DC 20036, USA
e-mail: kristie.kulinski@ncoa.org

This paper describes the history and rationale behind the development of a centralized data collection system for the national rollout of the Chronic Disease Self-Management Program (CDSMP) through the American Recovery and Reinvestment Act of 2009 Communities Putting Prevention to Work: CDSMP initiative. In addition to justifying the need for solutions to the burgeoning burden of chronic disease in the United States, this paper provides details about CDSMP and related self-management education programs, including their structure, facilitator training, and effectiveness. These topics set the stage for the processes and procedures to create and manage the database for use at the national, state, and local levels. Furthermore, this paper describes the processes related to selecting variables, coordinating data collection, and utilizing data to inform research and policy.

Keywords: chronic disease self-management, evidence-based program, data collection, intervention planning

RATIONALE

As more and more evidence-based interventions are being funded as multi-site programs by both federal agencies and major foundations, there is a growing need for uniform measures and protocols as well as centralized data collection systems. This paper describes one such data system developed in response to the national rollout of the Chronic Disease Self-Management Program (CDSMP) through the American Recovery and Reinvestment Act of 2009 Communities Putting Prevention to Work: CDSMP initiative (ARRA CDSMP) (1). In addition to describing the creation and management of the database used in this effort, we will discuss its uses at the national, state, and local levels as well as its utility for informing policy and research. Additionally, this paper will provide the necessary background for those wanting to understand the rationale behind this national initiative in terms of the burden of chronic conditions among older Americans and self-management (SM) as a core requirement for dealing with such conditions. As a case example, the processes related to selecting variables, developing a centralized data collection system, training, and managing data will be described for this grand-scale translational rollout of an evidence-based program.

BACKGROUND

BURDEN OF CHRONIC CONDITIONS

Chronic conditions have become endemic in the United States, with older adults bearing the greatest burden. Approximately 36% of adults age 18–34 have a chronic condition, compared to nearly 92% in the population aged 65 and over (2). This same trend is observed with regard to multiple chronic conditions, with a range of 14% among the population aged 18–34 to nearly 77% in the older adult population (2). Among Medicare beneficiaries, the most common chronic conditions include high blood pressure (58%), high cholesterol (45%), heart disease (31%), arthritis (29%), and diabetes (28%) (3).

Older adults with chronic conditions face a number of barriers in terms of coping with their illness and optimizing their health, which include lack of social support, low skill levels for symptom management, and low confidence in their abilities to manage their conditions (self-efficacy) (4). Increasingly, SM is being heralded as a key component in the improvement of health outcomes associated with chronic disease. According to the Institute of Medicine, SM is defined as "the tasks that individuals must undertake to live well with one or more chronic conditions." (5) Research demonstrates the positive impact of SM programs on these tasks, which include having the confidence to deal with the medical, role, and emotional management of their conditions (5, 6).

THE CHRONIC DISEASE SELF-MANAGEMENT PROGRAM

The CDSMP is perhaps the best known SM intervention (7). It was developed at Stanford University and is a peer-led, community-based intervention that helps individuals with chronic conditions learn skills and gain the confidence to manage and improve their health (7). The program focuses on challenges that are common to individuals living with any chronic condition, such as problem solving, decision making, symptom management, nutrition, exercise, medication use, emotions, and communicating with health care professionals. In addition to the standard CDSMP, Stanford offers a comprehensive suite of chronic disease self-management education (CDSME) programs, with disease-specific variants for people living with diabetes, chronic pain, HIV/AIDS, cancer survivors, and arthritis. Most of these also have culturally appropriate Spanish versions. The programs are available in over 30 countries and 25 languages.

Led by a pair of trained facilitators, many of whom also have chronic health conditions, these small, highly interactive workshops meet once a week for six consecutive weeks. During each 2.5-hour session, 10–15 participants focus on building the skills they need to manage their conditions. Fostering participant self-efficacy is at the core of the intervention, achieved through techniques such as skills mastery, peer modeling, reinterpretation of physiological symptoms, and social persuasion. Workshops are highly participative, with mutual success and support building participants' confidence in their ability to manage their health and maintain active, fulfilling lives. Participants create a weekly action plan and try new behaviors such as exercise monitoring. Each session includes an opportunity for feedback about progress and discussion of challenges. **Table 1** provides an overview of the topics and activities covered during each workshop session.

Workshop facilitator training and infrastructure

The program uses a train-the-trainer model consisting of Lay Leaders, Master Trainers, and T-Trainers (8). Lay Leaders can facilitate CDSMP workshops but cannot train others. They complete a structured training and must facilitate at least one workshop in the following year. Master Trainers can facilitate CDSMP workshops as well as train new Lay Leaders. As with CDSMP Lay Leaders, Master Trainers participate in a systematized training. After training, they must facilitate at least two CDSMP workshops within one year and conduct a Lay Leader training within 18 months. Finally, T-Trainers are authorized to facilitate workshops, train new Lay Leaders, and train new Master Trainers. This role involves the completion of an apprenticeship with a Stanford staff T-Trainer. Additionally, they must have facilitated at least three Lay Leader trainings prior to their apprenticeship, co-lead a Master Trainer training within 12 months of completing the apprenticeship, and conduct a Master Trainer training every two years.

Intervention effectiveness

The Chronic Disease Self-Management Program has been extensively evaluated through randomized controlled trials (9, 10). Workshop participants experience significant improvements across several domains, including physical activity, symptom management, communication with physicians, and general health. Additionally, the original research demonstrated that CDSMP participants spend fewer days in the hospital, as well as a trend toward fewer outpatient visits and hospitalizations (10).

Further cementing the value of CDSMP, the program has been successfully translated for implementation in a variety of community settings worldwide, with participants reporting results similar to the original research. A recent United States-based *National Study of CDSMP* encompassed over 1000 participants drawn from 145 workshops in 17 states (11). Sociodemographic, health status, and behavioral data were collected at baseline, 6, and 12 months, yielding a number of positive, significant improvements (12, 13). When aligned with the Institute for Healthcare Improvement's Triple Aim (13, 14), the following results are particularly noteworthy: better health – improvement in self-reported health, less depression, and better quality of life; *better care* – improved communication with physicians, medication compliance, and health literacy; and *lower health cost* – more than \$360 per person net savings after factoring in program costs (15). In addition to improving participant health and decreasing health care costs, the outcomes of this national study reinforce that CDSMP has been effectively translated from research to practice throughout the country.

NATIONAL INITIATIVES SUPPORTING CDSMP IMPLEMENTATION

Over the past decade, community-based implementation of CDSMP and its variants have received broad support through funding from federal agencies [e.g., the Administration on Aging (AoA), a program division within the Administration for Community Living, and the Centers for Disease Control and Prevention

Table 1 | CDSMP workshop overview by session.

	Week 1	Week 2	Week 3	Week 4	Week 5	Week 6
Overview of self-management and chronic health conditions	✓					
Making an action plan	✓	✓	✓	✓	✓	✓
Relaxation/cognitive symptom management	✓		✓	✓	✓	✓
Feedback/problem solving		✓	✓	✓	✓	✓
Difficult emotions		✓	✓			
Fitness/exercise		✓	✓			
Better breathing			✓			
Fatigue			✓			
Eating well				✓		
Advance directives				✓		
Communication				✓		
Medications					✓	
Making treatment decisions					✓	
Depression					✓	
Informing the health care team						✓
Working with your health care professional						✓
Future plans						✓

(CDC)], foundations (e.g., Atlantic Philanthropies, Archstone Foundation, Robert Wood Johnson Foundation, and Health Foundation of South Florida), and health care providers (e.g., Kaiser Permanente, Group Health Cooperative, and Dignity Health). Specific to the aging services network, AoA has supported states and community organizations in their efforts to develop infrastructure, workforce, and capacity to deliver CDSMP and other evidence-based programs. Since 2006, AoA has provided three major competitive grant programs to states to support dissemination of evidence-based programs. The 2006–2012 *Evidence-Based Disease and Disability Prevention Program* (EBDDP) grants were awarded to 24 states to support dissemination of CDSMP and evidence-based physical activity, fall prevention, nutrition, and behavioral health programs. The national program infrastructure was greatly expanded with the 2010–2013 *American Recovery and Reinvestment Act Communities Putting Prevention to Work: CDSMP* (ARRA CDSMP) grants awarded to 45 states, the District of Columbia, and Puerto Rico. The administration's current 2012–2015 *Empowering Older Adults and Adults with Disabilities through Chronic Disease Self-Management Education Programs* grant program, financed by the Prevention and Public Health Fund (PPHF), provides support to 22 states. Both the ARRA CDSMP and the PPHF grant programs have focused on not only chronic disease SM programs, including the generic CDSMP, but also programs developed for specific chronic conditions (arthritis, diabetes, HIV/AIDs, and chronic pain), for Spanish-speaking cultures, and in an online format. **Table 2A** highlights AoA funding history, although as previously noted a number of federal and other sources of funding have also supported these programs.

DATA COLLECTION

SELECTING STANDARDIZED MEASURES

The collection of standardized performance monitoring data has been a critical component of each of the aforementioned AoA initiatives. While the specific measures collected have evolved over time, the data collected by AoA grantees and their partners can be grouped within four categories: (1) workshop information; (2) participant information; (3) attendance; and (4) organization data. The current standardized measures, which were approved

Table 2 | Support, data requirements, and rationale for AoA-CDSMP initiatives.

A: EVOLUTION OF AoA-SUPPORTED CDSMP INITIATIVES

Year	Initiative	Reach
2003	Evidence-Based Prevention Program for the Elderly Model Communities Project	14 Communities
2006	Evidence-Based Disease Prevention and Disability Program	16 States
2006–2007	Evidence-Based Disease Prevention and Disability Program (funding made available to 24 states by AoA, plus three states funded by Atlantic Philanthropies)	27 States
2010	American Recovery and Reinvestment Act Communities Putting Prevention to Work: Chronic Disease Self-Management Program	47 States/Territories
2012	2012 Prevention and Public Health Funds: Empowering Older Adults and Adults with Disabilities through Chronic Disease Self-Management Education Programs	22 States

B: AoA GRANTEE DATA COLLECTION REQUIREMENTS

Data type	Elements collected
Workshop Information	Host organization and implementation site name/location, workshop leader names, workshop start/end dates, use of orientation session, workshop type, workshop language
Participant Information	Date of birth, ZIP Code, sex, race, ethnicity, chronic conditions, caregiver status, disability status, number of people in household, education level
Attendance	Sessions attended by participant
Organization Data	Organization type with regard to host organization and implementation site (list includes area agency on aging, county health department, health care organization, faith-based organization, workplace, residential facility, and library)

C: RATIONALE FOR SELECTING DATA TYPES

Data type	Rationale
Workshop Information	Map delivery infrastructure, identify type of workshop offered, identify diversity of languages, monitor start/end dates and number of workshop leaders as proxies for fidelity
Participant Information	Accurately describe participant population, ensure adequate reach to target population, monitor demographic elements that serve as proxies for health status and vulnerability (race/ethnicity, chronic conditions, caregiver status, disability status, education level, etc.)
Attendance	Track number of sessions attended by participant to determine completer status, identify organization and state successes/challenges with participant retention
Organization Data	Identify types of organizations involved in program delivery, monitor increase in delivery capacity and geographic reach

through the Office of Management and Budget (OMB) Paperwork Reduction Act, are listed in **Table 2B**.

RATIONALE FOR UNIFORM DATA COLLECTION AND MONITORING

Data elements for the ARRA CDSMP initiative were carefully and purposively chosen with the intent of balancing the critical need to monitor program operations and participant accrual with the desire to minimize data collection and reporting burden on program deliverers and participants (see **Table 2C**). Considering the myriad studies reinforcing the effectiveness of the program in the community when delivered with fidelity to the original model (6, 12), emphasis was placed on collecting reach data versus additional outcome data. Moreover, grantees and their partners were encouraged to invest their limited resources in program delivery, infrastructure, and sustainability to ensure ongoing access to CDSMP as opposed to engaging in costly outcomes measurement.

At the federal level, there is a strong emphasis on accountability and transparency to ensure that funds are being spent properly and the desired reach and impact are being achieved. Therefore, the uniform collection of appropriate measures ensures that due diligence is performed in this regard. For example, an overarching goal of the ARRA CDSMP initiative was to reach 50,000 program completers (i.e., those participants who attend four or more of the six workshop sessions), with a particular emphasis on engaging vulnerable and disadvantaged older adults (16). Because detailed attendance information was collected on each participant, it was easy to determine how many completers were reached. This attendance information was especially important because outcome measures were not collected in this initiative, thus workshop attendance served as a proxy variable indicating that participants received an adequate intervention dose. Additionally, because outcomes were not directly measured, demographic variables such as date of birth, living alone status, racial and ethnic status, education level, and number of chronic conditions served as proxies for health status and vulnerability. Collecting this participant and attendance information was deemed important for informing national and state leadership as to whether or not the target population was being reached/served by intervention workshops.

DATA COLLECTION TOOLS, COORDINATION, AND PROCESSES

Timely and efficient collection and reporting of programmatic data are critical to ensure the success and value of the national database. The following OMB-approved data collection forms accompany the national database: (1) Workshop Information Cover Sheet; (2) Attendance Log; (3) Participant Information Survey; and (4) Organization Data Form.

At a local level, workshop leaders complete the Workshop Information Cover Sheet. They are also responsible for using the Attendance Log to track participation at each session. During the first session (or an orientation session, if applicable), workshop leaders distribute a Participant Information Survey to each participant. The completion of these brief, 10-item surveys is optional and is not required for workshop participation. Completed surveys are collected from the participants and sent along with the Workshop Information Cover Sheet and Attendance Log to a person responsible for entering the information into the national database. Expected turnaround time for receiving the forms is generally two weeks after the conclusion of a workshop. While the structure for data entry varies by state, typically either (a) all data entry take place at the state level or (b) responsibility for data entry is divided regionally, with staff from selected organizations entering data on behalf of their peers. Decisions as to which model to use are generally based on adequacy of staffing for data entry/monitoring (e.g., is there sufficient staff time at a state level to devote to this task and keep up with demand, or does this task need to be parsed out regionally?). An additional consideration is the overall program management model, as some states centralize program management at the state level, whereas others take a decentralized approach with each region acting semi-autonomously.

DEVELOPING THE NATIONAL, ONLINE DATABASE

Prior to the ARRA CDSMP initiative, data were collected via paper forms, which were mailed to a centralized location and entered into an Excel spreadsheet. This spreadsheet was sent semi-annually by each grantee to a central repository, where the data were cleaned, analyzed, and shared back with AoA and their respective grantees. This system was rather burdensome with data transfers from multiple partners. There was also a considerable time lag that occurred between the submission of semi-annual data and the receipt of the analyzed data.

In 2010, with the advent of the ARRA CDSMP initiative and the major expansion, a more efficient data system was needed for tracking the national rollout of CDSMP and assessing whether initiative goals were being met. Thus, the National Council on Aging (NCOA), the designated resource center for chronic disease SM education programs, developed an online national database. A custom application was developed by NCOA on the Salesforce.com platform expressly for this purpose. Salesforce.com was selected for reasons that include NCOA's experience developing other data collection systems on the platform, cost-efficiency, web-based access, and data security.

Presently, the database is available as a free resource for all states implementing these programs, regardless of funding source. Upon request, users receive login information from NCOA, and can then enter workshop and participant data from any computer with Internet access. No software is required. All data are available in real-time, and data from any of the suite of in-person Stanford University CDSME programs can be entered. The data are stored securely and are de-identified at the participant level. The database does not contain participant names. Each participant is assigned a random unique identifier and is linked to a workshop though a separate unique identifier. Database users must view a recorded training webinar prior to accessing the system. Technical support related to database utilization and data entry is available via NCOA. Regular quality control activities, such as identifying erroneous duplicate workshops, are performed by NCOA and its database management partner, Senior Services. In addition, other quality measures are built into the system, such as prompting users to review workshop records with issues of concern such as workshop start and end dates that are fewer than 6 weeks apart and participant ages that are younger than 18 years (the minimum recommended participant age).

In addition to the ability to easily enter workshop and participant data, users have access to a variety of standard reports to inform program management and enhance quality assurance. These reports can be filtered by elements such as date, county, and host organization and offer a comparison to state and national data. Beyond the standard reports that are available to all database users, NCOA staff can develop custom reports in response to information and data requests from AoA leadership and other key stakeholders.

UTILITY OF COLLECTED DATA

The NCOA and AoA, as well as other program funders and stakeholders, use the information from the various data collection tools for numerous reasons, including to (1) comply with reporting requirements mandated by the authorizing statutes; (2) collect data for performance measures used in the justification of the budget to Congress and by program, state, and national decision makers; (3) effectively manage the program at the federal, state, and local levels; (4) identify program implementation issues and pinpoint areas for technical assistance activities; (5) identify best practices in program implementation and building sustainable program delivery systems and to develop resources to enable current and future program implementers to learn from and replicate these practices; and (6) provide information for reports to Congress, other governmental agencies, stakeholders, and to the public about grantee progress.

The uniform collection of these data elements using a coordinated online system has great practicality and utility for reporting and providing real-time monitoring and feedback. Using these data, AoA can perform state-based performance comparisons related to delivery site engagement, participant reach, participant retention, and program embedment/sustainability. These data can also enable program fidelity assessments to rapidly identify technical assistance needs and/or correct program drift.

Furthermore, these data can be used to develop webinars and other resources for state grantees and their partners (for the purposes of training, technical assistance, and/or strategic development) as well as generate standard and customized reports so grantees can identify local successes and opportunities for improvement. More specifically, these reports have been (and continue to be) used for quality control (e.g., identifying workshops that offered a "session zero," or introductory orientation session, to determine impact on participant retention), planning (e.g., identifying host organizations that are categorized as faith-based when looking to engage additional partners of this same type), and reach to a specific population (e.g., number of African American participants who indicate a diabetes diagnosis).

Beyond these data uses at a federal/national level, this uniformly collected data also provide great benefit to state grantees and their partners. These data serve to inform key stakeholders about progress and challenges, guide quality control and assurance efforts and forward planning, and help justify the need for, as well as attain, additional funding sources (through grant applications or other mechanisms). Furthermore, researchers have utilized these data to address a variety of topics, including program participation of older adults with diabetes (17).

CONCLUSION

Data collection for CDSMP and the suite of other Stanford University CDSME programs has been essential to nationwide program success and sustainability. With the inception of this database, states and community-based organizations offering CDSME had immediate, real-time access to their workshop and participant data for the first time. This proved to be an incredible value-add for the network. Not only does the data highlight program reach and inform program planning, it is also critical in terms of attaining additional resources to support implementation and infrastructure at national, state, and local levels. It is evident that the benefit gained from a national data collection system is certainly worth the investment in development, training, and maintenance. Future grand-scale initiatives delivering evidence-based programs are encouraged to use this ARRA CDSMP experience when creating data collection and monitoring systems.

REFERENCES

1. U.S. Department of Health and Human Services, Administration on Aging. *ARRA – Communities Putting Prevention to Work: Chronic Disease Self-Management Program 2012.* (2012). Available from: www.cfda.gov/index?s=program&mode=form&tab=step1&id=5469a61f2c5f25cf3984fc3b94051b5f
2. Machlin S, Cohen J, Beauregard K. *Health Care Expenses for Adults with Chronic Conditions, 2005. Statistical Brief #203.* Rockville, MD: Agency for Healthcare Research and Quality (2008).
3. Centers for Medicare and Medicaid Services. *Chronic conditions among Medicare Beneficiaries.* 2012 ed. Baltimore, MD: Chartbook (2012).
4. Bayliss EA, Ellis JL, Steiner JF. Barriers to self-management and quality of life outcomes in seniors with multimorbidities. *Ann Fam Med* (2007) **5**(5):395–402. doi:10.1370/afm.722
5. National Research Council. *1st Annual Crossing the Quality Chasm Summit: A Focus on Communities.* Washington, DC: The National Academies Press (2004).
6. Brady TJ, Murphy L, Beauchesne D, et al. *Sorting through the Evidence for the Arthritis Self-Management Program and the Chronic Disease Self-Management Program: Executive Summary of ASMP/CDSMP Meta-Analysis.* Atlanta, GA: Centers for Disease Control and Prevention (2011). Available from: http://www.cdc.gov/arthritis/docs/asmp-executive-summary.pdf
7. Chronic Disease Self-Management Program. (2014). Available from: http://patienteducation.stanford.edu/programs/cdsmp.html
8. Stanford School of Medicine. *Training Policies for Stanford Self-Management Programs.* (2014). Available from: http://patienteducation.stanford.edu/training/trnpolicies.html
9. Lorig KR, Sobel DS, Stewart AL, Brown BW Jr, Bandura A, Ritter P, et al. Evidence suggesting that a chronic disease self-management program can improve health status while reducing hospitalization: a randomized trial. *Med Care* (1999) **37**(1):5–14. doi:10.1097/00005650-199901000-00003
10. Lorig KR, Ritter P, Stewart AL, Sobel DS, Brown BW Jr, Bandura A, et al. Chronic disease self-management program: 2-year health status and health care utilization outcomes. *Med Care* (2001) **39**(11):1217–23. doi:10.1097/00005650-200111000-00008
11. National Study of the Chronic Disease Self-Management Program. *A Brief Overview.* Washington, DC: National Council on Aging (2013).
12. Ory MG, Ahn S, Jiang L, Lorig K, Ritter P, Laurent DD, et al. National study of the chronic disease self-management program: six month outcome findings. *J Aging Health* (2013) **25**(7):1258–74. doi:10.1177/0898264313502531
13. Ory MG, Ahn S, Jiang L, Smith ML, Ritter PL, Whitelaw N, et al. Successes of a national study of the chronic disease self-management program: meeting the triple aim of health care reform. *Med Care* (2013) **51**(11):992–8. doi:10.1097/MLR.0b013e3182a95dd1
14. Berwick DM, Nolan TW, Whittington J. The triple aim: care, health, and cost. *Health Aff* (2008) **27**:759–69. doi:10.1377/hlthaff.27.3.759
15. Ahn S, Basu R, Smith ML, Jiang L, Lorig K, Whitelaw N, et al. The impact of chronic disease self-management programs: healthcare savings through a

community-based intervention. *BMC Public Health* (2013) **13**(1):1141. doi:10.1186/1471-2458-13-1141

16. U.S. Administration on Aging. *American Recovery and Reinvestment Act Communities Putting Prevention to Work Chronic Disease Self-Management Program Announcement.* (2010). Available from: http://www.aoa.gov/AoARoot/Grants/Funding/2010.aspx
17. Erdem E, Korda H. Self-management program participation by older adults with diabetes. *Fam Community Health* (2014) **37**(2):134–46. doi:10.1097/FCH.0000000000000025

6

National dissemination of chronic disease self-management education programs: An incremental examination of delivery characteristics

Matthew Lee Smith[1]*, Marcia G. Ory[2], SangNam Ahn[2,3], Kristie P. Kulinski[4], Luohua Jiang[5], Scott Horel[2] and Kate Lorig[6]

[1] *Department of Health Promotion and Behavior, College of Public Health, The University of Georgia, Athens, GA, USA*
[2] *Department of Health Promotion and Community Health Sciences, Texas A&M Health Science Center, School of Public Health, College Station, TX, USA*
[3] *Division of Health Systems Management and Policy, School of Public Health, The University of Memphis, Memphis, TN, USA*
[4] *National Council on Aging, Washington, DC, USA*
[5] *Department of Epidemiology and Biostatistics, Texas A&M Health Science Center, School of Public Health, College Station, TX, USA*
[6] *Department of Medicine, Stanford Patient Education Research Center, Stanford School of Medicine, Palo Alto, CA, USA*

Edited by:
Sanjay P. Zodpey, Public Health Foundation of India, India

Reviewed by:
Aida Mujkic, University of Zagreb, Croatia
Ronit Elk, University of South Carolina, USA

***Correspondence:**
Matthew Lee Smith, Department of Health Promotion and Behavior, College of Public Health, The University of Georgia, 330 River Road, 315 Ramsey Center, Athens, GA 30602, USA
e-mail: health@uga.edu

With a near 20-year developmental history as an evidence-based program, the suite of Chronic Disease Self-Management Education (CDSME) programs were selected in 2010 for grand-scale dissemination in a federally supported initiative to improve the health of older Americans. The primary charge of this national effort was to establish a sustainable program delivery system for empowering American adults with one or more chronic conditions to better manage their health. The current study focused on a series of dissemination and implementation science research questions to: (1) examine the geographic distribution of participation in this initiative across the Unites States; (2) describe workshop characteristics engaged to reach program participants in various settings; and (3) describe personal characteristics of the first 100,000 participants. Each subsequent entering cohort was descriptively examined to indicate whether there was constancy or change in delivery sites and populations reached over time. Findings show a strengthening of the workshop delivery infrastructure in that it took 9.4 months to reach the first 25,000 participants in 853 counties compared to 5.4 months to reach the last 25,000 participants in 1,109 counties. The workshop delivery characteristics and participant characteristics remained relatively consistent across increments of 25,000 participants reached, although general trends were observed for some variables. For example, after reaching the first 25,000 participants, subsequent groups of 25,000 participants were reached more quickly. Additionally, workshops were increasingly delivered in ZIP Codes with higher percentages of families residing below the federal poverty line. As more participants were reached, more participants with chronic conditions were enrolled. This national translational study illustrates the rapid expansion of CDSME programs throughout the United States and capability to reach diverse populations in a variety of settings.

Keywords: chronic disease self-management, evidence-based program, older adults, sustainability, program implementation, program reach, evaluation

INTRODUCTION

Seen as a critical part of primary care for the past 20 years (1, 2), disease self-management programs have been associated with a plethora of positive health outcomes among middle-aged and older adults in the United States (3). While the healthcare system is increasingly expected to provide chronic care (1), chronic disease self-management initiatives outside of the physician's office are now widely recognized as an effective complement to improve health indicators and quality of life while reducing overall health-related complications and associated costs (4). One of the most extensively tested programs, the Stanford Chronic Disease Self-Management Program (CDSMP), is a 6-week program (5) that has strong evidence demonstrating its ability to improve participants' health status, modify their health behaviors, and reduce their healthcare utilization and associated costs (6–9). The interactive workshop sessions are designed to enhance three types of skills necessary for the everyday management of chronic conditions: medical management, emotional management, and social role management (6). While CDSMP remains the flagship program, Stanford has translated it to be delivered online, in multiple languages, and for specific diseases/conditions (e.g., diabetes, arthritis, chronic pain, HIV) (5). This collection of interventions (including CDSMP) comprises the suite of Chronic Disease Self-Management Education (CDSME) programs.

Building on a nascent evidence-based prevention initiative supported by the U.S. Administration on Aging (AoA) beginning in

2003 (10), funding was provided as part of the American Recovery and Reinvestment Act of 2009 (ARRA) to disseminate CDSME programs in 45 states, Puerto Rico, and the District of Columbia between 2010 and 2012 (11). Given the solid evidence base behind CDSMP, this jointly administered initiative of the AoA, the Centers for Disease Control and Prevention (CDC), and the Centers for Medicare and Medicaid Services (CMS) sought to bring these evidence-based programs to scale for the important goal of addressing the rapidly rising number of older adults struggling to manage their chronic conditions. The national goal of this ARRA-funded initiative was to reach at least 50,000 program completers (i.e., attend four or more of the six workshops sessions). Each participating state and entity was assigned a target goal for program completers based on the size of its population of older Americans. There was an expectation that certain delivery site types would be utilized (e.g., senior centers, healthcare organizations, residential facilities, educational institutions, faith-based organizations, and tribal centers), and special emphasis was placed on recruiting and enrolling racial/minority and other underserved populations.

The goal of having over 50,000 adults complete CDSME program workshops was accomplished within the first 24 months of this initiative across more than 1,000 United States counties (12). This accomplishment demonstrates the feasibility of a coordinated effort with the aging services network, the public health, and healthcare sectors. This study examined participant accrual of the first 100,000 participants enrolled in this national CDSME program roll out in four blocks (i.e., each representing 25,000 participants). Using this frame of progressing accrual blocks, the purposes of this study were to: (1) examine the geographic distribution of participation in this initiative across the Unites States; (2) describe workshop characteristics engaged to reach program participants in various settings; and (3) describe personal characteristics of the first 100,000 participants. Each subsequent entering cohort was descriptively examined to indicate whether there was constancy or change in delivery sites and populations reached over time.

MATERIALS AND METHODS

CHRONIC DISEASE SELF-MANAGEMENT EDUCATION (CDSME) PROGRAMS

As described previously, CDSMP falls within a suite of CDSME programs that have been widely disseminated in the U.S. as a method to empower patients with self-management skills to deal with their chronic conditions (12, 13). Drawing upon Social Learning Theory (14), CDSMP is an evidence-based, peer-led intervention consisting of six highly participative classes held for 2.5 h each, once a week, for six consecutive weeks (13). Additional details about the theory behind CDSME programs and their implementation can be found elsewhere (15).

DATA SOURCE AND STUDY POPULATION

This study reports findings based on cross-sectional data collected from the first 100,000 participants enrolled in the nationwide delivery of CDSME programs as part of the American Recovery and Reinvestment Act of 2009 (i.e., Recovery Act) *Communities Putting Prevention to Work: Chronic Disease Self-Management Program* initiative (12). Workshops were delivered in 45 states, Puerto Rico, and the District of Columbia (11). With support from AoA, a centralized online data system was developed by the National Council on Aging to collect data from participating organizations (15). Each state identified several database users at the state- and/or regional-level who were responsible for entering workshop and participant data.

MEASURES

In recognition of the importance of minimizing assessment burden, the data collection effort was limited to a short informational sheet about the delivery organization to be filled out by the delivery sites; a brief set of items describing participant characteristics such as age, sex, race/ethnicity, number and type of self-reported chronic conditions, living arrangements and ZIP Code (for participant residence and delivery site location); and attendance logs to document the specific sessions attended by each participant. While the expectation was that each organization would collect all the data referenced above, due to privacy and other concerns at some locations, all of the data elements were not collected at all of the sites (15). Further, because the completion of the participant questionnaire was not a pre-requisite for attending the workshop, some delivery sites chose not to collect all data points and some participants elected not to complete the questionnaire. However, to be counted as a "successful" completer (i.e., attending four of the six offered workshop sessions), the workshop information sheet and attendance roster was required.

ANALYSES

Statistical analyses for this study were performed using SPSS (version 21). Workshop and participant characteristics were compared between the first, second, third, and fourth group of 25,000 participants reached. Additionally, maps were generated to illustrate the cumulative geospatial distribution and accruement of CDSME program participants and workshops for the first 25,000 participants, 50,000 participants, 75,000 participants, and all 100,000 participants. Plots indicate workshop locations. Shading indicates the number of participants reached in each state (i.e., darker shade represents more participants reached). Hash markings represent the first year in which funding was received by state.

RESULTS

NATIONAL CDSME PROGRAM UPTAKE

Figure 1 depicts the cumulative geospatial distribution of the first 100,000 CDSME program enrollees by increments of 25,000 participants. As can be seen, the first 25,000 participants were reached by 2,226 workshops in 1,705 unique implementation sites over a 9.4-month period across 853 counties. At this stage in the intervention, only a few states had reached over 1,000 participants. Comparatively, the last 25,000 participants were reached by 2,154 workshops in 1,769 unique implementation sites over a 5.4-month period across 1,109 counties. At this stage in the intervention, only a few states had not reached over 1,000 participants.

CDSME PROGRAM WORKSHOP CHARACTERISTICS

Table 1 presents workshop characteristics for the first 100,000 CDSME program participants enrolled in the intervention. These

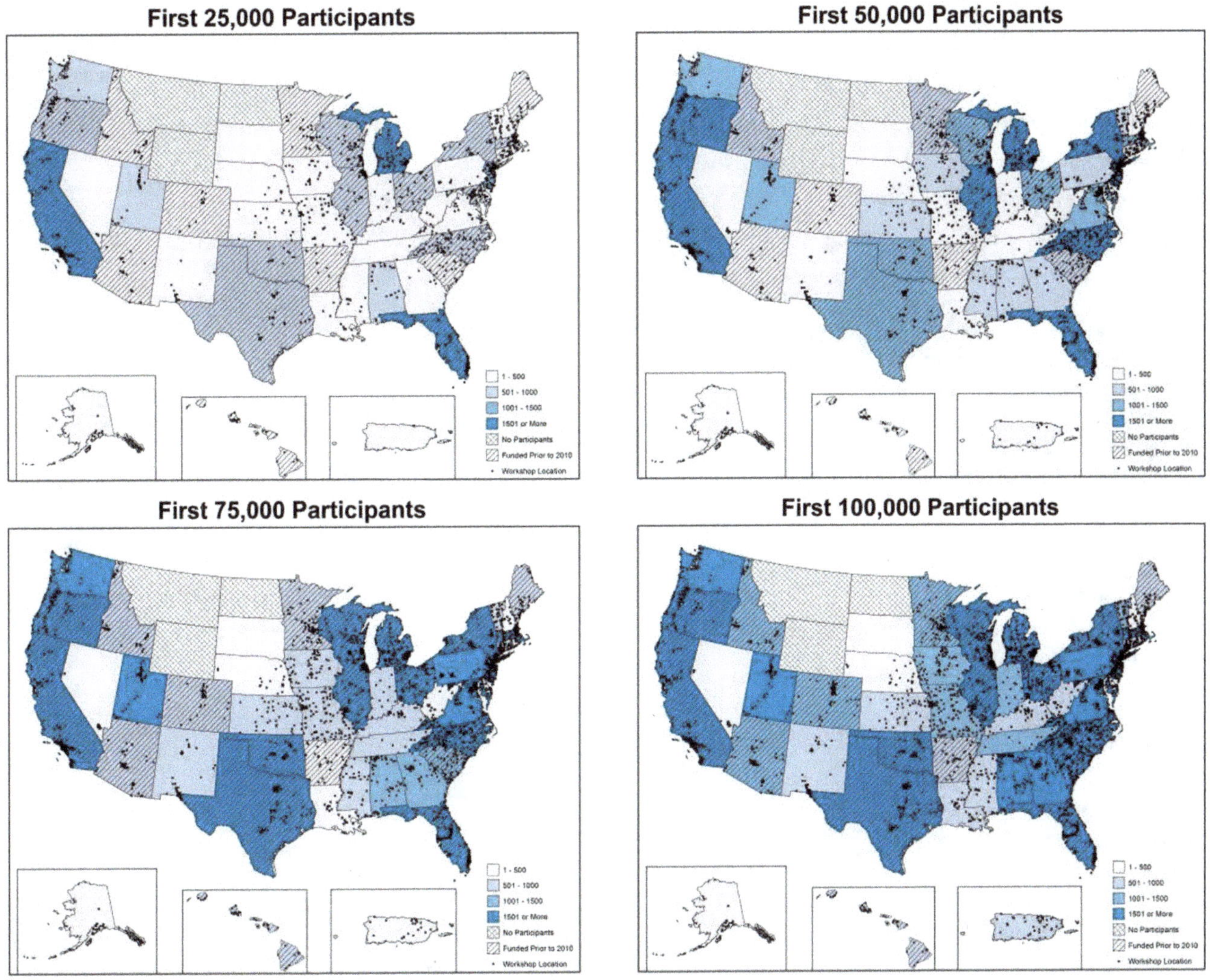

FIGURE 1 | Geospatial distribution of CDSMP workshops and participants by increments of 25,000 participants.

100,000 participants were reached by 8,702 workshops in 5,586 unique implementation sites over a 25.9 month period across 1,786 counties. The majority of participants enrolled in CDSMP workshops (78.4%), followed by Diabetes Self-Management Program (DSMP) workshops (10.3%) and Tomando Control de su Salud (Spanish CDSMP) workshops (8.9%). The largest proportion of participants attended workshops at senior centers or area agencies on aging (29.2%), followed by healthcare organizations (21.1%), residential facilities (17.6%), community/multi-purpose facilities (9.9%), faith-based organizations (8.4%), and other settings (e.g., correctional facilities malls, RV parks, fire departments, county administration buildings, private residences, casinos, career centers). The majority of participants attended workshops delivered in English (89.6%) and in metro settings (79.6%). On average, workshops included 12.69 (±4.18) participants, and participants attended 4.38 (±1.72) sessions. The workshop completion rate was 74.9%.

Workshop delivery characteristics remained relatively consistent across increments of 25,000 participants reached, although general trends were observed for some variables. For example, after reaching the first 25,000 participants, it took shorter amounts of time to reach subsequent groups of 25,000 participants (i.e., 9.37 months to reach the first 25,000 participants and 5.37 months to reach the last 25,000 participants). As more participants were reached, larger proportions participated in DSMP workshops (i.e., 8.3% for the first 25,000 participants and 12.0% for the last 25,000 participants) and fewer participated in Spanish-language workshops (i.e., 10.7% for the first 25,000 participants and 8.2% for the last 25,000 participants). Additionally, workshops were increasingly delivered in ZIP Codes with higher percentages of families residing below the federal poverty line (i.e., an average of 10.76 families below poverty for the first 25,000 participants and 11.46 for the last 25,000 participants).

CDSME PROGRAM PARTICIPANT CHARACTERISTICS

Table 2 presents participant characteristics of the first 100,000 CDSME program participants enrolled in the intervention. On average, the first 100,000 CDSME program participants were 67.09

Table 1 | Workshop characteristics by reach increments of 25,000 participants.

	Total	Participant 1–25,000	Participant 25,001–50,000	Participant 50,001–75,000	Participant 75,001–100,000
Number of unique counties served	1,786	853	1,048	988	1,109
Number of workshops delivered	8,702	2,226	2,138	2,184	2,154
Number of unique implementation sites	5,586	1,705	1,727	1,764	1,769
Time to enroll (in months)	25.91	9.37	6.00	5.17	5.37
Participants reached by CDSME workshop type					
Arthritis self-management program (ASMP)	0.5%	0.8%	0.4%	0.1%	0.5%
Chronic disease self-management program (CDSMP)	78.4%	80.2%	79.5%	75.6%	78.3%
Chronic pain self-management program (CPSMP)	0.5%	0.0%	0.6%	0.4%	1.0%
Diabetes self-management program (DSMP)	10.3%	8.3%	9.4%	11.3%	12.0%
Spanish ASMP	0.1%	0.3%	0.0%	0.0%	0.0%
Tomando control de su dabetes (Spanish DSMP)	1.4%	0.8%	1.1%	2.5%	1.2%
Tomando control de su salud (Spanish CDSMP)	8.9%	9.5%	8.9%	10.1%	7.0%
Delivery site types					
Senior center/AAA	29.2%	30.5%	27.4%	30.5%	28.3%
Healthcare organizations	21.1%	23.0%	20.5%	20.5%	20.5%
Residential facilities	17.6%	13.4%	18.5%	19.8%	18.8%
Community/multi-purpose facilities	9.9%	9.2%	10.2%	10.2%	10.0%
Faith-based organizations	8.4%	9.3%	8.9%	6.7%	8.7%
Educational institutions	2.3%	2.7%	2.1%	1.5%	2.8%
County health departments	1.3%	1.4%	1.3%	1.0%	1.4%
Tribal organizations	0.2%	0.2%	0.2%	0.1%	0.2%
Workplaces	0.5%	1.0%	0.6%	0.4%	0.2%
Other	9.5%	9.4%	10.2%	9.3%	9.1%
Workshop language					
English	89.6%	89.3%	90.0%	87.4%	91.8%
Spanish	10.4%	10.7%	10.0%	12.6%	8.2%
Number of participants enrolled in workshop	12.69 (±4.18)	12.61 (±4.22)	12.78 (±4.17)	12.66 (±4.18)	12.71 (±4.14)
Number of sessions attended	4.38 (±1.72)	4.36 (±1.75)	4.38 (±1.71)	4.40 (±1.68)	4.37 (±1.72)
Successful completion (attend 4+ sessions)					
No	25.1%	25.9%	25.3%	23.9%	25.4%
Yes	74.9%	74.1%	74.7%	76.1%	74.6%
Delivery site					
Metro	79.6%	78.6%	77.6%	82.6%	79.6%
Non-Metro	20.4%	21.4%	22.4%	17.4%	20.4%
Percent of families below poverty	1128 (±5.39)	10.76 (±4.11)	11.41 (±5.49)	11.48 (±15.67)	11.46 (±16.05)

(±14.58) years of age; 12.0% were under age 50 years, 42.7% were aged 65–79 years, and 19.9% were aged 80 years and older. The majority of participants was female (77.9%), non-Hispanic (82.6%), and white (66.0%). Approximately 22% of participants were African American, 4.5% were Asian or Pacific Islander, 1.6% American Indian or Native Alaskan, and 6.2% "other" or multiple races. The majority of participants resided with other individuals (84.4%) and lived in metro areas (78.2%). On average, participants self-reported 2.20 (±1.71) chronic conditions; 39.6% reported three or more co-morbidities.

Generally, participant characteristics remained consistent across increments of 25,000 participants reached; however, trends were observed for some variables. For example, as more participants were reached by CDSME programs, more participants with chronic conditions were enrolled, with the number of participants enrolling with three or more chronic conditions increasing from 34.3% for the first 25,000 participants to 42.0% for the last 25,000 participants (i.e., participant 75,001–100,000). Additionally, as more participants were reached, the program enrolled smaller proportions of participants who lived alone (i.e., decreasing from 21.9% for the first 25,000 participants to 11.3% for the last 25,000 participants).

DISCUSSION

Self-management education has been recognized as a critical factor in empowering adults to improve their health and functioning (3).

Table 2 | Sample characteristics by reach increments of 25,000 participants.

	Total	Participant 1–25,000	Participant 25,001–50,000	Participant 50,001–75,000	Participant 75,001–100,000
Age (average)	67.09 (±14.58)	67.37 (±14.31)	66.67 (±14.71)	67.28 (±14.62)	67.05 (±14.66)
Age group					
Under 50	12.0%	11.0%	12.7%	12.2%	12.2%
50–64	25.3%	26.0%	26.3%	24.2%	24.6%
65–79	42.7%	42.7%	41.6%	43.2%	43.4%
80+	19.9%	20.3%	19.5%	20.3%	19.7%
Sex					
Male	22.1%	21.9%	23.2%	21.1%	22.1%
Female	77.9%	78.1%	76.8%	78.9%	77.9%
Hispanic ethnicity					
No	82.6%	80.9%	83.3%	80.5%	85.6%
Yes	17.4%	19.1%	16.7%	19.5%	14.4%
Race					
White	66.0%	69.2%	65.0%	63.9%	66.3%
African American	21.7%	19.3%	22.4%	22.7%	22.1%
Asian/Pacific Islander	4.5%	5.2%	4.8%	4.2%	4.1%
American Indian/Alaska native	1.6%	1.4%	1.6%	1.8%	1.5%
Other/multiple races	6.2%	5.0%	6.3%	7.4%	6.0%
Number of chronic conditions (average)	2.20 (±1.71)	1.96 (±1.63)	2.25 (±1.17)	2.28 (±1.74)	2.31 (±1.73)
Number of chronic conditions					
0 Conditions	18.2%	22.5%	17.1%	17.0%	16.3%
1 Condition	20.9%	22.0%	21.0%	20.6%	19.8%
2 Condition	21.3%	21.2%	21.1%	20.9%	21.9%
3+ Condition	39.6%	34.3%	40.7%	41.5%	42.0%
Live alone					
No	84.4%	78.1%	86.0%	85.0%	88.7%
Yes	15.6%	21.9%	14.0%	15.0%	11.3%
Participant residence					
Metro	78.2%	77.8%	77.0%	80.9%	77.2%
Non-metro	21.8%	22.2%	23.0%	19.1%	22.8%

This study provides valuable dissemination and implementation insights into the nature and progression of the largest ever national roll out of CDSME programs (i.e., highly effective evidence-based programs designed to help middle-aged and older adults more effectively manage their chronic conditions). The aging services sector, in partnership with other healthcare, public health, community, and faith-based organizations, proved to be a coordinated, efficient, and diverse delivery system capable of rapidly reaching large numbers of older adults across the country. Exceeding programmatic goals of having 50,000 participants complete CDSME program workshops (12), over 100,000 participants were reached more quickly than in previous efforts (16). Further, with the exception of a predominant female participant population typically served with health promotion programs (16–18), participants were representative of the U.S. population and not just easy-to-reach subgroups.

The ability of this initiative to quickly reach 100,000 participants can be attributed to many factors. First, having each state set ambitious yet feasible and attainable goals (19) can help stimulate them to think differently about program planning, participant recruitment, and partnership development. Second, the stimulus money utilized in this initiative was essential for reaching this recruitment goal, but it was also leveraged by funds from other organizations with some non-traditional partners (e.g., healthcare partners), which fostered growth by adopting and promoting CDSME programs as an integral care practice. Third, capitalizing on the existing program delivery infrastructure established by previous AoA initiatives, the broad network of delivery and funding partners has resulted in widespread financing of CDSME programs by other government organizations. Fourth, workshops were available in many local communities largely because of the cooperation of the program developers to utilize and expand their training infrastructure (5). As seen in this initiative, the culmination of leveraging opportunities led to the rapid dissemination of CDSME programs by creating a highly collaborative community structure that accelerated the speed of scalability across the country to meet the needs of an increasingly diverse group of participants.

Past reports have shown CDSME programs have capacity to serve large numbers of heterogeneous adults via a growing network of delivery sites (8, 12, 20, 21). Success can be attributed, in part, to a community-driven delivery system that employed existing networks for recruiting participants of varied ages, race/ethnicity; disease status; geographic region; and socio-economic status (22). However, additional efforts are needed to help CDSME programs gain major penetration among the over 35 million older Americans estimated to have at least one chronic condition (23). As such, this study suggests several actions that can help make the dissemination of CDSME programs part of routine care.

First, we must further examine and strengthen referral systems to CDSME programs and the interconnectedness of the healthcare, public health, and aging services networks. Multi-institute funding initiatives that highly encourage/mandate multi-sectorial partnerships can set the stage for bridging such connections (11). Second, we need to embrace the paradigm shift in provider-patient communications that emphasizes the value of "informed and activated" patients working collaboratively with their prepared practice team (1). This theme, initially articulated in Wagner's chronic care model, is being revisited with the recent movement toward patient-centered care (24). Third, we need to be aware of the constraints facing today's healthcare providers in terms of shortened office visits and greater expectations for administrative paperwork (25). Thus, we recommend easy-to-employ methods and mechanisms (e.g., automated systems) to help health care providers know where evidence-based programs like CDSMP are offered. Also, guidelines are needed for identifying the types of patients who are best suited for specific programs (e.g., information about the pros and cons of generic self-care programs versus disease-specific programs). While clinicians and other allied health providers should be trained about these guidelines and referral processes, it is also important that program participants report back to their healthcare providers about their experiences and progress in such programs. Fourth, we must recognize that programmatic scalability needs to be paired with plans for achieving sustainability over time. Thus, we recommend that national, state, and local roll outs of evidence-based programs include sustainability planning as a core element. Successful sustainability plans are those that build upon and leverage existing resources, often employing champions for recognizing and promoting new models of care (26).

There are study limitations that must be acknowledged. While this national effort afforded large numbers of participants, specific data points were limited due to community concerns regarding burden. Additionally some data was missing due to local/regional constraints, and not necessarily individual refusal. Study data represented a "snapshot" of an ongoing evolving evaluation process at a particular time point. Underserved populations (e.g., African Americans) were overrepresented in this study because of the focus of the larger initiative to serve this subgroup of Americans. However, males were underrepresented in this study, as they traditionally are in evidence-based programs delivered through the aging services network (16–18). Despite these limitations inherent when using administrative records, we nevertheless believe this study represents a unique examination about how a national evidence-based dissemination rolls out over time, what infrastructure facilitates this type of grand-scale roll out, and what types of participants are reached.

Findings from this study capture the spread of CDSME programs during a national, government-funded roll out and show the ability of this intervention to rapidly reach a diverse set of participants using a well-coordinated delivery system. As of August 2014, over 196,700 participants reached by CDSME programs through 17,500 workshops in 1,200 counties across the United States. While this initiative capitalized and built upon previous efforts to create a delivery infrastructure for CDSME programs, this grand-scale dissemination has solidified the presence of CDSME programs with great potential for long-term sustainability. While this initiative has achieved impressive participant reach and completion, it should be noted that many other organizations throughout the United States offered the intervention despite not receiving this ARRA funding. Because data from these organizations are not represented in the databased used in the current study, these findings are even more encouraging in that they underrepresent the actual translation of CDSME programs nationwide. Continued efforts are needed to track the progression and proliferation of this suite of programs to empower patients with self-management skills to deal with their chronic conditions.

ACKNOWLEDGMENTS

The American Recovery and Reinvestment Act of 2009 (i.e., Recovery Act) Communities Putting Prevention to Work: Chronic Disease Self-Management Program initiative, led by the U.S. Administration on Aging in collaboration with the Centers for Disease Control and Prevention and the Centers for Medicare and Medicaid Services, allotted $32.5 million to support the translation of the Stanford program in 45 States, Puerto Rico, and the District of Columbia. The National Council on Aging served as the Technical Assistance Resource Center for this initiative and collected de-identified data on program participation.

REFERENCES

1. Wagner EH, Glasgow RE, Davis C, Bonomi AE, Provost L, McCulloch D, et al. Quality improvement in chronic illness care: a collaborative approach. *Jt Comm J Qual Improv* (2001) **27**(2):63–80.
2. Barr V, Robinson S, Marin-Link B, Underhill L, Dotts A, Ravensdale D, et al. The expanded Chronic Care Model: an integration of concepts and strategies from population health promotion and the Chronic Care Model. *Hosp Q* (2003) **7**(1):73. doi:10.12927/hcq.2003.16763
3. Brady TJ, Murphy L, O'Colmain BJ, Beauchesne D, Daniels B, Greenberg M, et al. A meta-analysis of health status, health behaviors, and healthcare utilization outcomes of the chronic disease self-management program. *Prev Chronic Dis* (2013) **10**:120112. doi:10.5888/pcd10.120112
4. Brady T, Murphy L, Beauchesne D, Bhalakia A, Chervin D, Daniels B, et al. *Sorting Through the Evidence for the Arthritis Self-Management Program and the Chronic Disease Self-Management Program: Executive Summary of ASMP/CDSMP Meta-Analysis.* Atlanta, GA: Centers for Disease Control and Prevention (CDC) (2011).
5. Stanford School of Medicine. *Chronic Disease Self-Management Program (Better Choices, Better Health® Workshop)* [cited 2014 July 12]. Available from: http://patienteducation.stanford.edu/programs/cdsmp.html
6. Bodenheimer T, Lorig K, Holman H, Grumbach K. Patient self-management of chronic disease in primary care. *JAMA* (2002) **288**(19):2469–75. doi:10.1001/jama.288.19.2469
7. Lorig KR, Sobel DS, Stewart AL, Brown BW Jr, Bandura A, Ritter P, et al. Evidence suggesting that a chronic disease self-management program can improve health status while reducing hospitalization: a randomized trial. *Med Care* (1999) **37**(1):5–14. doi:10.1097/00005650-199901000-00003

8. Ory MG, Ahn S, Jiang L, Smith ML, Ritter PL, Whitelaw N, et al. Successes of a national study of the chronic disease self-management program: meeting the triple Aim of health care reform. *Med Care* (2013) **51**(11):992–8. doi:10.1097/MLR.0b013e3182a95dd1
9. Ahn S, Basu R, Smith ML, Jiang L, Lorig K, Whitelaw N, et al. The impact of chronic disease self-management programs: healthcare savings through a community-based intervention. *BMC Public Health* (2013) **13**(1):1141. doi:10.1186/1471-2458-13-1141
10. Department of Health and Human Services. *AoA Evidence-Based Prevention Programs*. Washington, DC: Administration on Aging. (2013) [cited 2014 July 8]. Available from: http://www.aoa.gov/AoA_Programs/HPW/Title_IIID/index.aspx
11. U.S. Department of Health and Human Services, Administration on Aging. *ARRA – Communities Putting Prevention to Work: Chronic Disease Self-Management Program*. (2012) [cited 2014 June 14]. Available from: www.cfda.gov/index?s=program&mode=form&tab=step1&id=5469a61f2c5f25cf3984fc3b94051b5f
12. Ory MG, Smith ML, Kulinski KP, Lorig K, Zenker W, Whitelaw N. Self-management at the tipping point: reaching 100,000 Americans with evidence-based programs. *J Am Geriatr Soc* (2013) **61**(5):821–3. doi:10.1111/jgs.12239
13. Lorig K. *Living a Healthy Life with Chronic Conditions: Self-Management of Heart Disease, Arthritis, Diabetes, Asthma, Bronchitis, Emphysema & Others*. 3rd ed. Boulder, CO: Bull Pub. Company (2006). 382 p.
14. Bandura A. Social cognitive theory of self-regulation. *Organ Behav Hum Decis Process* (1991) **50**(2):248–87. doi:10.1016/0749-5978(91)90022-L
15. Kulinski KP, Boutaugh M, Smith ML, Ory MG, Lorig K. Setting the stage: measure seletion, coordination, and data collection for a national self-management initiative. *Front Public Health* (2015) **2**:206. doi:10.3389/fpubh.2014.00206
16. Smith M, Belza B, Altpeter M, Ahn S, Dickerson J, Ory M. Disseminating an evidence-based disease self-management program for older Americans: implications for diversifying participant reach through delivery site adoption. In: Maddock J, editor. *Rijeka*. Croatia: InTech (2012). p. 385–404.
17. Smith ML, Ory MG, Belza B, Altpeter M. Personal and delivery site characteristics associated with intervention dosage in an evidence-based fall risk reduction program for older adults. *Transl Behav Med* (2012) **2**(2):188–98. doi:10.1007/s13142-012-0133-8
18. Smith ML, Belza B, Braun KL, King S, Palmer RC, Sugihara NS, et al. National reach and dissemination of enhancefitness. *Health Behav Policy Rev* (2014) **1**(2):150–60. doi:10.14485/HBPR.1.2.7
19. The art of health promotion. *Am J Health Promot* (2004) **18**(4): TAH-1–TAH-12. doi:10.4278/0890-1171-18.4.TAHP-1
20. Erdem E, Korda H. Self-management program participation by older adults with diabetes: Chronic Disease Self-Management Program and Diabetes Self-Management Program. *Fam Community Health* (2014) **37**(2):134–46. doi:10.1097/FCH.0000000000000025
21. Korda H, Erdem E, Woodcock C, Kloc M, Pedersen S, Jenkins S. Racial and ethnic minority participants in chronic disease self-management programs: findings from the communities putting prevention to work initiative. *Ethn Dis* (2012) **23**(4):508–17.
22. Burdine JN, McLeroy K, Blakely C, Wendel ML, Felix MR. Community-based participatory research and community health development. *J Prim Prev* (2010) **31**(1):1–7. doi:10.1007/s10935-010-0205-9
23. Anderson GF. *Chronic Care: Making the Case for Ongoing Care*. Princeton, NJ: Robert Wood Johnson Foundation (2010).
24. Bojadzievski T, Gabbay RA. Patient-centered medical home and diabetes. *Diabetes Care* (2011) **34**(4):1047–53. doi:10.2337/dc10-1671
25. Ahn S, Tai-Seale M, Huber C Jr, Smith ML, Ory MG. Psychotropic medication discussions in older adults' primary care office visits: so much to do, so little time. *Aging Ment Health* (2011) **15**(5):618–29. doi:10.1080/13607863.2010.548055
26. Scheirer MA. Is sustainability possible? A review and commentary on empirical studies of program sustainability. *Am J Eval* (2005) **26**(3):320–47. doi:10.1177/1098214005278752

7

Methods for streamlining intervention fidelity checklists: An example from the Chronic Disease Self-Management Program

SangNam Ahn[1,2]*, Matthew Lee Smith[3], Mary Altpeter[4], Basia Belza[5], Lindsey Post[1] and Marcia G. Ory[2]

[1] *Division of Health Systems Management and Policy, School of Public Health, The University of Memphis, Memphis, TN, USA*
[2] *Department of Health Promotion and Community Health Sciences, Texas A&M Health Science Center, School of Public Health, College Station, TX, USA*
[3] *Department of Health Promotion and Behavior, College of Public Health, The University of Georgia, Athens, GA, USA*
[4] *Center for Health Promotion and Disease Prevention, The University of North Carolina at Chapel Hill, Chapel Hill, NC, USA*
[5] *School of Nursing, Biobehavioral Nursing and Health Systems, The University of Washington, Seattle, WA, USA*

Edited by:
Katherine Henrietta Leith, University of South Carolina, USA

Reviewed by:
Jay E. Maddock, University of Hawaii at Manoa, USA
Katherine Henrietta Leith, University of South Carolina, USA

****Correspondence:***
SangNam Ahn, Division of Health Systems Management and Policy, School of Public Health, The University of Memphis, 133 Robison Hall, Memphis, TN 38152-3530, USA
e-mail: sahn@memphis.edu

Maintaining intervention fidelity should be part of any programmatic quality assurance (QA) plan and is often a licensure requirement. However, fidelity checklists designed by original program developers are often lengthy, which makes compliance difficult once programs become widely disseminated in the field. As a case example, we used Stanford's original Chronic Disease Self-Management Program (CDSMP) fidelity checklist of 157 items to demonstrate heuristic procedures for generating shorter fidelity checklists. Using an expert consensus approach, we sought feedback from active master trainers registered with the Stanford University Patient Education Research Center about which items were most essential to, and also feasible for, assessing fidelity. We conducted three sequential surveys and one expert group-teleconference call. Three versions of the fidelity checklist were created using different statistical and methodological criteria. In a final group-teleconference call with seven national experts, there was unanimous agreement that all three final versions (e.g., a 34-item version, a 20-item version, and a 12-item version) should be made available because the purpose and resources for administering a checklist might vary from one setting to another. This study highlights the methodology used to generate shorter versions of a fidelity checklist, which has potential to inform future QA efforts for this and other evidence-based programs (EBP) for older adults delivered in community settings. With CDSMP and other EBP, it is important to differentiate between program fidelity as mandated by program developers for licensure, and intervention fidelity tools for providing an "at-a-glance" snapshot of the level of compliance to selected program indicators.

Keywords: intervention fidelity, quality assurance, Chronic Disease Self-Management Program, aging, evidence-based programs, expert consensus

INTRODUCTION

Chronic conditions have received nationwide attention because of their adverse impact on individuals' daily functioning, social interaction, and self-reported quality of life (1) as well as their association with rising healthcare costs (2). Self-management has been viewed as a key factor enabling patients to deal with the everyday challenges of chronic conditions through medical, emotional, and/or role management (3, 4). Despite national calls for more attention to public health strategies that empower Americans to be more involved in their own health (5), many Americans do not inherently possess the skills for actively engaging in self-management behaviors that can help ameliorate the effects of living with chronic diseases.

Evidence-based programs such as the Chronic Disease Self-Management Program (CDSMP) have gained national and international recognition for helping people with chronic conditions learn self-management skills (6, 7). While positive outcomes of CDSMP have been well documented (8), less is known about the actual implementation processes at the state or national level other than gross indicators of program completion or adherence to recommendations regarding class size (9, 10). Thus, the primary purpose of this project was to address intervention fidelity and describe a methodological approach to streamline a fidelity checklist. As a heuristic example, we used the fidelity checklist contained within the CDSMP Fidelity Toolkit (11). A secondary purpose of this project was to use this methodological process to evoke expert opinions about how leaders in the aging services field view the fidelity and quality assurance (QA) processes. As a note, we will consistently use "intervention" fidelity throughout the current study because we focus on a fidelity checklist assessing processes beyond the program itself (e.g., training, before the program, after the program, and evaluation).

PUBLIC HEALTH INITIATIVES AND EVALUATIONS

The U.S. Administration on Aging (AoA) Evidence-Based Disease Prevention Grant Programs, initiated in 2003, have stimulated the development and implementation of evidence-based programs (EBP) for seniors, which dispel earlier myths that health promotion efforts were futile in older populations (12). With this greater national appreciation for the potential of evidence-based health promotion programing for improving health and functioning among older adults, the research questions have shifted from "do we know what works?" to "can we do what is known to work?" This change in focus is now seen with service providers having ready access to a growing list of EBP, which have been widely tested in community and clinical settings and within the aging services network (13, 14).

Yet, the translation of scientifically tested research findings to community-based programs is often slow, fragmented, and subject to speculation by the practitioner community (15). As more EBP are offered by diverse host agencies in more diverse communities, evidence is mounting that their successful dissemination occurs sporadically (15–18). Translational research is coming of age, and models such as RE-AIM are being formulated to serve as guiding frameworks for planning implementation efforts and evaluating the public health impacts of EBP (19–21). More specifically, the RE-AIM framework seeks to identify and overcome the challenges facing program planners and practitioners when moving an EBP from the research setting in which it was developed to the less-than-perfect, resource-limited, and real-world practice environment (19–22).

The RE-AIM framework contains the following five key elements: reach, effectiveness, adoption, implementation, and maintenance (21, 23). Some studies examine all five elements, while others examine outcomes using one or two key elements (16). Our current study focuses on the "I" in RE-AIM, program implementation processes, specifically fidelity monitoring, which can be neglected because of funding and logistic issues in large-scale community-based disease prevention efforts for older adults.

INTERVENTION FIDELITY

As EBP become widely disseminated, there has been growing attention to program fidelity in implementation science (16). In terms of translational research, there has been a strong programmatic emphasis on fidelity, which can be defined as the adherence of actual treatment delivery to the protocol originally developed (24). A breach in intervention fidelity, defined as the adherent and competent delivery of an intervention by the interventionists (e.g., trainers, course leaders, and program coordinators) as set forth in the intervention manual (25), threatens licensure and makes it difficult to interpret study results. For example, if the program is not delivered as intended, it is difficult to know if the resulting health outcomes can be attributed to receipt of the intervention or to some other variation in the intervention's delivery (26).

While maintaining fidelity during program implementation is essential, ensuring the feasibility of monitoring fidelity is also important, especially for organizations with relatively limited capacity to administer the intervention (27). Fidelity to treatment or intervention delivery is one subset of overall treatment fidelity (28) and has often been monitored through observation, interviews, self-assessed fidelity checklists, and pairing of trained facilitators (26). Recent articles have highlighted the importance of having high resource commitment to better monitor fidelity in evidence-based health promotion programs such as CDSMP (29) or EnhanceFitness (30).

STRATEGIES FOR ENSURING CDSMP PROGRAM FIDELITY

Programmatic adherence to implementation aspects of CDSMP is supported by a centralized training and certification system that provides for scripted small-group and participatory workshops (2.5 h a week for 6 consecutive weeks) focused on self-management strategies that provide medical, emotional, and role management skills (4). In regard to the training and certification system, it is noted that there are three hierarchical levels of trainers (31). First, a person can be a certified (lay) leader when she or he completes 4-day Leader Training and facilitates one 6-week workshop within 12 months from the training date. Second, master trainer certification can be obtained when a person completes 4.5-day Master Training and facilitates two 6-week workshops within 12 months of completion of training. Third, a person can be a T-Trainer when she or he completes 4.5-day apprenticeship under supervision of a Stanford approved certifying T-Trainer and conducts at least one Master Training within 12 months completion. In addition, the program coordinator is another important workforce member who plays a key role in implementing CDSMP. The program coordinator, who may be a master trainer or lay leader, typically engages in a variety of tasks such as: identifying community partners, recruiting and supervising workshop leaders and participants, arranging for workshop sites, monitoring intervention fidelity, and evaluating program processes and outcomes (32).

A standardized resource material (e.g., the program guide "Living a Healthy Life with Chronic Conditions" revised in 2012) (4) helps provide general guidance behind the theory and activities. An implementation manual provides more detailed guidance to trainers (33), and a fidelity manual outlines mandatory program requirements. The 2010 CDSMP Fidelity Toolkit (11) contains a fidelity checklist with key aspects listed in the following link: http://patienteducation.stanford.edu/licensing/Fidelity_ToolKit2010.pdf. This fidelity checklist as part of the Toolkit is called "Must Do's Fidelity Checklist" and provides guidance for personnel with regard to the implementation of CDSMP (e.g., program coordinators, leaders, master trainers, or T-trainers). Personnel are advised to go through the list and check "Yes" for all the items they are currently doing, and are encouraged to incorporate these items with their fidelity plan for the future if they are not able to implement the entire fidelity task right away. These 157 items are chronologically categorized under 7 headings (16 subheadings or blocks): (1) personnel; (2) delivery before training; (3) fidelity during training; (4) fidelity after training; (5) fidelity during workshops; (6) fidelity for leaders and master trainer retention; and (7) fidelity after workshops. Each heading was further divided into a couple of subheadings.

Implementing EBP can require detailed monitoring and tracking information, placing substantial administrative burdens on program coordinators (15). As such, shorter fidelity tools were developed by some states implementing CDSMP including Missouri[1] and New Jersey[2]. However, none of these fidelity tools

[1] http://www.ncoa.org/chamodules/documents/MOCDSMPQITool.pdf

[2] http://www.ncoa.org/chamodules/documents/NJ_PeerLeaderChecklist.doc

Table 1 | Four rounds to streamline CDSMP fidelity checklists (original 157 items).

Round	Methods	Reduction criteria	Number of participants	Number of items left
One	Survey	Items related to master trainer training (T-training)/language literacy	114 master trainers	148
		Items that did not meet either statistical or practical approaches	114 master trainers	116
Two	Survey	Items not ranked "very high" in "feasibility" step and not selected as part of a predetermined number of items in "endorsement" step	47 master trainers	34/20/12
Three	Survey	Items not related to their perceptions about the most critical items for assessing program fidelity	7 experts	34
Four	Conference call	Version selection based on organizational resources	7 experts	34[a]/20/12

[a] *Most preferred.*

was systematically tested. In our role as technical advisors to the AoA Evidence-Based Disease Prevention Grant Programs, we were asked to explore methods for streamlining a fidelity checklist (e.g., CDSMP) and use these methodological processes to seek expert opinions about how leaders in the aging services field view the fidelity and QA processes.

MATERIALS AND METHODS

The expert consensus method refers to a multi-phase approach for statistically analyzing pooled opinions that minimizes biases inherent in other systems of summarizing expert viewpoints (34, 35). We used this method to gather and analyze expert opinion on streamlining the 157-item CDSMP fidelity checklist in 2010–2011. We employed three rounds of data collection using Qualtrics software (36) to streamline the original 157-item CDSMP fidelity checklist without losing essential fidelity items but improving feasibility of administration. As a final effort, we held a telephone conference to solicit expert opinion for making final recommendations regarding the use of fidelity checklists. **Table 1** displays these four rounds of checklist streamlining and the number of items remaining after each round. Human Subjects approval was obtained from the Texas A&M University Institutional Review Board.

PARTICIPANTS

As the credentialing unit, the Stanford University Patient Education Research Center compiles a list of all CDSMP master trainers and manages a listserv for exchange of information. Using this distribution list, we invited all active master trainers in 2010 to participate in our study. In Round One, we collected 119 responses (114 master trainers, 5 others), where 5 responses were eliminated from the final analysis since they were not master trainers. Twenty-six out of 114 were both master trainers and program coordinators. Out of these 114 master trainers, 47 agreed to participate in the second survey. In Round Two, 24 out of 47 master trainers responded to the survey (51% response rate). From this group, nine master trainers were willing to respond to the third survey. In Round Three, seven out of nine master trainers responded to the third survey (78% response rate). In Round Four, eight out of nine master trainers from Round Three agreed to participate in a telephone conference to obtain feedback, advice, and concerns from their experiences delivering and overseeing programs. In this last round, seven of out of eight experts were able to join the group-teleconference call with the study team. Each of the four rounds to streamline the CDSMP fidelity checklist contained multiple steps as shown below.

ROUND ONE: STREAMLINING THE ORIGINAL CDSMP BY "ENSURING" THE OVERALL FIDELITY OF CDSMP

Survey process

The survey in Round One was conducted in November and December 2010 with master trainers ($n = 114$) who identified through the Stanford CDSMP master trainer listserv. These experts helped us identify the items in the original 157-item CDSMP fidelity checklist, which they believed to be most important to ensuring the overall fidelity of the program. Participants were asked to rank statements on a scale of one (least important) to five (most important). During this initial step, we eliminated 8 items related to master trainer training and another item referring to language literacy, which resulted in an initial portfolio of 148 unique items to consider. To obtain the most relevant information from participants, the survey included skip patterns that presented participants with a list of items most appropriate to them based on their roles (i.e., master trainers or master trainers/program coordinators). Because of their universal relevance, some items were presented to every group.

Reduction criteria

To streamline the CDSMP fidelity checklist, we used both statistical and practical approaches based upon participants' ranking of each checklist item. First, the statistical approach involved eliminating items based on their distance from the mean score. Because of testing the statistical significance of multiple comparisons, we used the Bonferroni technique by adjusting the significance level (0.05) to avoid the risk of Type I error (37). Second, the practical version involved selecting only those responses that were rated as four or five in terms of importance. We eliminated any items that "failed" to meet criteria for either the statistical or practical cut-offs. For instance, there were 26 items in a question block (or subheading) asking the importance of fidelity before lay leader training. Relying on the statistical approach, the mean of these items was 4.15, and the adjusted significance level for this question block was 0.0019 (i.e., 0.05÷26). This process helped us identify six items that showed significantly lower importance ratings relative to the mean after adjusting multiple comparisons. In the same question block, the practical approach helped us identify another six items that were not rated as four or five. Of the 12 items identified for elimination, 2 items were mutually exclusive and 5 items were common to both the statistical and practical approaches. Thus, we were able to eliminate seven items that failed to meet the statistical or practical cutoff. In other question blocks (e.g., fidelity during workshops), we continued to use both approaches to eliminate items that failed to meet the statistical criteria or the practical criteria and we were able to delete 32 (22%) out of 148 checklist items. At the conclusion of Round One, we asked for volunteers to complete a second survey used to continue this expert consensus process.

ROUND TWO: STREAMLINING THE ORIGINAL CDSMP BY ASCERTAINING "FEASIBILITY" OF ADMINISTRATION AND "ENDORSEMENT" OF PREDETERMINED NUMBER OF ITEMS

Survey process

The second survey was conducted in June 2011. In this round, we solicited the opinions of the 47 master trainers who agreed to participate after Round One. Round Two involved asking participants to provide feedback via a two-step process that assessed both "feasibility" and "endorsement." The first step asked master trainers to rank how feasible they think it is to monitor each fidelity checklist item. Feasibility response categories included "not at all," "somewhat," and "very high." Based on the items identified as having "very high" feasibility in the first step, the master trainers were then asked to select a predetermined number of items (total 34) from each question block that they would endorse for inclusion in the final, shorter fidelity checklist versions. We had 24 master trainers respond to our second survey, resulting in a 51% response rate.

Reduction criteria

Employing the practical methodology based on the feasibility and endorsement responses, we were able to generate a shorter Fidelity-12 checklist (12 items), a medium-length Fidelity-20 checklist (20 items), and a longer version Fidelity-34 checklist (34 items). First, we calculated the percent of participants who endorsed each item relative to the total number of endorsements received for each question block (using a scale from 0 to 100%). We also calculated the percent of participants who endorsed each item received relative to the total number of feasibility ratings of "very high" (using a scale from 0 to 100%). The aggregate of this process was assessed on a combined scale of 0–200%. Fidelity-34 included 34 items that received the highest aggregate numbers of each question block (1, 2, or 3 items based on number of items in each question block). Due to our desire to streamline the checklist further, we selected only items with scores of 90 and 100 as cut-points on the combined 0–200 scale. Fidelity-20 (90 as a cut-off) included 20 items while Fidelity-12 (100 as a cut-off) included 12 items. At the conclusion of Round Two, 9 out of 24 master trainers agreed to participate in the survey in Round Three.

ROUND THREE: FINALIZING THE SHORTENED CDSMP FIDELITY CHECKLISTS

We surveyed nine experts to review the three shortened versions of the fidelity checklist and to help us address some remaining questions related to their perceptions about the most critical items for assessing intervention fidelity using Fidelity-34 as the referent. We had seven experts respond to the short survey, and the response rate was 78%. A report of findings was prepared indicating that Fidelity-34 was the one that experts felt best balanced the inclusion of key fidelity items with the feasibility of administration.

ROUND FOUR: CONFIRMING THE NECESSITY OF A SHORTER CDSMP FIDELITY CHECKLIST

We held a telephone conference with seven experts identified in Round Three to report on our findings and solicit expert opinion regarding the use of fidelity checklists. This conference call was critically important for obtaining feedback and advice from those with experience in delivering and overseeing programs. The experts confirmed a preference for Fidelity-34, but felt that the other two shorter versions should be available since the purpose and resources for administering the fidelity checklist might vary from one setting to another.

EXPERT CONSENSUS RESULTS: SUMMARY RECOMMENDATIONS

Table 2 displays the three versions of the CDSMP fidelity checklist (i.e., Fideity-12, Fidelity-20, and Fidelity-34). To sum up these streamlining processes, we included 14 question blocks out of the original 16 blocks (subheadings) that related to personnel to administer and the chronological tasks of CDSMP. In total, 36 items were included in three versions of fidelity checklist. Among these 36 items, 2 items were only included in the Fidelity-20 ("Have all Leaders facilitate at least once a year," and "Have trainees participate in two practice teaching activities during training"). Just like Fidelity-34, Fidelity-20 included at least one item of each question block. However, Fidelity-12, as the shortest version of CDSMP fidelity checklist, did not include any items from four question blocks: "Fidelity after lay leader training;" "Fidelity before master training;" "Fidelity when counseling out leaders/master trainers during training;" and "Fidelity during workshops: Physical environment and material resources." Although Fidelity-34 was highly recommended in Rounds Three and Four, CDSMP experts from the telephone conference also recommended providing organizational partners with all three versions and allowing them to select the best checklist based on their resources. For instance, organizations with time restraints and limited staffing may prefer shorter checklist versions to the longer version, whereas organizations with better staffing and time resources may want to utilize the more thorough version of the checklist.

DISCUSSION

Using the original CDSMP fidelity checklist as a case example, this research provides a methodology for streamlining fidelity checklists that have many unique items, making field implementation resource-intensive and challenging. We see the methodology described in this paper as our key contribution, which can be applied to different EBPs. It should be noted that these shortened checklists are for research only and require further field-testing

Table 2 | Streamlined fidelity checklists using expert consensus method: a CDSMP case study[a].

	Checklist version		
	Fidelity-12	Fidelity-20	Fidelity-34
Question block #1: program coordinator qualifications			
Ql They are very familiar with both the program fidelity and program implementation manuals	X	X	X
Q2 They have observed a Leader or Master Training	X	X	X
Question block #2: lay leader qualifications			
Q3 They are not afraid to speak in front of groups	–	–	X
Q4 They read, write, and speak the language of the workshop participants	X	X	X
Q5 They are able to attend all 4 days of training and complete two practice teachings during training as prospective leaders	X	X	X
Question block #3: fidelity before lay leader training			
Q6 Apply for, renew, or confirm receipt of organization's program license[b]	–	–	X
Q7 Adhere to recommended schedule for leader trainings (total of 4 days: recommended 2 days per week for 2 weeks)	–	X	X
Q8 Have two certified master trainers who are committed to conduct entire training sessions	X	X	X
Q9 Inform participants that their full attendance and participation is required on all training	–	–	X
Q10 Prepare a complete leader's manual for each participant	–	–	X
Question block #4: fidelity after lay leader training			
Q11 Have all leaders facilitate at least once a year	–	X	–
Q12 Not let those leaders with whom there are concerns facilitate workshops[b]	–	X	X
Question block #5: master trainer qualifications			
Q13 They are willing and available to attend a 4.5-day-master training	X	X	X
Q14 They either have led two workshops as a leader either before coming to master training or are willing and available to lead two workshops within 1 year after master training	–	–	X
Question block #6: fidelity before master training			
Q15 Prepare master trainer manuals and leader manuals for each participant	–	–	X
Q16 Determine the most recent training materials are being used for training (most current version are 3rd edition, living a healthier life with chronic conditions book and CDSMP manual (2006)	–	–	X
Q17 Follow the Stanford Patient Education Research Center's checklist for master trainings (obtained upon confirmation of training request)	–	–	X
Q18 Inform participants their full attendance and participation is required on all training days	–	X	X
Question block #7: fidelity during master training			
Q19 Have trainees participate in two practice teaching activities during training	–	X	–
Q20 Have trainees complete the second practice teaching session and demonstrate a minimum set of core competency as observed by a master trainer or T-trainer[b]	X	X	X
Q21 Make sure that training must be at least 27 h, usually over 4.5 days	–	–	X
Q22 Have training offered by two certified T-trainers	–	–	X
Q23 Understand and agree with the importance of program fidelity	–	–	X
Question block #8: fidelity after master training			
Q24 Conduct one leader training a year[b]	X	X	X
Question block #9: fidelity in judging trainee competence during training			
Q25 Adheres to the curriculum (also includes appropriate presentation of charts)	X	X	X
Q26 Facilitates group contributions particularly in the following types of activities: brainstorming, action planning, action plan feedback, and problem solving	–	X	X
Q27 Models activities appropriately	–	–	X
Question block #10: fidelity when counseling out leaders/master trainers during training			
Q28 Observe and document problem behaviors	–	–	X
Q29 Give the trainee specific reasons and examples of why they are concerned	–	–	X

(Continued)

Table 2 | Continued

	Checklist version		
	Fidelity-12	Fidelity-20	Fidelity-34
Q30 Tell the trainee what she/he did well, but also tell her/him clearly how they are expected to improve	–	–	X
Question block #11: fidelity for lay leader and master trainer retention			
Q31 Have defined protocols for resolution of potential personality conflicts, communication problems, improper behavior with participants and co-leaders or co-trainers is in place	X	X	X
Question block #12: fidelity during workshops: physical environment and material resources			
Q32 Have the necessary number and quality of educational materials and supplies	–	–	X
Q33 Offer the workshop 2.5 h a week over 6 weeks	–	X	X
Question block #13: fidelity during workshops: lay leader performance			
Q34 Have two leaders teach the workshops	X	X	X
Q35 Ensure that leaders use facilitation techniques appropriately and effectively	–	X	X
Question block #14: fidelity after workshops			
Q36 Track leader activity (i.e., programs they teach, retention rates)[b]	X	X	X

X, include; –, exclude.

[a]CDSMP sites must comply with licensure and fidelity requirements as defined by Stanford University Patient Education Research Center. The purpose of this research was to demonstrate the use of expert consensus method to streamline intervention fidelity monitoring checklists and to improve monitoring of evidence-based program fidelity. For the most current CDSMP licensure information, please visit Stanford University Patient Education Research Center (http://patienteducation.stanford.edu/licensing/).

[b]Some of these items represent a slight modification from the Stanford Self-Management Fidelity ToolKit (2010) to fit the current question format.

before specific endorsements can be made. The CDSMP fidelity checklist has been updated since the time of this study, and a new fidelity manual was developed that stresses the importance of setting intervention fidelity within an overall fidelity plan. These updated materials also distinguish "must do" fidelity strategies from those that are "nice to do" to strengthen program fidelity (33). For the most current requirements, please refer to the Stanford University Patient Education Center website[3].

Applying the expert consensus technique, we consolidated the 157-item CDSMP fidelity checklist into three abbreviated versions without sacrificing fidelity items deemed essential by master trainers. Due to its overall length, the original Stanford checklist was often used more as a self-assessment reminder rather than an actual fidelity checklist. Given the importance of program implementation as a core component of program evaluation (21, 23), we believe shorter fidelity checklists will prove beneficial to current and future program leaders and coordinators who are trying to implement EBP with limited financial or time resources.

Though the abbreviated checklists are likely less time-consuming than the original version, further improvements may be needed. First, any checklist should be seen as just one element in an overall QA plan (38). Additionally, one might explore different delivery modalities. For example, enabling users to access fidelity checklists online could further enhance their usefulness. An online monitoring system would allow for real-time review and feedback so that program coordinators and trainers can evaluate their progress and fidelity as implementation is occurring, making changes when necessary to adhere to program guidelines.

In addition to generating three abbreviated versions of CDSMP fidelity checklist, this study also demonstrated an effective use of expert consensus method for generating consensus from a broad field of CDSMP experts with varying experience and perspectives. When dealing with a diversity of opinions, problems may arise due to conflicting viewpoints, self-censorship due to lack of anonymity, incomplete feedback loops or poor communication, or lack of defined statistical methods for attributing quantitative values to subjective factors. Many of these potential pitfalls were avoided by using three iterative rounds of online surveys. Because respondents did not communicate directly, they were free to express their opinions. Statistical and practical methods were used to give each respondent's perspective equal weight in reaching consensus. In the Round Four telephone conference, expert participants did directly communicate, but because much of the work related to consolidating the list was already concluded, the participants were able to reach consensus easily.

At the end of the process, we were able to identify the most relevant and applicable items and garner experts' endorsement of the abbreviated checklists as useful. The methods employed in this study could be used as a model for administrators of other EBP aiming to reduce the length of a fidelity checklist for program monitoring. However, it is important to note that CDSMP sites must comply with licensure requirements and be familiar with the official CDSMP Implementation and Fidelity Manuals, which will need to be updated on a regular basis, if programmatic or licensure requirements change.

Several limitations should be considered. First, our relying on small-group processes should be understood for its lack of true representation of the general CDSMP master trainer population. Nevertheless, we believe the current study contributes to

[3]http://patienteducation.stanford.edu/licensing/

the literature related to streamlining a fidelity checklist because of the relative large sample size ($n = 114$) in Round One survey, and multiple rounds of survey, and a final telephone conference with content experts. Second, our study is potentially limited by focusing on one major stakeholder group, i.e., master trainers. The inclusion of various opinions from CDSMP completers, lay leaders, T-trainers, program developers, and researchers in academia in the Round Three survey could have ensured better representation by various CDSMP implementers and stakeholders. Third, the CDSMP program was revamped after the initiation of this study. While some aspects of the program have been improved upon, we believe the basic elements have remained consistent to ensuring fundamental intervention fidelity based on what is needed before, during, and after workshop delivery. Hence, the need for shortened fidelity checklists is still relevant. Fourth, the study was conducted within a specific time period when federal funding was available for CDSMP implementation. Such changes in the availability of resources and program demands may influence, which fidelity checklist items are most feasible to monitor. However, the ever-changing context and limited funding resources might make three short versions of the CDSMP fidelity checklist helpful and valuable. Fifth, there were noticeable dropouts between streamlining rounds. Since data were not collected from the purposive list of participants, it was not possible to make real comparisons between responders and non-responders. Sixth, we note that generating one intervention fidelity tool may not be the most effective or efficient way to capture all aspects of fidelity, which could be implementation fidelity for leaders or program fidelity for program coordinators and agency administrators. Last, we do not know the level of expertise and knowledge among participated master trainers since we did not collect this information. Nevertheless, we strongly believe master trainers are appropriate experts given the required level of training and experience with delivering CDSMP. To retain their certificates, master trainers are required to conduct 4-day Leader training within 18 months of original training and conduct either a 4-day Leader Training, a 6-week series of community workshops, or a Leader cross training (31).

CONCLUSION

Fidelity is critical to the successful dissemination of EBP. The challenge for the field is balancing resources for program delivery with those for assuring intervention fidelity. In this study we explore one avenue for reducing the administrative resources needed for maintaining fidelity. The study demonstrates the importance of finding ways to streamline intervention fidelity checklists for EBP, suggesting several key points. First, an expert consensus method is a viable approach to assessing the usability of fidelity checklists. Second, online software (e.g., Qualtrics) can be used for efficient data collection, analyses, and tracking of participant response with built-in reminder systems. Third, it is important to have input from stakeholders with various roles to have a comprehensive picture of intervention fidelity. We encourage researchers to apply this expert consensus model to other EBP, and to conduct further study of the reliability, validity, and practicability of fidelity checklists.

ACKNOWLEDGMENTS

This work was supported by the Administration on Aging [90OP0001/03]; and the National Institute of Child Health and Human Development [R01HD047143]. The opinions expressed are those of the authors and do not reflect those of the funding agency. The authors acknowledge the university members of the CDC's Prevention Research Centers Healthy Aging Research Network (PRC-HAN). The authors also thank Ms. Patti Smith, who helped to review this manuscript.

REFERENCES

1. Rothrock NE, Hays RD, Spritzer K, Yount SE, Riley W, Cella D. Relative to the general US population, chronic diseases are associated with poorer health-related quality of life as measured by the patient-reported outcomes measurement information system (PROMIS). *J Clin Epidemiol* (2010) **63**:1195–204. doi:10.1016/j.jclinepi.2010.04.012
2. Kaiser Family Foundation. *Health Care Costs: A Primer, Key Information on Health Care Costs and Their Impact.* Menlo Park, CA: The Henry J. Kaiser Family Foundation (2012).
3. Bodenheimer T, Lorig K, Holman H, Grumbach K. Patient self-management of chronic disease in primary care. *JAMA* (2002) **288**:2469. doi:10.1001/jama.288.19.2469
4. Lorig K, Holman H, Sobel D, Laurent D. *Living a Healthy Life with Chronic Conditions: Self Management of Heart Disease, Arthritis, Diabetes, Asthma, Bronchitis, Emphysema and Others.* Boulder, CO: Bull Publishing Company (2006).
5. Kulinski K, Smith ML, Ory MG. *The Chronic Disease Self-Management Program: Process, Organization, and Data Collection.* Washington, DC: National Council on Aging (2014).
6. Lorig K. *Chronic Disease Self-Management Program: Insights from the Eye of the Storm.* Stanford, CA: Patient Education Research Center, School of Medicine, Stanford University (2014).
7. Ory MG, Smith ML, Patton K, Lorig K, Zenker W, Whitelaw N. Self-management at the tipping point: reaching 100,000 Americans with evidence-based programs. *J Am Geriatr Soc* (2013) **61**:821–3. doi:10.1111/jgs.12239
8. Ory MG, Ahn S, Jiang L, Smith ML, Ritter PL, Whitelaw N, et al. Successes of a national study of the Chronic Disease Self-Management Program: meeting the triple aim of health care reform. *Med Care* (2013) **51**:992–8. doi:10.1097/MLR.0b013e3182a95dd1
9. Smith ML, Ory MG, Belza B, Altpeter M. Personal and delivery site characteristics associated with intervention dosage in an evidence-based fall risk reduction program for older adults. *Transl Behav Med* (2012) **2**:188–98. doi:10.1007/s13142-012-0133-8
10. Smith ML, Hochhalter AK, Cheng Y, Wang S, Ory MG. Programmatic influences on outcomes of an evidence-based fall prevention program for older adults: a translational assessment. *Transl Behav Med* (2011) **1**:384–93. doi:10.1007/s13142-011-0058-7
11. Stanford University Patient Education Research Center. *Stanford Self-Management Fidelity Tool Kit.* San Jose, CA: Stanford University Patient Education Research Center (2010).
12. Ory MG, Hoffman M, Hawkins M, Sanner B, Mockenhaupt R. Challenging aging stereotypes: designing and evaluating physical activity programs. *Am J Prev Med* (2003) **25**:164–71. doi:10.1016/S0749-3797(03)00181-8
13. National Council on Aging. *Evidence-Based Health Promotion Programs for Older Adults.* Washington, DC: NCOA (2012).
14. National Council on Aging. *Chronic Disease Self-Management Program Point of Contact Map.* Arlington, VA: NCOA (2014).
15. Glasgow RE, Emmons KM. How can we increase translation of research into practice? Types of evidence needed. *Annu Rev Public Health* (2007) **28**:413–33. doi:10.1146/annurev.publhealth.28.021406.144145
16. Gaglio B, Shoup JA, Glasgow RE. The RE-AIM framework: a systematic review of use over time. *Am J Public Health* (2013) **103**:e38–46. doi:10.2105/AJPH.2013.301299
17. Jernigan VBB. Community-based participatory research with Native American communities: the Chronic Disease Self-Management Program. *Health Promot Pract* (2009) **11**(6):888–99. doi:10.1177/1524839909333374

18. Green LW, Glasgow RE. Evaluating the relevance, generalization, and applicability of research: issues in external validation and translation methodology. *Eval Health Prof* (2006) **29**:126. doi:10.1177/0163278705284445
19. Belza B, Toobert DJ, Glasgow RE. *RE-AIM for Program Planning: Overview and Applications.* Washington, DC: National Council on Aging (2007).
20. Ory GM. *Evidence-Based Health Planning 101.* Arlington, VA: National Council on Aging (2011).
21. Glasgow RE, Vogt TM, Boles SM. Evaluating the public health impact of health promotion interventions: the RE-AIM framework. *Am J Public Health* (1999) **89**:1322–7. doi:10.2105/AJPH.89.9.1322
22. Ory MG, Altpeter M, Belza B, Helduser J, Zhang C, Smith ML. Perceived utility of the RE-AIM framework for health promotion/disease prevention initiatives for older adults: a case study from the U.S. evidence-based disease prevention initiative. *Front Public Health* (2015) **2**:143. doi:10.3389/fpubh.2014.00143
23. Glasgow RE, Klesges LM, Dzewaltowski DA, Estabrooks PA, Vogt TM. Evaluating the impact of health promotion programs: using the RE-AIM framework to form summary measures for decision making involving complex issues. *Health Educ Res* (2006) **21**:688–94. doi:10.1093/her/cyl081
24. Borrelli B. The assessment, monitoring, and enhancement of treatment fidelity in public health clinical trials. *J Public Health Dent* (2011) **71**:S52–63. doi:10.1111/j.1752-7325.2011.00233.x
25. Santacroce SJ, Maccarelli LM, Grey M. Intervention fidelity. *Nurs Res* (2004) **53**:63–6. doi:10.1097/00006199-200401000-00010
26. Frank JC, Coviak CP, Healy TC, Belza B, Casado BL. Addressing fidelity in evidence-based health promotion programs for older adults. *J Appl Gerontol* (2008) **27**:4–33. doi:10.1177/1090198114543007
27. Mowbray CT, Holter MC, Teague GB, Bybee D. Fidelity criteria: development, measurement, and validation. *Am J Eval* (2003) **24**:315–40. doi:10.1177/109821400302400303
28. Bellg AJ, Borrelli B, Resnick B, Hecht J, Minicucci DS, Ory M, et al. Enhancing treatment fidelity in health behavior change studies: best practices and recommendations from the NIH behavior change consortium. *Health Psychol* (2004) **23**:443–51. doi:10.1037/0278-6133.23.5.443
29. Tomioka M, Braun KL, Compton M, Tanoue L. Adapting Stanford's Chronic Disease Self-Management Program to Hawaii's multicultural population. *Gerontologist* (2012) **52**:121–32. doi:10.1093/geront/gnr054
30. Tomioka M, Braun KL. Implementing evidence-based programs a four-step protocol for assuring replication with fidelity. *Health Promot Pract* (2012) **14**:850–8. doi:10.1177/1524839912469205
31. Stanford University Patient Education Research Center. *Leader & Trainer Certification Guidelines.* San Jose, CA: Stanford University Patient Education Research Center (2013).
32. Stanford University Patient Education Research Center. *Implementation Manual.* San Jose, CA: Stanford University Patient Education Research Center (2008).
33. Stanford University Patient Education Research Center. *Program Fidelity Manual: Stanford Self-Management Programs 2012 Update.* San Jose, CA: Stanford University Patient Education Research Center (2012).
34. Karceski S, Morrell M, Carpenter D. The expert consensus guideline series: treatment of epilepsy. *Epilepsy Behav* (2001) **2**:A1–50. doi:10.1016/j.yebeh.2010.07.016
35. Frances A, Kahn DA, Carpenter D, Ross R, Docherty JP. The expert consensus practice guideline project: a new method of establishing best practice. *J Psychiatr Pract* (1996) **2**:295–306.
36. Snow J, Mann M. *Qualtrics Survey Software: Handbook for Research Professionals.* Provo, UT: Qualtrics Labs, Inc (2013).
37. Vogt WP. *Dictionary of Statistics & Methodology: A Nontechnical Guide for the Social Sciences.* Thousand Oak, CA: Sage Publications (2005).
38. National Council on Aging. *Checklist: Recommended Components for an "Ideal" Quality Assurance (QA) Plan.* Arlington, VA: NCOA (2014).

8

Building the older adult fall prevention movement – steps and lessons learned

***Ellen C. Schneider*[1]* *and (Bonita) Lynn Beattie*[2]**

[1] *Center for Health Promotion and Disease Prevention, University of North Carolina at Chapel Hill, Chapel Hill, NC, USA*
[2] *Falls Free® Initiative, National Council on Aging, Washington, DC, USA*

Edited by:
Matthew Lee Smith, The University of Georgia, USA

Reviewed by:
Elisa Beth Hutson McNeill, Texas A&M University, USA
Miruna Petrescu-Prahova, University of Washington, USA
Deborah Paone, Paone & Associates, LLC, USA

Correspondence:
Ellen C. Schneider, Center for Health Promotion and Disease Prevention, University of North Carolina at Chapel Hill, 1700 Martin Luther King Boulevard, CB 7426, Chapel Hill, NC 27599-7426, USA
e-mail: ecschnei@email.unc.edu

Background: Falls are the leading cause of older adult injuries and injury-related deaths. Until 2004, the growing public health issue of older adult falls received little national attention. To elevate and focus on the issue, the National Council on Aging launched the Falls Free® Initiative, a group of national and state agencies working collaboratively to address older adult falls with evidence-based solutions. Since then, attention to older adult falls has gained significant momentum.

Purpose: To describe the steps taken to create the momentum around fall prevention and lessons learned that could be applied to supporting other older adult health-related issues.

Method/objectives: The Falls Free® Initiative took key steps to promote the older adult falls prevention movement, including initiating organized advocacy and supporting the development of state coalitions through increasing awareness of the issue, promoting evidence-based programs, instituting evaluation, implementing systems change, and providing tailored technical assistance.

Results: Through the support of the Falls Free® Initiative and many partners, advocacy efforts have increased federal funding for fall prevention, the majority of states have fall prevention coalitions, and thousands of stakeholders are now engaged in fall prevention. Select lessons learned include leveraging compelling data, choosing passionate leaders for the movement, aligning the cause with partner missions, and being inclusive of all stakeholders.

Conclusion: Although much progress has been made in the fall prevention movement, the issue is growing along with the aging population. Efforts must continue to gain support from all affected stakeholders to reduce older adult falls and fall-related injuries.

Keywords: fall prevention, fall prevention movement, Falls® Free Initiative, awareness, advocacy

In 2012, over 2.4 million older adults were treated in emergency departments for falls; more than 722,000 or 30% of these patients had to be hospitalized (1). Every 29 min, an older adult in the United States dies from fall-related injuries (2). Direct medical costs for fall injuries total over $30 billion per year in the nation and account for 6% of all medical expenditures for this age group (3,4). The risk of falling increases with age, and accelerates after age 85 years due to issues such as declining muscle strength, increased frailty, poor eyesight, and limited movement (5). With an increased life expectancy among the growing baby boomer population, the problem of older adult falls has the potential to overwhelm resources required to address the needs.

Until 2004, the issue of older adult falls received little national attention in part due to its complexity and lack of readily available evidence-base interventions. As a growing public health issue, it clearly needed a national effort to promote awareness and action. Since then, attention to the issue of older adult falls has gained significant momentum through the work of many stakeholders around the country, primarily led through the National Council on Aging's (NCOA) Falls Free® Initiative (6).

Launched in 2005, the Falls Free® Initiative brought together national and state agencies to collaboratively address older adult falls with evidence-based solutions; the authors of this article were leaders in the effort. The Falls Free® Initiative has been particularly successful in advocacy at the national level and in supporting the creation and development of state fall prevention coalitions and local collaborative efforts across the country. The purpose of this paper is to describe the steps taken to create the momentum around fall prevention and lessons learned that could be applied to supporting other older adult health-related issues. Steps include creating a national initiative; initiating advocacy efforts; and developing and supporting coalitions to increase awareness of the issue, promote evidence-based programs, institute evaluation, and implement policy and systems change.

BACKGROUND OF THE FALLS FREE® INITIATIVE

In the early 2000s, the Archstone Foundation, a private grant-making organization based in California, began funding local fall prevention initiatives in the state. The Archstone Foundation was pleased with the growth of statewide activities and the subsequent development of a state fall prevention plan. The Foundation approached the NCOA to design a similar initiative on a national level. NCOA, with funding from the Archstone Foundation and the Home Safety Council, seated an advisory group of leading fall prevention experts to begin planning and conducted an environmental scan of organizations that were or should be working on fall prevention to identify key national stakeholders.

Concurrently, leading researchers were commissioned to develop review papers based on the best available evidence on fall prevention strategies targeted toward community-residing older adults. The review papers focused on the topics of physical mobility, medications management, home safety, environmental safety in the community, and additional cross-cutting areas for attention such as policy and advocacy.

With continued financial support from the Archstone Foundation and Home Safety Council, NCOA convened the national Falls Free® Summit in Washington, DC, USA in December 2004. Fifty-eight national organizations, professional associations, federal agencies, and leading fall prevention experts were invited to participate in this landmark summit to review the evidence and design a national blueprint for reducing falls among older adults.

As a result of the Summit, the National Action Plan (Plan available at http://www.ncoa.org/improve-health/center-for-healthy-aging/content-library/FallsFree_NationalActionPlan_Final.pdf) was created with 9 goals and 36 evidence-based strategies key to reducing older adult falls (7). Goals and strategies were offered for both providers and for older adults corresponding with the review papers on the evidence related to physical mobility, medications management, home and environmental safety, and cross-cutting issues. The long range vision of the Plan was that older adults would have fewer falls and fall-related injuries, maximizing their independence and quality of life (7). More than 8,000 print and CD ROM copies of the Plan were distributed; the Plan was also posted to the NCOA website where it has been downloaded over 125,000 times (personal communication, Emily Dessem, National Council on Aging, 2014 March 2). The purpose of the plan was to develop and enrich supplemental and complementary community-based programs and services to provide a continuum of care aimed at reducing falls and fall-related injuries, not to undermine medical interventions.

When the Plan was released, there was insufficient funding to mount a national campaign to promote action of its 36 strategies. However, in response to the participants' enthusiasm for the Summit process and the Plan itself, and in an effort to promote the strategies, the Falls Free® Initiative was created (6). This loose-knit collaborative of Summit attendees and their organizations was charged with working toward the progress of one or more of the strategies that resonated with their organizational missions. Since its inception, the Falls Free® Initiative has grown to over 70 national organizations, profession associations, and federal agencies (6).

The original 36 strategies remain relevant and evidence-supported. In 2008, the Falls Free® National Advisory Group convened to review progress made over its 3-year history. Group members engaged in a rich, broad-based exchange of ideas; this deliberation resulted in a number of recommendations and observations across the strategies presented in the National Action Plan, as well as emerging opportunities.

INITIATING ORGANIZED FALL PREVENTION ADVOCACY

In 2006, the Falls Free® Initiative recognized that the issue of older adult falls needed an active effort to advocate for appropriate national funding levels. Therefore, the National Falls Free® Advocacy Workgroup was formed and successfully advocated for the passage of the Keeping Seniors Safe from Falls Act, signed into law in April 2008 as PL 110-202 (8). The Act enfolded strategies taken directly from the National Action Plan authorizing research, demonstration programs, provider training, and public education to prevent older adult falls. Although the Act passed, no funding was appropriated with its enactment. The Workgroup continued its advocacy efforts and successfully doubled fall prevention funding for the Centers for Disease Control and Prevention's (CDC) National Center for Injury Prevention and Control (NCIPC) from $1 million in fiscal year 2008 to approximately $2 million in fiscal year 2009 and subsequent years.

Centers for Disease Control and Prevention has used those funds to translate and test evidence-based programs, conduct demonstration projects, and develop the STEADI (Stopping Elderly Accidents, Deaths and Injuries) Tool Kit for health care providers (9). In 2014, continued advocacy efforts led to the allocation of $5 million from the Affordable Act's Prevention and Public Health Fund for elder fall prevention to the Administration for Community Living/Administration on Aging (AoA) (10). Funds are to increase the availability of and accessibility to effective programs and services in communities.

DEVELOPING STATE FALL PREVENTION COALITIONS

In 2006, the Falls Free® Initiative accelerated with the addition of the State Coalitions on Fall Prevention Workgroup. At that time, only four states had fall prevention coalitions. These states approached Falls Free® leadership and asked to join the effort. The State Coalitions on Fall Prevention Workgroup was formed and designed to facilitate collaboration between states working on similar issues. The State Coalition Workgroup members reported that developing a state or large regional coalition to address falls and fall-related injuries offered a common forum for multidisciplinary organizations to address falls, deter duplication of efforts, raise awareness, and facilitate necessary roles of resource coordination, policy development, and systems change at the state level (11).

To encourage other states to develop their own fall prevention coalitions, the Falls Free® Initiative developed a tool kit, *Falls and Fall-Related Injuries Among Older Adults: A Practical Guide to State Coalition Building to Address a Growing Public Health Issue* (11). Based on available evidence for coalition building, it was designed to enfold the strategies, experiences, and lessons learned of the 10 fall prevention coalitions in existence by 2007 when the tool kit was created. It includes three stages and nine recommended steps, each with many subtasks, to initiate and build an effective Fall Prevention Coalition. The tool kit still serves as the basis of NCOA technical assistance to states and local communities seeking to build coalitions.

In addition to the tool kit, Falls Free® Initiative leadership provided individualized technical assistance to over 30 states that expressed interest in forming a fall prevention coalition. Technical assistance included structured calls or in-person meetings with coalition leads to walk them through the steps in the Coalition Building tool kit. Support was provided to answer questions about membership sectors, coalition structure, goals and objectives, funding, and evaluation. Formal quarterly calls were also held with the full State Coalitions on Fall Prevention Workgroup to problem solve and collaborate.

As new coalitions formed, they were added to the *State Coalitions on Fall Prevention: Working Collaboratively to Make a Difference Compendium of Initiatives* (12). This document was translated to an interactive map on the NCOA state fall prevention coalition website (13). The website features background and contact information for each coalition so that potential partners can join or have questions addressed about fall prevention activities in the state. Subsequently, NCOA worked with states to develop their own unique state profile of the impact of falls; the states included demonstrate a powerful visual for advocacy purposes (14).

In 2007, NCIPC and AoA entered into an interagency agreement to promote evidence-based fall prevention intervention including support of the Falls Free® Initiative. In the same year, NCIPC also named older adult falls as one of its top three priority areas. Making older adult falls a priority helped to engage the public health community and foster the development of fall prevention coalitions in states with CDC Core Violence and Injury Prevention Program grants; that funding could be used to support fall prevention activities and Injury Community Planning Groups with falls as a priority. From 2006 to 2014, the number of active or developing state fall prevention coalitions grew from 4 to 43 (see **Figure 1**).

SUPPORTING STATE FALL PREVENTION COALITIONS

As the number of coalitions grew, the NCOA continually collaborated with them to provide targeted technical assistance and assist them to enhance their individual and collective impact. The following discussion outlines the processes and tools NCOA's Falls Free® Initiative leadership, with support and input from coalitions and partners, developed to support and sustain their efforts.

INCREASING FALL PREVENTION AWARENESS

In 2008, the 10 state-member Falls Free® State Coalitions on Fall Prevention Workgroup (15) requested assistance in declaring a day of awareness; four states had already targeted the autumnal equinox, which NCOA and the remaining states adopted. In response, the National Advocacy Workgroup gained bipartisan sponsorship of the first annual National Falls Prevention Awareness Day (FPAD) resolution in the U.S. Senate and has obtained bipartisan sponsorship every year since then. The number of states observing FPAD grew from 4 in 2007 to 11 in 2008, 22 in 2009, 36 in 2010, 43 in 2011, 46 in 2012, and 47 in 2013, plus the District of Columbia (15).

According to a survey of state fall prevention coalition leads conducted by the NCOA, an estimated 2,076,041 older adults were reached during FPAD activities in 2013, more than 511,000 participated in evidenced-based fall prevention programs, over 17,000 were screened for falls risks, and more than 1.5 million older adults, family caregivers, professionals, and policymakers were reached through advocacy events and education and awareness campaigns (16). Since 2011, NCOA has offered an annual webinar in advance of FPAD to generate creative partnerships and activities across the country. Each year, webinar registration from across the country has exceeded 1,000.

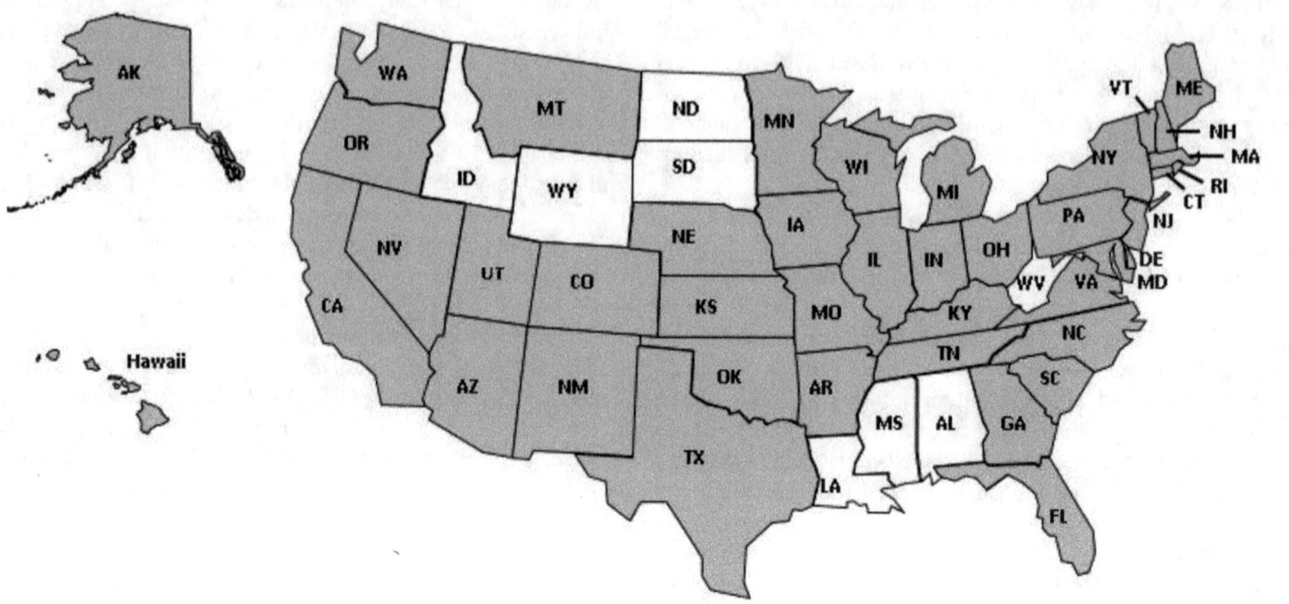

FIGURE 1 | States with active or developing fall prevention coalitions in 2014.

States indicated that increasing awareness of fall prevention was an important goal of their coalitions (11), and several implemented fall prevention awareness campaigns. To better understand the fall prevention awareness campaigns that the states and their fall prevention coalitions implemented and the lessons learned other states could apply to their awareness campaigns, Falls Free® leadership interviewed 10 state agencies and 1 national organization between October 2008 and February 2009. As a result of those interviews, *Falls Prevention Awareness: Lessons Learned from State Coalitions on Fall Prevention* (17) was developed to assist other states in developing fall prevention awareness campaigns. The document contains numerous lessons learned about target audiences, messaging, media and methods, and recommendations for FPAD activities.

PROMOTING EVIDENCE-BASED PROGRAMS

The Falls Free® Initiative is housed within the Center for Healthy Aging (CHA); CHA's mission is to promote evidence-based health promotion and disease prevention programs. The CHA has been working with a variety of state and local grantees since 2003 to adopt and sustain programs making a difference in the health, independence, and quality of life of older adults. These programs provide measurable improvements in patient outcomes and build patient knowledge skills and confidence to manage problems.

Since providers are increasingly being required by Centers for Medicare and Medicaid (CMS) to promote appropriate healthy behaviors, evidence-based programs can be a valuable asset for provider referrals. In alignment with this requirement, a key strategy of the Falls Free® Initiative is to increase access to quality programs and promote linkages and referrals from the health care community. A number of strategies within the *State Policy Toolkit for Advancing Falls Prevention* (discussed below) promote this effort to affect fall prevention.

There are a variety of evidence-based programs recognized as effective for fall prevention. A *CDC Compendium of Effective Fall Interventions: What Works for Community-Dwelling Older Adults, 2nd Edition* represents a significant CDC investment in providing access to programs that can work in a variety of community and home settings and have been shown through randomized trials to reduce falls (18). However, few of the 22 programs listed offer training, tools, and resources for successful implementation. Programs ready to implement include Stepping On, Tai Chi: Moving for Better Balance and Otago. In addition, ACL/AoA recognizes A Matter of Balance and others available for funding under the Older Americans Act, Title IIID (19).

Ongoing Falls Free® collaborative activities promote sharing among fall prevention coalitions of best practices, strategies, and funding opportunities for evidence-based programs. Active partnership-building strategies are used to link coalitions with national Falls Free® member organizations such as the American Physical Therapy Association through their state chapters and local activities.

INSTITUTING EVALUATION

State fall prevention coalitions expressed the need to demonstrate the impact of their coalition work to a variety of stakeholders, coalition partners, funding organizations, and policymakers. In response to those requests, NCOA organized an Evaluation Committee of the State Coalitions on Fall Prevention Workgroup to support state and local evaluation efforts. Members included state coalition leads, researchers, advisors, and CDC staff. The Evaluation Committee developed guidelines to help state fall prevention coalitions evaluate the impact of their efforts, and foster comparisons across states (20). The availability of a standard evaluation process and strategies helps to develop state baseline measures, promote consistency in evaluation efforts across states, and provide data for advocacy or funding opportunities.

The Evaluation Guidelines contain two important products for state coalitions, including the Falls Free® Logic Model and a standard set of survey questions (20). The Logic Model illustrates the causal assumptions linking coalition activities to long-term, measurable outcomes. State coalition leaders can choose to focus their efforts using the logic model (adaptable to states' specific needs) as a guide. The Logic Model articulates the relationship between the resources used to operate the coalition, the activities that the coalition conducts, and the outcomes and impact that the coalition will achieve. By demonstrating the progression, state coalitions can help stakeholders understand how their work leads to desired outcomes.

The standard set of survey questions measure progress of key stakeholders including older adults, children of older adults, primary care providers, and state legislators. The question sets were selected from validated surveys and research activities, and states were asked to use the questions as designed since the standard set of questions must be the same to allow comparisons across states and to demonstrate national impact. Three states (Kansas, New York, and New Hampshire) added a subset of questions from the standard set of survey questions to their state Behavioral Risk Factor Surveillance System (BRFSS) survey. In 2012, 94 people from across the country attended a webinar to learn how to use the Evaluation Guidelines (personal communication, Emily Dessem, National Council on Aging, 2014 March 2).

IMPLEMENTING FALL PREVENTION POLICY AND SYSTEMS CHANGE

Through these various efforts, significant progress was made in the areas of increasing fall prevention awareness, creating multidisciplinary networks, and identifying evaluation measures. However, to achieve systems change and long-term sustainability, state fall prevention coalitions recognized that implementing policy change was necessary, and subsequently requested assistance from Falls Free® leadership in identifying, implementing, and advancing a full array of fall prevention policies to pursue.

To assist the states in their policy development, Falls Free® leadership developed and released the *State Policy Toolkit for Advancing Falls Prevention*, which incorporates the previously discussed Falls Free® Logic Model as a framework to advance policy change (21). The tool kit was disseminated to the State Workgroup on Fall Prevention Coalition members and on the NCOA website. A webinar was held in 2013 to train over 250 attendees on how to use and implement policies in the policy tool kit. A survey of state fall prevention coalition leads was conducted prior to the webinar to ascertain policy implementation, and results indicate that coalitions are actively pursuing evidence-based policies (see **Figure 2**).

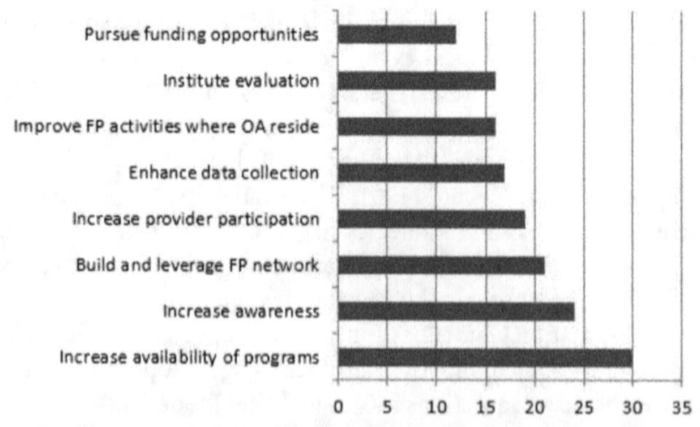

FIGURE 2 | Policy goals being "actively worked on" by state fall prevention coalitions are shown.

DISCUSSION AND LESSONS LEARNED

Although the Falls Free® Initiative played an important supportive role in the fall prevention coalition movement, progress would not have been possible without the work of thousands of people across the country, including the state fall prevention coalition leaders and members, public health community, aging services network, health care providers, researchers, and many, many others.

Creating a movement is not simple, but there are several lessons learned from the progress made thus far that could be applied to other older adult health care issues at the state or local level (11):

- Identify and promote the issue.
  - Use available data to define the issue, convey its impact, and design strategies.
  - Collect and share personalized stories of the impact of the issues and how programs and services are making a difference in the lives of older adults.
  - Advocate with legislators and decision-makers to promote your issue; if your organization is not permitted to advocate, find partners who can.
- Engage partners and leaders.
  - Find partners whose missions align in some way with your issue.
  - Choose engaged, passionate, determined leaders, and champions to promote the issue.
  - Clarify organizational relationships for lead roles and joint planning activities. Develop partnerships between health care, aging, public health, and research networks.
  - Promote collaboration in the cross-agency planning, design, implementation, and evaluation of programs for older adults.
  - Be inclusive; all stakeholders have a role to play.
- Identify solutions.
  - Seek out and adapt measurable, feasible, evidence-based solutions.
  - Increase the availability of tools, resources, and programs, so affected individuals will have methods to reduce their individual risks.
  - Keep trying if you fail. It can take time for a movement to take root, grow, and bloom.

While there has been significant progress in raising awareness of older adult falls, increasing the number of fall prevention coalitions, promoting evidence-based programs, instituting evaluation, implementing fall prevention policy and systems change, and enhancing federal funding for fall prevention efforts, much work still must be done. Older adults themselves and their caregivers need to take a more proactive role in fall prevention. Perhaps due to the stigma of falling, lack of understanding that many falls can be prevented, or limited knowledge on how to get involved, consumers are not yet well engaged in offering new goals for advancing this movement.

The escalating issue of older adult falls affects every state. As the Falls Free® Initiative has demonstrated, one effective approach is an inclusive, targeted coalition to bring partners together to address the issue. A successful rallying activity is the annual observance of FPAD. However, this one observance needs to be leveraged into a more comprehensive approach to community fall prevention.

Despite the states' request for coalition evaluation guidelines, uptake has been limited. States may not have embraced the guidelines due to lack of funding to conduct evaluations or lack of awareness that the guidelines are available.

Future research is needed to better understand how states and communities can implement policy and systems change to more effectively implement falls prevention initiatives within and across sectors such as health care, aging services, and public health. Additionally, the escalating issue of older adult falls is severely underfunded, so partners and stakeholders must continue to advocate for support.

With its growing network of dedicated champions, the Falls Free® Initiative will continue its collaborative efforts to address these areas of focus with the ultimate goal of reducing the number of falls and fall-related injuries, increasing life expectancy, and improving quality of life among older adults in the United States.

REFERENCES

1. Centers for Disease Control and Prevention. *Injury Prevention & Control: Data & Statistics (WISQARS).* (2014). Available from: http://www.cdc.gov/injury/wisqars/
2. Centers for Disease Control and Prevention. *Falls are a Major Threat for your Patients.* (2014). Available from: http://www.cdc.gov/HomeandRecreationalSafety/pdf/steadi/falls_are_a_major_threat.pdf
3. Guideline for the prevention of falls in older persons. American Geriatrics Society, British Geriatrics Society & American Academy of Orthopaedic Surgeons Panel on Falls Prevention. *J Am Geriatr Soc* (2001) **49**:664–72. doi:10.1046/j.1532-5415.2001.49115.x
4. Centers for Disease Control and Prevention. *Cost of Falls Among Older Adults.* (2014). Available from: http://www.cdc.gov/homeandrecreationalsafety/falls/fallcost.html
5. Centers for Disease Control and Prevention. *Falls Among Older Adults: An Overview.* (2013). Available from: http://www.cdc.gov/homeandrecreationalsafety/falls/adultfalls.html
6. National Council on Aging. *Falls Free® Initiative.* (2014). Available from: www.ncoa.org/FallsFreeInitiative
7. National Council on Aging. *Falls Free: Promoting a National Falls Prevention Action Plan.* (2005). Available from: http://www.ncoa.org/improve-health/center-for-healthy-aging/content-library/falls-free-promoting-a.html#sthash.mNlUg5yD.dpuf
8. Government Printing Office. *Public Law 110–202.* (2008). Available from: http://www.gpo.gov/fdsys/pkg/PLAW-110publ202/pdf/PLAW-110publ202.pdf

9. Centers for Disease Control and Prevention. *STEADI (Stopping Elderly Accidents, Deaths, & Injuries) Tool Kit for Health Care Providers.* (2014). Available from: http://www.cdc.gov/homeandrecreationalsafety/Falls/steadi/index.html
10. National Council on Aging. *Aging Program Funding.* (2014). Available at: http://www.ncoa.org/assets/files/pdf/public-policy–action/FY14-Request-v1.pdf?utm_source=FFEnews_1401&utm_medium=newsletter&utm_campaign=FFEnews)
11. National Council on Aging. *Falls and Fall-Related Injuries Among Older Adults: A Practical Guide to State Coalition Building to Address a Growing Public Health Issue.* (2014). Available from: www.ncoa.org/fallstoolkit
12. National Council on Aging. *State Coalitions on Fall Prevention: Working Collaboratively to Make a Difference – Compendium of Initiatives.* (2011). Available from: http://www.ncoa.org/improve-health/center-for-healthy-aging/content-library/State-Coalitions-Compendium-2011.pdf
13. National Council on Aging. *State Coalitions Map.* (2014). Available from: http://www.ncoa.org/improve-health/center-for-healthy-aging/falls-prevention/state-coalitions-map/
14. National Council on Aging. *Fall Prevention Profiles.* (2014). Available from: http://www.ncoa.org/improve-health/center-for-healthy-aging/content-library/falls-state-profiles/falls-prevention-state.html
15. National Council on Aging. *NCOA Leadership Making a Difference: The Falls Free® Initiative.* (2013). Available from: http://www.ncoa.org/assets/files/pdf/NCOA-Falls-Free-Overview-6-2014.pdf
16. National Council on Aging. *Falls Prevention Awareness Day 2013: A Compendium of State and National Activities.* (2013). Available from: http://www.ncoa.org/assets/files/pdf/center-for-healthy-aging/2013-FPAD-Compendium-FINAL.pdf
17. Schneider EC, Beattie BL. *Falls Prevention Awareness: Findings and Lessons Learned from State Coalitions on Fall Prevention.* (2009). Available from: http://www.ncoa.org/improve-health/center-for-healthy-aging/content-library/Falls_Prevention_Lessons_Learned1-27-10.pdf
18. Centers for Disease Control and Prevention. *CDC Compendium of Effective Fall Prevention Interventions: What Works for Community-Dwelling Older Adults.* 2nd ed. (2012). Available from: http://www.cdc.gov/HomeandRecreationalSafety/Falls/compendium.html
19. U.S. Administration on Aging. *Disease Prevention and Health Promotion Services (OAA Title IIID).* (2013). Available from: http://www.aoa.acl.gov/AoA_Programs/HPW/Title_IIID/index.aspx
20. National Council on Aging. *Evaluation Guidelines to Measure the Impact of State and Local Coalitions on Fall Prevention.* (2012). Available from: http://www.ncoa.org/improve-health/center-for-healthy-aging/content-library/evaluation-guidelines-1.html
21. Beattie BL, Schneider EC. *State Policy Toolkit for Advancing Fall Prevention.* (2012). Available from: www.ncoa.org/fallspolicy

9

Workshop characteristics related to Chronic Disease Self-Management Education program attendance

Matthew Lee Smith[1]*, Marcia G. Ory[2], Luohua Jiang[3], Kate Lorig[4], Kristie P. Kulinski[5] and SangNam Ahn[6,2]

[1] Department of Health Promotion and Behavior, College of Public Health, The University of Georgia, Athens, GA, USA
[2] Department of Health Promotion and Community Health Sciences, Texas A&M Health Science Center School of Public Health, College Station, TX, USA
[3] Department of Epidemiology, School of Medicine, University of California Irvine, Irvine, CA, USA
[4] Stanford Patient Education Research Center, Department of Medicine, Stanford University School of Medicine, Palo Alto, CA, USA
[5] National Council on Aging, Washington, DC, USA
[6] Division of Health Systems Management and Policy, School of Public Health, The University of Memphis, Memphis, TN, USA

Edited by:
Sanjay P. Zodpey, Public Health Foundation of India, India

Reviewed by:
Shridhar Murlidharrao Kadam, Public Health Foundation of India, India
Michael Elliott, Saint Louis University College for Public Health and Social Justice, USA

****Correspondence:***
Matthew Lee Smith, Department of Health Promotion and Behavior, College of Public Health, The University of Georgia, Health Science Campus, Wright Hall #345E, Athens, GA 30602, USA
e-mail: health@uga.edu

Using the national dissemination of Chronic Disease Self-Management Education (CDSME) programs, the purposes of this study were to (1) document intervention attendance rates as related to the number of participants enrolled in the workshop and (2) compare the relationship between workshop attendance and workshop size by delivery site rurality and type. Data were analyzed from the first 100,000 middle-aged and older adults who participated in CDSME workshops spanning 45 states, Puerto Rico, and the District of Columbia as part of the American Recovery and Reinvestment Act of 2009 *Communities Putting Prevention to Work: Chronic Disease Self-Management Program* initiative. Descriptive statistics are reported for all participants, then separately by each delivery site type. Ratios between the number of workshop participants and the number of workshop sessions attended were calculated and graphed based on the rurality of delivery and separately for the leading five delivery site types. Associations between the number of workshop participants and the number of sessions attended differed by delivery site rurality and type. Findings have implications for participant retention and workshop delivery costs, which can assist program deliverers to strategically plan implementation efforts in their areas.

Keywords: chronic disease self-management, evidence-based program, older adults, intervention dose, evaluation

INTRODUCTION

The recent movement toward evidence-based public health calls for a better understanding of the implementation and dissemination of evidence-based programs (EBP) for older adults delivered in real world settings (1–4). EBP are interventions based on research that were tested in clinical trials and translated into community-based models, which receive the same intended health benefits (5). EBP have common components, foremost of which are essential intervention elements, materials, and procedures (6). More specifically, implementation features must be considered, which include having a well-defined program structure and timeframe that enables the developers to track fidelity and others to uniformly deliver the program with replicable findings (7). Program developers often draw upon small group literature and adult learning principles to define the ideal class size for intervention (8–10), which is often 12–16 participants (11). From our experience working with program developers, determination of ideal class size is often more of an art than a science and is based on assumptions about ideal size to facilitate active group discussion. Secondary concerns often revolve around cost implications of different class sizes in intervention studies because per-participant costs are influenced by the total number of participants enrolled in workshops (12, 13).

With a desire to take EBP to scale in order to make a public health impact, there is a need for widespread penetration in the designated population of interest (14, 15). To counter recruitment challenges often seen in research studies (16–18), there is now a growing literature on strategies to increase recruitment by facilitating program adoption in a host of different delivery systems reflecting where the population of interest resides and frequently encounter in their daily lives.

Despite the assumed importance of structured program features such as class size or workshop delivery type, little is known about the programmatic impact of different delivery characteristics on achieving recommended intervention doses. This is, in part, because assumptions about ideal class size are often applied from prior literature without consideration of the specific intervention focus, population, or setting. Delivery sites may be seen as implementation issues rather than researchable variables, an attitude reinforced by the limited number of delivery site types included in most intervention studies.

The widespread availability of Chronic Disease Self-Management Education (CDSME) programs nationwide across a multitude of settings has provided opportunity to examine the programmatic impact of different delivery characteristics on participants receiving the recommended intervention dose. Using the national dissemination of CDSME programs, the purposes of this study were to (1) document intervention attendance rates as related to the number of participants enrolled in the workshop and (2) compare the relationship between workshop attendance and workshop size by delivery site rurality (i.e., metro, non-metro) and type (e.g., senior centers, healthcare organizations, residential facilities, faith-based organizations).

MATERIALS AND METHODS

PROGRAM DESCRIPTION

The Chronic Disease Self-Management Program (CDSMP) has been introduced and widely disseminated in the U.S. as a method to empower patients with self-management skills to deal with their chronic conditions (19). There is now a suite of CDSME programs licensed through the Stanford Patient Education Research Center, some of which are generic (e.g., CDSMP, Tomando Control de su Salud) and others that are disease specific (e.g., diabetes, arthritis, chronic pain). Drawing upon Social Learning Theory (20), CDSME programs are evidence-based, peer-led interventions consisting of six highly participative classes held for 2.5 h each, once a week, for six consecutive weeks (19). CDSME programs have resulted in improved health care and health (21, 22), while potentially saving healthcare costs (12).

DATA SOURCE AND STUDY POPULATION

Cross-sectional data for this study were obtained from a nationwide delivery of CDSME programs as part of the American Recovery and Reinvestment Act of 2009 (i.e., ARRA) *Communities Putting Prevention to Work: Chronic Disease Self-Management Program* initiative (15). The US Administration on Aging led this initiative in collaboration with the Centers for Disease Control and Prevention and the Centers for Medicare and Medicaid Services to support the translation of CDSME programs in 45 states, Puerto Rico, and the District of Columbia (23). Federal funding for this initiative enabled participants to enroll in CDSMP workshops free of charge. This initiative was originally designed to have 50,000 Americans complete at least four out of six CDSME workshop sessions between 2010 and 2012 and to embed CDSME program delivery structures into statewide systems (15). For this study, data were analyzed from the first 100,000 participants who attended CDSME program workshops and responded to all relevant survey questions. Workshops included in study analyses began between January 2010 and February 2012.

As described elsewhere (24), all states receiving ARRA funding for this initiative were assigned program completer target goals. It was expected that CDSME program workshops would be delivered through certain site (e.g., senior centers, healthcare organizations, residential facilities, educational institutions, faith-based organizations, and tribal centers). Each delivery site type recruited participants to enroll in workshops using their usual methods (e.g., flyers, emails, face-to-face). The majority of participants was introduced to the program during the first workshop session; however, some participants were introduced to the program during an optional pre-workshop session called a "session zero" (25).

MEASURES

Workshop attendance

Participants' attendance was recorded to determine if the recommended intervention dose was received. As defined by the program developers, a participant has "successfully" completed the program if they attended four or more of the six offered workshop sessions (15, 21, 22).

Class size

The number of participants enrolled in each CDSME workshop was recorded (i.e., ranging from 1 to 20 participants). The maximum number of participants allowed to be listed as enrollees in any single workshop was 20. As a point of reference, the program developers define the ideal class size as (i.e., between 10 and 15 participants) in the CDSMP fidelity manual (26).

Delivery site types

Data are presented for all 10 delivery site types (see **Table 1**), which were then assessed graphically based on the workshop rurality and independently for the leading five delivery site types based on participant enrollment (i.e., senior centers, healthcare organizations, residential facilities, community/multi-purpose facilities, and faith-based organizations). Data pertaining to CDSME program delivery site types were gathered administratively (24). Using the ZIP code information provided by each delivery site, workshops were categorized as metro or non-metro based on the rural–urban commuting area codes (RUCA) (27). The leading five CDSMP delivery site types included in analyses were senior centers or area agencies on aging (AAAs), healthcare organizations, residential facilities, community or multi-purpose centers (including libraries), and faith-based organizations.

Personal characteristics

Personal characteristics of the participants included age, gender, race/ethnicity, and self-reported number of chronic conditions (i.e., arthritis, cancer, depression, diabetes, heart disease, hypertension, lung disease, stroke, osteoporosis, and other chronic conditions).

ANALYSES

Descriptive statistics were calculated for all participants, then separately for each of the 10 delivery site types. Percentages are provided for categorical variables. Averages and standard deviations are provided for continuous and count variables. The average number of workshop sessions attended by the size of the workshop (i.e., the number of participants enrolled in each workshop) was calculated and graphed based on the rurality of delivery and separately for the leading five delivery site types.

RESULTS

CDSMP PARTICIPANT AND WORKSHOP CHARACTERISTICS BY DELIVERY SITE TYPE

Of the first 100,000 participants reached in this initiative, 29.2% attended workshops at senior centers/AAAs, 21.1% at healthcare organizations, 17.6% at residential facilities, 9.9% at community/multi-purpose facilities (including libraries), and 8.4% at faith-based organizations. Smaller proportions of participants attended workshops at educational institutions (2.3%), county health departments (1.3%), workplaces (0.5%), and tribal centers (0.2%). Approximately 9.5% of participants attended CDSME workshops at delivery sites classified as "other" (e.g., correctional facilities malls, RV parks, fire departments, county administration buildings, private residences, casinos, career centers).

Table 1 | Participant and workshop characteristics by delivery site type.

	Total ($n = 100{,}000$)	Senior Center/AAA ($n = 29{,}152$)	Healthcare Organization ($n = 21{,}136$)	Residential Facility ($n = 17{,}631$)	Comm/ Multi-Purp/ Library ($n = 9{,}891$)	Faith-Based Organization ($n = 8406$)	Educational Institution ($n = 2264$)	Health Department ($n = 1274$)	Tribal Center ($n = 189$)	Workplace ($n = 541$)	Other ($n = 9{,}516$)
PARTICIPANT CHARACTERISTICS											
Age	67.1 (±14.58)	71.1 (±11.76)	61.9 (±14.49)	73.5 (±12.96)	65.7 (±14.01)	65.7 (±13.71)	61.8 (±15.85)	64.2 (±14.59)	64.6 (±13.46)	60.8 (±14.80)	59.0 (±17.21)
Female	77.9%	80.5%	73.3%	82.7%	78.2%	78.9%	82.8%	79.6%	72.0%	81.7%	68.8%
Race/Ethnicity											
Latino/Hispanic	16.6%	12.4%	27.3%	10.4%	17.1%	13.0%	27.7%	7.7%	5.1%	5.4%	21.2%
Non-Hispanic White	54.4%	58.0%	51.7%	60.0%	49.9%	44.1%	58.6%	75.0%	24.3%	63.3%	48.6%
African-American	21.8%	23.6%	14.6%	23.7%	20.8%	34.0%	10.6%	9.4%	7.3%	13.5%	22.0%
Asian/Pacific Islander	4.6%	3.6%	3.2%	3.6%	10.1%	7.1%	2.3%	4.8%	0.0%	14.4%	4.2%
American Indian/ Alaska native	1.5%	1.2%	1.9%	1.0%	0.9%	0.8%	0.4%	1.5%	61.0%	1.7%	3.0%
Other race	1.2%	1.1%	1.3%	1.4%	1.1%	1.1%	0.6%	1.6%	2.3%	1.7%	1.0%
Average number of co-morbidities	2.2 (±1.71)	2.3 (±1.71)	2.1 (±1.68)	2.4 (±1.80)	2.1 (±1.70)	2.0 (±1.60)	2.0 (±1.66)	2.2 (±1.78)	2.7 (±1.80)	1.9 (±1.59)	2.0 (±1.63)
WORKSHOP CHARACTERISTICS											
Class size	12.7 (±4.18)	13.1 (±4.26)	12.1 (±4.13)	13.1 (±4.01)	12.5 (±4.18)	12.9 (±4.09)	12.9 (±4.10)	10.3 (±4.28)	9.6 (±2.74)	10.7 (±3.89)	12.8 (±4.12)
Number of sessions attended	4.4 (±1.72)	4.5 (±1.65)	4.2 (±1.78)	4.2 (±1.81)	4.4 (±1.70)	4.5 (±1.63)	4.5 (±1.70)	4.2 (±1.75)	4.2 (±1.69)	4.7 (±1.52)	4.7 (±1.66)
Successful completion	74.9%	77.0%	72.1%	70.2%	74.7%	78.7%	77.3%	69.2%	69.3%	82.6%	79.7%
Proportion of workshops in non-metro areas	20.4%	22.4%	17.7%	16.4%	17.1%	22.2%	25.8%	36.7%	13.8%	31.8%	25.7%

On average, participants were age 67.1 (±14.6) years and had 2.2 (±1.7) self-reported chronic conditions. The majority of participants were female (77.9%) and non-Hispanic white (54.4%). Almost 22% of participants were African-American and 16.6% were Hispanic. Workshops at senior centers/AAAs and residential facilities enrolled participants with older than average ages. Healthcare organizations, tribal centers, and sites categorized as "other" enrolled larger proportions of male participants. Healthcare organizations, community/multi-purpose facilities, educational institutions, and other sites enrolled larger proportions of Hispanic participants. Senior centers/AAAs, residential facilities, and faith-based organizations enrolled larger proportions of African-American participants. Healthcare organizations, residential facilities, community/multi-purpose facilities, and tribal centers enrolled more participants from metro areas. Workshops at senior centers/AAAs, residential facilities, and tribal centers enrolled participants with higher than average co-morbidities.

More than 20% of participants attended workshops delivered in non-metro areas. The workshops in non-metro areas had smaller average class size than those in metro areas, but no difference in class attendance. On average, workshops had 12.7 (±4.2) participants, and participants attended an average of 4.4 (±1.7) of the six workshop sessions. The majority of participants successfully completed the workshop (74.9%), indicating they received the recommended intervention dose. Senior centers/AAAs, faith-based organizations, educational institutions, and delivery sites categorized as "other" had higher than average workshop sizes and workshop attendance. Residential facilities also had higher than average workshop sizes. Workplaces also had higher than average workshop attendance.

ASSOCIATIONS BETWEEN WORKSHOP SIZE AND ATTENDANCE

As shown in **Figure 1**, associations between the number of workshop participants and the number of sessions attended differ by workshop rurality. More specifically, in workshops in metro areas, there was a negative correlation between participant number and session attendance for smaller workshops (i.e., workshops ≤ 8 participants). The average number of sessions attended in non-metro organizations had higher variability, especially for smaller workshops. Associations between the number of workshop participants and the number of sessions attended differed by delivery site type. More specifically, in senior centers/AAAs, there was a negative correlation between participant number and session attendance for smaller workshops (i.e., workshops ≤ 8 participants). Stated differently, the fewer the participants enrolled in a workshop, the higher the rate of session completion. For workshops with nine or more participants, the workshop size was not correlated with the average number of sessions attended. The relationships between participant number and session attendance in healthcare organizations and community/multi-purpose/libraries were similar to that observed in senior centers/AAAs. However, the average number of sessions attended in healthcare organizations had higher variability, especially for smaller workshops.

For delivery sites located in residential facilities, the number of workshop participants was negatively associated with session attendance. Generally, workshops with fewer participants had higher average workshop attendance. In faith-based organizations, however, there was no observed association between the number of workshop participants and workshop attendance.

DISCUSSION

As demonstrated in a previous study, workshop size was associated with workshop attendance in national dissemination efforts of EBP for older adults (13). As confirmed by other studies (15, 22), most delivery sites reported workshop sizes in the ideal range (i.e., between 10 and 15 participants) and large proportions of participants with successful completion rates. While general findings in the current study indicate that workshops with fewer participants had higher attendance rates, variability was noted by setting, especially among smaller workshops. Greater variability in smaller workshop as observed in workshops delivered in non-metro areas, healthcare organizations, and faith-based organizations. The strongest negative association was observed in residential facilities.

Consistent with the RE-AIM planning and evaluation framework (28, 29), wide-scale programmatic dissemination to diverse population subgroups often requires a multitude of community partnerships representing various settings. It is not surprising that senior centers/AAAs and healthcare organizations serve as the predominant sites, given the sponsorship of this initiative by the Administration on Aging (23). However, it is more interesting to consider the different delivery settings utilized in this initiative's program implementation and dissemination activities (e.g., senior centers, healthcare organizations, residential facilities, faith-based organizations). This study contributes to the emerging implementation science literature by identifying and documenting the wide variability in workshop size and attendance based on different setting types (30).

As seen elsewhere (31, 32), certain delivery site types are known to attract participants with certain characteristics, which make it difficult to disentangle the impact of workshop size and attendance from the types of participants who attend a particular delivery site type. Future research would benefit from qualitative research to better understand what drives participants to one setting or another. For example, is participant attendance related to the supply of programing at different settings? Is it that participants identify with a particular organizational setting and, therefore, attend workshops where they are most comfortable (33)? Or, is it simply a proximity issue in that participants attend workshops that are closes to their home or work (34)? Or, might it be a combination where participants are willing to travel further distances to attend workshops delivered in a setting of preference? These issues warrant further investigation at the individual-level based on preference and the workshop-level based on common characteristics associated with workshop size and attendance.

These study findings are illuminating in that they show the interconnectedness of and interaction between workshop size, delivery site type, and intervention dosage. Findings indicate that there is no "one size fits all" rule of thumb regarding ideal workshop size and that the recommended intervention dose can be obtained at different delivery settings in workshop of differing sizes. Additional research is needed to determine the influence of workshop

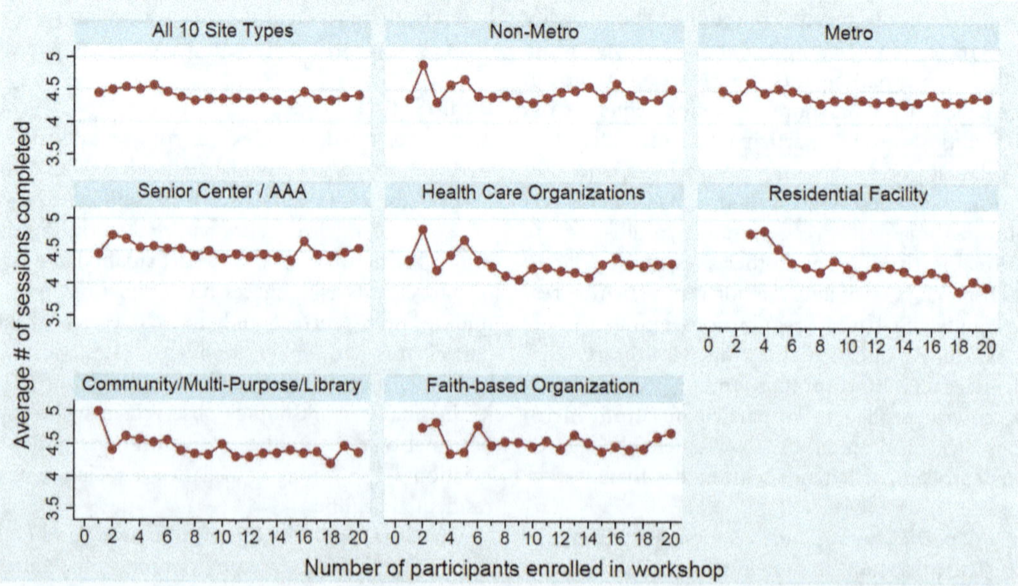

FIGURE 1 | Average number of workshop sessions attended by class size by workshop rurality and leading five delivery site type.

size and attendance on known health-related benefits associated with CDSME programs, controlling for workshop delivery site. Further, there is need for more sophisticated threshold analyses to determine the critical class size for optimal attendance and how that may differ by delivery site type.

Several study limitations can be noted. First, the cross-sectional nature of the study and lack of outcome data limited our ability to determine causality and associate workshop size and attendance with salient health outcomes. Second, there were a limited number of variables collected about the delivery sites and/or from participants; thus, we were unable to investigate the greater context of factors related to delivery site type selection, reasons for attendance, or reasons why certain delivery sites held workshops of certain sizes. However, the large number of workshops delivered and participants enrolled in this national initiative provides an initial glimpse into study questions and suggests areas needing more exploration. Third, this descriptive study was served as a preliminary examination of the relationship between workshop characteristics (delivery site type and number of participants) and class attendance. Future studies with more sophisticated, inferential statistics that include more predictor variables are needed to compare these relationships by other factors (e.g., self-reported chronic condition types) and health-related improvements resulting from intervention attendance.

This research has several practical implications. First, multi-pronged strategies are needed to improve participant retention so participants can receive the recommended intervention dose, despite workshop enrollment size. These strategies should be tailored approaches by delivery site types based on their specific participant characteristics and health-related status (35). Second, while class size may not always be associated with intervention dose, class size has implications for overall program costs (12, 36). This has been seen in our calculations of the cost savings that can be derived from CDSME programs based on variations in overall per-participant costs, which is highly dependent upon class size (12, 36). More specifically, based on a workshop cost of $3500 USD, per-participant costs can range from about $219 USD for larger workshops with 16 participants to $583 USD for smaller workshops with 6 participants (12). As such, because CDSME program workshops have a fair amount of fixed costs, regardless of workshop size (e.g., associated with site coordination, participant recruitment), hosting larger versus smaller workshops seems to be more fiscally beneficial to organizations implementing these programs. These cost-related variations have implications for program administrator and decision makers to finically plan future dissemination efforts and identify necessary resources and partners to achieve participant recruitment goals. Further, because of its small group approach using the social learning theory (19, 20), workshop size should be considered to ensure the program operates as intended and participants receive anticipated intervention benefits.

CONCLUSION

The implementation processes in a national rollout of evidence-based CDSME programs are necessarily complex. Previous assumptions about the ideal class size need to be weighed in terms of both programmatic and cost metrics, balancing the economies of "going to scale" with the benefits of smaller class sizes in some settings. Therefore, it is important to recognize how delivery sites cater to different types of participants, which may in turn influence program outcomes. Findings have implications for participant retention and workshop delivery costs, which can assist program deliverers to strategically plan implementation efforts in their areas.

ACKNOWLEDGMENTS

The American Recovery and Reinvestment Act of 2009 (i.e., Recovery Act) Communities Putting Prevention to Work: Chronic Disease Self-Management Program initiative, led by the US Administration on Aging in collaboration with the Centers for Disease Control and Prevention and the Centers for Medicare and Medicaid Services, allotted $32.5 million to support the translation of the Stanford program in 45 States, Puerto Rico, and the District of Columbia. The National Council on Aging served as the Technical Assistance Resource Center for this initiative and collected de-identified data on program participation.

REFERENCES

1. National Center for Chronic Disease Prevention and Health Promotion. *Healthy Aging Research Network: Putting Collective Wisdom to Work for Older Americans.* Atlanta, GA: Centers for Disease Control and Prevention (CDC) (2011). CS226787 p.
2. National Council on Aging. *Evidence-Based Health Promotion Programs for Older Adults: Key Factors and Strategies Contributing to Program Sustainability.* Washington, DC: National Council on Aging (2012).
3. Green LW, Ottoson JM, Garcia C, Hiatt RA. Diffusion theory and knowledge dissemination, utilization, and integration in public health. *Annu Rev Public Health* (2009) **30**:151–74. doi:10.1146/annurev.publhealth.031308.100049
4. Brownson RC, Colditz GA, Proctor EK. *Dissemination and Implementation Research in Health: Translating Science to Practice.* New York, NY: Oxford University Press (2012).
5. National Council on Aging Center for Healthy Aging. *About Evidence-Based Programs.* Washington, DC: (2014). Available from: http://www.ncoa.org/improve-health/center-for-healthy-aging/about-evidence-based-programs.html
6. Schulz R, Czaja SJ, McKay JR, Ory MG, Belle SH. Intervention taxonomy (ITAX): describing essential features of interventions. *Am J Health Behav* (2010) **34**(6):811–21. doi:10.5993/AJHB.34.6.15
7. National Council on Aging Center for Healthy Aging. *Module 2: What is Evidence-Based Health Promotion?: National Council on Aging.* (2014). Available from: http://www.ncoa.org/chamodules/series1/m2/module2.pdf
8. Northwest Center for Public Health Practice at the University of Washington School of Public Health. *Effective Adult Learning: A Toolkit for Teaching Adults.* Seattle, WA: Robert Wood Johnson Foundation (2014).
9. Burke SM, Carron AV, Patterson MM, Estabrooks PA, Hill JL, Loughead TM, et al. Cohesion as shared beliefs in exercise classes. *Small Group Res* (2005) **36**(3):267–88. doi:10.1177/1046496404267942
10. Carron AV, Spink KS. The group size-cohesion relationship in minimal groups. *Small Group Res* (1995) **26**(1):86–105. doi:10.1177/1046496495261005
11. National Council on Aging. *Center for Healthy Aging: Highlights.* Washington, DC: (2014). Available from: http://www.ncoa.org/improve-health/center-for-healthy-aging/
12. Ahn S, Basu R, Smith ML, Jiang L, Lorig K, Whitelaw N, et al. The impact of chronic disease self-management programs: healthcare savings through a community-based intervention. *BMC Public Health* (2013) **13**(1):1141. doi:10.1186/1471-2458-13-1141
13. Smith ML, Hochhalter AK, Cheng Y, Wang S, Ory MG. Programmatic influences on outcomes of an evidence-based fall prevention program for older adults: a translational assessment. *Transl Behav Med* (2011) **1**(3):384–93. doi:10.1007/s13142-011-0058-7
14. Ory MG, Altpeter M, Belza B, Helduser J, Zhang C, Smith ML. Perceptions about the community application of RE-AIM in the promotion of evidence-based programs for older adults. *Eval Health Prof* (2014). doi:10.1177/0163278714542335
15. Ory MG, Smith ML, Kulinski KP, Lorig K, Zenker W, Whitelaw N. Self-management at the tipping point: reaching 100,000 Americans with evidence-based programs. *J Am Geriatr Soc* (2013) **61**(5):821–3. doi:10.1111/jgs.12239
16. Levkoff S, Sanchez H. Lessons learned about minority recruitment and retention from the centers on minority aging and health promotion. *Gerontologist* (2003) **43**(1):18–26. doi:10.1093/geront/43.1.18
17. Levkoff SE, Prohaska TR, Weitzman PF, Ory MG. Minority populations: Recruitment and retention in aging research. In: Maddox GL, editor. *The Encyclopedia of Aging.* New York, NY: Springer Publishing Co (2000). p. 694–6.
18. Ory MG, Lipman PD, Karlen PL, Gerety MB, Stevens VJ, Singh MA, et al. Recruitment of older participants in frailty/injury prevention studies. *Prev Sci* (2002) **3**(1):1–22. doi:10.1023/A:1014610325059
19. Lorig K. *Living a Healthy Life with Chronic Conditions: Self-Management of Heart Disease, Arthritis, Diabetes, Asthma, Bronchitis, Emphysema & Others.* 3rd ed. Boulder, CO: Bull Pub. Company (2006). 382 p.
20. Bandura A. Social cognitive theory of self-regulation. *Organ Behav Hum Decis Process* (1991) **50**(2):248–87. doi:10.1016/0749-5978(91)90022-L
21. Ory MG, Ahn S, Jiang L, Lorig K, Ritter P, Laurent DD, et al. National study of chronic disease self-management six-month outcome findings. *J Aging Health* (2013) **25**(7):1258–74. doi:10.1177/0898264313502531
22. Ory MG, Ahn S, Jiang L, Smith ML, Ritter PL, Whitelaw N, et al. Successes of a national study of the chronic disease self-management program: meeting the triple aim of health care reform. *Med Care* (2013) **51**(11):992–8. doi:10.1097/MLR.0b013e3182a95dd1
23. U.S. Department of Health and Human Services, Administration on Aging. *ARRA – Communities Putting Prevention to Work: Chronic Disease Self-Management Program 2012.* (2014). Available from: www.cfda.gov/index?s=program&mode=form&tab=step1&id=5469a61f2c5f25cf3984fc3b94051b5f
24. Kulinski KP, Boutaugh M, Smith ML, Ory MG, Lorig K. Setting the stage: measure selection, coordination, and data collection for a national self-management initiative. *Front Public Health* (2015) **2**:206. doi:10.3389/fpubh.2014.00206
25. Jiang L, Smith ML, Chen S, Ahn S, Kulinski KP, Lorig K, et al. The role of Session Zero in successful completion of Chronic Disease Self-Management Program workshops. *Front Public Health* (2015) **2**:205. doi:10.3389/fpubh.2014.00205
26. Stanford Patient Education Research Center. *Program Fidelity Manual: Stanford Self-Management Programs 2012 Update.* Stanfrod, CA: Stanford School of Medicine (2012).
27. United States Department of Agriculture Economic Research Service. *Rural-Urban Commuting Area Codes: Overview.* (2014). Available from: http://www.ers.usda.gov/data-products/rural-urban-commuting-area-codes.aspx#.U-ObPmPqlZU
28. Glasgow RE, Klesges LM, Dzewaltowski DA, Bull SS, Estabrooks P. The future of health behavior change research: what is needed to improve translation of research into health promotion practice? *Ann Behav Med* (2004) **27**(1):3–12. doi:10.1207/s15324796abm2701_2
29. Glasgow RE, Vogt TM, Boles SM. Evaluating the public health impact of health promotion interventions: the RE-AIM framework. *Am J Public Health* (1999) **89**(9):1322–7. doi:10.2105/AJPH.89.9.1322
30. Israel BA, Schults AJ, Parker EA, Becker AB. BeckerReview of community-based research: assessing partnership approaches to improve public health. *Annu Rev Public Health* (1998) **19**:173–202. doi:10.1146/annurev.publhealth.19.1.173
31. Smith M, Belza B, Altpeter M, Ahn S, Dickerson J, Ory M. Disseminating an evidence-based disease self-management program for older americans: implications for diversifying participant reach through delivery site adoption. In: Maddock J, editor. *Public Health – Social and Behavioral Health.* Rijeka: InTech (2012). p. 385–404.
32. Smith ML, Ory MG, Ahn S, Belza B, Mingo CA, Towne Jr. SD, et al. Reaching diverse participants utilizing a diverse delivery infrastructure: a replication study. *Front Public Health* (2015) **3**:77. doi:10.3389/fpubh.2015.00077
33. Cooney SM, Small SA, O'Connor C. Strategies for recruiting and retaining participants in prevention programs. *What Works, Wisconsin Research to Practice Series, 2.* Madison, WI: University of Wisconsin–Madison/Extension (2007). Available from: http://whatworks.uwex.edu/attachment/whatworks_02.pdf
34. Salazar CI, Smith ML, Perez AG, Ahn S, Ory MG. Geospatial characteristics of the chronic disease self-management program: reaching diverse ethnic populations in San Antonio, Texas. *Tex Public Health J* (2011) **63**(1):16–20.
35. Smith ML, Wilson MG, DeJoy DM, Padilla H, Zuercher H, Corso P, et al. Chronic Disease Self-Management Program in the workplace: opportunities for health improvement. *Front Public Health* (2015) **2**:179. doi:10.3389/fpubh.2014.00179
36. Ahn S, Smith ML, Altpeter M, Post L, Ory MG. Healthcare cost savings estimator tool for chronic disease self-management program: a new tool for program administrators and decision makers. *Front Public Health* (2015) **3**:42. doi:10.3389/fpubh.2015.00042

10

Factors associated with successful completion of the Chronic Disease Self-Management Program among middle-aged and older Asian-American participants

SangNam Ahn[1,2]*, Matthew Lee Smith[3], Jinmyoung Cho[2,4], Luohua Jiang[5], Lindsey Post[1] and Marcia G. Ory[2]

[1] Division of Health Systems Management and Policy, School of Public Health, The University of Memphis, Memphis, TN, USA
[2] Department of Health Promotion and Community Health Sciences, School of Public Health, Texas A&M Health Science Center, College Station, TX, USA
[3] Department of Health Promotion and Behavior, College of Public Health, The University of Georgia, Athens, GA, USA
[4] Center for Applied Health Research, Baylor Scott & White Healthcare, Temple, TX, USA
[5] Department of Epidemiology, School of Medicine, University of California Irvine, Irvine, CA, USA

Edited by:
Shane Andrew Thomas, Monash University, Australia

Reviewed by:
Laura Rudkin, University of Texas Medical Branch, USA
Geraldine Sanchez Aglipay, University of Illinois at Chicago, USA

***Correspondence:**
SangNam Ahn, Division of Health Systems Management and Policy, School of Public Health, The University of Memphis, 133 Robison Hall, Memphis, TN 38152-3530, USA
e-mail: sahn@memphis.edu

Asian-Americans are a small but fast-growing population in the United States who are increasingly experiencing multiple chronic diseases. While the evidence-based Chronic Disease Self-Management Program (CDSMP) has been disseminated among various racial and ethnic populations, few studies specifically investigate participants with an Asian background. The study aims to identify characteristics of middle-aged and older Asian-American CDSMP participants (older than 50 years) and investigate factors related to successful workshop completion (i.e., attending 4+ of the 6 sessions) among this population. Data were analyzed from 2,716 middle-aged and older Asian-Americans collected during a 2-year national dissemination of CDSMP. Multilevel logistic regression analyses were conducted to identify individual- and workshop-level covariates related to successful workshop completion. The majority of participants were female, living with others, and living in metro areas. The average age was 71.3 years old (±9.2), and the average number of chronic conditions was 2.0 (±1.5). Successful completion of CDSMP workshops among participants was associated with their number of chronic conditions (OR = 1.10, P = 0.011), living in non-metro areas (OR = 1.77, P = 0.009), attending workshops from area agencies on aging (OR = 1.56, P = 0.018), and attending a workshop with higher completion rates (OR = 1.03, P < 0.001). This study is the first large-scale examination of Asian-American participants enrolled in CDSMP and highlights characteristics related to intervention attendance among this understudied minority population. Knowing such characteristics is important for serving the growing number of Asian-Americans with chronic conditions.

Keywords: Asian-Americans, chronic disease management, Chronic Disease Self-Management Program, evidence-based programs

INTRODUCTION

Almost three-quarters of Asian-American adults are foreign-born, representing many countries of origin, including China, India, and the Philippines (1). Collectively, these subgroups constitute the fastest-growing ethnic group in the country, representing almost 6% of the U.S. population (1). The Asian-American population in the U.S., which was estimated at 18.9 million in 2012 (2), grew by 46% from 2000 to 2010, and is outpacing the growth of other racial/ethnic groups. Between 2011 and 2012, the rate of population increase was 2.9% for Asian-Americans, 2.2% for Hispanics; 2.2% for Native Hawaiians and Other Pacific Islanders; 1.5% for American-Indians and Alaska Native; and 1.3% for African-Americans (2). This population growth warrants further study of health conditions among Asian-Americans. Although the prevalence rate of chronic conditions among Asian-Americans (42%) is lower than their African-American (77%), Latino (68%), and White (64%) counterparts, the burden of chronic conditions among Asian-Americans should be carefully scrutinized based on population projections (2–4). As the total population of Asian-Americans increases, it is expected that a greater number of Asian-Americans will suffer from chronic conditions.

The Chronic Disease Self-Management Program (CDSMP) has been introduced and widely disseminated in the U.S. as a method to empower patients with self-management skills to deal with their chronic conditions (5). Drawing upon social learning theory (6), CDSMP is an evidence-based, peer-led intervention consisting of six highly participative classes held for 2.5 h each, once a week, for six consecutive weeks (5). CDSMP has resulted in improved healthcare and health (7, 8), while potentially saving healthcare costs (9). While CDSMP has been successfully disseminated among diverse populations, there are few studies focusing specifically on the characteristics of middle-aged or older

Asian-Americans enrolled in CDSMP or examining the factors associated with completing CDSMP in this population. Previous studies have shown that Asian-Americans complete CDSMP at a somewhat higher rate than the general participant population and at about the same rate as White participants (10). Thus, the objective of the study was to analyze the dataset more closely to (1) identify characteristics of Asian-American CDSMP participants in the 2010–2012 national dissemination of CDSMP in the U.S.; and (2) identify the factors associated with CDSMP completion among middle-aged and older Asian-American participants.

METHODS

DATA SOURCE AND STUDY POPULATION

Cross-sectional data for this study were retrospectively obtained from a nationwide delivery of CDSMP as part of the American Recovery and Reinvestment Act of 2009 (i.e., Recovery Act) *Communities Putting Prevention to Work: CDSMP initiative* (11). The U.S. Administration on Aging led this initiative in collaboration with the Centers for Disease Control and Prevention and the Centers for Medicare and Medicaid Services to support the translation of CDSMP in 45 states, Puerto Rico, and the District of Columbia (12). This initiative was conducted between 2010 and 2012 with the goal of reaching the diverse population of the Americans embedding the delivery structures into statewide systems (11). Within the first 2 years of this initiative, there were more than 100,000 adults participating in 9,305 workshops in 1,234 U.S. counties (11). For this study, data were analyzed from 2,716 Asian-American participants (i.e., aggregate Asian ethnic groups) who aged 50 years or older and responded to all relevant survey questions.

MEASURES

DEPENDENT VARIABLE

Chronic Disease Self-Management Program workshop attendance was the dependent variable for this study. Successful completion was defined as attendance at four or more of the six workshop sessions, which is consistent with definitions used by the program developers and in a variety of other studies (7–9, 11).

INDIVIDUAL- OR NEIGHBORHOOD-LEVEL COVARIATES

As individual-level covariates, socio-demographic factors included age (in years), sex (male vs. female), and living arrangement (living with others vs. living alone). Health status was measured by the number of self-reported chronic conditions (i.e., arthritis, cancer, depression, diabetes, heart disease, hypertension, lung disease, stroke, osteoporosis, and other chronic conditions). As neighborhood-level covariates, median household income (in $10,000 units) was included based on the participants' ZIP Code. Rural–Urban Commuting Area Codes based on participants' ZIP Code information were used to categorize participants' residence (metro vs. non-metro) (13).

WORKSHOP-LEVEL COVARIATES

Workshop delivery sites included area agencies on aging (AAA)/senior centers, healthcare organizations, residential facilities, community or multi-purpose centers, faith-based organizations, educational institutions, recreational centers, tribal centers, and workplaces. The last four delivery sites made up <13% of the total and were coded as "other" for purpose of the study and their low distribution (<13%). Workshop composition varied in the proportion of Asian-Americans participating. We hypothesized that workshops with more racial/ethnic homogeneity might have higher completion rates due to shared culture and language (14, 15). Workshops with larger proportions of participants successfully completing the intervention might also signify greater social cohesion and support (i.e., higher completion workshop). We also hypothesized that Asian-American participants in workshops with higher overall completion rates would have higher completion rates themselves (16). As such, we computed the percentages of Asian-Americans and successful completers in each workshop. To avoid endogeneity issue, we excluded the current participant from their workshop when calculating the workshop completion rate. In other words, the resulting workshop completion rate represents the average completion rate among the classmates of each participant. The proportions of Asian-American participants and average workshop completion rates were included in analyses as workshop-level covariates.

STATISTICAL ANALYSIS

To compare the characteristics of the participants who completed the CDSMP workshop to those who did not, we used χ^2-tests for categorical independent variables and two-sample t-test for continuous independent variables. Multilevel logistic regression models were used to investigate the association between successful workshop completion and individual-level, as well as workshop-level covariates. First, all individual-level independent variables were introduced into a multilevel logistic regression model (Model 1). Then, we generated another multilevel logistic regression model after including workshop-level variables (Model 2). The proportion of variance explained (PVE) at the workshop level by different levels of variables was calculated as: $\text{PVE} = (V_0 - V_1)/V_0 \times 100$, where V_0 is the second-level variance of the Null Model, and V_1 is the second-level variance of the adjusted model (17). Multilevel analyses were conducted using the "gllamm" command in Stata 11 (18).

RESULTS

Table 1 shows frequency distributions of independent variables among the total population, and then divided by workshop completion status; 79.5% of participants successfully completed CDSMP workshops ($n = 2{,}159$) and 20.5% did not ($n = 557$). As a whole, Asian-American participants were predominantly female (73.1%), living with others (97.5%), and living in metro areas (91.3%). The average age was 71.3 years old (±9.2), and the average number of chronic conditions was 2.0 (±1.5).

Chronic Disease Self-Management Program completion was not significantly different in terms of age, sex, neighborhoods median income, or living arrangement. Considering individual-level variables, participants living in non-metro areas had significantly higher completion rates than their urban counterparts ($P = 0.009$). The number of chronic conditions was higher among those who completed CDSMP workshops relative to those who did not ($P = 0.009$). All workshop-level variables significantly differentiated between those who completed CDSMP workshops and who did not. Those who attended AAA delivery sites were

Table 1 | Characteristics of middle-aged and older Asian-American Chronic Disease Self-Management Program participants by CDSMP completion ($N = 2,716$).

	Total ($N = 2,716$)	CDSMP non-completion ($N = 557$)	CDSMP completion ($N = 2,159$)	
	N (%)	*N* (%)	*N* (%)	*P*-value*
Female	1,985 (73.1)	397 (71.3)	1,588 (73.6)	0.280
Living alone	68 (2.5)	19 (3.4)	49 (2.3)	0.124
Rural–urban commuting area codes				0.009
Metro	2,479 (91.3)	524 (94.1)	1,955 (90.6)	
Non-metro	237 (8.7)	33 (5.9)	204 (9.5)	
Workshop delivery site				0.010
Other	341 (12.6)	77 (13.8)	264 (12.2)	
Area agency on aging/senior centers	741 (27.3)	123 (22.1)	618 (28.6)	
Health care organization	379 (14.0)	77 (13.8)	302 (14.0)	
Residential facilities	431 (15.9)	111 (19.9)	320 (14.8)	
Community/multi-purpose	720 (26.5)	148 (26.6)	572 (26.5)	
Faith-based organization	104 (3.8)	21 (3.8)	83 (3.8)	
	Mean (±SD)	**Mean (±SD)**	**Mean (±SD)**	***P*-value[a]**
Age in years (from 50 to 101)	71.3 (±9.2)	71.2 (±9.5)	71.4 (±9.2)	0.670
Neighborhood median income in $10,000 unit (from 2.2 to 11.6)	6.2 (±1.4)	6.2 (±1.5)	6.2 (±1.3)	0.466
Number of chronic conditions (from 0 to 10)	2.0 (±1.5)	1.9 (±1.4)	2.1 (±1.5)	0.009
% Of Asian-Americans in the workshop	57.5 (±36.8)	53.2 (±36.7)	58.6 (±36.7)	0.002
Workshop completion rate (%)	74.9 (±18.7)	66.4 (±18.7)	77.1 (±18.0)	<0.001

**P-value for χ^2-test comparing the participants who completed the CDSMP workshop and who did not. Other workshop delivery sites include educational institutions, recreational centers, tribal centers, and workplaces.*

[a]P-value for two-sample t-test comparing the participants who completed the CDSMP workshop and who did not.

more likely to complete CDSMP workshops, whereas those who attended residential facilities or other sites had lower completion rates ($P = 0.010$). In addition, CDSMP workshop completion was positively associated with the percentage of Asian-American participants ($P = 0.002$) and the workshop completion rate in each workshop ($P < 0.001$).

Table 2 shows results of the multilevel logistic regressions including the Null Model (i.e., intercept-only model), Model 1 (only including individual-level variables), and Model 2 (including both individual-level and workshop-level variables). In Model 1, a higher number of chronic conditions and living in non-metro areas increased the odds of completing CDSMP workshops (OR = 1.09, $P = 0.030$; OR = 1.84, $P = 0.025$, respectively). In Model 2, the odds of completing CDSMP workshops increased among participants with a higher number of chronic conditions (OR = 1.10, $P = 0.011$), living in non-metro areas (OR = 1.77, $P = 0.009$), and those who attended a workshop with a higher completion rate (OR = 1.03, $P < 0.001$). Those who attended workshops from AAA (OR = 1.56, $P = 0.018$) were more likely to complete CDSMP workshops compared to those who attended CDSMP workshops from other delivery sites (i.e., educational institution, recreational center, tribal center, and workplace). The second-level variance explained by the individual-level variables (in Model 1) was $(1.45–1.41)/1.45 \times 100 = 2.8\%$, indicating that the individual-level variables explained 2.8% of the variability found at the second-level compared with the Null Model. Meanwhile, the second-level variance explained by the workshop-level variables (in Model 2) was $(1.41–0.16)/1.41 \times 100 = 88.7\%$, indicating that the workshop-level variables explained 88.7% of the variability found at the second-level compared with the Model 1.

DISCUSSION

This retrospective analysis is unique in that it identifies correlates significantly related to CDSMP completion at individual- and workshop-levels among Asian-American participants. The study findings are especially relevant given that Asian-Americans are the fastest-growing population in the U.S. The current study reveals that Asian-American participants are similar to other CDSMP participants in this national dissemination in terms of being predominantly female, living with others, residing in metro areas, and having multiple chronic conditions (7, 11). Workshop completion was positively associated with number of chronic conditions, attending workshops from AAA, attending higher completion workshops, and rural residence. These factors independently or in combination contributed to the 80% CDSMP completion rate among Asian-American participants. Recent studies utilizing the same dataset reported that the average CDSMP completion rate was 75% ($n = 89,861$) (10, 11), which is slightly lower than that (i.e., 80%) of the Asian-American participants shown in the current study. They also found no significant difference in completion rates between Asian-American and White participants (10).

Table 2 | Individual and workshop characteristics associated with successful completion of Chronic Disease Self-Management Program (CDSMP) among middle-aged and older Asian-American participants ($N = 2,716$).

	Empty model	Model 1	Model 2
	Adjusted OR (95% CI)	Adjusted OR (95% CI)	Adjusted OR (95% CI)
Individual characteristics			
Age	–	1.00 (0.99–1.01)	1.00 (0.99–1.02)
Sex			
Male	–	Ref.	Ref.
Female	–	1.12 (0.88–1.43)	1.08 (0.86–1.35)
Number of chronic conditions	–	**1.09 (1.01–1.18)**	**1.10 (1.02–1.18)**
Neighborhood median income	–	1.06 (0.96–1.18)	1.04 (0.96–1.12)
Living arrangement			
Living with others	–	Ref.	Ref.
Living alone	–	0.69 (0.36–1.31)	0.71 (0.40–1.27)
Rural–urban commuting area codes			
Metro	–	Ref.	Ref.
Non-metro	–	**1.84 (1.08–3.15)**	**1.77 (1.15–2.71)**
Workshop characteristics			
Workshop delivery site			
Other	–	–	Ref.
Area agency on aging/senior centers	–	–	**1.56 (1.08–2.25)**
Health care organization	–	–	1.42 (0.94–2.15)
Residential facilities	–	–	1.12 (0.76–1.67)
Community/multi-purpose	–	–	1.35 (0.91–2.00)
Faith-based organization	–	–	1.21 (0.64–2.27)
% Of Asian-Americans in the workshop	–	–	1.00 (0.99–1.01)
Workshop completion rate (%)	–	–	**1.03 (1.02–1.03)**
Between-area variation (SE)	1.45 (0.30)	1.41 (0.30)	0.16 (0.14)

Other workshop delivery sites include educational institutions, recreational centers, tribal centers, and workplaces.
OR are printed in bold if $P < 0.05$.
OR, odds ratio; 95% CI, 95% confidence interval; Ref., referent.

However, there has been no further analysis of the factors that might influence completion rates among Asian-Americans.

The positive association between the participants' health status (i.e., represented by the number of chronic conditions) and their likelihood of completing the program is consistent with recent CDSMP evaluations (8). This result is relatively encouraging given that an earlier study found those with chronic conditions had lower attendance rates of behavioral interventions in the community (19). Mobility issues related to chronic conditions have been cited as probable barriers to intervention adherence (20, 21). There is little evidence to help us disentangle the positive association between severe health conditions and workshop completion. However, when study participants engage in highly participative workshops focusing on goal setting and problem solving skills needed by those coping with multiple chronic conditions, their motivations to attend these workshops may outweigh other factors, which would limit attendance, such as pain, depression, or mobility issues. As such, this research highlights the importance of recognizing the value of prevention across the disease continuum and especially targeting those with multiple chronic conditions for CDSMP.

Rural residence seems to be an important factor related to CDSMP completion among Asian-Americans. The current study reveals 8.7% of participants reported living in non-metro areas, which is two times greater than the 2010 Census estimates of rural-residing Asian-Americans (4.3%) (22). In the current study including both individual- and workshop-level variables, Asian-American participants who lived in non-metro areas were 77% more likely to complete CDSMP compared to those who lived in metro areas. There are multiple potential explanations for this finding. First, there could be more social integration in rural communities so that participants could be more likely to know leaders, organizers, and participants, leading to a natural support system for encouraging attendance. Similarly, it could be easier to "get the word out" to participants in rural communities once rural informants were reached. Alternatively, if fewer participants are enrolled in rural workshops, it might be easier for leaders to provide reminders about workshop sessions and communicate with participants outside of workshop time. In our additional analysis, average number of participants enrolled in rural workshops (i.e., 11.7) was significantly lower than that of urban workshops (i.e., 14.2) ($P < 0.001$). Second, the general lack of access to healthcare in rural areas (23, 24) might encourage participants in rural areas to take advantage of available behavioral interventions like CDSMP. More in-depth analysis is needed to reveal which aspects of the non-metro CDSMP facilitated more successful completion. Along this line, future studies should further investigate the extent to which rural residence affects completion of evidence-based programs among Asian and other smaller racial/ethnic groups.

When workshop-level variables were included in the analysis, one of the interesting results was the significant association between program completion and specific delivery site. Asian-American CDSMP participants were more likely to complete CDSMP when they attended workshops from AAA. In a sense, AAAs or senior centers are especially advantaged in delivering evidence-based programs to minority groups because AAAs have had a longer experience of providing educational services or congregate meals that have attracted diverse populations (25). This early advantage is strengthened by new mandates for AAAs to deliver evidence-based programs for diverse groups of seniors (25). Nevertheless, the association between delivery sites and CDSMP completion requires another look while considering participants' residence (metro vs. non-metro). In an additional analysis, we found that AAA (28.2%) and community/multi-purpose centers (28.8%) were the two most common delivery sites in metro areas, whereas other (i.e., educational institution, recreational center, tribal center, and workplace) (35.2%) and residential facilities (19.0%) were two most common delivery sites in non-metro areas. This may indicate that adding the workshop characteristics in Model 2 does not seem to confound the relationship between rural residence and workshop completion anymore when looking at the relatively small changes of odds ratios of rural residence covariate (from 1.84 in Model 1 to 1.77 in Model 2). Nevertheless, these results may require additional study to address unanswered questions: which delivery sites can reach out to diverse populations? What factors related to delivery sites might be associated with more successful completion of CDSMP (e.g., rural residence or specific delivery sites or both)?

As part of the workshop-level variables, Asian-American participants who attended workshops with higher completion rates were more likely to complete the program. There are very few studies explaining variation of completing interventions in terms of percentage of intervention completers among specific racial and ethnic groups. One of the plausible explanations would be related to efficient or engaging CDSMP leaders. These leaders may instruct workshops in a way that provides participants with more enjoyment or educational benefit from each session, thereby increasing participants' motivation to complete the program. Alternatively, when a large portion of participants in a workshop were diligently engaging in each session, other "less-interested" participants may have been effectively encouraged to complete the program through a form a positive peer pressure. These factors independently or together, coupled with an assumption that Asian people feel more comfortable in a group (i.e., collectivism rather than individualism) and tend to follow the group (26) might boost attendance and increase complete rates of CDSMP. While it was assumed that Asian-American participants in classes with higher proportions of Asian-Americans would be more likely to complete CDSMP, this *a priori* hypothesis was not supported. Moreover, the current study also found that utilizing the multilevel analysis (i.e., individual- and workshop-levels) is highly recommended since including workshop-level variables explained more than 88% of the second-level variance.

Despite the study's unique contribution to the literature, some limitations should be considered. First, these results were based on cross-sectional data, which limit our ability to determine a causal relationship between any of the variables and CDSMP completion. Second, the study participants are not nationally representative, which limits the generalizability of these study findings. Third, our data relied on program participants' self-reported measurements that may generate recall bias or social desirability bias. However, we were not able to find problematic patterns related to this concern. Third, and most importantly, it is over-simplistic to lump all Asian-Americans together in one category. Because of the multiplicity of nationalities and unique cultures in Asia, it is difficult to make generalizations or draw conclusions about such a broadly defined, diverse population. Additionally, we did not include measures, which would clarify participants' level of acculturation that likely influence the variables' effects on program participation or workshop completion. Unfortunately, the available data did not allow distinctions among different Asian-Americans; however, we recommend that sub-classifications of Asian-American participants be collected and analyzed in future studies. Nevertheless, the primary purpose of this study was to explore the characteristics of Asian-American CDSMP participants and contributing factors related to program completion, and as such offer initial insights that can be explored further.

CONCLUSION

The underlying value of our study is the potential to improve the implementation and dissemination of successful evidence-based programs among Asian-Americans. A major study conclusion is that completion rates among Asian-American CDSMP participants were high (approximately 80% of participants), but they could be improved with careful targeting of these populations based on health status, participant's residence, and workshop delivery sites. In this way, our findings can inform policy makers, program coordinators, and workers in the field who want to expand CDSMP utilization among Asian-Americans. The crucial next step will be focusing on improving implementation and dissemination of CDSMP among diverse segments of Asian-Americans. Such actions can help the growing population of Asian-Americans achieve improvements in health and health care outcomes.

ACKNOWLEDGMENTS

This work was supported by the Administration on Aging (90OP0001/03); and the National Institute of Child Health and Human Development (R01HD047143). The authors also thank Ms. Patti Smith, who helped to review this manuscript.

REFERENCES

1. Pew Research Center. *Pew Research Social & Demographic Trends: The Rise of Asian Americans* (2013). Available from: http://www.pewsocialtrends.org/2012/06/19/the-rise-of-asian-americans/
2. Census Bureau US. *Asians Fastest-Growing Race or Ethnic Group in 2012, Census Bureau Reports* (2013). Available from: http://www.census.gov/newsroom/releases/archives/population/cb13-112.html

3. Collins KS, Fund C. *Diverse Communities, Common Concerns: Assessing Health Care Quality for Minority Americans.* New York, NY: Commonwealth Fund (2002).
4. National Center for Health Statistics. *Older Americans 2012: Key Indicators of Well-being* (2012). Available from: http://www.agingstats.gov/Main_Site/Data/2012_Documents/Docs/EntireChartbook.pdf
5. Lorig K, Holman H, Sobel D, Laurent D. *Living a Healthy Life with Chronic Conditions: Self Management of Heart Disease, Arthritis, Diabetes, Asthma, Bronchitis, Emphysema and Others.* 3rd ed. Boulder, CO: Bull Publishing Company (2006).
6. Bandura A. Social cognitive theory of self-regulation. *Organ Behav Hum Decis Process* (1991) **50**(2):248–87. doi:10.1016/0749-5978(91)90022-L
7. Ory MG, Ahn S, Jiang L, Lorig K, Ritter P, Laurent DD, et al. National study of chronic disease self-management six-month outcome findings. *J Aging Health* (2013) **25**(7):1258–74. doi:10.1177/0898264313502531
8. Ory MG, Ahn S, Jiang L, Smith ML, Ritter PL, Whitelaw N, et al. Successes of a national study of the chronic disease self-management program: meeting the triple aim of health care reform. *Med Care* (2013) **51**(11):992–8. doi:10.1097/MLR.0b013e3182a95dd1
9. Ahn S, Basu R, Smith ML, Jiang L, Lorig K, Whitelaw N, et al. The impact of chronic disease self-management programs: healthcare savings through a community-based intervention. *BMC Public Health* (2013) **13**(1):1141. doi:10.1186/1471-2458-13-1141
10. Erdem E, Korda H. Self-management program participation by older adults with diabetes: chronic disease self-management program and diabetes self-management program. *Fam Community Health* (2014) **37**(2):134–46. doi:10.1097/FCH.0000000000000025
11. Ory MG, Smith ML, Patton K, Lorig K, Zenker W, Whitelaw N. Self-management at the tipping point: reaching 100,000 Americans with evidence-based programs. *J Am Geriatr Soc* (2013) **61**(5):821–3. doi:10.1111/jgs.12239
12. U.S. Department of Health and Human Services Administration on Aging. *ARRA – Communities Putting Prevention to Work: Chronic Disease Self-Management Program* (2012). Available from: http://www.cfda.gov/?s=program&mode=form&tab=step1&id=5469a61f2c5f25cf3984fc3b94051b5f
13. U.S. Department of Agriculture Economic Research Service. *ERS/USDA Briefing Room: Measuring Rurality: Rural-Urban Commuting Area Codes* (2014). Available from: http://www.ers.usda.gov/data-products/rural-urban-commuting-area-codes.aspx
14. Barrera M Jr, Castro FG, Strycker LA, Toobert DJ. Cultural adaptations of behavioral health interventions: a progress report. *J Consult Clin Psychol* (2013) **81**(2):196. doi:10.1037/a0027085
15. Cardemil EV. Cultural adaptations to empirically supported treatments: a research agenda. *Sci Rev Mental Health Pract* (2010) **7**(2):8–21.
16. Burke BL, Vassilev G, Kantchelov A, Zweben A. Motivational interviewing with couples. In: Miller WR, Rollnick S, editors. *Motivational Interviewing.* New York, NY: The Guilford Press (2002). p. 347–61.
17. Sanz-Barbero B, García LO, Hernández TB. The effect of distance on the use of emergency hospital services in a Spanish region with high population dispersion: a multilevel analysis. *Med Care* (2012) **50**(1):27–34. doi:10.1097/MLR.0b013e31822d5e03
18. StataCorp. *Stata Statistical Software: Release 11.* College Station, TX: StataCorp LP (2009).
19. Virgil KM. *Community-Based Exercise Program Attendance and Exercise Self-Efficacy in African American Women.* Indianapolis: Indiana University – Purdue University Indianapolis (2013).
20. Jerant AF, Friederichs-Fitzwater MM, Moore M. Patients' perceived barriers to active self-management of chronic conditions. *Patient Educ Couns* (2005) **57**(3):300–7. doi:10.1016/j.pec.2004.08.004
21. Jones F. Strategies to enhance chronic disease self-management: how can we apply this to stroke? *Disabil Rehabil* (2006) **28**(13–14):841–7. doi:10.1080/09638280500534952
22. Housing Assistance Council. *Rural Research Brief: Race & Ethnicity in Rural America* (2012). Available from: http://www.ruralhome.org/storage/research_notes/rrn-race-and-ethnicity-web.pdf
23. Rosenthal TC, Fox C. Access to health care for the rural elderly. *JAMA* (2000) **284**(16):2034–6. doi:10.1001/jama.284.16.2034
24. Chan L, Hart LG, Goodman DC. Geographic access to health care for rural Medicare beneficiaries. *J Rural Health* (2006) **22**(2):140–6. doi:10.1111/j.1748-0361.2006.00022.x
25. Smith LA, McCaslin R. Enhancing baccalaureate student learning in research and gerontology through partnership with an area agency on aging. *J Teach Soc Work* (2011) **31**(1):79–88. doi:10.1080/08841233.2010.539149
26. Power D, Schoenherr T, Samson D. The cultural characteristic of individualism/collectivism: a comparative study of implications for investment in operations between emerging Asian and industrialized Western countries. *J Operat Manage* (2010) **28**(3):206–22. doi:10.1016/j.jom.2009.11.002

11

Implementing a chronic disease self-management program into China: The Happy Life Club™

Colette Joy Browning[1,2]*, Hui Yang[2], Tuohong Zhang[3], Anna Chapman[2], Shuo Liu[4], Joanne Enticott[2] and Shane Andrew Thomas[2,5]

[1] Royal District Nursing Service Institute, St Kilda, VIC, Australia
[2] School of Primary Health Care, Monash University School of Primary Health Care, Monash University, Melbourne, VIC, Australia
[3] Research Center for Ageing and Health Services, Department of Global Health, Peking University, Beijing, China
[4] Department of Social Medicine and Management, School of Public Health, Peking University, Beijing, China
[5] The University of Adelaide, Adelaide, SA, Australia

Edited by:
Matthew Lee Smith, The University of Georgia, USA

Reviewed by:
Martin Dempster, Queen's University Belfast, UK
Emily Joy Nicklett, University of Michigan, USA

***Correspondence:**
Colette Joy Browning, School of Primary Health Care, Building 1 270 Ferntree Gully Road, Notting Hill, VIC 3168, Australia
e-mail: colette.browning@monash.edu

China is experiencing population aging, increased prevalence of chronic diseases, and reductions in the frequency of healthy lifestyle behaviors. In response to these significant transitions, China is implementing major reforms in health care services with a focus on strengthening primary health care. In this paper, we describe a 12-month diabetes management program, the Happy Life Club™ (HLC™), implemented in a primary health care setting in Beijing, that uses doctor and nurse health coaches trained in behavior change techniques and motivational interviewing (MI). This paper reports the results of this pilot study and discusses issues involved in the implementation of Chronic Diseases Self-Management Programs in China. The intervention group showed improvements in HbA1c levels at 6 months and both the control and intervention groups showed reductions in waist circumference over time. Systolic blood pressure improved over time in the intervention group. The intervention group showed improvement in quality of life across the intervention period and both groups showed decreases in psychological distress across the intervention. Doctor visits increased between baseline and 6 months, but there was no change in doctor visits between 6 and 12 months for both groups. The effects were modest, and further investigations are required to evaluate the long-term impact of health coach approaches in China.

Keywords: chronic disease self-management, motivational interviewing, diabetes, older people, China

INTRODUCTION

China is now following the trajectory of many Western countries in terms of population aging, increased prevalence of chronic diseases and reductions in the population frequency of healthy lifestyle behaviors. For example, over the period 1998–2008, the incidence of diabetes mellitus (DM) tripled in China and, from 1991 to 2006, physical activity levels decreased by 32% (1, 2). In response to these significant transitions, China is implementing major reforms in health care services for its 1.4 billion citizens. The primary health care reforms, first announced in 2009, aim to deliver basic chronic disease care through community health services with referral of complex cases to the tertiary hospital system (3, 4). Chronic illness management approaches in China are neither typically patient centered nor do they include a central role for the patient in the self-management of their condition (5). Furthermore, patients are often dissatisfied with the medical services they receive while doctors focus on providing medications to manage chronic diseases rather than the facilitation of behavior change to moderate or control these conditions (6, 7).

Our work in China has focused on designing diabetes management programs that can be delivered effectively and efficiently in primary health care settings. Over the last decade the number of cases of DM in China has increased to the extent that China now has the highest number of DM cases globally. Xu et al. (8) estimated that in 2010, the prevalence of DM was 11.6%, representing 113.9 million adults. The prevalence of DM increases with age in Chinese adults: in those aged 70 years and over it is estimated that 21.8% of women and 22% of men have diabetes (9). The Chinese government has recognized the need for new approaches to the management of DM including self-care education and the incorporation of healthy lifestyle interventions into routine care (10, 11). However, such approaches need a trained workforce of health professionals who understand and embrace patient-centered care and who possess the requisite skills in behavior change and counseling principles and practice. Such an approach, involving the training of doctors and nurses in patient-centered care and behavior change techniques, has been piloted and developed into a diabetes self-management program in Beijing, China: the Happy Life Club™ (HLC™). This program is based on a similar program developed in Australia (12).

The HLC™ program involves nurses and doctors in primary care settings, trained in motivational interviewing (MI) and behavior change techniques, delivering face-to-face and telephone coaching to patients with T2DM. MI is a way of communicating with patients that is collaborative in style and focused on how patients talk about change (13). In order to facilitate change, it is assumed that the patient needs to elicit their own ideas about change as they will then be more likely to act. MI is founded upon an attitude of acceptance and compassion. It aims to strengthen the patient's motivation to achieve a goal by resolving ambivalence. MI is linked to the stages of change approach whereby the coach assists the patient to work through stages of change, from no intention to change to a commitment to change and action (14). The MI approach has been shown to be effective in achieving glycemic control in adults with T2DM but to date the approach has not been tested widely in the Chinese context (15). Therefore, the purpose of this paper is to report findings from the pilot HLC™ study and discuss issues involved in implementing a CDSMP developed for Western primary care in a Chinese setting.

MATERIALS AND METHODS

SAMPLE AND PROGRAM SETTING

The data reported in this article are based on a 12-month pilot study of $n = 100$ patients of age 55 years and over with Type 2 Diabetes Mellitus (T2DM). The pilot study was conducted in Fangzhuang. The Fangzhuang community is located in the south of Beijing and has a resident population of 110,000; 21.4% of which are aged 60 years and above. The community has an established community health service system that includes a large Community Health Center (CHC) or community hospital which, administrated by the local government, functions as the main primary health care provider. The CHC includes five community health stations (CHSs), which aim to serve the health needs of the local communities. Participants were approached consecutively as they attended their usual diabetes appointment and asked if they wished to participate in the study. Recruitment continued until 100 patients had agreed to participate. The patients were randomly allocated to the intervention group or the control group (see below). Health professionals in the CHC and the CHSs are government employed doctors and nurses. The pilot study was subsequently expanded into a pragmatic cluster randomized controlled trial (16). The study was approved by the Monash University Human Research Ethics Committee.

THE INTERVENTION

The HLC program uses trained health coaches. In the pilot study, the control group received usual care provided by a family physician where patients are typically referred to diabetes specialists and/or Traditional Chinese Medicine (TCM) practitioners. The intervention group received telephone and face-to-face coaching in addition to usual care. The key components of the intervention were patient-centered care and the use of MI (13) to help effect change in diet, physical activity, and general chronic disease self-management behaviors. In the first 3 months, participants received two face-to-face and two telephone coaching sessions per month after which, as the participants gained confidence in self-management, the frequency diminished. Overall, the intervention group received a maximum of 19 telephone coaching and 18 face-to-face coaching sessions. The intervention ran for 12 months.

COACH TRAINING

The health coaches (experienced doctors and nurses) received a certified training program. Doctors and nurses were chosen to deliver the intervention as they are by far the main providers of health care in China. Other health professionals such as diabetes educators are virtually non-existent in the Chinese health system (17). The training program consists of a self-learning package and health coach skills workshops. The self-learning package included key concepts in patient-centered care, health psychology and behavior change approaches, the epidemiology of diabetes, and the role of MI in behavior change. The self-learning package was followed by a 2-day intensive MI workshop. This workshop covered the concepts and spirit of MI including: promoting a patient-centered approach and a collaborative coach style that focused on the stage of behavior change of targeted lifestyle behaviors relevant to chronic disease management; eliciting patient's intrinsic motivation to change; promoting client choice; building self-efficacy; and resolving patient ambivalence. The workshop included the application and practise of MI core skills: the use of open-ended questions; affirmation; reflection, and summarizing across the behavior change process. During the implementation of the HLC™, refresher workshops were conducted and, 1 month after the initial training, the coaches participated in a further half-day advanced training workshop.

MEASURES AND STATISTICAL PROCEDURES

Clinical, self-reported health, and well-being measures, and health service use were collected at baseline, 6 and 12 months. Clinical measures included HbA1c, blood pressure, waist circumference, and BMI. Quality of life was measured using the WHOQOL-BREF (18). Psychological well-being was measured using the Kessler Psychological Distress Scale (K10) (19). Participants were asked how often they had visited the doctor in the last 6 months. Differences between the control and intervention groups at baseline, 6, and 12 months were assessed using repeated measures ANOVA with the control and intervention groups as between-subjects factors. Effect sizes were calculated.

RESULTS

Table 1 shows the baseline characteristics of the participants ($n = 100$). At the 6-month follow-up, $n = 5$ participants were lost to follow-up: one participant died and four participants moved house and could not be contacted. There were no differences between the groups in terms of key demographic variables at baseline except that the control group participants were more highly educated. Sixty-seven percent of the total sample was women.

Table 1 | Baseline characteristics of participants.

Baseline characteristics	Control	Intervention	Total
Participants, *n*	50	50	100
Age in years, mean ± SD	63.3 ± 7.8	65.8 ± 7.5	64.2 ± 7.7
Female	33	34	67
Married (including *de facto*)	47	44	91
Retired	44	46	90
Education			
Primary or less	7	13	20
Secondary/high school	25	34	59
Tertiary/technical	18	3	21
Duration of diabetes in years, mean ± SD	8.2 ± 6.1	9.0 ± 6.3	8.6 ± 6.2

Table 2 | Mean scores and SD for clinical, self-reported health, and well-being measures and doctor visits at baseline, 6 and 12 months for the control and intervention groups ($n = 100$).

Measure	Baseline ($N = 100$)		6 months ($N = 95$)		12 months ($N = 95$)		Effect Size from group (partial eta squared)	Effect Size from time (partial eta squared)
	Control	Intervention	Control	Intervention	Control	Intervention		
HbA1c	7.00 ± 0.81	7.16 ± 1.11	6.96 ± 0.92	6.88 ± 1.10	7.16 ± 1.16	6.88 ± 0.88	0.036 (small effect)	0.029 (small effect)
Systolic blood pressure (mmHg)	128.2 ± 12.7	132.0 ± 15.4	128.6 ± 15.0	129.2 ± 12.1	129.1 ± 12.6	125.0 ± 12.4	0.054 (small effect)	0.026 (small effect)
Diastolic blood pressure (mmHg)	76.5 ± 6.9	77.6 ± 8.1	75.9 ± 6.7	76.6 ± 6.9	76.5 ± 7.8	76.2 ± 7.4	0.008	0.007
Waist circumference (cm)	91.82 ± 7.10	90.56 ± 9.19	89.86 ± 7.25	89.02 ± 8.89	89.13 ± 7.14	88.59 ± 9.26	0.004	0.088 (small-medium effect)
BMI (kg/m2)	25.37 ± 2.64	25.60 ± 3.40	25.47 ± 2.35	25.63 ± 3.27	25.44 ± 2.39	25.60 ± 3.41	0.001	0.001
WHOQOL-BREF	3.40 ± 0.85	3.34 ± 0.67	3.40 ± 0.74	3.44 ± 0.77	3.36 ± 0.49	3.83 ± 0.81	0.047 (small effect)	0.044 (small effect)
K10	19.0 ± 6.4	17.3 ± 6.3	16.9 ± 6.7	15.1 ± 6.2	15.9 ± 5.0	13.8 ± 3.7	0.001	0.159 (medium effect)
Number of community doctor visits	5.38 ± 3.33	5.17 ± 2.49	5.70 ± 4.21	6.88 ± 4.95	5.68 ± 3.87	6.98 ± 4.97	0.016	0.032 (small effect)

Partial eta squared values: small effects indicated by 0.02, medium effects by 0.13, and large by 0.26.

Table 2 shows a comparison between the control and intervention groups at baseline, 6, and 12 months on key clinical and health measures.

There was a significant interaction effect between HbA1c and group over the period baseline to 6 months ($F = 7.098$, $p = 0.009$). The intervention group showed significant improvement in HbA1c levels between baseline and 6 months. However, the effect size was small. Neither group showed changes in HbA1c over the period 6–12 months. There was a significant interaction effect between systolic blood pressure and group ($F = 5.194$, $p = 0.006$), indicating that the intervention group significantly improved over time compared to the control group. Again, the effect size was small. Diastolic blood pressure and BMI did not change across the intervention period for either group; however, waist circumference decreased for both groups over time ($F = 8.591$, $p < 0.001$). There was no significant difference between the groups in terms of decrease in waist circumference. The effect size was small to medium.

There was a significant interaction effect between quality of life and group ($F = 4.612$, $p = 0.011$). The intervention group showed improvement in quality of life across the intervention. The effect size was small. The control group showed no significant change in quality of life across the intervention period. Both groups showed a decrease in scores on the K10 between baseline and 6 months ($F = 11.306$, $p < 0.001$) and between 6 and 12 months ($F = 4.577$, $p = 0.035$), but there were no significant differences between the groups. The effect size for changes over time was medium. In terms of visits to the community doctor in the last 6 months, both groups showed a significant increase in doctor visits between baseline and 6 months ($F = 4.844$, $p = 0.030$), but no change between 6 and 12 months. The effect size for changes over time was small.

DISCUSSION

The pilot study demonstrated that a CDSMP using Western concepts of behavior change and MI has an effect on the management T2DM particularly in terms of the key physiological parameters of HbA1c levels and systolic blood pressure. However, the effect sizes were small. By 6 months, the intervention group had achieved the goal of an HbA1c <7% and this may have contributed to no further significant reductions in HbA1c at 12 months. The intervention group also showed improvements in quality of life across the intervention and both groups showed reductions in psychological distress.

Both groups showed improvements in some of the clinical and health indicators. This may be due to participation effects, with no differential effect due to the intervention. In China, people with T2DM do not regularly monitor their condition, including HbA1c levels, due to cost. The control group received feedback about their HbA1c levels and this may have motivated them to implement self-management approaches (Hawthorne effect). The study was conducted in a residential area where there was the potential for contamination between the groups. The participants lived in the same building or residential area and potentially had close interaction when shopping or participating in community activities. Participants in the intervention group may have discussed their coaching with other residents. While the coaches were asked not to use MI with their other patients, it is difficult to control this. Coaches may have used the techniques with patients outside the intervention group.

While one of the aims of a CDSMP is to reduce hospital-based specialists' visits in order to reduce health care costs, in our pilot community, doctor (general practitioner) visits increased. We concluded that this increase was largely due to an improvement in doctor–patient relationships. In China, dissatisfaction with the services provided by hospital-based doctors is very high (20). The HLC pilot may have increased the participant's confidence in gaining a higher quality of care from their community doctors thus increasing primary health service use.

There are few trials of behavioral and psychological approaches to the management of T2DM in China. One recent but small 12-week intervention ($n = 40$) that used cognitive behavior therapy (CBT), found that the CBT group showed reductions in fasting glucose, HbA1c, and depression compared to the usual care group (21). A systematic review of lifestyle interventions aimed at preventing T2DM in developing countries (22) identified only one Chinese study (23). There is a pressing need to rigorously evaluate the different behavioral and psychological approaches to the management of T2DM in China, particularly when interventions that have only been proven effective in Western settings are used.

We have attempted to address the issues raised by this pilot study in the full pragmatic cluster randomized controlled trial (11) where there is more geographical separation between the groups. The full trial is also sufficiently powered to detect differences between the groups. The pilot study was conducted in a relatively high SES urban area in Beijing. Its applicability in rural and low SES areas is unknown and requires further testing. In the full trial, which includes sampling across SES groups, the influence of SES will be examined.

CDSM approaches require a health workforce that is highly trained in communication skills, patient-centered approaches, and behavior change frameworks and skills. Traditionally, there has been little focus on these skills in health care practitioner training in China (24). Behavior change and psychological approaches to the prevention and management of chronic illnesses are limited in China as there are only 2.4 professionals with psychology training per 1 million of the population (25) compared to 3500 nurses and physicians per 1 million of the population (17). Consequently, psychological and behavioral approaches to health and illness have not been widely endorsed either by medical practitioners, policy makers, or the general population. We were therefore interested in whether a Western model of CDSM would successfully translate into a Chinese setting. It would seem that health literacy concerning chronic illnesses in China is improving, especially among women and those with higher SES ("a long illness turns a patient into a doctor") (26). In addition, the holistic mind–body approach embodied in TCM, where it is assumed that health is governed by emotion and thoughts, is actually consistent with CDSM approaches (27). Despite the modest effects found in this pilot study, we were pleasantly surprised by how well our CDSMP was adopted by both the coaches and the patients. We could not put it better than one of our coaches:

> MI is a powerful tool. Since using it, both me and the patient have opened our mouths, and have more conversations... We work together and start talking about what small steps to take, and what is the easiest way to go... Patients then have their ideas of targets and a plan. I encourage them constantly... It does not work immediately, but several months later, I find they really get success... if one can maintain a new behavior for 3–6 months, the behavior seems to be a stable life habit.

The patients showed similar positive views about their experiences of the intervention:

> Before this project, I was quite negative about my disease and for everything I just relied on my doctors. But now, I can manage the disease by myself. If my blood sugar level is high I will try to find the reason by myself first ... because I am the person who knows me better. I do not feel the disease is a huge burden to me anymore and that is really good. (Female, 61 years old, duration of T2DM 8 years)

Our qualitative results support the view that patients appear to have benefited from the approach in terms of changing health behaviors and gaining confidence in managing their T2DM. Patients in the intervention group were also able to reach the HbA1c goal of 7% and improve systolic blood pressure. However, we need stronger evidence to conclude that our approach will lead to long-term changes in T2DM management.

REFERENCES

1. Yang G, Kong L, Zhao W, Wan X, Zhai Y, Chen LC, et al. Emergence of chronic non-communicable diseases in China. *Lancet* (2008) **372**(9650):1697–705. doi:10.1016/S0140-6736(08)61366-5
2. Ng SW, Norton EC, Popkin BM. Why have physical activity levels declined among Chinese adults? Findings from the 1991-2006 China health and nutrition surveys. *Soc Sci Med* (2009) **68**(7):1305–14. doi:10.1016/j.socscimed.2009.01.035
3. Editorial. China must not neglect reform of primary care. *Lancet* (2005) **365**(9468):1362. doi:10.1016/S0140-6736(05)66346-5
4. Liu Q, Wang B, Kong Y, Cheng KK. China's primary health-care reform. *Lancet* (2011) **377**:2064–6. doi:10.1016/S0140-6736(11)60167-0
5. Yang H, Thomas SA, Browning CJ. Chronic disease management in community health. In: Li ZX, Zhang Y, Yang H, editors. *Community Health Services Management*. Beijing: People's Military Medicine Publisher (2010). p. 65–97.
6. Bhattacharyya O, Dulu Y, Wong S. Evolution of primary care in China 1997-2009. *Health Policy* (2011) **100**(2011):174–80. doi:10.1016/j.healthpol.2010.11.005
7. Browne D. The long march to primary health care in China: from collectivism to market economics. *Public Health* (2001) **115**:2–3. doi:10.1038/sj.ph.1900742
8. Xu Y, Wang L, Bi Y, Li M, Wang T, Wang L, et al. Prevalence and control of diabetes in Chinese adults. *JAMA* (2013) **310**(9):948–59. doi:10.1001/jama.2013.168118
9. Yang W, Lu J, Weng J. Prevalence of diabetes among men and women in China. *N Engl J Med* (2014) **362**:1090–101. doi:10.1056/NEJMoa0908292
10. International Diabetes Federation. *New Diabetes Figures in China: IDF Press Statement*. IDF (2010). Available from: http://www.idf.org/press-releases/idf-press-statement-china-study
11. Pan XR, Yang WY, Li GW, Liu J. Prevalence of diabetes and its risk factors in China, 1994, national diabetes prevention and control cooperative group. *Diabetes Care* (1997) **20**(11):1664–9. doi:10.2337/diacare.20.11.1664

12. Kelly J, Menzies D, Taylor S. The good life club: methodology and study design – a discussion. *Aust J Prim Health* (2003) **9**(2&3):186–91. doi:10.1071/PY03045
13. Miller WR, Rollnick S. *Motivational interviewing: Helping people change.* New York: Guilford Press (2013).
14. Prochaska JO, Velicer WF. The transtheoretical model of health behavior change. *Am J Health Promot* (1997) **12**(1):38–48. doi:10.4278/0890-1171-12.1.38
15. Ismail K, Winkley K, Rabe-Hesketh S. Systematic review and meta-analysis of randomised controlled trials of psychological interventions to improve glycaemic control in patients with type 2 diabetes. *Lancet* (2004) **363**(9421):1589–97. doi:10.1016/S0140-6736(04)16202-8
16. Browning CJ, Chapman A, Cowlishaw S, Li Z, Thomas SA, Yang H, et al. The happy life club™ study protocol: a cluster randomised controlled trial of a type 2 diabetes health coach intervention. *BMC Public Health* (2011) **11**:90. doi:10.1186/1471-2458-11-90
17. Hou J, Michaud C, Li Z, Dong Z, Sun B, Zhang J, et al. Transformation of the education of health professionals in China: progress and challenges. *Lancet* (2014) **384**(9945):819–27. doi:10.1016/S0140-6736(14)61307-6
18. World Health Organization. *WHO Quality of Life-BREF (WHOQOL-BREF).* (1991). Available from: http://www.who.int/substance_abuse/research_tools/whoqolbref/en/
19. Kessler RC, Anderws G, Colpe LJ, Hiripi E, Mroczek DK, Normand SLT, et al. Short screening scales to monitor population prevalence and trends in non-specific psychological distress. *Psychol Med* (2002) **32**:959–76. doi:10.1017/S0033291702006074
20. Thomas SA, Yang H, Browning C, Zhang T, Xiaofei L, Ren Y, et al. Quality of care in different community health facilities in China: from the patient's point of view. *J Chin Gen Pract* (2007) **10**(27):1760–4. doi:10.3969/j.issn.1007-9572.2007.21.002
21. Sun H, Zhang Q. Effects of psychological interventions on depression and glucose metabolism of low-income people with type 2 diabetes. *Chin Clin Pract Med* (2009) **3**(11):96–7. doi:10.3760/cma.j.issn1673-8799.2009.11.62
22. Rawal LB, Tapp RJ, Williams ED, Chan C, Yasin S, Oldenburg B. Prevention of type 2 diabetes and its complications in developing countries: a review. *Int J Behav Med* (2012) **19**:121–33. doi:10.1007/s12529-011-9162-9
23. Li G, Zhang P, Wang J, Gregg EW, Yang W, Gong Q, et al. The long-term effect of lifestyle interventions to prevent diabetes in the China Da Qing diabetes prevention study: a 20-year follow-up study. *Lancet* (2008) **371**:1783–9. doi:10.1016/S0140-6736(08)60766-7
24. Qian M, Juhua M. Problems and solutions to the teaching of a doctor-patient communication course. *Res Med Educ* (2012) **9**(8):1047–9. doi:10.3760/cma.j.issn.2095-1475.2010.08.012
25. Han B, Kan Z. Psychology in China. *Psychologist* (2007) **20**:734–6. Available from: http://www.thepsychologist.org.uk/archive/archive_home.cfm/volumeID_20-editionID_154-ArticleID_1280-getfile_getPDF/thepsychologist/1207chin.pdf
26. Song Y, Ma W, Yi X, Wang S, Sun X, Tian J, et al. Chronic diseases knowledge and related factors among the elderly in Jinan, China. *PLoS One* (2013) **8**(6):e68599. doi:10.1371/journal.pone.0068599
27. Tan C, Chen W, Wu Y, Chen S. Chinese medicine for mental disorder and its applications in psychosomatic diseases. *Altern Ther Health Med* (2013) **19**(1):59–69. Available from: http://todayspractitioner.com/wp-content/uploads/2013/11/Chinese-Medicine-for-Mental-Disorder-and-its-Applications-in-Psychosomatic-Diseases-191_ATM_p59_69tan.pdf

12

Cost-effectiveness of the chronic disease self-management program: Implications for community-based organizations

Rashmita Basu[1]*, Marcia G. Ory[2], Samuel D. Towne Jr.[2], Matthew Lee Smith[3], Angela K. Hochhalter[1] and SangNam Ahn[4]

[1] *Baylor Scott & White Health, Temple, TX, USA*
[2] *Department of Health Promotion and Community Health Sciences, School of Public Health, Texas A&M Health Science Center, College Station, TX, USA*
[3] *Department of Health Promotion and Behavior, College of Public Health, The University of Georgia, Athens, GA, USA*
[4] *Division of Health Systems Management and Policy, School of Public Health, The University of Memphis, Memphis, TN, USA*

Edited by:
Sue Ellen Levkoff, University of South Carolina, USA

Reviewed by:
Sharyl Kidd Kinney, University of Oklahoma College of Public Health, USA
Sue Ellen Levkoff, University of South Carolina, USA

****Correspondence:***
Rashmita Basu, Baylor Scott & White Health, 2401 South 31st Street, Temple, TX 76508, USA
e-mail: rbasu@sw.org

Chronic conditions are the leading cause of growing healthcare spending, disability, and death in the U.S. In the wake of national health reform, policy makers and healthcare professionals are becoming increasingly concerned in containing healthcare costs while improving quality of patient care. A basic policy question is whether the Chronic Disease Self-Management Program (CDSMP), a widely distributed evidenced-based self-managed program, can be cost-effective in managing chronic conditions while improving quality of life. Utilizing data from the *National Study of CDSMP*, the primary objective of the current study is to estimate cost-effectiveness of the CDSMP program among individuals with at least one chronic condition. The second objective is to determine how cost-effectiveness ratios vary by depression status. EuroQol-5D (EQ-5D) was used to measure health-related quality of life (HRQOL) of CDSMP participants, which was then converted to quality-adjusted life years (QALYs) for cost-effectiveness analysis. Participants who completed the CDSMP program experienced higher EQ-5D scores from baseline to 12-month follow-up (increased from 0.736 to 0.755; $p < 0.001$). The incremental cost-effectiveness ratio (ICER) ranges from $83,285 to $31,285 per QALYs, which can be comparable to the common benchmark of $50,000/QALYs. ICER by baseline depression status indicates that it will cost more per QALYs gained for those diagnosed with depression based on their Patient Health Questionnaire-8 score. However, cautions should be taken while considering this point estimate too literally because the average cost for CDSMP participants was a rough estimate and based on several simplifying assumptions. Identifying cost-effective strategies that can lower the burden of chronic disease among community-dwelling adults is critical for decision makers in allocating limited resources. Policy makers and community organizations can use this information to guide funding decisions and delivery of CDSMP programs for individuals with multiple chronic health conditions.

Keywords: chronic disease self-management, cost-effectiveness analysis, health-related quality of life, older adults, EQ-5D and quality-adjusted life years

INTRODUCTION

With the rapid aging of the baby boomer cohort, it is estimated that one in five Americans will be 65 years or older by 2030 (1). Simultaneously, the existence of multiple chronic conditions among Americans 65 years or older is becoming increasingly prevalent, with 60–75% of older adults having at least two chronic conditions (2), many of which are preventable (1). Moreover, the number of Americans with chronic conditions is projected to increase by 37% by the year 2030 (3). More than 75% of total healthcare costs are attributable to the treatment of chronic illnesses (3). Furthermore, chronic conditions among older adults are associated with lower quality of life and increased limitations in activities of daily living (4–7).

With a mission to promote health and the quality of life in Americans, the U.S. Department of Health and Human Services' Center for Disease Control and Prevention (CDC) has supported population surveillance of health-related quality of life (HRQOL) (8). HRQOL is a multi-dimensional measure, which is defined as "perceived physical and mental health over time" (9). It can be considered as a part of a person's overall quality of life that is determined by his or her health status. Because HRQOL addresses physical and mental health of a large number of individuals, it can offer current health data that public health agencies need to assess population health. In light of the growing prevalence of chronic illness, healthcare burdens, and concerns for promoting population health, service providers and policy makers are pursuing cost-effective ways to design self-management programs that can improve the health and well-being of the population (10, 11). As healthcare costs continue to rise for treating chronic diseases, identifying ways to manage the progression of multiple chronic conditions among older adults is critical and time-sensitive (12, 13).

To promote health and the quality of life of community-dwelling older adults, federal, state, and local stakeholders are implementing evidence-based initiatives to engage individuals in managing chronic health conditions while improving health outcomes (14, 15). One such approach is the implementation of self-management programs that improve health and quality of life while simultaneously reducing costly healthcare utilization (16–20). These self-management programs have the potential to embrace the triple aim goals of healthcare (better care, improved patient care experience, and lower cost of care) that will enhance population health (21).

The Chronic Disease Self-Management Program (CDSMP), one of the well-studied evidence-based programs, improves health status and chronic illness symptoms while showing promise for lowering healthcare spending through the reduction in hospitalization (22, 23). Although evidence suggests that CDSMP can improve health outcomes among patients with chronic diseases (24–26), little is known about the *cost-effectiveness* of improving HRQOL among CDSMP participants. Moreover, program effectiveness may vary when chronic diseases are accompanied by depression because individuals with depression are less likely to complete the self-management education programs than those without depression (27). Thus, the current study has two goals: (1) to perform an economic evaluation of the CDSMP by utilizing a cost-effectiveness analysis of HRQOL among CDSMP participants from baseline to 6-month and 12-month follow-up; and (2) to examine how the intervention effectiveness varies for participants with or without depression at baseline.

MATERIALS AND METHODS

NATIONAL STUDY OF CDSMP AS STUDY BASIS

The current study utilized a change in HRQOL measures at three time points (baseline, at 6-month, and at 12-month) to examine the cost-effectiveness of the intervention among middle-aged and older adults enrolled in the *National Study of the Chronic Disease Self-Management Program (CDSMP)*. Data were analyzed from workshops delivered nationwide by 22 licensed sites in 17 states across the nation from August 2010 to April 2011. CDSMP workshops were supported by various federal, state and local sources, healthcare organizations, and community agencies. The eligibility criteria and recruitment, intervention delivery, and referral activities are described elsewhere (22). Sites already licensed to deliver CDSMP were selected and then agreed to participate in the *National Study*, delivering the manualized workshops following standardized intervention protocols and submitting data for study purposes. Data were collected in person before the start of the intervention (baseline) and at 6 and 12 months post-intervention by mail/phone. Investigators had no role in leader training, workshop recruitment, or program implementation. Each CDSMP delivery site recruited people for workshops in their usual fashion, which included referrals from organizations serving older adults (e.g., senior centers, healthcare facilities, and social service organizations as well as self-referrals from other recruitment activities including flyers, brochures, and health fairs). The intervention was designed to focus on content areas including (a) techniques to manage typical responses to chronic health problems such as frustration, fatigue, pain, and isolation: (b) improving healthy behavior such as physical exercise for maintaining and improving strength, flexibility, and endurance; and (c) appropriate use of medications, effective communication with healthcare professionals (24, 28). For the purpose of this study, participants with complete information on indicators of HRQOL at baseline, 6-month, and 12-month follow-up were included.

Study sample

As a part of translating this intervention, CDSMP included 1,170 community-dwelling individuals at baseline, 6 months, and 12 months across the nation. A total of 825 (71%) participants completed 12-month follow-up assessment including HRQOL measures and approximately 77% ($n = 903$) participants completed 6-month follow-up (29). While attrition was minimal for a community-based translational research study, HRQOL information at the 6-month follow-up data was missing for 77 participants ($N = 748$ contributed to the final analyses). Few differences were observed based on data attrition. Participants who completed follow-up assessments at 6-month and 12-month tended to be older, and completers of the 6-month assessment were more likely to be non-Hispanic White (15). Institutional Review Board approval for the *National Study* was obtained at Stanford University and Texas A&M University.

MEASURES

Health-related quality of life measures

In the current study, we focus on the healthy-days measure of HRQOL because it captures the key concepts of population health and well-being. This construct is aligned with one of CDSMP's main objectives of empowering program participants to better manage their chronic conditions and experience a higher quality of life. Healthy-days measures are important components that assess HRQOL. The HRQOL includes a set of four questions (8):

1. Would you say that in general your health is; Excellent, Very good, Good, Fair, or Poor?
2. Now thinking about your physical health, which includes physical illness and injury, for how many days during the past 30 days was your physical health not good?
3. Now thinking about your mental health, which includes stress, depression, and problems with emotions, for how many days during the past 30 days was your mental health not good?
4. During the past 30 days, for about how many days did poor physical or mental health keep you from doing your usual activities, such as self-care, work, or recreation?

In the current study, we utilize an "unhealthy days" summary measure, which is based on the second and third questions, estimates the overall number of days when physical and mental health was not good. We then calculate the number of days estimated to be healthy, which is the complement to unhealthy days measure (total number of "healthy days" limits to maximum of 30 days as this is the maximum possible value that this measure could possibly take). These items have been extensively used for evaluating program objectives in other studies (8, 30–33) and the validity of these measures has been confirmed in population based samples. Participants responded to each item with the number of days ranging from 0 to 30.

Cost measures

The average cost per CDSMP participant varies by the number of enrolled participants per workshop with the estimated per-participant cost ranging from \$219 to \$583 (23). In the *National Study of CDSMP,* 145 workshops had an average size of 12.7 (±4.18) participants, with the majority of workshops (66.2%) having between 8 and 16 participants. A detailed description of the cost measures reported by CDSMP delivery sites appears elsewhere (23). Based on extant literature confirmed by experts in the delivery field, we estimated program costs at \$350 per participant, assuming an average of 10 participants in each CDSMP workshop (23). These program costs typically include licensure costs, trained peer personnel, materials, and any space rental costs (34). Because the CDSMP was a community-based program and goal that this type of self-management program is to provide evidence regarding resources needed to deliver within the community, cost data are collected at the aggregate level. In the case of CDSMP, per-participant costs were aggregated at the workshop level. Individual-level cost data are less valuable for the effective implementation of this type of community-based program.

Other participant-level measures

Participants' demographic characteristics measured at baseline included age, gender, race/ethnicity, and number of chronic conditions. Measures and a sample questionnaire can be found in English and Spanish (35). Depressive symptoms were measured using the Patient Health Questionnaire (PHQ) (36). Self-rated items (9 DSM-IV criteria) scored from 0 (not at all) to 3 (nearly everyday) were added to determine overall PHQ score of study participants at baseline. A score greater than or equal to 10 was considered clinically depressed because this cut-off point of 10 has a sensitivity and specificity of 88% in detecting a diagnosis of major depression in primary care patients (36). The reliability of the PHQ-9 is high, with a Cronbach's α of 0.89 and test–retest reliability of 0.84 (37). We used an eight-item version of the PHQ (38), which excludes the item that asks patients if they have been bothered by "thoughts that you would be better off dead or of hurting yourself in some way." Scores for the eight-item version of the PHQ range from 0 to 24, and are highly correlated with scores on the nine-item version ($r = 0.997$) (38).

ANALYSIS

HRQOL, EQ-5D, and QALYs

The CDC-derived measure of HRQOL is one of the most commonly used outcome measures for evaluating burden of disease in public health research. However, a single measurement such as quality-adjusted life year (QALY) is considered as a more useful measure for cost-effectiveness analyses (38–40). This is because QALY uses preference-based measures of HRQOL, which uses summary scores (i.e., utility values) to represent population preferences for different health states. Because the number of unhealthy days are not preference-based measures of HRQOL (as asked in the CDSMP survey), the CDC "healthy days" measures cannot be used directly in the cost-effectiveness analyses (41). Since the CDSMP survey did not include preference-based measure of EQ-5D, the non-preference-based scores of "healthy days" measure was converted to preference-based EuroQol 5D (EQ-5D) utilizing the method proposed by Jia and Lubetkin (42). The EQ-5D is an internationally developed preference-based (29, 43) method that provides a measure of utility scores to calculate QALYs which is used in cost-effectiveness analyses (44). EQ-5D estimates are obtained from healthy days by matching the cumulative distributions of the two HRQOL measures and EQ-5D from Behavioral Risk Factor Surveillance System and Medical Expenditure Panel Survey datasets (42). For example, we obtained EQ-5D utility score corresponding to number of "healthy days" measures in our sample. Detail description of the estimation method including underlying assumptions can be found in Jia and Lubetkin (42). Utility values range from 1 (best possible health state) through 0 (death) (44). We then used EQ-5D scores to calculate QALY for the calculation of cost-effectiveness ratios.

Estimation of participant specific QALYs was based on partitioning the study period into the number of follow-up assessments and weighting each time interval by the individual's utility score during that period of time (45). It is assumed that changes in utility values are linear over time, which is the most commonly used method in cost-effectiveness analysis. Individual-level QALYs are then estimated by applying the area-under the curve approach. Details of this method can be found elsewhere (42). The general expression for calculating QALYs using individual data that are fully observed (i.e., no censoring) can be written as follows (45):

$$\text{QALY} = \sum_{t=0}^{n} \left[\frac{(Q_t + Q_{t+1})}{2} \times \frac{(T_{t+1} + T_t)}{T} \right] \quad (1)$$

where, n is the number of utility measurements over the study period (i.e., 1 year), Q_t is the individual utility score (i.e., EQ-5D score) obtained in the tth measurement, T is the total duration of study period expressed in terms of total number of time units in a year (e.g., months), T_t is the time period in which the tth measurement takes place (expressed as number of time units in a year). In our case, $n = 2$ (i.e., first interval from baseline to 6-month and second interval from 6-month to 12-month), $T = 12$ (i.e., number of months in a year), and three time points as $T_0 = 0$, $T_1 = 6$, and $T_2 = 12$. For example, in our current study, QALYs are obtained by substituting mean EQ-5D scores and controlling for baseline utility (45):

$$\text{Incremental QALY} = \sum_{t=0}^{n} \left[\frac{(0.743 - 0.736)}{2} \times \frac{6}{12} + \frac{(0.743 - 0.736)}{2} \times \frac{6}{12} + \frac{(0.755 - 0.743)}{2} \times \frac{6}{12} \right] = 0.007 \quad (2)$$

Cost-effectiveness analysis

The strong need to control healthcare costs for the treatment of chronic diseases led us to search for interventions that produce greatest value, based on comparative economic evaluation (46). Cost-effectiveness analysis (CEA) is a type of economic evaluation method that can be utilized to assess whether money is well spent in a particular health promotion program (47). Funding agencies may continue to support programs on the basis of this information or may find additional interventions that can produce the best outcomes with available resources. The most widely used method for CEA is the incremental cost-effectiveness ratio (ICER), which compares differences in cost to differences in effectiveness between two competing interventions and therefore relevant for policy making decisions. In the absence of a control group, we are comparing health gains compared to no intervention (i.e., "doing nothing"). Therefore, in this case, ICER was calculated compared to baseline and measures the effectiveness of CDSMP in improving QALYs compared to "doing nothing."

An important first step of calculating ICER is to quantify its average cost of a program in order to relate the cost to specific measures of the program (48). Considering zero cost for "no intervention," the numerator of ICER is the average cost and denominator includes the mean effectiveness of the program (48, 49). In our case, the numerator is the mean program cost spent per CDSMP participant and denominator is QALYs estimates. The QALYs is particularly useful in quantifying program effectiveness and is the most commonly used measure of treatment effectiveness in CEA literature (50, 51). The ICER for each outcome measure was calculated by dividing per person CDSMP workshop costs by the QALYs. Therefore ICER can be indicated as:

$$\text{ICER}=\frac{\text{Average cost spent per CDSMP participant} - \$0}{\text{QALYs gained adjusted for baseline utility score}} \quad (3)$$

RESULTS

Table 1 describes participants' characteristics at baseline. In total, 1,170 participants completed the baseline assessment. On average, participants were 65 years old, nearly 83% were female, and had an average of 13 years of education. Ethno-racial composition included 55% non-Hispanic white, 16% African American, 22% Hispanic, and 6.5% others. About 79% reported two or more conditions and 79.1% of participants attended four or more workshop sessions.

Table 1 | Sample characteristics at baseline ($N = 1170$).

Variables	% Mean (SD)
Age (in years)	65.4 (14.3)
Female	82.7
Race/ethnicity	–
Non-Hispanic White	55.2
African American	16.0
Hispanic	22.3
Other	6.5
Workshop completion rate	79.1
Education (1–23)	12.9 (3.8)
At least two chronic conditions	79.0
PHQ-8 depression (0–24)	6.6 (5.5)
Healthy days (0–30)	17.9 (11.5)
EQ-5D (0–1)[a]	0.736 (0.156)

[a] *In our sample, EQ-5D value ranges from 0.411 to 0.995.*

Table 2 represents summary statistics for healthy days and corresponding EQ-5D measures at baseline, 6-month, and 12-month during the study. Both healthy days (17.9–19.2) and corresponding EQ-5D scores (0.743–0.755) were significantly improved from baseline to 12-month) period (with a p-value <0.001); however, no significant improvement was observed for these measures from baseline to 6-month.

Table 3 presents the similar statistics by baseline depression status. Changes in mean healthy days and EQ-5D scores were examined by utilizing paired t-test by baseline depression status. On average, participants with depression at baseline reported lower number of healthy days and their corresponding EQ-5D scores were also lower than participants who had no depression at baseline. However, both groups (depression versus no depression at baseline) showed significant improvement in healthy days and EQ-5D scores from baseline to the12-month period. These results indicate that CDSMP improves population health status among individuals with multiple chronic conditions through better disease self-management strategies.

Table 4 shows the cost-effectiveness results for the CDSMP intervention. Incremental cost-effectiveness ratios (ICER) are calculated for the overall group as well as by baseline depression status. These ratios explain how much each additional QALYs gained with CDSMP will cost. Overall, ICER ranges from $83,285 to $31,285 per QALYs gained for participants in the CDSMP program with the median of $50,000/QALYs. ICER by baseline depression status indicates that it will cost more per QALYs gained for those diagnosed with depression based on PHQ-8 score.

DISCUSSION

Prior evidence suggests that CDSMP can significantly improve health outcomes for individuals with a variety of chronic conditions (21, 24). However, economic efficacy of the CDSMP on HRQOL is not well known. The current study developed a preference-based EQ-5D measure of HRQOL from healthy days to quantify the cost-effectiveness of a CDSMP program for improving QALYS gained for individuals with multiple chronic conditions. Although there is no universally acceptable threshold value for cost-effectiveness ratio (52), costs range from $50,000 to $75000 per QALYs gained have been considered as an acceptable value for resources expended (48).

Health-related quality of life is recognized as an important measure in public health as well as clinical research because it includes a population-based approach that addresses physical and mental health of a large number of individuals over time. Moreover, converting non-preference-based measures of HRQOL to a preference-based measure provides a way to compare the efficacy of CDSMP to other evidenced-based disease management programs in the literature. As shown in the current study, the economic value of CDSMP, as measured in dollars per QALYs gained, may have far reaching effects when magnified across the U.S. Thus, finding ways to improve the reach of the CDSMP among especially vulnerable individuals (e.g., rural, minority, low income) is a critical path of research for future studies.

Policy makers are interested in finding ways to improve the health of individuals with multiple chronic conditions as a significant share of healthcare dollars are attributed to the

Table 2 | Changes in mean (SD) of healthy days and EQ-5D scores among CDSMP participants during the study period.

HRQOL measures	Baseline	6 months	12 months	*p*-value for the change	
				Baseline and 6 months	Baseline and 12 months
Healthy days (0–30)	17.9 (11.5)	18.5 (11.4)	19.2 (11.1.)	0.25	<0.001
EQ-5D (0–1)	0.736 (0.156)	0.743 (0.156)	0.755 (0.152)	0.32	<0.001

Table 3 | Changes in mean (SD) of healthy days and EQ-5D scores by depression status at baseline.

HRQOL measures	Depression at baseline (PHQ-8 ≥10)						Difference in scores: baseline and 6-months		Difference in scores: baseline and 12-months	
	Yes			No			Yes	No	Yes	No
	Baseline	6-months	12-months	Baseline	6-months	12-months				
Healthy days	16.4 (11.5)	17.3 (11.4)	17.9 (11.2)	24.1 (8.8)	24.9 (8.8)	27.2 (6.9)	0.33	0.52	0.01	0.001
EQ-5D	0.721 (0.15)	0.728 (0.15)	0.737 (0.15)	0.825 (0.11)	0.830 (0.13)	0.861 (0.10)	0.29	0.96	0.007	0.005

treatment of chronic medical conditions. Deploying resources with the goal of population-based health management will facilitate efficient allocation of resources in such a way that will lower overall healthcare cost, and improve quality of care experience (50). The CDSMP provides a mechanism to deliver cost-effective evidence-based strategies to those who may benefit most (e.g., being older and having co-morbid conditions). Poor quality of life and other mental health concerns has broader effects than immediate impacts on individuals with chronic conditions.

LIMITATIONS

This study builds upon an existing translational *National Study of CDSMP*, which was not originally designed as an economic cost-effectiveness study. Hence, several variables typically included in economic analyses were not present (e.g., a comparison group or individual cost measures). While there was some participant attrition over time, the impacts appear minimal in terms of the diversity of participants in the study.

As an accommodation to available data, our study has assumed a standard per-participant costs now cited in the CDSMP literature (23). Although ICER values seem very attractive, cautions should be used to interpret too literally because these values can change substantially depending on changes in cost estimates assumption and point estimates. We acknowledge that this is a rough estimate that excludes a full consideration of all potential costs. One consideration is whether to include the opportunity cost of participating in the CDSMP program. Here, the opportunity cost would be the value of participation time in the workshop and which could be calculated based on wage forgone or the value of leisure time forgone. Since the majority of CDSMP participants are older adults, we can make the assumption that there is limited (if any) opportunity cost involved in terms of forgone wages as they are likely to be out of labor force. So, the value of leisure time could be the only way to calculate the opportunity cost of participating in the program. However, there is evidence that people do not always value the use of leisure time and it is also hard to estimate the value given the availability of survey instruments. The theoretical notion is that high motivation and retirement lower the time cost of participating in this type of health promotion program. Literature also suggests excluding time cost of participants in physical activity interventions (51).

Another limitation is that the calculation of QALYs was not adjusted for possible confounding factors which could potentially influence cots and outcome measures (45). Although the use of multiple regression method would control for this imbalance, the lack of a control group of CDSMP intervention makes this method infeasible in the current study. There are many more unmeasured benefits of the CDSMP that are not captured in the outcomes presented in the current study. For example, participants typically report many positive aspects of their participation including new social interactions. As such, the complete value of this evidence-based program is not fully measured in the current analysis and may be targeted for future study.

Using the generally accepted cost-effectiveness ratio of $50,000/QALYs, results of this study indicate that CDSMP is potentially cost-effective for individuals with multiple chronic conditions. Utilizing the most widely used generic measure of HRQOL from a population-based health days measure, the current study quantifies cost-effectiveness of CDSMP. However, due to the fact that CERs evaluate how a program's costs compare to its outcomes, judgments about whether the outcomes achieved are worth than the cost are subjective and dependent on several factors (e.g., current needs and resources).

Nevertheless, we feel that this study makes a major contribution as one of the first studies to quantify the benefits of CDSMP in terms of a preference-based quality of life measure and examine the impacts for those with co-morbid depressive symptomatology. It provides a foundation for future cost-effectiveness studies of self-management programs for adults with multiple chronic conditions.

Table 4 | ICER for QALYs for CDSMP participants.

Overall						ICER by depression status based on PHQ-8 score											
QALYs = 0.007						Depressed at baseline QALYs = 0.006[a]						Not depressed at baseline QALYs = 0.026[b]					
Average cost-ranges			ICER = average cost/QALYs			Average cost-ranges			ICER = average cost/QALYs			Average cost-ranges			ICER = average cost/QALYs		
Max	Median	Min	Max	Median	Min	Max	Median	Min	Max	Median	Min	Max	Median	Min	Max	Median	Min
$583	$350	$219	$83,285	$50,000	$31,285	$583	$350	$219	$97166	$58333	$36500	$583	$350	$219	$22423	$13461	$8423

[a] $Incremental\ QALY_{depression=yes} = \left[\frac{(0.728-0.721)}{2} \times \frac{6}{12} + \frac{(0.728-0.721)}{2} \times \frac{6}{12} + \frac{(0.737-0.728)}{2} \times \frac{6}{12}\right] = 0.006.$

[b] $Incremental\ QALY_{depression=no} = \left[\frac{(0.861-0.825)}{2} \times \frac{6}{12} + \frac{(0.861-0.825)}{2} \times \frac{6}{12} + \frac{(0.861-0.830)}{2} \times \frac{6}{12}\right] = 0.026.$

ACKNOWLEDGMENTS

The American Recovery and Reinvestment Act of 2009 (i.e., Recovery Act) Communities Putting Prevention to Work: Chronic Disease Self-Management Program initiative, led by the U.S. Administration on Aging in collaboration with the Centers for Disease Control and Prevention and the Centers for Medicare and Medicaid Services, allotted $32.5 million to support the translation of the Stanford program in 45 States, Puerto Rico, and the District of Columbia. This research was supported by a grant to the National Council on Aging, with subcontracts to Texas A&M University and Stanford University.

REFERENCES

1. Centers for Disease Control and Prevention. *The State of Aging and Health in America 2013. Atlanta (GA): CDC.* (2013). Available from: http://www.cdc.gov/aging/pdf/state-aging-health-in-america-2013.pdf
2. Ralph NL, Mielenz TJ, Parton H, Flatley AM, Thorpe LE. Multiple chronic conditions and limitations in activities of daily living in a community-based sample of older adults in New York City, 2009. *Prev Chronic Dis* (2013) **10**:E199. doi:10.5888/pcd10.130159
3. Anderson GF. *Chronic Care: Making the Case for Ongoing Care.* Princeton, NJ: Robert Wood Johnson Foundation (2010). Available from: http://www.rwjf.org/content/dam/farm/reports/reports/2010/rwjf54583
4. Barile JP, Thompson WW, Zack MM, Krahn GL, Horner-Johnson W, Bowen SE. Multiple chronic medical conditions and health-related quality of life in older adults, 2004–2006. *Prev Chronic Dis* (2013) **10**:E162. doi:10.5888/pcd10.120282
5. Dominick KL, Ahern FM, Gold CH, Heller DA. Relationship of health-related quality of life to health care utilization and mortality in older adults. *Aging Clin Exp Res* (2002) **14**:499–508. doi:10.1007/BF03327351
6. Unutzer J, Donald LP, Diehr P, Simon G, Grembowski SD, Katon W. Quality adjusted life years in older adults with depressive symptoms and chronic medical disorders. *Int Psychogeriatr* (2000) **12**:15–33. doi:10.1017/S1041610200006177
7. Fortin M, Lapointe L, Hudon C, Vanasse A, Ntetu AL, Maltais D. Multimorbidity and quality of life in primary care: a systematic review. *Health Qual Life Outcomes* (2004) **2**:51. doi:10.1186/1477-7525-2-51
8. Moriaty DG, Zack MM, Kobau R. The centers for disease control and prevention's healthy days measures – population tracking of perceived physical and mental health over time. *Health Qual Life Outcomes* (2003) **1**:37. doi:10.1186/1477-7525-1-37
9. Centers for Disease Control and Prevention. *Measuring Healthy Days: Population Assessment of Health-Related Quality of Life [Internet].* Atlanta (GA): CDC (2000). Available from: http://www.cdc.gov/hrqol/pdfs/mhd.pdf
10. Harris JR, Wallace RB. The Institute of Medicine's new report on living well with chronic illness. *Prev Chronic Dis* (2012) **9**:E148. doi:10.5888/pcd9.120126
11. Parekh AK, Barton MB. The challenge of multiple comorbidity for the US health care system. *JAMA* (2010) **303**:1303–4. doi:10.1001/jama.2010.381
12. Parekh AK, Goodman RA, Gordon C, Koh HK. Managing multiple chronic conditions: a strategic framework for improving health outcomes and quality of life. *Public Health Rep* (2011) **126**(4):460–71. Available from: http://www.publichealthreports.org/cphce/126_4_460.pdf
13. Patient Protection and Affordable Care Act of 2010. *Pub L. 111-148. 124 Stat. 119.* (2010). Available from: http://www.gpo.gov/fdsys/pkg/PLAW-111publ148/pdf/PLAW-111publ148.pdf
14. Barlow J, Turner A, Edwards R, Gilchrist M. A randomised controlled trial of lay-led self-management for people with multiple sclerosis. *Patient Educ Couns* (2009) **77**:81–9. doi:10.1016/j.pec.2009.02.009
15. Ory MG, Ahn S, Jiang L, Smith ML, Ritter PL, Whitelaw N, et al. Successes of a national study of the chronic disease self-management program: meeting the triple aim of health care reform. *Med Care* (2013) **51**:992–8. doi:10.1097/MLR.0b013e3182a95dd1
16. Brady TJ, Murphy L, O'Colmain BJ, Beauchesne D, Daniels B, Greenberg M, et al. A meta-analysis of health status, health behaviors, and health care utilization outcomes of the chronic disease self-management program. *Prev Chronic Dis* (2013) **10**:120112. doi:10.5888/pcd10.120112

17. Bodenheimer T, Lorig K, Holman H, Grumbach K. Patient self-management of chronic disease in primary care. *JAMA* (2002) **288**:2469–75. doi:10.1001/jama.288.19.2469
18. Reeves D, Kennedy A, Fullwood C, Bower P, Gardner C, Gately C, et al. Predicting who will benefit from an expert patients programme self-management course. *Br J Gen Pract* (2008) **58**:198–203. doi:10.3399/bjgp08X277320
19. Labrecque M, Rabhi K, Laurin C, Favreau H, Moullec G, Lavoie K, et al. Can a self-management education program for patients with chronic obstructive pulmonary disease improve quality of life. *Can Respir J* (2011) **18**: e77–81.
20. Ahmed S, Bartlett SJ, Ernst P, Paré P, Kanter GM, Perreault R, et al. Effect of a web-based chronic disease management system on asthma control and health-related quality of life: study protocol for a randomized controlled trial. *Trials* (2011) **12**:260. doi:10.1186/1745-6215-12-260
21. Berwick DM, Nolan TW, Whittington W. The triple aim: care, health and cost. *Health Aff (Millwood)* (2008) **27**(3):759–69. doi:10.1377/hlthaff.27.3.759
22. Lorig KR, Sobel DS, Stewart AL, Brown BW Jr, Bandura A, Ritter P, et al. Evidence Suggesting that a chronic disease self-management program can improve health status while reducing hospitalization: a randomized trial. *Med Care* (1999) **37**(1):5–14. doi:10.1097/00005650-199901000-00003
23. Ahn S, Basu R, Smith ML, Jiang L, Lorig K, Whitelaw N, et al. The impact of chronic disease self-management programs: healthcare savings through a community-based intervention. *BMC Public Health* (2013) **13**:1141. doi:10.1186/1471-2458-13-1141
24. Ory MG, Ahn S, Jiang L, Lorig K, Ritter P, Larent DD, et al. National study of chronic disease self-management six-month outcome findings. *J Aging Health* (2013) **25**:1258–74. doi:10.1177/0898264313502531
25. Lorig K, Holman H, Sobel D, Laurent DD. *Living a Healthy Life with Chronic Conditions: Self Management of Heart Disease, Arthritis, Diabetes, Asthma, Bronchitis, Emphysema and Others.* 3rd ed. Boulder, CO: Bull Publishing Company (2006).
26. Lorig K, Ritter PL, Pifer C, Werner P. Effectiveness of the chronic disease self-management program for persons with a serious mental illness: a translation study. *Community Ment Health J* (2013) **50**:96–103. doi:10.1007/s10597-013-9615-5
27. Erdem E, Korda H. Self-management program participation by older adults with diabetes: chronic disease self-management program and diabetes self-management program. *Fam Community Health* (2014) **37**:134–46. doi:10.1097/FCH.0000000000000025
28. Smith ML, Ory MG, Larsen R. Older women in a statewide evidence-based falls prevention program: who enrolls and what benefits are obtained? *Womens Health Issues* (2010) **20**:427–34. doi:10.1016/j.whi.2010.07.003
29. Rabin R, de Charro F. EQ-5D: a measure of health status from the EuroQol Group. *Ann Med* (2001) **33**:337–43. doi:10.3109/07853890109002087
30. Smith ML, Ory MG, Ahn S, Bazzarre TL, Resnick B. Older adults' participation in a community-based falls prevention exercise program: relationships between the EASY tool, program attendance, and health outcomes. *Gerontologist* (2011) **51**:809–21. doi:10.1093/geront/gnr084
31. Smith ML, Ahn S, Sharkey JR, Horel S, Mier N, Ory MG. Successful falls prevention programming for older adults in Texas: rural-urban variations. *J Appl Gerontol* (2012) **31**:3–27. doi:10.1177/0733464810378407
32. Smith ML, Ahn S, Mier N, Jiang L, Ory MG. An evidence-based program to reduce fall-related risk among older adults: a comparison of program efficacy by ethnicity. *Calif J Health Promot* (2012) **10**:28–43.
33. NCOA. *About Evidence-Based Programs.* Available from: http://www.ncoa.org/improve-health/center-for-healthy-aging/about-evidence-based-programs.html
34. Page TF, Palmer RC. Cost analysis of chronic disease self-management programs being delivered in South Florida. *Health Educ J* (2014) **73**:228–36. doi:10.1177/0017896912471047
35. Stanford School of Medicine. *Training Policies for Stanford Self-Management Programs.* Palo Alto, CA: Patient Education Research Center (2014). Available from: http://patienteducation.stanford.edu/training/trnpolicies.html
36. Kroenke K, Spitzer RL. The PHQ-9; a new depression diagnostic and severity measure. *Psychiatr Ann* (2002) **32**(9):509–15.
37. Kroenke K, Spitzer RL, Williams JB. The PHQ-9: validity of brief depression severity measure. *J Gen Intern Med* (2001) **16**:606–13. doi:10.1046/j.1525-1497.2001.016009606.x
38. Kroenke K, Strine TW, Spitzer RL, Williams JB, Berry JT, Mokdad AH. The PHQ-8 as a measure of current depression in the general population. *J Affect Disord* (2009) **114**:163–73. doi:10.1016/j.jad.2008.06.026
39. The Secretary's Advisory Committee on National Health Promotion and Disease Prevention Objectives for 2020. *Phase I Report: Recommendations for the Framework and Format of Healthy People 2020 [Internet].* (2008). Available from: http://www.healthypeople.gov/sites/default/files/PhaseI_0.pdf
40. Metzler M, Kanarek N, Highsmith K, Straw R, Bialek R, Stanleyl J, et al. Community health status indicators project: the development of a national approach to community health. *Prev Chronic Dis* (2008) **5**:A94.
41. Jia H, Lubetkin EI. Trend in quality-adjusted life-years lost contributed by smoking and obesity. *Am J Prev Med* (2010) **38**:138–44. doi:10.1016/j.amepre.2009.09.043
42. Jia H, Lubetkin EI. Estimating EuroQol EQ-5D scores from population healthy days data. *Med Decis Making* (2008) **28**:491–9. doi:10.1177/0272989X07312708
43. Kind P, Dolan P, Gudex C, Williams A. Variations in population health status: results from a United Kingdom national questionnaire survey. *BMJ* (1998) **316**:736–41. doi:10.1136/bmj.316.7133.736
44. Goldsmith KA, Dyer MT, Buxton MJ, Sharples LD. Mapping of the EQ-5D index from clinical outcome measures and demographic variables in patients with coronary heart disease. *Health Qual Life Outcomes* (2010) **8**:54. doi:10.1186/1477-7525-8-54
45. Manaca A, Hawkings N, Sculpher MJ. Estimating mean QALYs in trial-based cost-effectiveness analysis: the importance of controlling for baseline utility. *Health Econ* (2005) **14**:487–96. doi:10.1002/hec.944
46. Cellini SR, Kee JE. Cost-effectiveness and cost-benefit analysis. In: Wholey JS, Hatry HP, Newcomer KE, editors. *Handbook of Practical Program Evaluation.* San Francisco, CA: John Wiley & Sons Inc (2010). 493 p.
47. Haddix A, Teutsch SM, Corso PS. *Prevention Effectiveness: A Guide to Decision Analysis and Economic Evaluation.* 2nd ed. Oxford: Oxford University Press (2003). 264 p.
48. Ory MG, Smith ML, Kulinski KP, Lorig K, Zenker W, Whitelaw N. Self-management at the tipping point: reaching 100,000 Americans with evidence-based programs. *J Am Geriatr Soc* (2013) **61**:821–3. doi:10.1111/jgs.12239
49. Drummond MF, Stoddart GL, Torrance GW. *Methods for the Economic Evaluation of Healthcare Programmes.* Oxford: Oxford University Press (1987).
50. Brownson CA, Hoerger TH, Fisher EB, Kilpatrick KE. Cost-effectiveness of diabetes self-management programs in community primary care settings. *Diabetes Educ* (2009) **35**:761–9. doi:10.1177/0145721709340931
51. Woolf SH. A closer look at the economic argument for disease prevention. *JAMA* (2009) **301**:536–8. doi:10.1001/jama.2009.51
52. Boheler C, Milton KE, Bull FC, Fox-Rushby JA. The cost of changing physical activity behavior: evidence from a "physical activity pathway" in a primary care setting. *BMC Public Health* (2011) **11**:370. doi:10.1186/1471-2458-11-370

13

Fall prevention in community settings: Results from implementingTai Chi – Moving for Better Balance in three states

Marcia G. Ory[1]*, Matthew Lee Smith[2], Erin M. Parker[3], Luohua Jiang[4], Shuai Chen[5], Ashley D. Wilson[1], Judy A. Stevens[3], Heidi Ehrenreich[3] and Robin Lee[3]

[1] *Department of Health Promotion and Community Health Sciences, Texas A&M Health Science Center School of Public Health, College Station, TX, USA*
[2] *Department of Health Promotion and Behavior, The University of Georgia College of Public Health, Athens, GA, USA*
[3] *National Center for Injury Prevention and Control, Centers for Disease Control and Prevention, Atlanta, GA, USA*
[4] *Department of Epidemiology and Biostatistics, Texas A&M Health Science Center School of Public Health, College Station, TX, USA*
[5] *Department of Statistics, Texas A&M University, College Station, TX, USA*

Edited by:
Michal Grivna, United Arab Emirates University, United Arab Emirates

Reviewed by:
Milka Dančević-Gojković, Public Health Institute of Federation of Bosnia and Herzegovina, Bosnia and Herzegovina
Pankaja Desai, University of Illinois at Chicago, USA

****Correspondence:***
Marcia G. Ory, Department of Health Promotion and Community Health Sciences, Texas A&M Health Science Center, 1266, College Station, TX 77843–1266, USA
e-mail: mory@srph.tamhsc.edu

Tai Chi: Moving for Better Balance (TCMBB) is an evidence-based fall prevention exercise program being disseminated in selected communities through state injury prevention programs. This study: (1) describes the personal characteristics of TCMBB participants; (2) quantifies participants' functional and self-reported health status at enrollment; and (3) measures changes in participants' functional and self-reported health status post-intervention. There were 421 participants enrolled in 36 TCMBB programs delivered in Colorado, New York, and Oregon. Of the 209 participants who completed both baseline enrollment and post-intervention surveys, the average age of participants was 75.3 (SD ± 8.2) years. Most participants were female (81.3%), non-Hispanic (96.1%), White (94.1%), and described themselves as in excellent or very good health (52.2%). Paired *t*-test and general estimating equation models assessed changes over the 3-month program period. Pre- and post-assessment self-reported surveys and objective functional data [Timed Up and Go (TUG) test] were collected. On average, TUG test scores decreased ($p < 0.001$) for all participants; however, the decrease was most noticeable among high-risk participants (mean decreased from 18.5 to 15.7 s). The adjusted odds ratio of reporting feeling confident that a participant could keep themselves from falling was five times greater after completing the program. TCMBB, which addresses gait and balance problems, can be an effective way to reduce falls among the older adult population. By helping older adults maintain their functional abilities, TCMBB can help community-dwelling older adults continue to live independently.

Keywords: Tai Chi: Moving for Better Balance, fall prevention, fall prevention program, community setting, older adults

INTRODUCTION

Tai Chi is a Chinese form of exercise that uses slow, flowing body movements. It had been practiced for centuries in Asia before being introduced to the United States in the early twentieth century (1). The physical and mental health benefits of Tai Chi are well documented (2–4), and in the 1990s, Tai Chi was rigorously tested by the National Institute on Aging as a fall prevention intervention (5, 6). A Cochrane review and meta-analysis concluded that Tai Chi reduced the risk of falling 28%, with greater effectiveness among those with lower initial fall risk (7). Today Tai Chi is widely recognized as an effective fall intervention (8–10).

The Tai Chi: Moving for Better Balance (TCMBB) program is an evidence-based fall prevention exercise program that was developed by researchers at the Oregon Research Institute with partial funding from the Centers for Disease Control and Prevention (CDC). The original 26-week intervention used 24 Tai Chi forms or sequences of controlled movements, and it was shown in a randomized controlled trial to be effective in reducing falls (11, 12). TCMBB consists of eight forms that progress from easy to difficult to improve older adults' postural stability, balance, and coordination (13). Classes consist of 10–15 participants led by a trained instructor. One-hour classes are held twice a week for 12 weeks (24 total classes) (13). Feasibility testing has demonstrated that this program is well accepted by older adults and can be implemented with fidelity in community settings (14, 15).

In 2011, the CDC launched a 5-year project to implement TCMBB in selected communities in Oregon, Colorado, and New York. This was part of a larger project to reduce falls and fall-related injuries by engaging fall prevention coalitions, healthcare organizations, and other partners to integrate clinical and evidence-based community fall prevention programs in selected communities (16). TCMBB is intended for relatively healthy older adults with few functional limitations.

This study describes the results of implementing TCMBB during the first 2 years of the project. The purposes of the study were to: (1) describe the personal characteristics of TCMBB participants; (2) quantify participants' functional and self-reported health status at enrollment; and (3) measure changes in participants' functional and self-reported health status after completing the program.

MATERIALS AND METHODS

TCMBB IMPLEMENTATION

The three states offered TCMBB in a variety of settings including YMCAs, healthcare organizations, residential facilities, faith-based organizations, recreational facilities, and senior centers. State grantees hosted 30 TCMBB trainings from 2011 to 2013 at which Master Trainers from the Oregon Research Institute trained 400 instructors. In addition, the YMCA of the USA (Y-USA) engaged the Oregon Research Institute to train 10 YMCA faculty trainers to be TCMBB instructors.

The target audience for TCMBB is community-dwelling older adults aged 60 and older who can walk easily with or without assistive devices. In each state, participants were recruited by staff at member organizations, through family and friends, and through advertisements aimed at older adults. Methods of recruitment and referral varied across states and were based on existing partnerships. For example, Colorado and New York were most likely to recruit at YMCAs whereas Oregon recruited through senior centers and health care organizations since there were no YMCAs in their service delivery areas. As a program implemented through existing traditional community settings, there were limited exclusionary criteria and medical clearance was not required for participation. While no age restrictions were placed on enrollment, our analyses were restricted to people aged 60 years and older to reflect the study target population.

DATA COLLECTION

Data for this project were collected from multiple sources. Attendance was obtained from attendance logs collected at each class. A 20-question self-administered survey was used to collect pre- and post-TCMBB program data. The first was administered at the initial TCMBB class (enrollment or baseline survey) and the second at the final class (course completion or post-intervention survey). The surveys took approximately 15 minutes to complete and assistance was provided to participants who needed help filling out the forms. Questions included socio-demographic characteristics (e.g., age, sex, race, and ethnicity), whether the participant had been referred to the program by a healthcare provider, self-reported health status (excellent, very good, good, fair, or poor), satisfaction with their current activity levels (very, mostly, somewhat, or not at all satisfied), and confidence in their ability to keep themselves from falling (four-point scale ranging from strongly agree to strongly disagree). Self-reported functional ability was assessed by the reported level of difficulty in performing various activities (e.g., climbing one flight of stairs) on a four-point scale ranging from no difficulty (scored 1) to unable to do (scored 4) (17). Class completion was defined as attending at least 70% of the classes (i.e., 17 out of 24 classes).

The Timed Up and Go (TUG) test was used to measure functional status at enrollment and completion. This test has been widely used to assess functional mobility and predict fall risk and has been validated among community-dwelling older adults (18–20). The test measures the time in seconds required for participants to "rise from a standard arm chair, walk at [their] typical or normal pace to a line on the floor 3 meters away, turn, return, and sit down again" (21). Participants who completed the TUG in <12 seconds were classified as low risk and those who took 12 or more seconds were classified as high risk (22).

STATISTICAL ANALYSES

Baseline characteristics (demographic characteristics, class attendance, and TUG results) were compared for those who completed both the baseline and post-intervention questionnaires to those who completed only the baseline questionnaire using chi-square tests to identify potential biases from loss to follow-up. Changes in TUG test times between baseline and post-intervention were compared using two-tailed paired t-tests; results were examined for all participants combined and stratified by baseline risk level. General estimating equations (GEE) models using a logit link function were used to compare differences in self-reported functional and health status at baseline and post-intervention; models were run using SAS version 9.3 GENMOD procedure (SAS Institute Inc., Cary, NC, USA) and adjusted for gender, age, race, and state. GEE models are longitudinal data models that use all available data in model estimation (i.e., do not require paired data) and can account for the correlation among repeated measures from the same participant (23).

The Texas A&M University Institutional Review Board granted approval to analyze data on program participants and outcomes collected using survey instruments and functional assessments.

RESULTS

PARTICIPANT CHARACTERISTICS AND COURSE ATTENDANCE

Between September 1, 2011 and December 31, 2013, the three states offered 36 TCMBB programs and enrolled 537 people aged 60 and older. Of these enrollees, baseline data were collected from 421 (78.4%); 20.2% of participants were in Oregon, 39.9% in Colorado, and 39.9% in New York (**Table 1**). Of the 421 participants who provided a baseline questionnaire, 209 also completed a post-intervention questionnaire (**Table 1**).

The average age of participants was 75.3 (SD ± 8.2) years. Most participants were female, non-Hispanic, and White. About half of the participants attended at least 70% of classes (17 out of 24), with participants attending on average 13.6 (SD ± 8.0) of the 24 possible classes. Only 16 participants (8.5%) reported they were referred to TCMBB by a healthcare provider.

The 212 participants who "dropped out" or were lost to follow-up were not significantly different from those who completed the program in terms of gender, race, ethnicity, self-reported health status, or provider referral to class. However, dropouts were significantly older (average age 76.1 vs. 74.1) and more likely to have been classified as high risk based their TUG time at baseline.

PARTICIPANT FUNCTIONAL PERFORMANCE

Of 421 participants with baseline data, 199 (47.3%) completed the TUG test at both baseline and post-intervention (**Table 2**).

Table 1 | Characteristics of Tai Chi: Moving for Better Balance (TCMBB) participants.

	All enrolled participants[a]	Participants who completed both the baseline enrollment and post-intervention surveys	Participants who completed only the baseline enrollment survey	X^2	*P*-value
	N = 421	*N* = 209	*N* = 212		
	n (%)	*n* (%)	*n* (%)		
Location				3.24	0.197
Oregon	85 (20.2)	35 (16.8)	50 (23.6)		
Colorado	168 (39.9)	85 (40.7)	83 (39.2)		
New York	168 (39.9)	89 (42.6)	79 (37.3)		
Age group				8.96	0.011
60–69	115 (27.3)	61 (29.2)	54 (25.5)		
70–79	177 (42.0)	98 (46.9)	79 (37.3)		
80+	129 (30.6)	50 (23.9)	79 (37.3)		
Gender				0.22	0.639
Female	335 (80.3)	169 (81.3)	166 (79.4)		
Male	82 (19.7)	39 (18.8)	43 (20.6)		
Missing	4	1	3		
Race				0.11	0.742
White	388 (93.7)	192 (94.1)	196 (93.3)		
Non-White	26 (6.3)	12 (5.9)	14 (6.7)		
Missing	7	5	2		
Ethnicity (Hispanic/Latino)				0.06	0.807
Yes	15 (3.7)	8 (3.9)	7 (3.4)		
No	395 (96.3)	198 (96.1)	197 (96.6)		
Missing	11	3	8		
Self-reported health status				3.86	0.145
Excellent/very good	211 (50.7)	108 (52.2)	103 (49.3)		
Good	165 (39.7)	85 (41.1)	80 (38.3)		
Fair/poor	40 (9.6)	14 (6.8)	26 (12.4)		
Missing	5	2	3		
Referred by healthcare provider					
Yes	35 (8.5)	18 (8.7)	17 (8.3)	0.03	0.872
No	378 (91.5)	189 (91.3)	189 (91.7)		
Missing	8	2	6		
Timed up and go (TUG) time at enrollment				5.65	0.017
Low risk (baseline TUG < 12 s)	279 (71.7)	154 (77.0)	125 (66.1)		
High risk (baseline TUG ≥ 12 s)	110 (28.3)	46 (23.0)	64 (33.9)		
Missing	32	9	23		
Participants who completed 70%+ classes	209 (49.6)	163 (78.0)	46 (21.7)	133.41	<0.001

[a]*Enrolled participants include all persons 60 years and older who filled out the baseline enrollment survey on the first day of the program (421/537 participants). Individual survey questions may have had missing data.*

Of these, 45 (22.6%) were categorized as high risk. After completing TCMBB, the proportion of participants categorized as high risk decreased significantly to 14% ($n = 28$; data not shown). On average, TUG test scores decreased significantly for all participants but the change was most evident among high risk participants where the average TUG time decreased from 18.5 to 15.7 seconds.

SELF-REPORTED OUTCOME IMPROVEMENTS

Table 3 compares self-reported outcome measures at baseline and post-intervention. Results are presented as percentages and as odds ratios adjusted for gender, age, race, and state. Significant improvements from baseline to post-intervention were observed for all outcomes except self-reported difficulty in walking across the room.

Table 2 | Changes in Tai Chi: Moving for Better Balance (TCMBB) participants' timed up and go (TUG) times from baseline enrollment to post-intervention[a].

Changes in TUG times (in seconds)	TUG at baseline		TUG at post-intervention		Change in TUG from baseline to post-intervention[b]		
	N	Mean (±SD)	*N*	Mean (±SD)	*N*	Mean (±SD)	*P*-value
TUG times for all participants	199	11.2 (±6.7)	199	9.9 (±6.0)	199	−1.3 (±2.7)	<0.001
Low risk (enrollment TUG time < 12 s)	154	9.1 (±1.4)	154	8.2 (±1.6)	154	−0.8 (±1.3)	<0.001
High risk (enrollment TUG time ≥ 12 s)	45	18.5 (±11.2)	45	15.7 (±10.5)	45	−2.7 (±4.9)	0.001

SD, standard deviation.

[a]While 389 participants completed the TUG at enrollment, this table highlights the 199 participants who completed the TUG at both baseline and post-intervention.

[b]Paired t-tests with an alpha of 0.05 were used to compare changes in participants' TUG times between baseline and post-intervention. A reduction in time indicates a positive functional improvement.

Table 3 | Changes in Tai Chi: Moving for Better Balance (TCMBB) participants' self-reported health and functional outcomes from baseline to post-intervention[a].

Health outcome	Baseline ($N = 209$)[b]	Post-intervention ($N = 209$)[b]	Adjusted change from baseline to post-intervention[c]	
	N (%)	*N* (%)	Odds ratios from logistic models	*P*-value
Health status, satisfaction, and confidence				
Excellent or very good health status	108 (52.2)	123 (58.9)	1.35 (1.03, 1.77)	0.031
Very/mostly satisfied with physical activity levels	126 (60.9)	160 (76.9)	2.21 (1.60, 3.05)	<0.001
Feel confident not falling (strongly agree or agree)	149 (74.9)	196 (93.8)	6.16 (3.48, 10.89)	<0.001
Self-reported functional status				
No difficulty in walking across room	178 (86.4)	183 (88.4)	1.30 (0.83, 2.02)	0.249
No difficulty in walking one block	149 (77.2)	166 (83.0)	1.60 (1.19, 2.17)	0.002
No difficulty in stooping, crouching, and kneeling	71 (34.8)	85 (41.3)	1.32 (1.04, 1.68)	0.023
No difficulty in getting out of a straight back chair	141 (73.4)	163 (81.1)	1.67 (1.14, 2.44)	0.008
No difficulty in climbing one flight of stairs	133 (64.6)	144 (72.0)	1.42 (1.03, 1.68)	0.034

SD, standard deviation.

[a]Data are reported for $n = 209$ participants who completed both the baseline and post-intervention surveys.

[b]The sample size is slightly smaller than 209 for some health outcomes due to missing data. The amount of missing data ranges from 0 to 8% for different outcomes.

[c]Adjusted odds ratios from GEE logistic regression modeling the probability of response = 1 at an alpha of 0.05. All models account for repeated measures from the same participant and are adjusted for gender, age, race, and state. An odds ratio > 1 represents a positive improvement in self-reported health.

The GEE model results showed that the adjusted odds ratio (aOR) of reporting excellent or very good health status increased by 35% (aOR = 1.35, 95% CI 1.03–1.77). The odds of being very or mostly satisfied with physical activity levels also increased significantly (aOR = 2.21, 95% CI 1.60–3.05). The odds of feeling confident that a participant could keep themselves from falling was five times greater after completing TCMBB (aOR = 6.16 95% CI 3.48–10.89).

Among the five items assessing functional status, the aORs for participants who reported "no difficulty" significantly increased for walking one block (aOR = 1.60, 95% CI 1.19–2.17); stooping, crouching, kneeling (aOR = 1.32, 95% CI 1.04–1.68); getting out of a straight back chair (aOR = 1.67, 95% CI 1.14–2.44); and climbing one flight of stairs (aOR = 1.42, 95% CI 1.03–1.68). About 86% of participants reported no difficulty walking across the room at baseline, and this proportion did not increase significantly at post-intervention.

DISCUSSION

This study examined 2 years of evaluation data collected from older adults age 60+ who participated in TCMBB programs offered in selected communities across three states. Comparing data collected at enrollment and course completion, TCMBB was associated with significant improvements in self-reported health status, satisfaction with physical activity levels, fall-related confidence, ability to perform basic functional tasks (e.g., walking one block, climbing a flight of stairs), and in the TUG test. Similar positive results have been seen in earlier studies of Tai Chi (14, 24), and provide additional evidence that Tai Chi is a useful fall prevention program for older adults.

Recruitment of participants is a concern for most fall prevention programs. While the distribution of TCMBB participants' race and ethnicity was similar to the populations from which they were recruited, the percentage of male participants was low. Retaining TCMBB participants was also challenging.

Participants attended on average 57% of the 24 classes. While it was not possible in this study to monitor falls, those who did not attend regularly may not have received an adequate intervention dose for reducing their fall risk. The reasons for low attendance are unknown. However, anecdotal reports from the state health departments implementing TCMBB suggest that some older adults may have considered the Tai Chi program a "drop-in" activity instead of an ongoing program. Those who did not complete the course were somewhat older and took longer to complete the TUG at enrollment, which suggests that health issues may have contributed to their not finishing the program.

Barriers to the success of TCMBB, as for other community-based fall prevention programs, include maintaining regular attendance and encouraging participants to continue activities after the program ends. Although the participants in this study demonstrated positive outcomes, one 12-week program is unlikely to provide long-term benefits without booster classes. Tai Chi, like other strength and balance exercises, is most effective when it is practiced for 50 hours or more (11). Therefore, older adults would benefit from having an ongoing Tai Chi program in their community, if they attended regularly. Some participating sites are now offering an introductory 12-week TCMBB followed by an ongoing program.

Another challenge has been the limited availability of community Tai Chi classes. State health departments have been able to address this by developing public–private partnerships with organizations that have existing infrastructure to offer classes to older adults. For example, the Y-USA now endorses a modified version of TCMBB called Y-Moving for Better Balance (Y-MFBB) that is being offered in local YMCAs (25). State health departments are also beginning to implement and support other Tai Chi programs (e.g., Tai Chi for Arthritis) that have been shown to be effective for fall prevention (26).

Ideally all older adults would have access to a wide range of evidence-based fall prevention programs that could meet their varied needs. Thus, in the larger fall prevention project, TCMBB was offered along with Stepping On (27) and Otago (28), which are designed for older adults with some functional limitations who are at moderate and high fall risk, respectively. As the availability of Tai Chi and other fall prevention programs expands, it will be important to ensure that fidelity to the key elements of the original interventions is maintained so that the programs remain effective in preventing falls.

LIMITATIONS

This study has number of limitations. First, sampling and dropout issues limit the generalizability of the results. Participants were self-selected from participating communities and may not be representative of the older adult population either in those communities or in the participating states. Program effectiveness was based on comparing assessments from participants who attended both the first and last class. These participants were slightly younger and had fewer functional limitations, as measured by better TUG times at baseline, compared to participants who were not available for the post-intervention assessment. However, because the results are for those who provided both baseline enrollment and post-intervention assessments, we can be confident we are comparing the same population before and after the intervention. We did not take into account differences in total attendance among people who provided baseline and post-intervention assessments, so the effectiveness of the full intervention may be underestimated.

Second, the program was delivered in a multitude of settings, and outcomes may have been influenced by variability in instructor and site. Although all instructors were certified trained instructors, we recommend more attention be given to treatment fidelity monitoring in future research and practice. The CDC Guide for Program Implementation (13) has examples of a class observation form for monitoring instructor adherence to core program elements.

Third, in order to limit the reporting burden on the program delivery personnel, we used a limited number of self-reported outcomes and one timed functional assessment (i.e., the TUG). Although there was training provided for conducting the TUG, including available step-by-step online videos, this training was limited. Therefore, results may not be comparable to standardized TUG tests administered by trained professionals. Finally, while TCMBB participants reported improved functional status and demonstrated better TUG scores, we do not know if this led to a reduction in falls, since falls were not monitored during or after the program.

CONCLUSION

Tai Chi: Moving for Better Balance, which addresses gait and balance problems, can be an effective way to reduce falls among the older adult population. Various forms of Tai Chi have been shown to be most appropriate for younger and healthier older adults who are at relatively low risk of falling. By helping older adults maintain their functional abilities, TCMBB can help community-dwelling older adults continue to live independently.

In this study, TCMBB participants reported positive effects on their functional and health status. However, the high dropout rates among program participants highlight a major challenge to implementing effective community-based fall prevention programs. Community-based programs are a promising approach for older adult fall prevention, but there are ongoing challenges to ensuring that high quality programs are available for – and attended by – older adults who can benefit from such programs.

ACKNOWLEDGMENTS

We thank the Colorado, New York, and Oregon State Injury Prevention Centers for coordinating Tai Chi: Moving for Better Balance, a Community-Based Older Adult Fall Prevention Program and collecting the study data and Margaret Kaniewski with the Centers for Disease Control and Prevention for her programmatic support and critical review of the manuscript. Funding Source: This research was supported in part by the Centers for Disease Control and Prevention, Prevention Research Centers Special Initiative Project funding for the State Fall Prevention Program under 5U48DP001924, and the Research Participation Program at the Centers for Disease Control and Prevention administered by the Oak Ridge Institute for Science and Education through an interagency agreement between the U.S. Department of Energy and CDC.

REFERENCES

1. National Center for Complementary and Alternative Medicine (NCCAM). *Tai Chi: An Introduction.* National Institute of Health (2010) [cited 2014 Aug 11]. Available from: http://nccam.nih.gov/health/taichi/introduction.htm#overview
2. Leung DP, Chan CK, Tsang HW, Tsang WW, Jones AY. Tai chi as an intervention to improve balance and reduce falls in older adults: a systematic and meta-analytical review. *Altern Ther Health Med* (2011) **17**(1):40–8.
3. Lee MS, Ernst E. Systematic reviews of t'ai chi: an overview. *Br J Sports Med* (2012) **46**(10):713–8. doi:10.1136/bjsm.2010.080622
4. Kuramoto AM. Therapeutic benefits of Tai Chi exercise: research review. *WMJ* (2006) **105**(7):42–6.
5. Ory MG, Schechtman KB, Miller JP, Hadley EC, Fiatarone MA, Province MA, et al. Frailty and injuries in later life: the FICSIT trials. *J Am Geriatr Soc* (1993) **41**(3):283–96.
6. Province MA, Hadley EC, Hornbrook MC, Lipsitz LA, Miller JP, Mulrow CD, et al. The effects of exercise on falls in elderly patients. A preplanned meta-analysis of the FICSIT trials. Frailty and injuries: cooperative studies of intervention techniques. *JAMA* (1995) **273**(17):1341–7. doi:10.1001/jama.273.17.1341
7. Cameron ID, Murray GR, Gillespie LD, Robertson MC, Hill KD, Cumming RG, et al. Interventions for preventing falls in older people in nursing care facilities and hospitals. *Cochrane Database Syst Rev* (2010) **20**(1):CD005465. doi:10.1002/14651858.CD005465.pub2
8. Michael YL, Whitlock EP, Lin JS, Fu R, O'Connor EA, Gold R, et al. Primary care-relevant interventions to prevent falling in older adults: a systematic evidence review for the U.S. preventive services task force. *Ann Intern Med* (2010) **153**(12):815–25. doi:10.7326/0003-4819-153-12-201012210-00008
9. Stevens JA. *A CDC Compendium of Effective Fall Interventions: What Works for Community-Dwelling Older Adults.* Atlanta, GA: Centers for Disease Control and Prevention. National Center for Injury Prevention and Control. Division of Unintentional Injury Prevention (2010).
10. National Council on Aging. *Falls Free: Promoting a National Falls Preventions Action Plan* (2005) [cited 2014 Aug 11]:[1-51 p.]. Available from: http://www.ncoa.org/improve-health/center-for-healthy-aging/content-library/FallsFree_NationalActionPlan_Final.pdf
11. Sherrington C, Tiedemann A, Fairhall N, Close JCT, Lord S. Exercise to prevent falls in older adults: an updated meta-analysis and best practice recommendations. *N S W Public Health Bull* (2011) **22**(3–4):78–83. doi:10.1071/NB10056
12. Li F, Harmer P, McAuley E, Duncan TE, Duncan SC, Chaumeton N, et al. An evaluation of the effects of Tai Chi exercise on physical function among older persons: a randomized controlled trial. *Ann Behav Med* (2001) **23**(2):139–46. doi:10.1207/S15324796ABM2302_9
13. National Center for Injury Prevention and Control. *Tai chi: Moving for Better Balance A guide for program Implementation* (2011) [cited 2014 Aug 6]:[1-146 p.]. Available from: http://api.ning.com/files/lpWX79eu*NgqhrxYqum3lrPOm6Dp4GRQCK9J1qwtJylSBPaJ2W38NVNJNcBqszLkRplWB9ee-lwV4PIN-hUoPujtn*zU9vRw/TCManual_Compiled__v19.pdf
14. Li F, Harmer P, Glasgow R, Mack KA, Sleet D, Fisher KJ, et al. Translation of an effective tai chi intervention into a community-based falls-prevention program. *Am J Public Health* (2008) **98**(7):1195–8. doi:10.2105/AJPH.2007.120402
15. Li F, Harmer P, Mack KA, Sleet D, Fisher KJ, Kohn MA, et al. Tai Chi: moving for better balance – development of a community-based falls prevention program. *J Phys Act Health* (2008) **5**(3):445–55.
16. Kaniewski M, Stevens JA, Parker EM, Lee R. An introduction to the Centers for Disease Control and Prevention's efforts to prevent older adult falls. *Front Public Health* (2015) **2**:119. doi:10.3389/fpubh.2014.00119
17. Wallace RB, Herzog AR. Overview of the health measures in the health and retirement study. *J Hum Resour* (1995) **30**:S84–107. doi:10.2307/146279
18. Bohannon RW. Reference values for the timed up and go test: a descriptive meta-analysis. *J Geriatr Phys Ther* (2006) **29**(2):64–8. doi:10.1519/00139143-200608000-00004
19. Hutton I, Gamble G, McLean G, Butcher H, Gow P, Dalbeth N. Obstacles to action in arthritis: a community case-control study. *Int J Rheum Dis* (2009) **12**(2):107–17. doi:10.1111/j.1756-185X.2009.01392.x
20. Shumway-Cook A, Brauer S, Woollacott M. Predicting the probability for falls in community-dwelling older adults using the timed up & go test. *Phys Ther* (2000) **80**(9):896–903.
21. Podsiadlo D, Richardson S. The timed "up & go": a test of basic functional mobility for frail elderly persons. *J Am Geriatr Soc* (1991) **39**(2):142–8.
22. Bischoff HA, Stahelin HB, Monsch AU, Iversen MD, Weyh A, von Dechend M, et al. Identifying a cut-off point for normal mobility: a comparison of the timed 'up and go' test in community-dwelling and institutionalised elderly women. *Age Ageing* (2003) **32**(3):315–20. doi:10.1093/ageing/32.3.315
23. Hardin JW. Generalized Estimating Equations (GEE). *Encyclopedia of Statistics in Behavioral Science.* Hoboken, NJ: John Wiley & Sons, Ltd. (2005). doi:10.1002/0470013192.bsa250
24. Rogers CE, Larkey LK, Keller C. A review of clinical trials of tai chi and qigong in older adults. *West J Nurs Res* (2009) **31**(2):245–79. doi:10.1177/0193945908327529
25. Ehrenreich H, Pike M, Hohman K, Kaniewski M, Longjohn M, Myers G, et al. CDC and YMCA: a promising partnership for delivering fall prevention programming. *Front Public Health* (2015) **2**:235. doi:10.3389/fpubh.2014.00235
26. Stevens JA, Voukelatos A, Ehrenreich H. Preventing falls with Tai Ji Quan: a public health perspective. *J Sport Health Sci* (2014) **3**(1):21–6. doi:10.1016/j.jshs.2013.10.002
27. Ory MG, Smith ML, Jiang L, Lee R, Chen S, Wilson AD, et al. Fall prevention in community settings: results from implementing Stepping On in three states. *Front Public Health* (2015) **2**:232. doi:10.3389/fpubh.2014.00232
28. Shubert TE, Smith ML, Ory MG, Clarke CB, Bomberger SA, Roberts E, et al. Translation of the Otago Exercise Program for adoption and implementation in the United States. *Front Public Health* (2015) **2**:152. doi:10.3389/fpubh.2014.00152

14

Linking evidence-based program participant data with Medicare data: The consenting process and correlates of retrospective participant consents

Philip Lloyd Ritter[1]*, Marcia G. Ory[2], Matthew Lee Smith[3], Luohua Jiang[4], Audrey Alonis[1], Diana D. Laurent[1] and Kate Lorig[1]

[1] *Stanford Patient Education Research Center, Stanford School of Medicine, Stanford, CA, USA*
[2] *School of Public Health, Texas A&M University, College Station, TX, USA*
[3] *College of Public Health, The University of Georgia, Athens, GA, USA*
[4] *Department of Epidemiology & Biostatistics, School of Public Health, Texas A&M Health Science Center, College Station, TX, USA*

Edited by:
Roger A. Harrison, University of Manchester, UK

Reviewed by:
Shu-Chun Chuang, National Health Research Institutes, Taiwan
Daniel Francis Fahey, California State University San Bernardino, USA

***Correspondence:**
Philip Lloyd Ritter, 1000 Welch Road, Suite 204, Palo Alto, CA 94304, USA
e-mail: philr@stanford.edu

As part of a nation-wide study of the Chronic Disease Self-Management Program (*National Study*), older participants were asked to consent to have their Medicare data matched with study data. This provided an opportunity to examine the consenting process and compare consenters, refusers, and non-responders. We compared the three groups on a large number of variables. These included demographic, *National Study* participation, health indicator, health behavior, and health-care utilization variables. We assessed differences in 6-month change scores for time-varying variables. We also examined whether asking participants to consent prior to the final questionnaire impacted completion of that questionnaire. Of 616 possible participants, 42% consented, 44% refused, and 14% failed to respond. Differences by ethnicity were found, with Hispanics more likely to consent. There was a consistent tendency for those who participated most in the *National Study* to consent. With the exception of number of chronic diseases, there was no evidence of health indicators or health behaviors being associated with consenting. Participants with more physician visits and more nights in the hospital were also more likely to consent. Those asked to consent before the 12-month follow-up questionnaire were less likely to complete that questionnaire than those who were asked after. Fewer than half consented to link to their Medicare data. The greater willingness to consent by those who participated most suggests that willingness to consent may be part of program engagement. Consenters had more diseases, more MD visits, and more nights in the hospital, suggesting that greater contact with the medical system may be associated with willingness to consent. This indicates that examinations of Medicare data based only on those willing to consent could introduce bias. Asking for consent appears to reduce participation in the larger study.

Keywords: chronic disease self-management, patient education, Medicare, consenting, cost analysis

INTRODUCTION

Most of what we know about the effectiveness of evidence-based chronic disease self-management programs (CDSMP) comes from self-reports of health and health-care outcomes experienced by participants (1). In 2010, the National Council on Aging (NCOA), the Stanford Patient Education Research Center and Texas A&M Health Science Center's Program on Healthy Aging initiated a major longitudinal nation-wide U.S. study of participants in a dissemination of the Stanford CDSMP (2). The primary purposes of the project were to inform NCOA's technical assistance work and assessing the impact of the program when offered in a variety of "real world" settings across the nation. Baseline enrollment of study participants began in August 2010 and ended in April 2011, with subsequent collection of 6- and 12-month follow-up survey data. That study is known as the *U.S. National Study of the CDSMP* (referred to as the *National Study*), and details of the intervention and the self-reported outcomes have been published elsewhere (3, 4, 5, Ory et al. in prepartion).

After completion of the initial intervention and during the collection of follow-up questionnaires, the Centers for Medicare & Medicaid Services (CMS) contracted with NCOA for a pilot study to examine the feasibility of matching *National Study* participants with their CMS data. Linking with administrative claims data would provide an alternative and potentially more precise method for examination of health-care utilization and associated costs savings attributed to program participation.

Because consent to match study data with CMS data was not obtained at the beginning of the *National Study*, all potential subjects had to provide supplemental consent for the specific purposes of having their CDSMP data linked to CMS Medicare Administrative Data. A subset of *National Study* participants who were at least 65.5 years of age at the beginning of the *National Study* were invited to enroll in the CMS study. This paper reports about this consenting process and how consenters differed from: (a) those who actively declined to participate (refusers); and (b) those who did not respond (non-responders). Institutional Review Board (IRB) approval was obtained at Stanford University and Texas A&M University for the initial National Study and for the subsequent consenting study reported in this paper.

MATERIALS AND METHODS

CONSENTING PROTOCOL

There were several steps to the consenting process. We started by mailing consent requests to 188 participants who had recently completed their 6-month questionnaires and had been 65.5 or older at the beginning of the *National Study.* The process would continue as other participants completed or would have completed 6- or 12-month follow-up questionnaires. These first mailings occurred in August and September 2011. Potential participants were asked to provide the last four digits of their social security number (SSN) and to consent to allow their study identifying information to be used to obtain Medicare claims data. There was an initial assumption that having a partial SSN would accelerate the matching process. After 3 weeks and several follow-up or attempted follow-up contacts by telephone, only 23% of the initial 188 potential participants had consented. Feedback from participants revealed some concerns about providing SSNs. We therefore suspended the consenting process and modified the protocol for those who had not yet responded and for subsequent mailings. In the revised protocol, we asked participants for permission to match their study identifying data with their Medicare data using name, gender, address, and date of birth – four identifiers that we hypothesized would yield fairly accurate matches with CMS records. Detailed information on processes for linking various administrative data sets can be found elsewhere (6, 7). Given the low initial response rate and stated concerns among older adults about revealing such highly identifiable information, requests for any part of participants' SSNs were dropped. The following six-step protocol was followed for the remainder of the study.

Step 1: Each potential participant received a short hand-addressed note explaining the CMS study and telling them that in a few days they would receive a gray envelope containing the study details, consent forms, and a small gift. The gray envelope was used so that the mailing could not be confused with the *National Study* questionnaires, which were sent out in white envelopes.
Step 2: Three days later consent forms were mailed along with a gift of four "forever" stamps.
Step 3: Five to 10 days later at least two calls were made. Messages were left on the second calls if participants were not yet reached.
Step 4: Two weeks later those who had not responded received a post card reminder.
Step 5: One month after the first mailing, those who had not responded received a second consent-form mailing.
Step 6: Approximately 6 weeks after the initial mailing, phone calls were made to participants. At least three attempts were made to reach each participant. Consents could be obtained on the phone if study participants allowed the research assistant to read the entire five-page consent statement prior to accepting via verbal consent.

DATA ANALYSES

Primary analyses compare those who consented to participate in the CMS study with those who were eligible to participate (were enrolled or likely to be enrolled in Medicare) but did not consent. The latter group consisted of two subsets, those who actively declined to participant and those who did not respond to consent requests. Consequently, two additional sets of comparisons were conducted comparing: (1) those who consented to those who actively declined; and (2) those who either consented and/or declined (responded) to those who did not respond to the mailings and phone calls. Given the study emphasis on who would actively consent to have their data linked, only those able to give consents (e.g., living participants) were included in these analyses.

Comparisons between groups of individuals (consenters, refusers, and non-responders) were made using demographic, CDSMP workshop participation, health indicator, health behavior, and health-care utilization variables (described below). Differences between groups were tested using independent sample t-test for continuous variables, chi-squares for categorical variables, and non-parametric (Wilcoxon) tests for low frequency medical utilization variables.

The consent forms were first mailed to all potential participants after they had the opportunity to complete 6-month or, in the case of the earliest *National Study* recruitment cohorts, 12-month follow-up questionnaires. Thus, we were also able to examine whether 6-month changes were related to whether participants consented, refused, or did not respond. We compared mean changes on two health indicators, three health behaviors, and three health-care utilization measures.

MEASURES

Demographic variables included age, gender, number of years of education, and ethnic identification (African-American, Hispanic, or non-Hispanic white). CDSMP program participation was measured in a number of ways. Both the mean number of workshop sessions attended (out of a possible six) and completion of the program (defined as having attended at least four of the six sessions) were tabulated. Assuming that those who had previously consented to be in a sub-study might differ from those who had not, we calculated the percentage of National Study participants who were also participating in a sub-study for people with Type 2 diabetes and had agreed to furnish blood samples for testing hemoglobin A1c levels (8). Finally, we tabulated the proportions of participants who completed 6- and 12-month follow-up questionnaires as part of the larger *National Study.*

Three health indicators were measured. These consisted of the mean number of comorbid conditions reported, PHQ-8 depression, and self-reported general health. The PHQ-8 consists of eight items, which are summed resulting in a range of 0–24 (9). The self-reported general health measure consists of a single-item ranging from one (excellent) to five (poor) and was originally used in the National Health Interview Survey (10). For each of the three measures, a higher score is less desirable (more conditions, greater depressive symptoms, and worse overall health).

The three health behaviors were whether exercised during the past week, communication with physician and medication adherence. The exercise measure was a single-item that asked if the participant had participated in physical activity or exercise within the last week. Communication with physician scale is a 3-item, 6-point scale and was developed to evaluate the CDSMP and related programs and has been described by Lorig and colleagues (11). Medication adherence was the sum of four questions regarding medication use (12). A higher score indicates less medication adherence.

We also examined three measures of health-care utilization: physician visits, emergency department visits, and nights of hospitalization in the previous 6-months. These self-report measures have been found to be relatively unbiased when compared to health provider records in an earlier study (13).

We calculated completion rates of 12-month follow-up questionnaires for those who were asked to consent before 12-month follow-up and those with consent forms sent after the 12-month follow-up period. This was to help ascertain if the consent process might have affected participation in follow-up within the larger study.

RESULTS

PARTICIPANTS

At the time CMS consent requests and forms were mailed, there were a total of 639 *National Study* participants who were the appropriate age to have Medicare (65.5 or older). These people were mailed CMS consent requests between August and December 2011 (**Figure 1**). Of the 639, 21 subsequently indicated that they were not participating in Medicare for a variety of reasons but mainly because they were still employed and/or had other medical insurance, including veterans' benefit. This left 618 participants with Medicare. An additional two had died before receiving the mailing, as had 6 participants who were known to have died before the mailing. The eight deceased individuals (six who were never sent consent forms and two who were) are not included in these analyses. Thus, there were 616 participants (618 minus the 2 who were discovered to have been deceased) who could have actively consented to participate. Of these, 260 consented, 169 by mail, and 91 by phone. Two-hundred sixty-nine actively declined, while 87 did not respond. In summary, of the 616 eligible participants, 42% consented to participate, 44% declined to participate, and 14% did not respond.

NON-RESPONDERS

Of the 87 who did not respond, 12 indicated they did not want to be called or hung up and were put on a "do-not-call" list. There were 20 participants who were contacted and indicated they would return the forms but never did. These included seven who mentioned being ill and seven who indicated they were very busy, including two with deaths in the family. Two thought they had returned the forms, four said they had not received the forms and four requested we call back but were not reached. The remaining 45 were never contacted (failed to respond to mail or phone messages, had no or full answering machines, or had no or disconnected phone numbers).

DIFFERENCES BETWEEN CONSENTERS, REFUSERS, AND NON-RESPONDERS AT BASELINE

Table 1 shows the mean of continuous measures or the percentage of categories at baseline for each of the three groups of

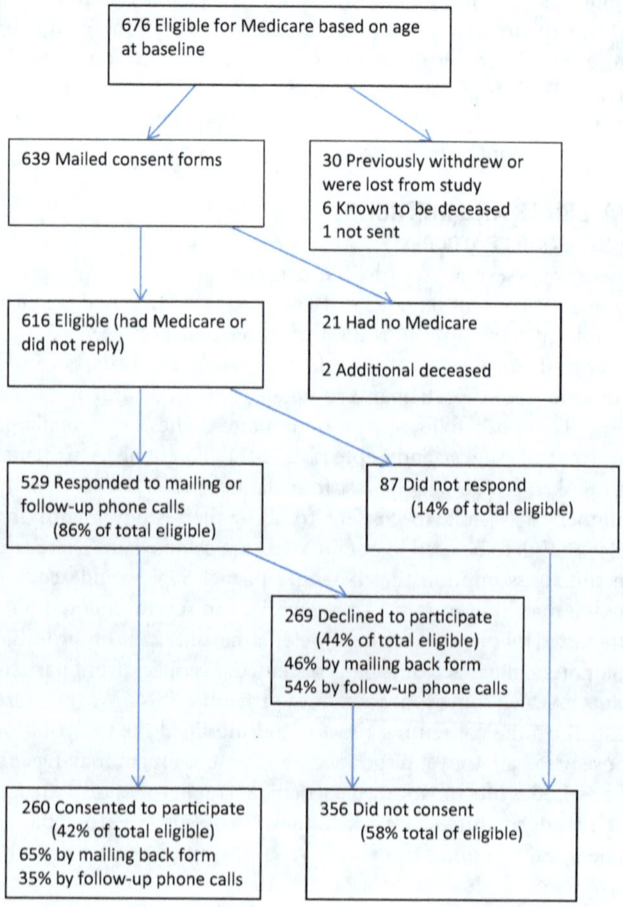

FIGURE 1 | Status of CDSMP participants invited to participate in Medicare cost study.

potential CMS study participants. The last three columns present the P-values for three sets of comparisons. The first column compares those who consented with all those who did not consent (both refusers and non-responders). The second column shows results from the comparison of those who consented with those who actively declined to consent. The last column examines the comparison of those who responded with those who did not respond.

Among the demographic variables, there was little difference in age, education, or gender. The non-response group had higher proportions of African-Americans and Hispanics. In addition, among those who responded, the consenters had greater proportions of African-Americans and Hispanics than did the refusers, although the differences were only marginally significant for African-Americans ($p = 0.057$). The proportion Hispanic was significantly higher for consenters when compared to both refusers and to all others. Described in another way (not shown in the table), Hispanics were more likely to consent than non-Hispanics (53 versus 40%, $p = 0.026$). African-Americans were more likely to not respond than non-African-Americans (22 versus 13%, $p = 0.027$). Non-Hispanic whites had the lowest level of non-response (11 versus 20% for others, $p = 0.002$).

Table 1 | Baseline participant and workshop characteristics among CDSMP national study participants by consented, refused, or failed to respond to invitation to participate in Medicare cost study.

Baseline characteristic	Consented ($N = 260$)	Refused ($N = 269$)	No response ($N = 87$)	*P*-value (A) consent versus no consent	*P*-value (B) consent versus decline	*P*-value (C) response versus no response
DEMOGRAPHIC CHARACTERISTICS						
Mean age	73.7 (5.07)	74.2 (5.08)	73.7 (5.17)	0.419	0.315	0.707
Mean years of education	13.1 (3.97)	13.2 (3.23)	12.6 (4.4)	0.997	0.623	0.261
Percent male	16.5%	16.7%	16.1%	0.991	0.953	0.900
Percent African-American	15.0%	12.6%	23.0%	0.388	0.432	0.057
Percent Hispanic	18.9%	9.29%	21.8%	*0.031*	*0.002*	0.098
Percent non-Hispanic White	61.5%	68.3%	47.6%	0.660	0.104	0.002
WORKSHOP PARTICIPATION						
Mean number of sessions attended (0–6)	4.92 (1.61)	4.23 (1.96)	4.13 (1.89)	*<0.001*	*<0.001*	*0.037*
Completed program (4+)	85.5%	72.9%	69.0%	*<0.001*	*<0.001*	*0.033*
Participated in HbA1c study	12.7%	9.29%	5.75%	0.084	0.211	0.137
Completed 6-month questionnaire	95.0%	90.0%	48.3%	*<0.001*	*0.029*	*<0.001*
Completed 12-month questionnaire	92.3%	80.3%	35.6%	*<0.001*	*<0.001*	*<0.001*
HEALTH INDICATORS						
Number of Chronic diseases	3.03 (1.55)	2.78 (1.45)	2.44 (1.18)	*0.005*	0.052	*0.001*
PHQ depression	5.35 (4.56)	4.79 (4.43)	6.06 (5.10)	0.513	0.155	0.061
General health	3.07 (0.882)	2.99 (0.916)	3.14 (0.904)	0.516	0.282	0.302
HEALTH BEHAVIORS						
% Exercised (past week)	76.5%	76.1%	71.3%	0.809	0.908	0.313
Communication with MD	2.66 (1.33)	2.81 (1.32)	2.57 (1.46)	0.421	0.202	0.276
Medication adherence	0.808 (1.05)	0.732 (0.971)	0.779 (1.04)	0.440	0.392	0.935
HEALTH-CARE UTILIZATION						
# of physician visits	3.80 (3.54)	3.29 (3.20)	2.52 (3.07)	0.012	0.081	*0.009*
# ED visits	0.142 (0.411)	0.205 (0.610)	0.118 (0.359)	0.658	0.486	0.526
# of hospital nights	0.946 (4.08)	0.300 (1.02)	0.977 (4.90)	*0.045*	0.063	0.468

For means, standard deviations are given in parentheses. Percentages are the percent within each of the three categories (consenters, refusers, and non-responders) that belong to the variable (e.g., 16.5% of consenters were male compared to 16.7% of refusers).

P-values are from chi-square test for categorical variables and from independent sample t-tests for continuous variables, except number of ED visits and number of hospital nights, which are from Wilcoxon rank sum tests. P(A) compares those who consented ($N = 260$) with all who did not consent ($N = 356$). P(B) compares those who consented ($N = 260$) with those who actively declined to consent ($N = 269$). P(C) compares those who responded ($N = 529$) with those who did not respond ($N = 87$).

P-values less than 0.05 are shown in italics.

There were a number of significant differences in workshop participation indicators. Consenters attended more sessions, were more likely to have completed the program and more likely to return 6- and 12-month questionnaires. Those who had already consented to participate in the diabetes A1c study were also more highly represented among consenters than non-consenters, but the difference was not statistically significant ($p = 0.084$).

The mean number of comorbid chronic conditions was greater among those who consented and lower among those who did not respond. The other two health indicators (depression and self-reported overall health) did not differ significantly among the three groups. Similarly, there were no statistical differences among baseline health behaviors.

There were two significant differences in baseline self-reported health-care utilization. Consenters had a higher mean number of physician visits in the last 6 months compared to all non-consenters and to non-responders. Consenters also had a higher number of hospital nights than those who did not consent.

SIX-MONTH CHANGES IN HEALTH INDICATORS, BEHAVIORS, AND UTILIZATION

No significant differences were found in 6-month changes in the two health indicators (depression and self-reported overall health) and three health behaviors (exercise, communication with physician, and medication adherence) among the three groups (**Table 2**). Among health-care utilization measures, those who consented had a 6-month increase in emergency department visits compared to those who refused to consent or did not consent overall. Although not significant, non-responders had greater reductions in hospitalizations than did consenters, while those who actively refused slightly increased their nights of hospitalization. As

Table 2 | Six-month changes, among CDSMP national study participants by consented, refused, or failed to respond to invitation to participate in Medicare cost study.

Baseline measure	Consented ($N = 246$)	Refused ($N = 241$)	No response ($N = 42$)	P-value (A) consent versus no consent	P-value (B) consent versus decline	P-value (C) response versus no response
HEALTH INDICATORS						
PHQ depression	−0.614 (3.85)	−0.575 (4.05)	−0.610 (4.28)	0.923	0.914	0.981
General health	−0.069 (0.721)	−0.575 (4.05)	−0.095 (0.932)	0.805	0.721	0.799
HEALTH BEHAVIORS						
% Exercised (past week)	0.094 (0.465)	0.075 (0.450)	0.122 (0.557)	0.762	0.644	0.620
Communication with MD	0.122 (1.14)	0.201 (1.15)	−0.283 (0.986)	0.922	0.466	*0.023*
Medication adherence	−0.036 (1.01)	−0.074 (1.04)	0.214 (1.18)	0.958	0.682	0.107
HEALTH-CARE UTILIZATION						
No. of physician visits	0.150 (3.55)	0.148 (3.82)	0.366 (3.00)	0.925	0.995	0.713
No. ED visits	0.029 (0.602)	−0.113 (0.196)	0.0 (0.392)	*0.046*	*0.032*	0.754
No. of hospital nights	−0.154 (5.77)	0.188 (2.38)	−0.50 (2.39)	0.835	0.696	0.518

Standard deviations are given in parentheses. P-values are from independent sample t-tests, except number of ED visits and number of hospital nights, which are from Wilcoxon rank sum tests. P (A) compares those who consented (N= 246) with all who did not consent (N= 281). P (B) compares those who consented (N= 246) with those who actively declined to consent (N= 241). P (C) compares those who responded (N= 487) with those who did not respond (N= 40). P-values less than 0.05 are shown in italics.

noted above, non-response for consents was associated with lower return of 6-month questionnaires – only 48% of non-responders had completed 6-month questionnaires compared to 92% of responders ($p < 0.001$). Thus, the reduction in hospitalizations among the non-responders may reflect a biased subset of all non-responders.

DIFFERENCES BETWEEN TIMING OF THE CONSENT REQUESTS

There were 356 participants who were asked to consent after completing the 6-month study period but before being asked to complete 12-month questionnaires. These consisted of all those who had entered the *National Study* in 2011. There were 251 participants who were asked to consent after completing the 12-month follow-up period (those who entered the study during 2010). Of those who were asked to consent after 12 months in the study, 84% had completed 12-month questionnaires. In contrast, only 76% of those who were asked to consent before 12 months eventually completed a 12-month questionnaire ($p = 0.020$ from chi-square).

There were no statistically significant associations between the proportions of participants who consented and when participants were asked. Among those who responded, the proportion who consented was 49.5% for those asked before 12 months and 48.6% for those who had completed the 12-month follow-up period (not shown in tables).

DISCUSSION

RESULTS

These data present a unique opportunity to examine factors associated with older adults' willingness to consent to have their programmatic data linked to administrative claims data. This information is important for identifying potential systematic biases in assessing programmatic impacts using administrative data and guiding future initiatives desiring to link data sources *post hoc*.

The most notable differences between consenters and non-consenters were among the workshop participation variables. Consenters (versus non-consenters) and responders (versus non-responders) attended more sessions and were more likely to complete the program and both 6- and 12-month follow-up questionnaires. This is not unexpected and suggests that those more engaged with the program or with their health-care are more likely to be willing to share their Medicare information.

There were little differences in demographic conditions between the three groups, with the exception of ethnicity. Hispanic and African-Americans were less likely to respond. In contrast, among those who responded, members of these two minority groups were more likely to consent. While non-Hispanic white participants were more likely to respond, they were also more likely to decline to consent.

Although few statistically significant differences in health indicators and health behaviors were found between consenters and non-consenters, participants who consented reported more illnesses or more contact with the medical system. The consenters had higher mean number of self-reported conditions and physician visits at baseline as well as less decreases in ED visits at 6 months than those who did not consent.

While non-responders had a mean of 0.5 days decrease in hospital nights at 6-months, over 50% of the 6-month data was missing for that group. Thus, in our case, any attempt to estimate possible changes in medical expenditures for non-respondents would be subject to bias resulting from the high attrition rate. The likelihood that consenters were both more engaged with their health-care self-management and were likely to have greater numbers of chronic conditions would introduce further bias into studies of Medicare utilization.

IMPLICATIONS: THE CONSENTING PROCESS

There is increased concern about the third arm of the Triple Aims for Health-Care, e.g., wanting to document that effective interventions can be provided for better value (14) and lower costs. Thus, cost effectiveness of interventions is becoming more important. To determine costs and cost effectiveness, at least for older adults, examining Medicare claims data is treated as a "gold standard." To gain such access, participants must usually sign an informed consent. Little is known about the population that consents to examination of their claims data as opposed to those who decline. This study opens a window into these differences.

The best variable for matching data is SSN or at least the last four digits of this number. In our study, only 23% of the initial potential participant population was willing to disclose this number within 3 weeks involving multiple contacts. Even after exhaustive follow-up involving as many as eight attempted contacts, only 42% of the population was willing to consent to having any data used for matching to Medicare data, while 44% actively refused consent.

Of equal importance, we found several significant differences between those who consented and those who did not. Of particular interest are both the baseline differences and 6-month differences in changes in self-reported health-care utilization. If these differences are mirrored in Medicare claims data, it brings to question conclusions regarding the cost effectiveness of these evidence-based interventions. We must acknowledge that such conclusions represent only those who consent and that consenters may represent less than half the population. Furthermore, this population differs in several ways from those who do not consent.

This study highlights limitations in using Medicare or claims data as the sole standard for assessing cost outcomes, if consent is required. Unfortunately, in a free society without a nationalized health service database, it is almost impossible to secure unbiased estimates of costs. It is beyond the scope of this paper to discuss the problems with self-report, billing, or insurance payments. All have well-known problems. We would suggest that the solution to this conundrum is to use two or more methods of estimating costs and triangulating outcomes.

There are at least two other disadvantages for a retrospective consenting process for seniors enrolled in evidence-based programs. First, the personnel costs must be considered. In the case of this study, it took one-and-one-half full-time positions over more than 3 months to attempt to consent just over 600 people.

The second disadvantage is the potential of people opting not to participate in studies, programs, or treatment when consent to examine claims data is required. In the fall of 2013, the Agency for Community Living (ACL) began asking participants in evidence-based community programs funded by the agency to voluntarily consent to having their ZIP Codes and birth dates matched with Medicare data. While it is not known if people did not attend programs because of this request, ACL did receive many complaints from sites and the consenting process was dropped when CMS decided the data would not be needed.

In the study presented here, we estimate that at least 7% of those who had completed 6-month questionnaires and were contacted by phone with a request to consent, both refused to consent and asked to be dropped from the original *National Study* before completing 12-month questionnaires (12 participants). In addition, 6% of the 87 non-respondents refused further contact (5 participants who were put on the do-not-call list) and subsequently did not complete 12-month questionnaires after having completed 6-month questionnaires. Thus, we are aware of at least 17 specific participants in the ongoing study who were likely lost to follow-up as a result of being contacted with a request to consent. Of those who were asked to consent after completion of the 12-month follow-up period, 84% had completed 12-month questionnaires. In contrast, only 76% of those who were asked to consent before 12 months eventually completed a 12-month questionnaire. This suggests that as many as 28 out of 356 participants did not complete 12-month questionnaires and likely would have if they had not been asked to consent. It appears clear that the consenting process contributed to attrition in the larger study. For the *National Study*, where consenting at recruitment was no longer an option, there likely would have had less effect on participation in follow-up questionnaires if we had delayed the consent process for all participants until after all follow-up was completed.

LIMITATIONS

The study to match Medicare data with *National Study* data was conceived and initiated after the *National Study* was well underway. Thus, we lost the opportunity to learn if consent rates might have been different had participants been asked to consent at the time of enrollment in the larger intervention and study. There were little differences in rates of consenting between those who were asked 6 months after entering the study versus those who were asked to consent after the 12-month follow-up period, but it is possible consent rates would have been higher at baseline. However, based on the greater attrition rate among those who were asked to consent before the final follow-up questionnaire, it is likely that asking for consent to match to Medicare data earlier might have reduced participation rates during the initial enrollment in the overall study.

This study was limited to the consenting process and comparing consenters versus others. As noted in the Section "Materials and Methods," we do not address the actual matching of participant data with CMS Medicare data for those who consented to allow such matching. The matching process is described elsewhere (6). Nor do we attempt to offer solutions for several issues raised. The findings suggest the need for future research on the problem of increased attrition among those asked to allow matching, and on the problem of differences between consenters and non-consenters resulting in bias.

We present a large number of comparisons in **Table 1**. Because of the exploratory nature of this study, we have not attempted to adjust for multiple comparisons. Thus caution should be exercised in drawing conclusions from any single statistically significant result. Of more importance are the patterns in the results, specifically the tendency of consenters to be more involved with the medical system and to be more involved or engaged in the intervention and larger *National Study*. Further study of the ethnic differences in consenting would be highly desirable.

CONCLUSION

Fewer than half the eligible participants consented to link their name, gender, age, and ZIP Code to Medicare data. Those who consented were significantly different in several ways from those who chose not to consent or who did not respond. In particular, consenters may have had more contact with the medical system and more illness. This suggests that data based only on those who consent may be biased toward greater medical utilization and costs. The findings also suggest that asking participants to consent to match Medicare data may reduce participation in an intervention study. These findings have a potential to affect the use of data for policy decisions based on linking Medicare data with specific interventions.

ACKNOWLEDGMENTS

Support was provided by the Centers for Medicare and Medicaid Services through contract # HHSM-500-2011-00088C. Nancy Whitelaw of the National Council on Aging was a principal investigator for the *National Study.* Mirna Sanchez of the Stanford Patient Education Research Center assisted in the management of that study and the consenting process.

REFERENCES

1. Brady TJ, Murphy L, O'Colmain BJ, Beauchesne D, Daniels B, Greenberg M, et al. Meta-analysis of health status, health behaviors, and health care utilization outcomes of the chronic disease self-management program. *Prev Chronic Dis* (2013) **10**:120112. doi:10.5888/pcd10.120112
2. Lorig KR, Sobel DS, Stewart AL, Brown BW, Bandura A, Ritter P, et al. Evidence suggesting that a chronic disease self-management program can improve health status while reducing hospitalization: a randomized trial. *Med Care* (1999) **37**(1):5–14. doi:10.1097/00005650-199901000-00003
3. Ory MG, Ahn S, Jiang L, Lorig K, Ritter P, Laurent DD, et al. National study of chronic disease self-management: six-month outcome findings. *J Aging Health* (2013) **25**:1258. doi:10.1177/0898264313502531
4. Ory MG, Ahn S, Jiang L, Smith ML, Ritter PL, Whitelaw N, et al. Successes of a national study of the chronic disease self-management program: meeting the triple aim of health care reform. *Med Care* (2013) **51**(11):992–8. doi:10.1097/MLR.0b013e3182a95dd1
5. Ahn S, Basu R, Smith ML, Jiang L, Lorig K, Whitelaw N, et al. The impact of chronic disease self-management programs: healthcare savings through a community-based intervention. *BMC Public Health* (2013) **13**:1141. doi:10.1186/1471-2458-13-1141
6. Lorden AL, Radcliff TA, Jiang L, Horel SA, Smith ML, Lorig K, et al. Leveraging administrative data for program evaluations: a method for linking datasets without unique identifiers. *Eval Health Prof* (2014). doi:10.1177/0163278714547568
7. National Council on Aging. *Pilot Report of the Chronic Disease Self-Management Program, Contract HHSM-500-2011-00088C.* Washington, DC: Report submitted to the Centers for Medicare and Medicare Services (CMS) (2013).
8. Lorig K, Ritter PL, Ory MG, Whitelaw N. Effectiveness of the chronic disease self-management program for with type 2 diabetes: a translation study. *Diabetes Educ* (2013) **39**(5):655–63. doi:10.1177/0145721713492567
9. Kroenke K, Strine TW, Spritzer RL, Williams JB, Berry JT, Mokdad AH. The PHQ-8 as a measure of current depression in the general population. *J Affect Disord* (2009) **114**(1–3):163–73. doi:10.1016/j.jad.2008.06.026
10. Idler EL, Angel RJ. Self-rated health and mortality in the NHANES-I epidemiologic follow-up study. *Am J Public Health* (1990) **80**:446–52. doi:10.2105/AJPH.80.4.446
11. Lorig K, Stewart A, Ritter P, González V, Laurent D, Lynch J. *Outcome Measures for Health Education and Other Health Care Interventions.* Thousand Oaks CA: Sage Publications (1996).
12. Morisky DE, Green LW, Levine DM. Concurrent and predictive validity of a self-reported measure of medication adherence. *Med Care* (1986) **24**:67–74. doi:10.1097/00005650-198601000-00007
13. Ritter PL, Stewart AL, Kaymaz H, Sobel DS, Bloch DA, Lorig KR. Self-reports of health care utilization compared to provider records. *J Clin Epidemiol* (2001) **54**:136–41. doi:10.1016/S0895-4356(00)00261-4
14. Berwick DM, Nolan TW, Whittington J. The triple aim: care, health, and cost. *Health Aff* (2008) **27**:759–69. doi:10.1377/hlthaff.27.3.759

15

Factors supporting implementation among CDSMP organizations

Deborah Paone*

Paone & Associates, LLC, Minneapolis, MN, USA

Edited by:
Matthew Lee Smith, The University of Georgia, USA

Reviewed by:
Samuel D. Towne, The University of South Carolina, USA
Danice Brown Greer, The University of Texas at Tyler, USA

****Correspondence:***
Deborah Paone, Paone & Associates, LLC, 10413 Rhode Island Circle, Minneapolis, MN 55438, USA
e-mail: deborahpaone@paoneandassociates.com

Reaching individuals who can benefit from evidence-based health promotion and disability prevention programs is a goal of federal, state, and local agencies as well as researchers, providers, community agencies, and other stakeholders. Implementation effectiveness at the organizational level must be achieved in order to reach these individuals and sustain the program. This mixed methods study examined eight organizations within two states that successfully implemented the Chronic Disease Self-Management Program (CDSMP) and sustained it from 4 to 10 years. There were two types of organizations: aging services and health care. Internal and external implementation factors and influences were explored. Additional examination of state activities (as a key external agent supporting CDSMP implementation) was conducted. The examination found agreement among the eight organizations regarding why they had adopted the CDSMP – citing the alignment between the program and their organizations' mission and purpose to improve health status and promote better self-care, and the demonstrated value (benefits) of the program. Organizations were also alike in that they described the importance of an internal champion and supportive senior leader. Organizations differed in how they experienced and valued peer support and collaborative networks. Organizations also differed in how they filled their CDSMP workshops. Internal drivers and capability were more often discussed as facilitating successful implementation than external factors. However, state activities and external support enabled successful adoption – particularly funding and training. The primary challenges identified by this set of organizations included difficulty in recruiting participants (filling workshops) and irregular or insufficient funding sources. These challenges were identified as significant and represented barriers to sustaining the program.

Keywords: implementation, evidence-based health promotion, organizational capacity, implementation factors, sustainability, chronic disease self-management program

INTRODUCTION

Reaching individuals who can benefit from evidence-based health promotion (EBHP) and disability prevention programs is an important goal for public health. Stakeholders for successful EBHP program dissemination and implementation include: the individual/consumer, program manager or champion within an organization, the organizational executive, a purveyor or external agent such as the state department of health or of aging, funding organizations, national program centers maintaining fidelity-monitoring, federal agencies, and policymakers. Decisions made at each level can change the landscape for effective implementation.

Evidenced-based programs can be viewed as complex innovations – those requiring multiple inputs within an organization or system. The path from adoption to sustainability of evidence-based programs is often characterized by a series of fits and starts, with internal and external forces affecting progress. For example, Fixsen, Blasé, and colleagues place special emphasis on *human capability and systems* [emphasis added] that support the practitioner/worker implementing the program (1). Because implementation is so dependent on human behavior, successful and sustained implementation will require ongoing training, coaching, feedback, data, and other systems working in tandem to regularly maintain the desired behavior [(1), p. 4]. Durlak and DuPre focus on environment/context and implementation structure and factors that influence the implementation process including: community participation/collaboration, provider characteristics, innovation characteristics, organizational capacity, and technical assistance/training (2). Greenhalgh and colleagues describe a good "innovation to system fit" as a key factor where the existing values, norms, strategies, goals, skill mix, supporting technologies, and ways of working are aligned (3).

Other internal factors influencing implementation success at the organizational level include: organizational leadership, organizational climate, staff capability, staff buy-in, and acceptability to the consumer, patient, or client (4–8). External factors found to be important to include: technical assistance and availability of adequate resources (9, 10). Community-based organizations, in particular, may have additional challenges or constraints requiring adaptation to the type or level of technical assistance, or to the protocol itself (10, 11). For example, one study of community-based organizations found that barriers to EBHP program adoption included: resource constraints, program adaptation challenges, and conflicts with organizational culture (12).

CHRONIC DISEASE SELF-MANAGEMENT PROGRAM

The Chronic Disease Self-Management Program (CDSMP) is an evidence-based program for adults with chronic disease to encourage these individuals to better manage and maintain their health status. The development of the CDSMP evolved from knowledge and practice experience gained from the Arthritis Self-Management Program [(13), p. 680]. The CDSMP is designed to build on the strengths and capability of individuals – including belief in their own abilities, knowledge of what to do regarding their condition, and behavior skills to address situations that arise (13). The program was tested in a randomized controlled trial of 952 subjects receiving the CDSMP from community-based program sites in the 1990s followed by another study of 831 subjects followed over several years through a longitudinal trial. In both trials, CDSMP proved to have significant positive effects on participants' self-efficacy, levels of exercise, self-reported health, and other health status measures (14). The participant group also had fewer hospital days (14, 15).

One estimate puts a dollar value of potential medical care cost savings at over $4.2 billion – savings that could be realized from better health management if just 10% of persons with chronic conditions participated in the CDSMP (16, 17). In addition to the medical cost savings, there are quality of life benefits for individuals who are more actively engaged in their health management. A study of the health-related outcomes of a sample of 687 CDSMP participants found that significant improvements were observed for health outcomes such as depression, self-assessed health, and unhealthy physical days (18).

The CDSMP follows a 6-week, 2.5 h/week group format and is guided by a tightly scripted protocol that is delivered by certified instructors. Each week, the workshop focuses on a specific self-care management and educational topic. Instructors (two instructors are required for every workshop) follow guidelines and participants set a goal each week to pursue. Participants report on progress they have made, week by week, to the other participants in the group. The format includes facilitated interaction and group sharing. Participants often encourage each other and offer insights into the way they have managed their own conditions.

Dissemination of the CDSMP was fostered through a collaborative initiative (called "Communities Putting Prevention to Work: CDSMP") funded under the American Reinvestment and Recovery Act (ARRA). Two-year grants (2010–2012) totaling $27 million were awarded to 45 states. A program evaluation of this national dissemination initiative for CDSMP was conducted in 2012–2013 (19). This process evaluation focused primarily on the states' (purveyors') activities. The state units on aging and the state or local public health departments most often performed this role. These external agents provided technical assistance, training, fidelity-monitoring, marketing, and other support for a defined period to implementing organizations (19).[1] Such external support is one factor that was examined in the study described in this article.

[1]It should be noted that organizations do not have to be a part of a federal initiative to implement CDSMP.

Given the multiple program components and requirements for both instructors and organizational sponsors of CDSMP, the need for specific marketing or referral methods to attract participants into the program, and the specific funding needed to sustain it, this EBHP program can be considered a complex innovation. Embedding the program and sustaining it requires ongoing commitment by the organization to continue to invest in the training, materials, and outreach to keep the workshops filled and facilitated by instructors who meet the protocol requirements.

STUDY PURPOSE

The ARRA-funded national dissemination and implementation effort for CDSMP provides an opportunity to study the experiences of organizations and a dataset, which can be mined. This study uses that dataset as a starting point to identify a set of organizations that effectively implemented and sustained the CDSMP. To be considered successful, the organizations had to have offered at least four workshops in the 2-year timeframe, with a completion rate of 65% or higher. All organizations had to continue to offer the program at the time of the interviews (2013).

Key informant interviews with organizational managers responsible for the program provided qualitative data. Using a set of internal and external factors that previously have been identified in the literature as important facilitators, this study examined commonalities and differences among two different types of organizations implementing the CDSMP. It focused on common internal facilitators and also explored the type and perceived value of external support provided by a key state agent – the department charged with dissemination of the program.

The research question was:

- "What affected implementation success of the evidence-based CDSMP among eight organizations located in two states – examining a defined set of implementation factors (internal and external)?"

The purpose of this article is to offer insight on implementation of CDSMP from the organizational perspective. Understanding more about what factors or influences positively support organizations on the CDSMP implementation "journey" from adoption to sustainability can help identify what needs to be enhanced, what barriers exist, how some organizations have overcome these barriers, and what lessons they have learned. Such insight can help enhance external supports, such as policy, technical assistance, public health marketing, or fidelity-monitoring as well as clarify internal organizational elements that were important. This knowledge may help increase the likelihood that organizations will effectively implement and sustain the program.

MATERIALS AND METHODS

This mixed methods study examined implementation of CDSMP by eight organizations located in two states (identified as State #1 and State #2) and the support offered by their state agency to facilitate dissemination and implementation. The two states remain unnamed to protect the identity of the respondents. There were two types of organizations included in this sample: aging services organizations (ASOs), including three area agencies on aging and one other aging services provider, and health care organizations (HCOs), including three hospital/clinic systems and one health care center.

DATA SOURCES AND SAMPLE SELECTION

The ARRA dataset (secondary data) and results from an electronic survey (primary data) were used to conduct several iterations of review in order to select the study sample of organizations. The ARRA dataset provided information, by state, on the number and type of organizations that participated in CDSMP implementation from 2010 to 2012 through the ARRA network. States were selected that had participated in a previous national EBHP initiative (from 2006 to 2007). This was done in order to maximize the likelihood that the state had invested time and resources to create structures or processes that fostered dissemination and implementation of these EBHP programs.

There were 24 states that participated in both the prior EBHP initiative and the ARRA grant. The pool was further narrowed to seven states that had at least six ASOs and HCOs. The ARRA dataset was then used to find organizations that met a set of criteria indicating implementation effectiveness for CDSMP. These criteria were: the organization offered at least four workshops within the 2 years of the ARRA initiative, had at least a 65% completion rate, and continued to offer the workshop in 2013. In addition, the CDSMP program manager within the organization had to have institutional memory of the implementation process. Institutional memory is defined as knowledge of the organization's motivation, climate, and/or steps to beginning the program by virtue of being employed by the organization during the timeframe when this occurred.

KEY INFORMANTS AND INTERVIEW PROTOCOLS

The qualitative data source was comprised of 10 semi-structured interviews conducted by telephone by the investigator. The two types of key informants were: (1) state representatives who were the responsible managers for the CDSMP in their state, and (2) organizational representatives who were the managers of the CDSMP within their implementing organizations.

Two semi-structured interview protocols were designed with questions probing a set of pre-defined implementation factors, drawing from the work of Durlak and DuPre, Fixsen, Greenhalgh, and Damschroder (1–3, 20). The investigator pilot-tested the instrument with a CDSMP manager who did not participate in the study. The investigator also had the instrument reviewed by a national program manager providing technical support to CDSMP implementing organizations.

Many of the items on the interview protocol had adjectival responses scaled (best to worst) with a corresponding weight from +2 to −2. This five-point scale is consistent with the scale used by Damschroder (20).

Training in interview techniques was not required as the investigator was a seasoned interviewer, having conducted more than 100 interviews over 20 years of experience in health services evaluation – of both health services professionals as well as laypersons. Key informants provided verbal and written consent. The questions were provided to each key informant at least 1 week prior to the scheduled interview. Each interview took about an hour to conduct. Interviews were recorded and transcribed. The study was submitted to the University of North Carolina Institutional Review Board and determined to be exempt.

Factors probed in the state representative interviews were:

- Drivers of CDSMP dissemination and implementation in the state.
- Type and level of assistance provided to implementing organizations in the state.
- Peer support and communication – whether and how this was fostered within the state.

Factors probed in the organizational interviews included:

- Drivers for adoption within organization – the "will" to do this.
- Program fit.
- Ease of use of the protocol.
- Value.
- External support (particularly state agency support and peer networking).

State agency representatives were interviewed first (April/May 2013). This allowed the investigator to ask questions about the external context in which the implementing organizations had been operating. It provided a picture of the state's activities in fostering CDSMP from the state's perspective, prior to hearing from the organizations. The aging services division was the entity responsible for CDSMP dissemination within State #1. Two representatives from this agency participated in the key informant interview, including the program coordinator who had been in that role for 3 years and the director of the division. One representative from State #2 participated in the key informant interview. This individual had served as the program coordinator since 2007 and was from the department of public health.

Organizational representatives were interviewed second. There were eight organizational key informants (one per organization) who participated in interviews between June and August, 2013. All had been involved in the implementation of CDSMP for their organizations for at least 3 years and all were CDSMP Master Trainers.

RESULTS

The results from the state key informant interviews provide context and background to the organizational data and therefore are offered first.

STATES' PERSPECTIVES – ADOPTION AND EARLY EFFORTS

The technical assistance and dissemination support to implementing organizations from State #1 focused on building the capacity and infrastructure for CDSMP. Drivers for the state included interest in helping elders to stay active and healthy-support for CDSMP and other EBHP programs were included in the State Plan. The state began offering "mini-grants" to aging services providers interested in CDSMP through a competitive application process. The state tapped into the existing network of Area Agencies on Aging. The primary support provided to implementing organizations were start-up grants (to cover workshop direct costs), Master Trainer and Peer Leader training sessions, and the CDSMP workbooks, which were to be given or loaned to participants. This state focused on having a corps of Master Trainers trained by Stanford University. The Master Trainers would then train workshop leaders.

Drivers for CDSMP came from the public health department in State #2. The attraction was the evidence base and the defined purpose/focus for this program, which emphasized personal engagement in one's own health. This state contracted with external agencies to provide technical assistance and support to implementing CDSMP organizations. Through these agencies, the state provided training, workshop materials, marketing support, and fidelity-monitoring. The state also required implementing organizations to participate in peer collaboration and information sharing. Initially, this state paid for the license cost of each funded organization under ARRA. With state support the number of Master Trainers grew substantially.

Comments by these state representatives about early dissemination efforts included:

> We had programs that encouraged health and wellness of seniors – but before 2006 people were not aware of CDSMP. We did not have this evidence-based program. There was only 1 Master Trainer in the whole state. We needed to build capacity and infrastructure. We started with natural partners who had an interest.
>
> We included this kind of focus in our State Plan. There were major goals around empowering older people to stay active and healthy.
>
> We had several organizations that were committed to evidence-based programing and knew about CDSMP. In fact our first training session was led by one of them. We created partnerships with these organizations and partnered with them very closely.
>
> We found interest among organizations that had already had a successful track record of offering the program. It then grew very organically from one organization to another. As it [funding] was made available [for implementing organizations] we worked with organizations all over the state – rural, metro, etc.

One of these states contracted separately with a consultant agency to identify data elements for tracking and monitoring the program. Each funded CDSMP provider organization was required to submit data to the state office on these elements. In 2010, this state adopted a name for CDSMP to be used consistently statewide – this name was branded. In that same year, the state purchased a multi-organizational license for CDSMP for their state. This meant that many organizations that with their own single-organization licenses through Stanford switched to operate under the state's license.

When asked about how information sharing was fostered among CDSMP implementing organizations, these state representatives described their role as conveners and facilitators – providing forums for these organizations to gather and communicate. This included regional meetings, newsletters, and electronic list-serves.

STATES' PERSPECTIVES – IMPLEMENTATION ISSUES AND SUSTAINABILITY

Since the ARRA funding ended, one state has focused on supporting the Master Trainers and ensuring fidelity-monitoring. This state also includes a calendar of workshop offerings on their government website as well as all the forms that CDSMP providers need. With the ARRA funding ended, the other state does not pay license costs for CDSMP providers, nor does it compensate organizations for training costs. The state representative explained that it has a philosophy of local authority and control and also that program sustainability requires embedding at the organizational level. Each organization is expected to create its own business plan to address CDSMP (as well as to support other health promotion, disability prevention programing). The state still provides some funding support to the external agency providing technical assistance and peer collaboration facilitation and marketing assistance. This state also maintains policy support for CDSMP (e.g., it is in the State Plan).

The state representatives offered the following insights about organizational implementation of CDSMP and sustainability:

> I think that an across-the-board issue in implementation is staff turnover and agency redirection as a result . . . Any time [senior] management changes there is a question – will they see the value?
>
> There is a very high investment upfront to become a CDSMP provider organization – heavy staff or volunteer training and certification, etc. That is also an ongoing issue – keeping the volunteers certified and active. They have many reasons why they might drop out including their own health issues.
>
> One thing I've seen is if the organization doesn't truly have the buy-in of the higher level administration, it will struggle when the funding ends. Grants are good for start-up, but a sustainability plan is needed.

ORGANIZATIONAL PERSPECTIVES

The results from the electronic survey showed that most of the eight organizations (75%) had begun offering CDSMP between 2006 and 2009 (one began before 2006 and one started in 2010). All of the organizations had offered at least four CDSMP workshops in the 2-year time period. The range in number of workshops offered spanned from a low of 5 to a high of 21 in this time period. All eight organizations had an overall completion rate[2] of 65% or higher, with a range from 66 to 78%. In addition, all of the organizations reported that they followed the program with fidelity. Thus the electronic survey confirmed these eight organizations met the criteria for inclusion – they represented a group of successful implementers with extensive experience.

Adoption and fit

The examination found agreement among the eight organizations on why the organization had adopted the CDSMP – citing alignment between the program and the organization's purpose related to improving health and promoting better self-care. Many

[2]Completion was defined as the participant completing 4 of the 6 sessions of CDSMP.

organizations had begun implementing the program prior to the ARRA grant funding in 2010 – thus the grant facilitated the work that this set of organizations had already begun (it was not the reason that they adopted the program). Informants frequently discussed the organizational leadership and internal champion for the program. This strong champion for the program (sometimes it was the respondent) was instrumental in getting their organization to adopt and implement CDSMP. For example, this comment was offered:

> I was the champion for the program and then I influenced others. I think the evidence-based nature and availability of the training was what attracted me to CDSMP.

From the beginning and continuing through the time of the interviews – organizational respondents said that CDSMP was seen as a good fit. Even so, CDSMP was often discussed as being somewhat unusual compared to the organization's other services. The structured protocol of CDSMP was what set this program apart from the organizations' usual health education and wellness services.

> This program is a great fit – it fits extremely well. However I would also say that (especially in the beginning) – in some ways it was new. It was outside the norm (the group workshop with a structured protocol) of what we typically did, how we typically provided education.

> The program fits well with the organization. This is because the core concept of CDSMP is one of promoting the individual's self-management.

> Really this is a perfect fit with our organization. All of our volunteers are 55 and older and this program is designed around the idea of peer leaders. That fit perfectly.

Figure 1 provides a side-by-side comparison of the respondents' ratings on "Fit" of CDSMP with their organizations.

Implementation of CDSMP requires a number of components (e.g., organizational licensure, instructor training and use of prescribed guidelines, session scripts and materials, and recruitment of participants). Despite this complexity, the program was often described by informants as relatively easy to adopt. This was true even though many of these organizations had not had any prior experience implementing an EBHP program.

All informants mentioned that the heavily scripted workshop sessions, well-developed content of CDSMP, and required training assisted in implementation. This ease of use was noted by both experienced informants (e.g., community health educators who said they had used evidence-based protocols extensively) and by informants who said they had never used evidence-based protocols. **Figure 2** provides a side-by-side comparison across the eight organizations on "ease of use" of the CDSMP protocol.

> Even though we had never done an evidence-based class, I would say the protocol was very easy to follow. The guidelines were very clear.

> I would say the protocol was very easy because of the partnership we had. When we first started we were under another license-holder's license ... they provided us with technical support and trainings, and the manuals. That made it easy.

> This was somewhat easy in that it was scripted and heavily directed.

Value

Comments about value focused on the participants and benefits they received from the program. Respondents talked about seeing participants make progress on their personal health goals and maintain a commitment to a healthier lifestyle. Respondents also discussed program value in terms of alignment with the future direction for the organization – many mentioned health care reform and the growing awareness of the need to achieve better population health management, prevent disability or decline (**Figure 3**). Comments are offered below:

> This program is of extremely high value. It has proven results. It also attracts volunteers ...

> As we go down the health care reform path, I think this kind of program will be even more valued.

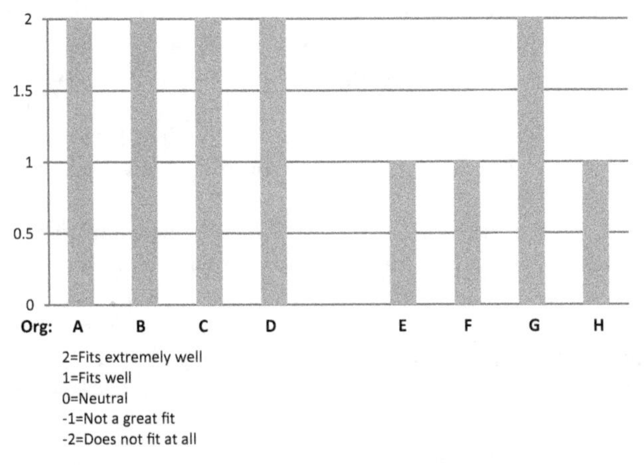

FIGURE 1 | Organizational respondents' rating of CDSMP program "Fit" with their organization.

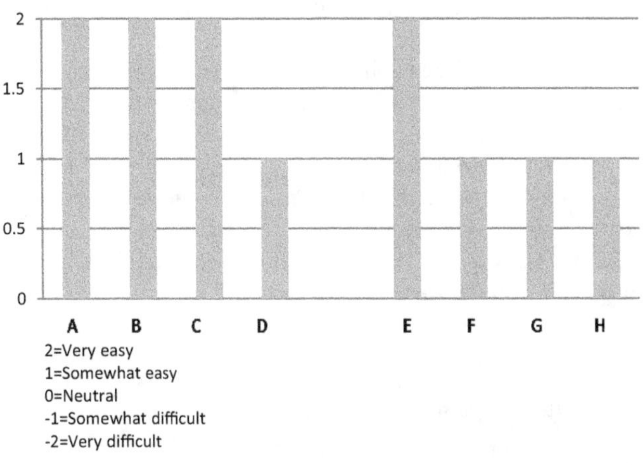

FIGURE 2 | Organizational respondents' rating of "ease of use" of CDSMP protocol during their implementation experience.

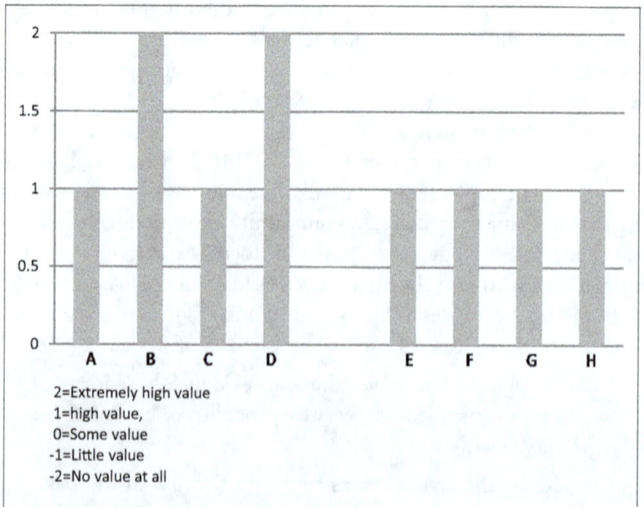

FIGURE 3 | Organizational respondents' rating of "value of CDSMP" to their organizations.

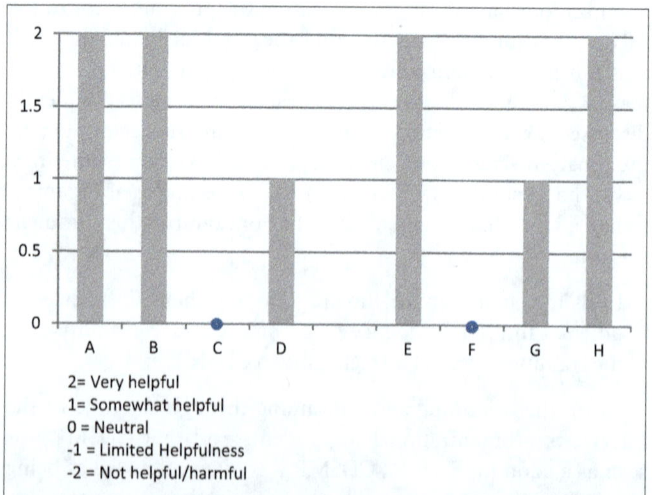

FIGURE 4 | Organizational respondents' rating of "level of external support and helpfulness" during their implementation experience.

External support

One objective of this research was to assess the importance of external support to the organizations implementing CDSMP. The support from the state agency disseminating CDSMP was particularly probed, as the state department responsible for CDSMP dissemination was considered a key purveyor of the program.

Most of the informants indicated that their state agency had assisted with: funding, marketing, training, fidelity-monitoring, supplies, and peer networking. However, the way that these informants valued this support differed from "very helpful" to "neutral." One reason given for the lukewarm rating given by a respondent was that the support from the state had diminished over time.

In addition to the support provided by the state, organizations named other sources of external support including: Stanford University (served as a source of information, provided supplies/materials, and guided fidelity-monitoring), local organizations such as libraries, senior housing facilities, senior centers and hospitals (helped with logistics, provided space, and helped with marketing), and the county health department (helped with peer leader training).

Respondents differed in how they experienced or perceived the level of peer support/collaboration their organizations received. Several remarked they did not receive much of this type of external support. A few said that there was extensive support and collaboration with similar organizations. This may indicate differences in the type or level of support offered – or it may be a function of the individual's or organization's commitment to and efforts around engaging in peer networks and collaborative activities. Comments included:

> The peer collaboration is not growing. It was initially high, but as the program grew, it became minimal.
>
> We have had modest peer collaboration.
>
> There is extensive peer collaboration ... We meet monthly via conference calls and share information and strategies ... We've worked at making this CDSMP operate consistently across the state. We are doing fidelity monitoring the same way across the state and have set up a method to do that, as a peer group. We communicate regularly.

A graphic depiction of the ratings from all eight organizations on the level and helpfulness of external support (a combined score from −2 to +2, corresponding to the adjectival responses) is shown in **Figure 4**.

CHALLENGES

Organizational key informants were asked about their implementation challenges. There was substantial consistency among this set of eight respondents about the challenges they faced in implementing CDSMP and in sustaining the program.

Recruitment/lack of demand

Recruiting participants and filling workshops was the number one challenge described by five of the eight organizational informants. Seven of the eight organizational informants said that it took "very significant effort" (−2) or "significant effort" (−1) to fill the workshops. Stanford fidelity guidelines recommend that class size be from 8 to 16 participants to optimize peer support and problem-solving. Six of the eight organizational representatives said that they have had to cancel a class at some point in time due to insufficient registration. These findings are consistent with other studies (19, 21).

The lack of demand for CDSMP was seen as being an effect of at least two things. First, very few individuals with chronic disease self-identify as needing the program – that is the individual hearing or reading about CDSMP does not interpret the program as being relevant for them. Marketing to consumers directly was challenging. This group of organizational managers instead often sought out other collaborative agencies, such as seniors center managers, senior housing facility managers, case managers, or health coaches to describe and promote the program as well as encourage participation among their clientele. Second, there was a lack of awareness on the part of physicians and other clinical providers about CDSMP and its' benefit. The organizational informants said that they rarely had direct referrals from physicians to the CDSMP workshops (except where the program was a referral option within the health system's medical information system).

Informants described extensive efforts to market the program and educate adults about the benefits of the program. The four aging service organizations more often described their "sales" and "outreach" efforts – going to senior centers, retirement housing facilities, doctor's offices and putting up fliers, including information in newsletters, and networking with local social services agencies. The four HCOs more often described their internal health system connections as sources of referrals, including physicians working in the health system and health coaches.

> Getting the workshops/classes filled is difficult – getting the number of participants we need to hold the class. They need it, but they don't understand that – it has to be sold.
>
> It takes significant effort – marketing and recruitment to fill the workshops.
>
> We have a system of referrals within the clinic. If a provider wants to refer he or she can click on the classes we are offering through our electronic system – then we get the referral and follow-up.

A side-by-side comparison across the eight organizations of ratings on the "Demand/Recruitment" factor is shown in **Figure 5**.

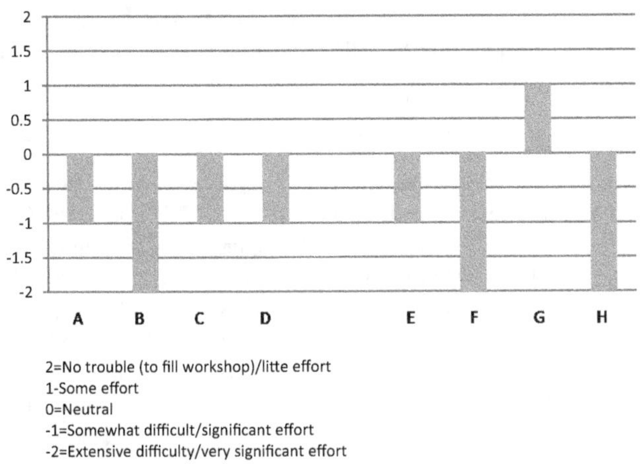

FIGURE 5 | Organizational respondents' ratings on "demand/recruitment factor" – pertaining to the level of effort to fill CDSMP classes during their implementation of this program.

was covering the costs entirely out of their core operational budget – which also relies heavily on grants.

Three of the HCOs talked about the lack of external funding and hospital budget issues. These organizations discussed the shorter-term focus of their organizations where community health education is not seen as core – more of a community benefit. Therefore CDSMP and other health promotion, disease prevention programs are vulnerable to budget cuts. Despite this, one HCO respondent saw the potential for CDSMP. She said it was becoming more relevant for where the health care system is going in terms of accountability for population health. Despite their lack of current external funding, there was some optimism around the growing awareness and support for this type of program among the health care organizational respondents.

> Without additional funding we can't do this on an ongoing basis . . . I only expect to do 1 or 2 [workshops] this year. This is down from the 18 workshops we did in 2011 and 2012.
>
> Hospitals are under a lot of budget restrictions. They are less able to provide this kind of community benefit now. We've had some reductions in staff in community health education. I don't think this is self-sustaining – not so far.
>
> I think there is some potential demand for this – under ACOs there is a commitment to population health and every member within their population. There is a basic level of service to be provided. CDSMP could be part of that.

ORGANIZATIONAL ADVICE

Organizational informants reflected on lessons learned. They used various strategies to address implementation challenges or enhance their programs.

Strategies and advice included:

- Have a strong program champion internally.
- Build and maintain support at all levels internally especially senior administration and managers or clinical professionals who can serve as referral sources internally.
- Pursue a variety of ways to extend reach and improve visibility of CDSMP in order to build external referral sources and tap into collaborative resources (e.g., volunteers, building space for workshop locations, etc.).
- Recruit, train, and retain strong workshop leaders (staff or volunteers).
- Conduct ongoing marketing and outreach to make target population groups (potential participants) aware of the program.
- Measure results. Present a "return on investment" or value proposition to key stakeholders.

DISCUSSION

A study of eight organizations, purposively selected because of long-term successful experience with CDSMP, revealed that internal drivers and capability were more often discussed as facilitating successful implementation than external factors.

FACILITATING FACTORS

Common facilitating factors for adoption and successful implementation of the CDSMP included:

- Program-to-organization fit.
- Organizational leadership.
- Training and well-developed materials.

These factors are consistent with other studies examining program implementation and sustainability. For example, a review of 19 empirical studies of health-related programs found the following factors to be important to the organizations (the study focused on organizations continuing the program at least 2 years following the ending of external funding): program champion, program fit with organizational mission, perceived value/benefits to clients, and support of stakeholders (22).

Program-to-organization fit

These eight organizational informants discussed alignment between the focus and purpose of CDSMP and the overall purpose or mission of their organizations as a facilitating factor in adoption and implementation effectiveness. Others studying implementation success have discussed the importance of fit between the innovation (program) and the organization – particularly the fit with the purpose or *values* of the organization (3, 4). This may be an important baseline criterion for an organization to consider when considering an EBHP program to adopt.

Organizational leadership

The managers responsible for CDSMP discussed both their own leadership as internal champions of the program, and the leadership from their supervisors, department directors, or senior executives – who demonstrated their support for CDSMP adoption and the implementation process. These administrators remained committed to offering the program even with limited funding.

Supportive leadership has been identified elsewhere as an organizational characteristic linked to successful implementation (23). The importance of champions and organizational leadership has been found to be a facilitator to health promotion practices being adopted, implemented, and maintained. For example, in a study of five Canadian provincial efforts to adopt a chronic disease prevention initiative, the research team found that there was "remarkable consistency in the top factors identified as facilitators and barriers to health promotion capacity building" [(7), p. 470]. Internal organizational factors were *most frequently mentioned* as facilitating implementation (more than external factors). Organizational respondents particularly noted the importance of having skilled, committed staff and supportive senior leadership (7). This may be another baseline criterion for organizations when considering EBHP program adoption.

Training and materials

Among these organizations, the CDSMP protocol and training materials were described as well-developed, easy-to-use, and excellent guides. These materials and training sessions worked well for both staff members and volunteers. Researchers of implementation effectiveness have discussed the importance of having quality tools and training (e.g., manuals, guides, worksheets, education, skills development, etc.) to support organizational performance and implementation effectiveness (23).

External support

External support also facilitated implementation among these eight organizations. Key external supports described as "very helpful" by these eight organizations were: (1) funding, (2) training and workshop materials, and (3) fidelity-monitoring. The value of peer support and collaboration varied among this set of respondents – for some organizations this type of support had been (and continued to be) very important. Other organizations had not participated and/or did not rely on peer support very much. These findings are consistent with other research identifying key supports for implementation, including the perceived benefits of using the EB program and collaborative technical assistance or program supports that are matched or tailored to the organization (12). This external support may be particularly important to the organization in the adoption and early implementation phases.

BARRIERS AND THREATS TO SUSTAINABILITY

Common barriers and threats to sustainability included difficulties in recruiting participants, and lack of funding for the program – including lack of participant health insurance coverage for this type of EBHP program. It is likely that these challenges are linked.

Lack of demand

Recruiting participants to the workshops was a key challenge among the organizations in this study. Seven of the eight organizations said that getting participants into the workshops was the number one challenge. Organizations said that there is low awareness of the program among both the lay public and physicians – a key referral source.

The need for better marketing and distribution systems for public health programs has been identified elsewhere. In a study of 32 community-based prevention programs only modest penetration occurred in the marketplace, which limited impact. The researchers called for more effective approaches that "employ a reinforcing combination of both high-risk (targeting) and population-wide strategies" [(24), p. 571]. Others working in public health have pointed out the stark contrast between the sophistication of marketing and distribution systems for products and services in the business sector and the "unassigned, underemphasized, and underfunded" dissemination strategies in the public health sector [(25), p. 215].

Lack of funding/insurance

Since many people with chronic conditions have Medicare as their primary insurance, the fact that CDSMP is not covered by Medicare is an impediment.[3] Medicare beneficiaries (and physicians) may believe that if a service or program is not covered by Medicare, then that service has not been shown to have enough benefit to the patient/consumer to warrant coverage. This has been shown to be true in other studies where the lack of insurance coverage contributed to underuse of proven services, such

[3]The Medicare program does provide coverage for patient education and rehabilitation, most commonly for specific defined time periods and usually related to a new diagnosis, illness, surgical procedure, or injury, or an exacerbation of an existing condition/issue.

as secondary prevention programs in cardiac rehabilitation (26). Other researchers studying implementation and sustainability have noted that fiscal support is a critical external factor in some or all stages of adoption, implementation, and sustainability (6, 27).

While the focus or mission of health care and ASOs may be to assist individuals to improve or maintain health, they are reimbursed largely for addressing problems (after-the-fact), not preventing them. HCOs' reimbursement comes primarily from illness care/treatment not prevention (28). For social service organizations such as area agencies on aging that provide direct services to elders, provision of services is primarily based on an older individual requesting help for an existing problem or need (relying on grant and OAA funding and skewed to those financially vulnerable). Thus, the CDSMP runs into the same challenge that many public health interventions face: lack of funding for prevention.

It is the author's opinion, that without a regular source of funding or payment for service, the "value" of CDSMP has to be demonstrated one person and one provider at a time. The lack of payment for EBHP programs such as CDSMP may be interpreted by the lay public or by physicians as a signal that the program does not provide sufficient value in terms of health status improvement or effect. Given these forces at work, participation remains low and each referral/registration to a CDSMP workshop is hard-won. Organizations expend extra effort to get the program costs covered for those who do elect to participate. Without demand, there is little pressure to pay for these programs. Thus, the cycle perpetuates.

This issue goes beyond what the single manager within an implementing organization can address alone or even what a program coordinator at the state level can solve. It calls for a systems approach – where the stakeholders are aware of common overall objectives, their roles and boundaries in producing results, and the accountability of component parts to one another (29–31).

It is also important that policy and technical assistance is informed by and supportive of practice in the field. The Centers for Medicaid and Medicare Services (CMS) has commissioned studies of EBHP programs that include CDSMP, but notes challenges, particularly how to directly fund community-based wellness and prevention programs for this and other programs (32). CMS calls for more research to: "develop a sustainable framework for supporting a health ecosystem of community-based providers, while not exposing the Medicare program to undue risk" [(32), p. 72].

Meanwhile the infrastructure to support CDSMP may be eroding. The infrastructure investment under ARRA facilitated regional and local training, grew state, and organizational expertise on how to run these programs, fostered fidelity-monitoring peer collaboration and shared learning, produced Master Trainers and peer workshop leaders in every state, and engaged implementing organizations to commit to and market the program. As evidenced by the response from these eight organizations in just two states, these external supporting and infrastructure components seem to be shrinking.

LIMITATIONS

The primary limitation of this study is due to there being a single investigator. A second researcher to review and confirm the categorization and coding of comments and to interpret the findings would add strength to this examination. This limitation was addressed into some degree by: (1) conversations with experts in the field who are familiar with CDSMP and its implementation history and challenges, (2) careful crafting of the key informant interview instruments, (3) feedback from the national dataset program manager familiar with organizations implementing this program and with state agents, and (4) review of published studies about CDSMP, particularly recent program evaluations to identify important external factors. Other limitations include the small sample size of organizations and the exclusive focus on "successful" implementing organizations. This research would be strengthened by examining additional organizations of many types, located within other states, and having variable success in implementation – using the same interview protocol including the scaled response options.

CONCLUSION

Reflecting on the lessons learned from these eight successful CDSMP organizations, recommendations related to enhancing internal and external supports are offered.

Supportive elements for adoption and early implementation efforts that drove these organizations were very consistent, especially organizational leadership and the perceived value and fit of CDSMP with the mission and purpose of the organizations. Advice by this set of successful organizations included clarifying the benefit of the program using both participant and organizational metrics. Thus recommendations to enhance *internal* capability to support effective implementation include:

- Identify an internal program champion who has the ability to help drive adoption and ensure senior level buy-in and commitment to the program;
- Make the case that the program is a good fit with the organization's mission and purpose;
- Clearly identify the value of the program in terms that make sense to key stakeholders – e.g., to the participant, organization, funders, and policymakers. Measure and report this value consistently and repeatedly to enhance demand and solidify the foundation of support – which will help raise awareness of the value and benefits of CDSMP in the local area and should help in referrals to the program.

External supports were also clearly important for adoption and early implementation efforts among these organizations. Training and fidelity-monitoring were especially noted, as was funding to get the program up and running. Organizations noted that they could have also used help building awareness of the program. Therefore, recommendations for program sustainability in terms of *external supports* include:

- Enhance supportive policy at the federal and state level for CDSMP and programs like it that focus on improving prevention and self-management behaviors of individuals with chronic conditions and engaging individuals in their own care through fostering organizational readiness;
- Maintain support for training and fidelity-monitoring as a funded external support that appears to be key to both implementation and sustainability;

- Improve visibility/public awareness of the program through national campaigns or other methods to lessen the burden on each organization to make this program known;
- Accelerate efforts to make benefit changes to the Medicare program to include CDSMP as a defined benefit for persons with chronic conditions to reduce the barriers around funding the program and to embed it in the fabric of the organizations that have done the hard work of adopting and implementing it.

Reaching individuals who can benefit from EBHP and disability prevention programs is an important public health goal. As health care and social support "systems" within the U.S. move haltingly forward toward more accountability for producing outcomes in health status among defined population (patient/client) groups, programs like CDSMP will become more relevant as a strategy for population health management. At that time, perhaps the program will be seen as a fundamental service of these organizations, with funding allocated through internal budgeting processes.

Until that time, organizations willing to adopt such programs must be supported effectively. Key external supports, such as training, materials, and funding provide the bedrock for dissemination and implementation [(11), p. 46]. National marketing campaigns or other external marketing supports are clearly needed. These findings are consistent with a more extensive review of activities at the state (intermediary agent) level on CDSMP diffusion and dissemination. In a final evaluation report about CDSMP to the Administration on Aging (focusing on states' activities), the authors also recommended a "centralized or coordinated process for recruitment, intake, referral, and registration/enrollment" [(19), p. 97]. Both studies call for a coordinated, systems approach. Without this greater effort, individuals with chronic conditions, medical providers, and potential referral organizations within a given region are likely to remain unaware of the program and its value. This is a tremendous missed opportunity for public health and disability prevention.

Chronic disease represents one of the top public health issues domestically and globally. Stronger public policy to ensure there is an infrastructure to support EBHP programs that have demonstrated effectiveness with chronic disease populations should be a public health priority.

ACKNOWLEDGMENTS

The author would like to thank the state and organizational representatives who shared their insights and implementation experiences and Kristie Kulinski from the National Council on Aging for her data support. The author thanks Nancy Whitelaw, Ph.D., and Mary Altpeter, Ph.D., for their review and suggestions on this manuscript and for serving on the doctoral dissertation committee, which guided the development and execution of this study. Finally, thanks to faculty members from the Health Policy and Management Department of the Gillings School of Public Health from the University of North Carolina-Chapel Hill for their guidance throughout the doctoral program.

REFERENCES

1. Fixsen D, Naoom S, Blase K, Friedman R, Wallace F. *Implementation Research: A Synthesis of the Literature.* Tampa, FL: The National Implementation Research Network, Louis De La Parte Florida Mental Health Institute, University of Florida (2005).
2. Durlak JA, DuPre EP. Implementation matters: a review of research on the influence of implementation on program outcomes and the factors affecting implementation. *Am J Community Psychol* (2008) **41**(3):327–50. doi:10.1007/s10464-008-9165-0
3. Greenhalgh T, Robert G, Macfarlane F, Bate P, Kyriakidou O. Diffusion of innovations in service organizations: systematic review and recommendations. *Milbank Q* (2004) **82**(4):581–629. doi:10.1111/j.0887-378X.2004.00325.x
4. Klein KJ, Sorra JS. The challenge of innovation implementation. *Acad Manage Rev* (1996) **21**(4):1055–80. doi:10.2307/259164
5. Simpson DD. A conceptual framework for transferring research to practice. *J Subst Abuse Treat* (2002) **22**(4):171–82. doi:10.1016/S0740-5472(02)00231-3
6. Simpson DD. A framework for implementing sustainable oral health promotion interventions. *J Public Health Dent* (2011) **71**(s1):S84–94. doi:10.1111/j.1752-7325.2011.00234.x
7. Robinson K, Driedger M, Elliott S, Eyles J. Understanding facilitators of and barriers to health promotion practice. *Health Promot Pract* (2006) **7**:467–576. doi:10.1177/1524839905278955
8. Aarons G, Horowitz J, Dlugoz L, Ehrhart M. The role of organizational processes in dissemination and implementation research. In: Brownson R, Colditz G, Proctor E, editors. *Dissemination and Implementation Research in Health: Translating Science to Practice.* (Vol. Chapter 7), New York, NY: Oxford University Press (2012). p. 128–53.
9. Mitchell R, Florin P, Stevenson J. Supporting community-based prevention and health promotion initiatives: developing effective technical assistance systems. *Health Educ Behav* (2002) **29**:620–39. doi:10.1177/109019802237029
10. Wilcox S, Dowda M, Leviton L, Bartlett-Prescott J, Bazzare T, Campbell-Voytal K, et al. Active for life: final results from the translation of two physical activity programs. *Am J Prev Med* (2008) **35**(4):340–51. doi:10.1016/j.amepre.2008.07.001
11. Whitelaw N. System change and organizational capacity for evidence-based practices: lessons from the field. *Generations* (2010) **34**(1):43–50.
12. Ramanadhan S, Crisostomo J, Alexander-Molloy J, Gandelman E, Grullon M, Lora V, et al. Perceptions of evidence-based programs among community-based organizations tackling health disparities: a qualitative study. *Health Educ Res* (2011) **27**(4):717–28. doi:10.1093/her/cyr088
13. Lorig K. Chronic disease self-management a model for tertiary prevention. *Am Behav Sci* (1996) **39**(6):676–83. doi:10.1177/0002764296039006005
14. Lorig KR, Sobel DS, Stewart AL, Brown BW Jr, Bandura A, Ritter P, et al. Evidence suggesting that a chronic disease self-management program can improve health status while reducing hospitalization: a randomized trial. *Med Care* (1999) **37**(1):5. doi:10.1097/00005650-199901000-00003
15. Lorig KR, Ritter P, Stewart AL, Sobel DS, Brown BW Jr, Bandura A, et al. Chronic disease self-management program: 2-year health status and health care utilization outcomes. *Med Care* (2001) **39**(11):1217–23. doi:10.1097/00005650-200111000-00008
16. Ory M, Ahn S, Jiang L, Ritter PL, Whitelaw N, Lorig K. Successes of a national study of the chronic disease self-management program: meeting the triple aim of health care reform. *Med Care* (2013) **51**(11):992–8. doi:10.1097/MLR.0b013e3182a95dd1
17. Ahn S, Basu R, Smith M, Jiang L, Lorig K, Whitelaw N, et al. The impact of chronic disease self-management programs: Healthcare savings through a community-based intervention. *BMC Public Health* (2013) **13**:1141. doi:10.1186/1471-2458-13-1141
18. Ory M, Ahn S, Jiang L, Whitelaw N, Lorig K, Matthew LS. National study of chronic disease self-management program (CDSMP): one year changes in health outcomes for older adults. *Presentation Session #289097 at 141st APHA Annual Meeting and Exposition.* Boston, MA (2013).
19. Woodstock C, Korda H, Erdem E, Pedersen S, Kloc M, Tollefson E. *Chronic Disease Self-Management Program Process Evaluation.* Washington, DC: Administration for Community Living (2013).
20. Damschroder LJ, Aron DC, Keith RE, Kirsh SR, Alexander JA, Lowery JC. Fostering implementation of health services research findings into practice: a consolidated framework for advancing implementation science. *Implement Sci* (2009) **4**(1):50. doi:10.1186/1748-5908-4-50

21. Frank J, Lau C. *Empowering Older People to Take More Control of Their Health Through Evidence-Based Prevention Programs: A Capping Report.* Washington, DC: National Council on Aging (2013).
22. Scheirer MA. Is sustainability possible? A review and commentary on empirical studies of program sustainability. *Am J Eval* (2005) **26**(3):320–47. doi:10.1177/1098214005278752
23. Wandersman A, Chien V, Katz J. Toward an evidence-based system for innovation support for implementing innovations with quality: tools, training, technical assistance, and quality assurance/quality improvement. *Am J Community Psychol* (2012) **50**:445–59. doi:10.1007/s10464-012-9509-7
24. Merzel C, D'Afflitti J. Reconsidering community-based health promotion: promise, performance, and potential. *Am J Public Health* (2003) **93**(4):557–74. doi:10.2105/AJPH.93.4.557
25. Krueuter M, Casey C, Bernhardt J. Enhancing dissemination through marketing and distribution systems: a vision for public health. In: Brownson R, Colditz G, Proctor E, editors. *Dissemination and Implementation Research in Health: Translating Science to Practice.* (Vol. Chapter 11), New York, NY: Oxford University Press (2012). p. 213–22.
26. Balady GJ, Ades PA, Bittner VA, Franklin BA, Gordon NF, Thomas RJ, et al. Referral, enrollment, and delivery of cardiac rehabilitation/secondary prevention programs at clinical centers and beyond: a presidential advisory from the American heart association. *Circulation* (2011) **124**:2951–60. doi:10.1161/CIR.0b013e31823b21e2
27. Aarons G, Hurlburt M, Horwitz S. Advancing a conceptual model of evidence-based practice implementation in public service sectors. *Adm Policy Ment Health* (2011) **38**:4–23. doi:10.1007/s10488-010-0327-7
28. McGinnis JM, Williams-Russo P, Knickman J. The case for more active policy attention to health promotion. *Health Aff* (2002) **21**(2):78–93. doi:10.1377/hlthaff.21.2.78
29. Churchman CW. *The Systems Approach.* New York, NY: Dell Publishing Co (1968).
30. Deming WE. *The New Economics for Industry, Government, Education.* Cambridge, MA: MIT Center for Advanced Engineering Study (1993).
31. Ulrich W. Some difficulties of ecological thinking, considered from a systems perspective: a plea for critical holism. *Syst Pract* (1993) **6**:583–611. doi:10.1007/BF01059480
32. Centers for Medicare & Medicaid. *Report to Congress: The Centers for Medicare & Medicaid Services' Evaluation of Community-Based Wellness and Prevention Programs under Section 4202(b) of the Affordable Care Act.* (2013). Available from: http://innovation.cms.gov/Files/reports/CommunityWellnessRTC.pdf

16

Examining sustainability factors for organizations that adopted Stanford's Chronic Disease Self-Management Program

Michiyo Tomioka* and Kathryn L. Braun

Office of Public Health Studies, University of Hawai'i at Mānoa, Honolulu, HI, USA

Edited by:
Matthew Lee Smith, The University of Georgia, USA

Reviewed by:
Angie Hochhalter, Scott & White Healthcare, USA
Lynda Anderson, Centers for Disease Control and Prevention, USA

****Correspondence:***
Michiyo Tomioka, Office of Public Health Studies, University of Hawai'i at Mānoa, 1960 East-West Road, Biomed D-209, Honolulu, HI 96822, USA
e-mail: mtomioka@hawaii.edu

In 2006, funds were received to replicate Stanford's Chronic Disease Self-Management Program (CDSMP) among eldercare providers in Honolulu. This case study, conducted 1 year after the close of the initial 3-year replication grant, explored factors for sustaining the delivery of CDSMP, with an aim to create guidelines for cultivating sustainability. Face-to-face semi-structured interviews were conducted with one representative from each of eight eldercare agencies, with the representative specified by the agency. Representatives discussed the presence and strength (low, medium, or high) of sustainability factors, including readiness, champions, technical assistance, perceived fit of CDSMP with their agency, CDSMP modifiability, perceived benefits of CDSMP, and other. Only three of the eight agencies (38%) were still offering CDSMP by the end of 2010. Agencies who sustained CDSMP rated higher on all sustainability factors compared to those that did not sustain the program. Additional factors identified by representatives as important were funding and ongoing access to pools of elders from which to recruit program participants. When replicating evidence-based programs, sustainability factors must be consciously nurtured. For example, readiness must be cultivated, multiple champions must be developed, agencies must be helped to modify the program to best fit their clientele, evaluation findings demonstrating program benefit should be shared, and linkages to funding may be needed.

Keywords: chronic disease, health promotion, evidence-based, minority groups, sustainability

INTRODUCTION

Demand for preventing, delaying the onset, and managing chronic diseases has escalated. Attention is being given to expanding replication of evidence-based health promotion programs, those proven to work, to address chronic disease (1). Several federal agencies recommend that service providers adopt evidence-based health promotion programs rather than "reinvent the wheel" in efforts to help older adults maintain health and independent living for as long as possible (2, 3). Yet, studies on how organizations learn about, adapt, and sustain such programs are limited (4, 5).

In replicating an evidence-based program, organizations need adequate knowledge and skills in adapting the program to fit local circumstances while maintaining fidelity and evaluating the program to assure that it achieves the outcomes promised in the original research (6–8). Much of the extant literature outlines the many challenges of translating scientific knowledge to community practice (9–13). These include: (1) resistance to new practice modalities; (2) lack of organizational buy-in; (3) lack of specific goals and standards in translating the evidence; and (4) rigidity of evidence-based practice that cannot be molded to meet specific needs of the applied setting or target population (4, 6, 14).

These adaptation barriers also influence the long-term continuation of evidence-based programs, and more attention is being focused on ways to assure widespread availability of evidence-based programs (15–18). Useful models such as RE-AIM (Reach, Effectiveness, Adoption, Implementation, and Maintenance) help guide replication processes and evaluation (19).

At the same time, researchers have summarized and advanced definitions of program sustainability, identified factors associated with sustainability, and developed conceptual frameworks to understand program sustainability (15, 17, 20–22). According to literature review of sustainability research by Wiltsey-Stirman et al. (18), one of the most cited definitions of sustainability evolved from work of Scheirer (15) and Shediac-Rizhallah and Bone (17) and is: "the integration of the new program into ongoing organizational systems."

Scheirer's framework for program sustainability posits four phases of program adoption: (1) initiation; (2) implementation; (3) level of use (full or partial); and (4) sustainability (sustained, discontinued, or replaced) (15). Based on her literature review, agencies that sustain new programs likely agree that the program can be modified to fit their organization, see the program as fitting their organization's mission, perceive program benefits, have champions for the program, and have access to technical assistance while adopting the program.

The purpose of this study was to describe and determine the important factors that supported or hindered sustainability of the Stanford's Chronic Disease Self-Management Program (CDSMP) among eldercare service providers in Hawai'i. CDSMP was developed to empower people with various chronic diseases to take control of their health (23). Participants attend six 2.5-h sessions (one per week). Facilitators share knowledge and use motivational interviewing techniques to engage participants, who make weekly action plans to help themselves take small steps toward changing a behavior of their choice. Numerous studies of CDSMP have shown that people who participate in this program feel better, have better control over the symptoms of their chronic diseases, and are better able to talk to their physicians (23, 24). Although the original test of CDSMP was conducted with Caucasians (25), it has been successfully adapted to fit Hawai'i's multicultural communities (26).

The implementation of CDSMP in Hawai'i was supported by Hawai'i Healthy Aging Partnership (HHAP), formed in 2003 to increase access to health promotion programs among Hawai'i older adults with chronic conditions. HHAP members include professionals from government offices for aging and public health, elder care agencies, and the university. The process of CDSMP adaptation began in August 2006 when HHAP was awarded a 3-year grant from the Administration on Aging (AoA). HHAP members developed CDSMP implementation and evaluation plans, assessed readiness to implement CDSMP, and coordinated training for CDSMP leaders. Implementation in two of Hawai'i's four counties began in July 2007. It was expanded statewide in 2008 with funds from the National Council on Aging (NCOA). The sustainability phase began in 2009, when the original implementation funding ended. The purpose of this study, guided by Scheirer's sustainability framework, was to better understand the process and factors associated with sustainability of CDSMP in Hawai'i.

MATERIALS AND METHODS

DESIGN, SETTINGS, PARTICIPANTS

Although CDSMP was implemented statewide, the findings reported here were gathered as a part of the Honolulu case study, which was conducted to understand the process of organizational change for CDSMP adoption. In the Honolulu case study, data from state and county government, community organizations, and older adults were examined to investigate "how" and "why" organizations in Honolulu adapted, implemented, and sustained CDSMP successfully or unsuccessfully (27). The Honolulu case study was approved by University of Hawai'i Institutional Review Board. This paper reports on a portion of data collected, specifically from the eight service providers in Honolulu that started to replicate CDSMP in 2007.

For the Honolulu case study, we identified three phases of the CDSMP adoption path. The first 6 months of 2007 was considered as the Initiation Phase, when HHAP began planning replication and training agency personnel in CDSMP delivery. The Delivery Phase ran from June 2007 to June 2009, during which time staff members from multiple agencies were trained and then delivered CDSMP to older adults and participated in ongoing fidelity monitoring and evaluation. The Sustainability Phase began in July 2009, when original funding ended. This paper reports on the Sustainability Phase of new-program adoption.

The eight providers included multi-purpose social service organizations (designated as A and D), community health centers (designated as B, F, G, and H), a community college (designated as E), and a community meals program (designated as C). Four providers (A, B, C, and D) had a closer relationship with the Honolulu County Area Agency on Aging than the other four (E, F, G, and H), because they had been funded by the Honolulu County Area Agency on Aging for other programs. Five providers (A, B, C, E, and G) were involved with HHAP during the statewide planning of CDSMP adoption, whereas three providers (D, F, and H) joined HHAP when CDSMP training was held. Each provider chose the employee to be interviewed in this study.

MEASURES

The investigators developed an interview guide that asked about the five sustainability factors identified by Scheirer (15): (1) champions; (2) technical assistance; (3) perceived fit of the program; (4) program modifiability; and (5) perceived benefits of the program. A sixth factor, readiness to replicate, was added, as it was considered important to HHAP partners. After discussing each factor, participants were asked to rate its importance to sustainability as low, medium, or high. Finally, they are asked to identify other sustainability factors (**Table 1**).

Readiness refers to an individual's and agency's sense of preparedness to replicate the program. A champion is an agency employee who plays a key role in adapting, delivering, and/or sustaining CDSMP in the agency. Technical assistance refers to help employees could access when they had questions or encountered problems in CDSMP implementation and sustainment. Perceived fit of the program implies a similarity between the new intervention and the parent organization's mission and culture. Program modifiability refers to the level of satisfaction that the agency has with the modifications that it can make to the evidence-based program (e.g., to better fit its clientele and agency structure) without jeopardizing the behavior-changing components of the program. Perceived benefits of the program include feelings of staff and clients (which may or may not be based on evaluation data) that the program is making a positive impact.

These factors were identified by Scheirer (15), with the exception of readiness (item 1). Readiness as a sustainability factor was identified through our review of the sustainability literature and discussion with funders, who considered organizational readiness an important first step in adoption of CDSMP.

Although providers continue to offer CDSMP, data for this study of sustainability factors were collected in late 2010. At that time, the first author (MT) conducted face-to-face, semi-structured interviews with the eight community provider representatives in Honolulu. The interview questions were sent to the representatives ahead of the interview to help them prepare. All eight representatives provided a written consent. Interviews were held at the representatives' offices and took about an hour. Six individuals allowed their interviews to be audio taped and, for two, hand notes were made. All interviews were transcribed into text files.

ANALYSIS

Ratings of low, medium, or high were noted for each respondent for each sustainability factor. The discussion of each factor and the discussion of other possible factors were read independently by two researchers. For the most part, discussion of *a priori* sustainability factors served to give examples of, expand on, and contextualize each factor, which was useful in understanding its

Table 1 | Summary of sustainability factors assessed.

Sustainability factors	Sample questions
1. Readiness	Describe your "readiness" to replicate CDSMP. For example, how adequate was training in the program, data collection, and program monitoring forms? How prepared was your agency?
2. Champions[a]	Describe your experience with program champions for CDSMP? Who and how many people from your organization were helping with CDSMP, and in what ways? What did these champions do? Comment on their effectiveness.
3. Technical assistance[a]	How does your organization have access to technical assistance to sustain the program? Comment on the availability and usefulness of technical assistance as you replicated CDSMP.
4. Program-organization fit[a]	How does CDSMP match your organization's culture or mission? Comment on the level of "fit" between CDSMP and your agency.
5. Program modifiability[a]	Describe your ability to change or modify CDSMP that fit your clients and your agency. Describe your experience making program modifications while trying to maintain fidelity to the original CDSMP design.
6. Perceived program benefits[a]	How did organizational leaders and worker feel CDSMP impacted your clients? How do you think CDSMP benefited the people you served? In what ways has your involvement in CDSMP benefited clients, staff, and your organization?
7. Other (open-ended)	How do you think CDSMP will be sustained by your agency? What are the major factors that contributed to long-term sustainability?

[a]*Identified by Scheirer (15).*

ranking (low, medium, or high). Analysis of responses to the open-ended question about other possible factors required the two researchers to discern themes in the data and then code responses into themes. These were discussed in a meeting, and differences were resolved by re-reading the interview transcript together and having further discussion until consensus was reached. There were no major disagreements during the analysis process.

RESULTS

The progress of the eight providers who volunteered to replicate CDSMP in Honolulu is shown in **Figure 1**. One provider (H) dropped out during the Initial Phase (the first 6 months) because of the organization decided that it could not dedicate staff time to deliver CDSMP. Thus, only seven of the eight organizations entered the 2-year Delivery Phase. Two providers (E and F) dropped out before the end of that phase. For Provider E, two staff members completed CDSMP training and offered it twice in the community, but the organization felt that it was too time consuming to recruit and track clients and chose to discontinue. Provider F was not able to fully implement the program with its fidelity monitoring and evaluation requirements. Of the five entering the Sustainment Phase in mid-2009, only three providers (A, B, D) were still sustaining CDSMP in late 2010. Provider G had replaced CDSMP with another program, and Provider C discontinued the program. Provider F decided to reengage with CDSMP at this time.

During the analysis process, it became clear that organizations that sustained CDSMP had more supports throughout the process than the organizations that were unable to sustain CDSMP. **Table 2** shows a summary of rating results from the interview.

READINESS

Thinking back to the Delivery Phase, providers described and rated their level of readiness to replicate CDSMP. The five providers (63%) who scored their organization as "high" had noted in their discussion of readiness that their staff had spent time learning about the concept of evidence-based programing prior to program adoption, felt well trained in CDSMP and data collection, were motivated to pilot CDSMP in their community, had identified potential CDSMP participants, had established policies and procedures related to CDSMP, and had purchased a CDSMP license. The three providers who scored medium or low remembered some uncertainty within their organization and perhaps some miscommunication with HHAP as to the costs associated with CDSMP licensing, the coordination of CDSMP workshops, and the need to participate in fidelity monitoring and evaluation.

CHAMPIONS

Respondents agreed that having champions was very important to sustainability, and the organizational representatives that reported high champion effectiveness were most likely to be from organizations that sustained CDSMP. The transcript-analysis process, however, distinguished three types of champions, including program champions, participant champions, and supervisor champions.

Respondents defined a program champion as someone who had been trained to lead CDSMP, had a passion for it, was very committed, was able to promote it, and had the drive to expand it. Although all organizations had staff trained in CDSMP, not all could identify a program champion at the time of the interview, while some agencies reported as many as three program champions. The three sustained programs reported having more than one program champion at their organization.

Interview findings suggested that the most successful program champions had relatively flexible schedules, which allowed them to offer CDSMP during or outside of work hours, and their job descriptions included CDSMP. They had strong skills in teamwork and took time to educate other branches of the organization in CDSMP to increase organizational buy-in. They advocated for

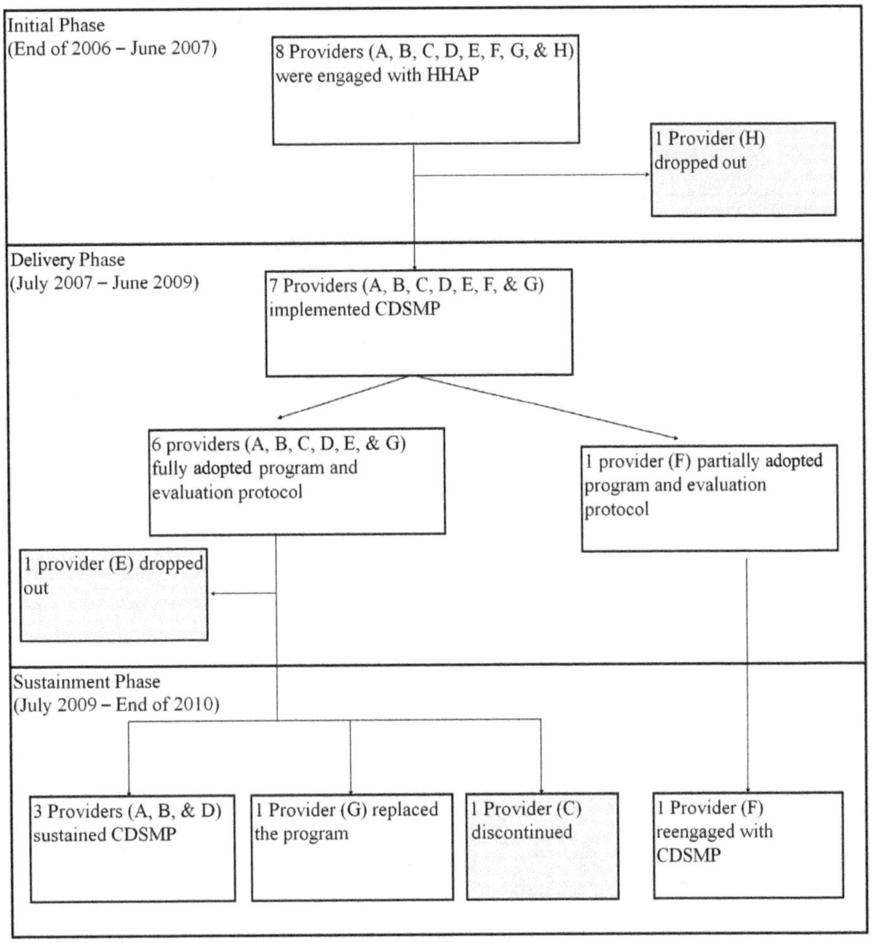

FIGURE 1 | Providers progress over the 4 years.

other staff in the agency to attend CDSMP leader training. They networked with CDSMP leaders at other agencies, which helped them find a substitute or second workshop leader when needed. They also were seen as role models by program participants and provided support to CDSMP leaders at other organizations. As one provider noted: "*Both champions have been enthusiastic and . . . try to promote, try to get more funding, try to get more people, are involved . . . and they wish they were able to do more.*"

The two providers who reported no program champion might have had a program champion initially, but this person changed jobs or became too busy to lead and advocate for CDSMP. One provider said: "*We don't have a champion because we had to take care of other things. . . Champion requires that one person constantly pushes CDSMP.*" Sustained organizations reported that they would be able to continue to sustain the program as long as they had leaders and trainers on board. To facilitate this, HHAP continues to provide CDSMP leader trainings and encourage organizations to continuously send new staff or volunteers to training so that they could keep enough leaders within their organizations.

A participant champion was described as someone who had graduated the CDSMP (attending four or more sessions out of six), realized benefits from the program, and was willing to share their story about CDSMP. By talking about the benefits they received, they helped to recruit other participants for the program. Many providers felt that the word-of-mouth strategy was the most effective approach to attract new participants.

A supervisor champion was described as a manager who supported the delivery of CDSMP within the organization and supported the program champions in leading CDSMP sessions. Supervisor champions always sent an agency representative to the statewide HHAP meetings and saw CDSMP as a valuable service to offer agency clients. Interview analysis suggested that all sustained agencies had a supervisor champions. Respondents for the other four agencies felt that their supervisors were not strong champions. Two of them said that their supervisors oversaw a variety of projects and remained relatively uninvolved with CDSMP replication efforts. The other two providers reported that they did not get any support from their supervisors because their supervisors had unrealistic expectations of CDSMP, for example, that it would take less time than it did, would be more modifiable that it was, or would generate revenue. The discrepancy between the expectations of these supervisors and those of the staff trained in CDSMP discouraged staff from championing the program in their agencies.

Table 2 | Summary of interview rating results.

Outcome	Org	Readiness	Champions				Program-organization fit	Program modifiability	Perceived benefits	Technical assistance
			No. of prog champ	Effectiveness	Supervisor support	Participants champ				
Sustained	A	H	2	H	H	Yes	H	H	H	H
	B	H	3	H	H	Yes	H	H	H	H
	D	H	2	H	H	Yes	H	H	H	H
Replaced	G	H	1	H	H	?	H	H	H	H
Discontinued	C	M	0	L	L	No	L	H	H	H
Reengaged	F	L	1	M	L	No	L	H	M	H
Dropped out in implementation phase	E	L	0	L	M	No	L	M	M	M
Dropped out in initial phase	H	L	0	L	L	No	L	M	–	M

H, high; M, medium; L, low; ?, unknown.

PROGRAM-ORGANIZATION FIT

Five providers (63%) reported that CDSMP fit well with their organizational mission and goals. They valued the program's concept of empowerment and its goal to help clients improve health and maintain independence through self-management. They also felt that their participants would appreciate the program's motivational interviewing approach.

Two providers rated program-organizational fit as medium. They felt that CDSMP fit their general mission – to improve the well-being of older adults – but not the type of service they provided, in this case meal delivery and college courses.

PROGRAM MODIFIABILITY

Five out of eight providers (63%) reported that the modifications of CDSMP by HHAP (with permission of Stanford) to fit Hawai'i's multicultural population helped them attract enrollees. This was done by including local examples and expressions of local culture in the curriculum (26). One provider gave this example: "*. . . our participants are not fluent English speakers . . . so it takes double the time to explain things. . . . We serve local food that they like or fit with their culture, they feel happy even though they work hard during the session. We also offer certificate of completion with leis.a little recognition for their hard work and they were very happy about it.*" Providers who reported high program modifiability also spent time to develop local marketing tools that included pictures of local older adults and symbols that resonated with Hawai'i's cultures. The three providers who rated medium or low in program modifiability noted disappointment that the program materials were not available in the languages of their target groups (e.g., the various Pacific Islander languages, like Samoan, Chuukese, and Marshallese) and that the program required two leaders to deliver each workshop. They also reported that the structured outline and scripted format of the workshop were too foreign for their clients.

PERCEIVED BENEFITS

One agency was not able to rate this factor because it dropped out prior to implementing CDSMP. Of the seven remaining providers, five rated CDSMP benefit to clients as "high" and perceived CDSMP was a good investment. They reported seeing improvements in the health of their clients and related success stories of participants who had lost weight, were exercising more, and/or were keeping better track of their health. One provider noted: "*I see them really change and keep hearing their stories . . . We had a quite a few that really struggled with making action plans. Boy, when they get it, they get it and they got so excited, you know, the first time they come back, they were so proud that they got something accomplished. I just think . . . you know, to me, it's really had a big impact on people's lives.*" They also saw benefits for their staff, many of whom had incorporated CDSMP tools (e.g., problem solving and developing action plan) into their daily activities and had gained confidence in public speaking. One provider used some of the CDSMP tools for staff training. They also mentioned the benefit of receiving evaluation results from HHAP specific to their agency to share with supervisors and funders. Hearing good stories from their participants and seeing the positive evaluation data further boosted their confidence in replicating CDSMP. The two providers who were rating this factor as "medium" noted that some of the agency's staff and clients were unable to grasp or apply CSDMP self-management strategies.

TECHNICAL ASSISTANCE

Six of the eight providers (63%) reported that the technical assistance that they received from HHAP was very useful. Technical assistance was provided through HHAP's monthly meetings, from the evaluation team, and from Stanford. At monthly meetings, providers were able to exchange ideas on how to leverage resources, to recruit and retain participants and leaders, and to carry-out the evaluation protocol. Meeting attendance also helped providers to develop strong skills in working with other providers. These relationships were useful when they needed to find a substitute leader for a CDSMP session or borrow books and other program materials for a workshop. A provider said: "*We are fortunate to have partners for CDSMP. I can call [Agency name], if I have questions. They also helped us and clarify things for us. One time, we did not have CDSMP books, and I called them... It was very helpful.* "Some providers reported that the Stanford website and email listserv were useful and helped motivate them to continue offering CDSMP. The providers who rated technical assistance as medium indicated that they wanted more support to recruit participants and more clarification of program requirements.

OTHER SUSTAINABILITY FACTORS

Interviewees were asked to identify other factors related to sustainability. Two were identified – having access to potential participants (four providers) and having access to additional funding (seven providers).

Because most of the providers were offering CDSMP to their existing clientele, they initially did not encounter problems finding participants. However, at some point they had provided CDSMP to all willing clientele. For the most part, agency clients were willing to participate in the program, and attendance was high (26), but "*once we went through all of the participants, then we did not have any more new participants... we do not have a large turnover in our clients, so we could not expand our numbers.*" Provider B noted that their organization was established to serve a specific community. After all willing clients completed CDSMP, their organization had to consider the advantages and disadvantages to enrolling people from other communities. Provider A felt that the CDSMP was important enough to continue because it fit so well with their program. This provider's solution was to conduct CDSMP workshop with a combination of participants who have done it before and any new participants that they could find.

Additional funding was also a critical factor to sustain CDSMP. One provider stated "*in the long-term, always funding is needed, things cost money and staff time, plus money for licensing [and] when the new books come out... all of those things cost something.*" Although most of the providers were able to access additional funding through the HHAP's awarded grants, sustained organizations' interviewees also wrote proposals to other funders to support CDSMP. They also used cost-saving strategies, such as holding workshops at no-cost sites and creating a library of workshop materials that could be loaned to (rather than purchased for or by) participants.

DISCUSSION

Evidence-based health promotion programs are developed in research settings, and replicating them in real-world settings can be challenging (4, 5). This study examined factors related to sustainability of CDSMP by Honolulu County providers a year after initial funding ended. Depending on presence and strength of these factors, providers varied in their sustainment of CDSMP as shown in **Figure 1**.

As Scheirer (15) proposed, new-program sustainability can be enhanced by having many champions (and several types of champions), ensuring program fit with the organizational mission, allowing some modifications to the program so it can better fit clientele, seeing benefits of the program, and having access to technical assistance. In addition to these five factors, this study identified three more factors that appear to contribute to sustainability of CDSMP – readiness, access to additional funding, and access to potential participants.

Readiness can be cultivated by providing training about evidence-based programing, fidelity monitoring, and program evaluation, along with training in the intervention to be adopted (13). For non-profit organizations, external funding to support added programs is essential, especially in light of cutback to social services and the piloting of the "reimbursement-for-service" model by many eldercare service providers. Although continued funding was not cited explicitly by the majority of studies of program sustainability reviewed by Scheirer (15), she noted that many of these programs had in fact found alternative funding to maintain new programs.

Exhausting potential clients can occur in agencies that work within small geographic areas, have a fixed number of clients that they are allowed to serve, and/or have low client turnover (28). This is especially true in Hawai'i, where providers receiving funds through the AAAs are contracted to serve a specified number elders, often in a defined target area. With low turnover in clientele, all willing participants can participate in CDSMP over the course of several years. Also, some service providers in Hawai'i serve elders who speak languages for which CDSMP is not available. It may be that CDSMP is more sustainable in Hawai'i's health maintenance organizations that serve thousands of clients, as a portion of their clients would likely be diagnosed with chronic disease each year. Meanwhile, HHAP members have expressed a desire to learn about and replicate other evidence-based programs that could benefit their clientele. Already, a number of providers in the state are replicating EnhanceFitness with good success (29).

This study explored CDSMP sustainability among eight eldercare providers in one of Hawai'i's four counties, and only one representative from each organization was interviewed. Although organizations selected to be interviewed the individual most closely involved in CDSMP adaptation, the interviewee may not represent the whole organization.

Also, because the interview asked about sustainability after initial funding ended, the results may have been compromised by inability to recall events, especially for those organizations that discontinued CDSMP, and by social desirability bias. Future examination of new-program sustainability would benefit from prospective study and inclusion of multiple representatives of an organization.

Despite the limitations, this study was able to confirm the importance of the sustainability factors proposed by Scheirer (15), and added three more, which may be specific to the Hawai'i context of CDSMP replication. The clear message from this study is that planning for sustainability should start before replicating evidence-based programs. It requires tremendous effort to translate evidence-based programs, to build provider capacity, to implement a new program (or new practice) in real-world setting, and to sustain it. These findings can help guide healthcare workers and organizations to plan and sustain the adoption of evidence-based programs.

ACKNOWLEDGMENTS

This study was based on the doctoral thesis of the first author. We acknowledge the Hawai'i Healthy Aging Partnership, a coalition of the Hawai'i Executive Office on Aging, the Area Agencies on Aging, the Hawai'i State Department of Health, the University of Hawai'i, and service providers dedicated to expand health promotion options for older adults in Hawai'i. Funding for the Hawai'i Health Aging Partnership has been received from U.S. Administration on Aging, National Council on Aging, State of Hawai'i, County of Kaua'i, and County of Maui.

REFERENCES

1. Altpeter M, Bryant L, Schneider E, Whitelaw N. Evidence-based health practice: knowing and using what works for older adults. *Home Health Care Serv Q* (2006) **25**(1–2):1–11. doi:10.1300/J027v25n01_01
2. Brownson RC, Baker EA, Leet TL, Gillespie KN, True WR. *Evidence-Based Public Health*. 2nd ed. Oxford, UK: Oxford University Press (2011). 293 p.
3. U.S. Administration on Aging. *Facts AoA Evidence-Based Prevention Program*. Washington, DC: U.S. Department of Health and Human Services, Administration on Aging (2010). Available from: http://www.aoa.gov/AoARoot/Press_Room/Products_Materials/pdf/fs_EvidenceBased.pdf
4. Glasgow RE, Lichtenstein E, Marcus AC. Why don't we see more translation of health promotion research to practice? Rethinking the efficacy-to-effectiveness transition. *Am J Public Health* (2003) **93**(8):1261–7. doi:10.2105/AJPH.93.8.1261
5. Green LW, Glasgow RE. Evaluating the relevance, generalization, and applicability of research: issues in external validation and translation methodology. *Eval Health Prof* (2006) **29**(1):126–53. doi:10.1177/0163278705284445
6. Alkema GE, Frey D. Implications of translating research into practice: a medication management intervention. *Home Health Care Serv Q* (2006) **25**(1–2):33–54. doi:10.1300/J027v25n01_03
7. Glasgow RE, Klesges LM, Dzewaltowski DA, Bull SS, Estabrooks P. The future of health behavior change research: what is needed to improve translation of research into health promotion practice? *Ann Behav Med* (2004) **27**(1):3–12. doi:10.1207/s15324796abm2701_2
8. Dusenbury L, Brannigan R, Falco M, Hansen W. A review of research on fidelity of implementation: implications for drug abuse prevention in school settings. *Health Educ Res* (2003) **18**(2):237–56. doi:10.1093/her/18.2.237
9. Doig GS, Simpson F. Efficient literature searching: a core skill for the practice of evidence-based medicine. *Intensive Care Med* (2003) **29**(12):2119–27. doi:10.1007/s00134-003-1942-5
10. Dunn AL, Blair SN. Translating evidenced-based physical activity interventions into practice: the 2010 challenge. *Am J Prev Med* (2002) **22**(4):8–9. doi:10.1016/S0749-3797(02)00432-4
11. Elliott DS, Mihalic S. Issues in disseminating and replicating effective prevention programs. *Prev Sci* (2004) **5**(1):47–53. doi:10.1023/B:PREV.0000013981.28071.52
12. Goodman RM. Community-based participatory research: questions and challenges to an essential approach. *J Public Health Manag Pract* (2001) **7**(5):v–vi.
13. Simpson DD, Flynn PM. Moving innovations into treatment: a stage-based approach to program change. *J Subst Abuse Treat* (2007) **33**(2):111–20. doi:10.1016/j.jsat.2006.12.023
14. Grol R. Successes and failures in the implementation of evidence-based guidelines for clinical practice. *Med Care* (2001) **39**(8):II.46–54. doi:10.1097/00005650-200108002-00003
15. Scheirer MA. Is sustainability possible?: a review and commentary on empirical studies of program sustainability. *Am J Eval* (2005) **26**(3):320–47. doi:10.1177/1098214005278752
16. Scheirer MA, Dearing JW. An agenda for research on the sustainability of public health programs. *Am J Public Health* (2011) **101**(11):2059–67. doi:10.2105/AJPH.2011.300193
17. Shediac-Rizkallah MC, Bone LR. Planning for the sustainability of community-based health programs: conceptual frameworks and future directions for research, practice and policy. *Health Educ Res* (1998) **13**(1):87–108. doi:10.1093/her/13.1.87
18. Wiltsey-Stirman SW, Kimberly J, Cook N, Calloway A, Castro F, Charns M. The sustainability of new programs and innovations: a review of the empirical literature and recommendations for future research. *Implement Sci* (2012) **7**(17):1–19. doi:10.1186/1748-5908-7-17
19. Ory MG, Evashwick CJ, Glasgow RB, Sharkey JR. *Pushing the Boundaries of Evidence-Based Research: Enhancing the Application and Sustainability of Health Promotion Programs in Diverse Populations. In Behavioral change: An Evidence-Based Handbook For Social and Public Health*. Edinburgh: Elsevier (2005). p. 267–93.
20. Akerlund KM. Prevention program sustainability: the state's perspective. *J Community Psychol* (2000) **28**(3):353–62. doi:10.1002/(SICI)1520-6629(200005)28:3<353:AID-JCOP9>3.0.CO;2-6
21. Johnson K, Hays C, Center H, Daley C. Building capacity and sustainable prevention innovations: a sustainability planning model. *Eval Program Plann* (2004) **27**(2):135–49. doi:10.1016/j.evalprogplan.2004.01.002
22. Mancini JA, Marek LI. Sustaining community-based programs for families: conceptualization and measurement. *Fam Relat* (2004) **53**(4):339–47. doi:10.1111/j.0197-6664.2004.00040.x
23. Stanford Patient Education Research Center. *Selected Publications [Internet]*. Palo Alto, CA: School of Medicine Patient Education Research Center (2013). Available from: http://patienteducation.stanford.edu/bibliog.html
24. Ory MG, Smith ML, Kulinski KP, Lorig K, Zenker W, Whitelaw N. Self-management at the tipping point: reaching 100,000 Americans with evidence-based programs. *J Am Geriatr Soc* (2013) **61**(5):821–3. doi:10.1111/jgs.12239
25. Lorig KR, Sobel DS, Stewart AL, Brown BW Jr, Bandura A, Ritter P, et al. Evidence suggesting that a chronic disease self-management program can improve health status while reducing hospitalization: a randomized trial. *Med Care* (1999) **37**(1):5–14. doi:10.1097/00005650-199901000-00003
26. Tomioka M, Braun KL, Compton M, Tanoue L. Adapting Stanford's chronic disease self-management program to Hawaii's multicultural populations. *Gerontologist* (2012) **52**(1):121–32. doi:10.1093/geront/gnr054.U.S
27. Tomioka M. *Organizational Change in the Aging Network to Whom it May Concern: Promote Evidence-Based Programs [Dissertation]*. Honolulu (HI): University of Hawaii (2014). 186 p.
28. Freedman AM, Kuester SA, Jernigan J. Evaluating public health resources: what happens when funding disappears? *Prev Chronic Dis* (2013) **10**:130130. doi:10.5888/pcd10.130130
29. Tomioka M, Sugihara N, Braun KL. Replicating the enhance fitness physical activity program in Hawai'i's multicultural population: 2007-2010. *Prev Chronic Dis* (2012) **9**:110155. doi:10.5888/pcd9.110155

17

Meeting the challenge of cancer survivorship in public health: Results from the evaluation of the chronic disease self-management program for cancer survivors

Betsy C. Risendal[1]*, Andrea Dwyer[1], Richard W. Seidel[2], Kate Lorig[3], Letoynia Coombs[4] and Marcia G. Ory[5]

[1] Community and Behavioral Health, Colorado School of Public Health, Aurora, CO, USA
[2] Carilion Clinic, Virginia Tech Carilion School of Medicine, Roanoke, VA, USA
[3] School of Medicine, Stanford University, Stanford, CA, USA
[4] Colorado Health Outcomes, University of Colorado, Aurora, CO, USA
[5] Health Promotion and Community Health Sciences, Texas A&M Health Science Center School of Public Health, College Station, TX, USA

Edited by:
Matthew Lee Smith, The University of Georgia, USA

Reviewed by:
Diane Elliot, Oregon Health and Science University, USA
Miruna Petrescu-Prahova, University of Washington, USA

***Correspondence:**
Betsy C. Risendal, Community and Behavioral Health, Colorado School of Public Health, 13001 E. 17th Place, MS F538, Aurora, CO 80045, USA
e-mail: betsy.risendal@ucdenver.edu

Introduction: Self-management has been identified as an important opportunity to improve health outcomes among cancer survivors. However, few evidence-based interventions are available to meet this need.

Methods: The effectiveness of an adapted version of the Chronic Disease Self-Management Program for cancer survivors called Cancer Thriving and Surviving was evaluated in a randomized trial. Outcomes were assessed at baseline and 6-months post program via written survey among 244 participants in Colorado. Repeated measures analysis was used to analyze pre/post program change.

Results: Statistically significant improvement was observed among those in the intervention in the following outcomes: Provider communication (+16.7% change); depression (−19.1%); energy (+13.8%); sleep (−24.9%) and stress-related problems (−19.2%); change over time was also observed in the controls for energy, sleep, and stress-related outcomes though to a lesser degree. Effect sizes of the difference in change over time observed indicate a net beneficial effect for provider communication (0.23); and decreases in depression (−0.18); pain (−0.19); problems related to stress (−0.17); and sleep (−0.20).

Conclusion: Study data suggest that the self-management support from adaptation of the CDSMP can reach and appeal to cancer survivors, improves common concerns in this population, and can fill an important gap in meeting the ongoing need for management of post-diagnosis issues in this growing segment of the U.S. population.

Keywords: cancer survivorship, self-management support, patient education, community-based research, effectiveness trial

INTRODUCTION

The estimated lifetime risk of developing cancer is 45% among men and 38% among women, with an expected total of 1.6 million new cancer cases in 2012 (1). More individuals are living longer due to improvements in early detection and treatment, and therefore, the number of cancer survivors in the U.S. has dramatically increased. Current estimates suggest that there are over 13 million survivors alive today in the U.S., with an estimated 18 million at the end of the decade; an estimated 65% of all survivors live 5 years or more. This dramatic increase in the survivor population has consequences for both the health of survivors and the healthcare system. For example, many survivors experience late and long-term effects from cancer and its treatment. Pain, fatigue, depression, impaired physical function, and fear of recurrence are among the most common consequences of cancer as described in the landmark report by the Institute of Medicine, "From Cancer Patient to Cancer Survivor: Lost in Transition" (2). This Report also concluded that the care of cancer survivors is fragmented and poorly coordinated and that self-management support can help promote the delivery of quality care and improved health outcomes in this population. Further, cancer survivors die from non-cancer causes at a rate higher than the general population (3, 4) likely due to the long-term side effects of cancer and its treatment and risk factors common to both cancer and non-cancer causes of death.

The Chronic Care Model [CCM; (5)] is a rigorously evaluated and widely adopted approach to care management for chronic conditions and features self-management support as one of the key components for assuring quality healthcare. Self-management is defined as comprehensive engagement of the patient in problem solving, decision making, and daily health-related behaviors in partnership with their healthcare provider and community (6). A 2007 review by Nolte et al. (7) found many benefits from self-management programs are also relevant to survivorship such as:

improved knowledge, acquisition of skills, symptom management, and ability to self-monitor health and healthcare needs.

The Chronic Disease Self-Management Program (CDSMP) is one of the few evidence-based interventions available across a variety of health-related conditions for comprehensive self-management support (8). While there are now specialized versions for some chronic conditions such as diabetes, chronic pain, HIV/AIDS, and arthritis[1], an adapted version for cancer survivors has only recently been developed for use and testing in the U.S. The purpose of the current paper is to describe the findings from the 6-month outcome evaluation of cancer thriving and surviving (CTS) among over 200 cancer survivors in the post-treatment phase who participated in a randomized trial in Colorado between 2011 and 2013. In this paper, we report the effectiveness of the evidence-based CDSMP translated to cancer survivors by comparing the magnitude of the effect observed in the intervention vs. control group over time.

MATERIALS AND METHODS

INTERVENTION

Developed by researchers from the Stanford Patient Education Research Center at Stanford University, the model for the CDSMP program entails a series of six weekly small-group sessions led by trained facilitators. The model is based on social cognitive theory (9) to focus on building skills, sharing experiences, and support among the participants to maximize engagement. Sessions follow a standardized curriculum detailed in a program manual to promote fidelity to the following program elements: brainstorming, action plan formulation, action plan feedback, problem solving, and decision making (10).

In brief, adaptations to the CDSMP for cancer survivors were guided by the research of Foster et al. (11) and the subsequent conceptual model (12) to include restoration of self-confidence, adjustment to changed self, and confidence to self-manage cancer-related problems. The resultant CTS curriculum was initially developed by Macmillan Cancer support in the U.K and subsequently modified by the Stanford Patient Education Center to incorporate language more common to the U.S.

Researchers at the Colorado School of Public Health (CSPH) partnered with the Consortium for Older Adult Wellness (COAW) to deliver the program. COAW is a community-based agency with state-wide license to deliver the evidence-based CDSMP. Individuals who were already trained and licensed to provide the CDSMP workshops and who were also cancer survivors completed a 2-day cross-training program led by the Stanford Patient Education Center to ensure fidelity to the model.

RECRUITMENT

Cancer survivors throughout the "Front Range" of Colorado, where roughly two-thirds of state's population resides, were approached in a variety of outreach methods including: interactions with cancer center staff and brochures left at medical offices, mailed to homes using mailing lists from local cancer survivor programs, distributed at cancer survivor local events, and media. Potential respondents identified from these routes were contacted by COAW personnel (located in Denver, also within the Front Range) to assess interest and eligibility for participation in the program. Participants were allocated to the intervention or control groups for the analytic evaluation. Inclusion in the program required participants to be over the age of 21 years and diagnosed with cancer that required radiation, surgical, or adjuvant chemotherapy treatment, but not to be in active treatment at the time of enrollment. Persons currently receiving maintenance therapies for cancer delivered after completion of primary treatment (such as anti-hormonal treatments) were eligible. Support persons/caregivers of the above were also allowed to attend. All persons had to speak and read/write in English, and also agree to attend in-person classes and arrange transportation to attend classes. Persons in end-of-life care or currently undergoing active treatment for cancer were excluded, as were individuals over the age of 79 years. Approval to conduct the research was obtained by the Colorado Multiple Institutional Review Board; participants provided signed informed consent. No incentives were offered to potential participants.

INTERVENTION DELIVERY

Twenty-seven workshops were delivered in Colorado between August 2011 and January 2013. Each workshop consisted of six 2.5 h sessions led by two facilitators as described above. Facilitators were periodically observed by Master Trainers and provided written feedback to monitor fidelity and quality assurance.

DATA COLLECTION

Written self-administered surveys were collected from participants at baseline and for final follow-up measure (6 months after program completion). Instruments were from the Stanford CDSMP Evaluation[2] and have been widely used in many health and aging studies (13, 14) and are viewed as pragmatic measures (15). Participants were asked at baseline to self-report demographic characteristics (age, gender, marital status, race/ethnicity) as well as cancer-related history (caregiver, time since diagnosis, type of cancer, co-morbid conditions).

STUDY DESIGN

This study deployed a randomized controlled trial design, where participants were randomized in a 2:1 ratio following consent to the intervention vs. control group. Since the purpose of this study was to evaluate effectiveness rather than efficacy, we intentionally sought to maximize the number of participants receiving the intervention so that we could gain more experience to inform implementation and also to improve the generalizability of the results by broadening the characteristics and delivery while still utilizing a valid comparison group. Participants were randomized to group assignment using a random number generator by the research coordinator who was separate from the intervention delivery. Caregivers/support persons were randomized as a pair with their survivor so they could attend sessions together, and therefore, not counted toward the 2:1 ratio. Persons who consented and were randomly assigned to the control group were offered to attend the CTS workshops after the final evaluation assessment was

[1] http://patienteducation.stanford.edu/programs/cdsmp.html

[2] http://patienteducation.stanford.edu/research

collected at 6-months following consent; thus their data served as the control for those randomized to the intervention group. This design was chosen to facilitate retention of controls over the 6-month time period between consent and assessment of the main outcome measures at 6 months post-program (in order to mirror the CDSMP evaluation plan), and to gain more experience with intervention delivery.

OUTCOMES

Our hypothesis was that the intervention would produce improvement in outcomes directly related to health beliefs and behaviors related to physical activity (days active/minutes active), self-efficacy, and communication with providers. Secondary outcomes of interest included self-reported health and symptoms (health status, depression, energy, pain, sleep, and stress).

The following describes measures employed in this study:

- Days active, minutes active: days active, minutes active: respondents were asked how many days in the past week they were physically active or exercising for at least 30 min and how many total minutes in the past week they were physically active or exercising, including brisk walking, running, dancing, bicycling, water exercise, etc., that may cause faster breathing or heartbeat, or feeling warmer. For the current analyses, we are using continuous count data for number of minutes exercised and number of days exercised. Respondents were asked how many days in past week they were physically active or exercising for at least 30 min and how many total minutes in the past week they were physically active or exercising (including brisk walking, running, dancing, bicycling, water exercise, etc.) that may cause faster breathing or heartbeat, or feeling warmer. For the current analyses, we are using continuous count data for number of minutes exercised and number of days exercised.
- Participant care seeking behaviors (communication with physicians): communication with a physician was measured using a three-item scale, which asked participants if they did the following things when visiting a physician: prepare a list of questions, ask questions about things they want to know or do not understand, and discuss personal problems. Scores for these items ranged from never (0) to always (5). If respondents answered at least two of these items, the scale was calculated as the mean of the non-missing items. Higher scores represent better communication with a physician. An increase or positive change is desirable.
- Self-efficacy: this was measured using a six-item scale, which asked participants how confident they were keeping fatigue, physical discomfort, pain, emotional distress, and other symptoms and health problems caused by cancer diagnosis and treatment from interfering with the things they want to do; they were also asked about their confidence doing different tasks and activities needed to manage their cancer diagnosis and treatment to reduce their need to see a doctor. Responses to these items ranged from Not at all confident to (1) to Totally confident (10). If respondents answered at least four of these items, the scale was calculated as the mean of the non-missing items. Higher scores represented greater confidence. An increase or positive change was desired.
- Health status: we asked respondents to rate their health on a scale of excellent (1) to poor (5). A low value on this scale indicates better health; a decrease or negative change from the base-line period to the final period for this variable.
- Health symptomatology:
    - o Energy: we asked patients five questions about their level of energy: (1) Do you feel worn out?, (2) Did you have a lot of energy?, (3) Did you feel tired?, (4) Do you have enough energy to do the things you wanted to do?, and (5) Did you feel full of pep?. Responses to these items range from none of the time (0) to all of the time (5). If the respondent replied to at least three of these five items, the scale was calculated as the mean of the non-missing items with the two negatively worded items (1 and 3) reversed coded. A high score on this scale represents more energy. An increase or positive change for scale is desirable.
    - o Pain, stress, and sleep problems: these three visual scales ranged from no problem (0) to very big problem (10). A high score on these scales represents more problems. A decrease or negative change on this scale was desired.
- Depression: participants completed the eight-item Personal Health Questionnaire Depression Scale (16). The items' responses ranged from Not at all (0) to Nearly Everyday (3). Sum scores ranged from 0 to 24. Higher scores indicate more severe depression. A decrease or negative change in these items was desired.

STATISTICAL ANALYSIS

Pearson Chi Square and Fisher exact tests were used in **Table 1** to compare the demographic characteristics of the intervention and control groups.

In order to determine if the outcome variables showed the change in the desired direction over time, we used repeated measures analysis with an unstructured variance covariance matrix. This method models the correlations between repeated observations from the same individual. It also utilizes available data for all participants, regardless of final measure completion allowing for a form of intent to treat analysis, which reduces potential drop-out bias. A case is only excluded if they did not answer a sufficient number of items on both the pre- and the post-test. If they have enough data for either time period, they were included in the sample. Data from participants were only excluded if they did not supply an adequate number of responses required for each instrument; if they had enough responses for either time point the data were included in the analysis. Each of the 10 outcomes described above served as dependent variables in models with no intercepts and a time period (baseline, final) by group assignment interaction as the independent variable. Parameters resulting from this model include an estimated mean for each group at each time period (17). Contrasts were estimated to determine change from baseline to final and differences between groups.

We conducted additional analyses to determine if the effect of the intervention was moderated by age. These models were similar to the models described above except a three-way interaction of age group (<65, 65+), treatment group (intervention vs. control), and time period since diagnosis replaced the two-way interaction. No interaction effect was observed, so the original analyses are presented.

Table 1 | Characteristics at baseline among study participants*, by treatment group (*n*, %).

Characteristic	Intervention (*n* = 169*)	Control (*n* = 89*)	*p*-Value
Age (years)			
<50	33 (19.5)	19 (21.4)	0.93
50–64	81 (47.9)	41 (46.1)	
65+	55 (32.5)	29 (32.6)	
Sex			
Male	38 (22.5)	9 (10.1)	0.01
Female	131 (77.5)	80 (89.9)	
Marital status			
Married/partner	106 (62.7)	47 (52.8)	0.19
Single	62 (36.7)	42 (47.2)	
	1 (0.6)		
Hispanic ethnicity	13 (7.7)	6 (6.7)	0.78
Race			
White	145 (85.8)	74 (83.2)	0.57
Black	14 (8.3)	5 (5.6)	0.43
Other**	11 (6.5)	11 (12.4)	0.11
Insurance			
Medicaid	10 (5.9)	3 (3.4)	0.55
Medicare	83 (49.1)	31 (34.8)	0.03
HMO (Kaiser)	28 (16.6)	8 (9.0)	0.09
Private	63 (37.3)	34 (38.2)	0.88
VA/Other	4 (2.4)	2 (2.3)	1
None	6 (3.6)	3 (3.4)	1
Employment			
Working	47 (27.8)	38 (42.7)	0.04
Not working	49 (29.0)	15 (16.9)	
Retired	49 (29.0)	25 (28.1)	
Other	11 (6.5)	2 (2.3)	
Missing	13 (7.7)	9 (10.1)	
Self-rated health			
Excellent	13 (7.7)	8 (9.0)	0.76
Very good	52 (30.8)	29 (32.6)	
Good	77 (45.6)	35 (39.3)	
Fair	25 (14.8)	15 (16.9)	
Poor	2 (1.2)	1 (1.1)	
Missing	0 (0.0)	1 (1.1)	
Years since diagnosis	18 (10.7)		
<1	73 (43.2)	7 (7.9)	0.87
1–3	44 (26.0)	41 (46.1)	
4–9	29 (17.2)	24 (27.0)	
10+	5 (3.0)	13 (14.6)	
Missing		4 (4.5)	
Cancer type			
Breast	66 (39.1)	66 (74.2)	<0.0001
Lymph./Hodgkins	27 (16.0)	4 (4.5)	0.01
Prostate	12 (7.1)	4 (4.5)	0.41
Colorectal	11 (6.5)	2 (2.3)	0.23
Endometrial/uterine	7 (4.1)	1 (1.1)	0.27
Ovary	9 (5.3)	0 (0.0)	0.03
Multiple myeloma	6 (3.6)	2 (2.3)	0.72
Lung	9 (5.3)	1 (1.1)	0.17
Leukemia	6 (3.6)	4 (4.5)	0.74
Melanoma	4 (2.4)	1 (1.1)	0.66
***Other	43 (25.4)	6 (6.7)	0.0003

(Continued)

**Includes persons diagnosed with cancer (excludes participating caregivers).*

***Anyone who did check black or white including those who checked Asian, Native American, or other.*

****Including cancer of the cervix, bladder, bone, brain, esophagus, kidney, liver, pancreas, thyroid, or other.*

Effect sizes were calculated using Cohen's *d* (18), which is defined as the difference between two means divided by the pooled SD of the groups. Analysis was conducted using the Mixed Procedure of SAS 9.4. Unlike statistical significance, effect size is not dependent on sample size for interpretation. Effect size is a quantitative measure of the relative strength of the intervention whereby a larger absolute effect size value always indicates a stronger effect.

RESULTS

RECRUITMENT AND RANDOMIZATION

The activities described above resulted in 493 referrals (see Consort Diagram, **Figure 1**). Since this was an effectiveness study, the eligibility criteria were quite broad and only 12 of these individuals were ineligible (reasons included: did not receive treatment for cancer, over age 79, and still in treatment). A total of 158 subjects ultimately did not enroll as follows: did not show for first session to sign consent form ($n = 37$); not interested after learning more ($n = 31$); unreachable/voicemail left ($n = 38$); bad timing/inconvenient time/location ($n = 34$); in cancer treatment because cancer returned following initial outreach ($n = 18$). This resulted in a total of 323 eligible subjects enrolled, including 267 persons diagnosed with cancer and 56 caregivers/supporters. Randomization resulted in 169 survivors (and 29 of their caregivers) assigned to the intervention and 89 survivors (and 15 of their caregivers) assigned to the control. Only the survivors (not caregivers) in each group were utilized for the comparisons described in this paper (see below).

PARTICIPATION/COMPLETION

The average number of participants in each workshop was 8.2 ± 2.7; half the sessions had 7–9 participants (48.2%) with the remainder of workshops approximately evenly split between 5and 6 (29.6%) or 10 or greater participants (22.2%). The majority of participants (84%) completed four or more of the six sessions in each workshop (data not shown). Of the 169 persons diagnosed with cancer who were assigned to the intervention, 117 completed the final program measure (69.2%). A similarly high percentage of persons diagnosed with cancer and assigned to the control group ($n = 89$) completed the final measure ($n = 72$; 81.0%). Baseline characteristics of completers and non-completers were compared (data not shown) with only one factor (gender) significantly different between groups (more women in the intervention group); differences by intervention vs. control group in regard to completion were not observed. Baseline characteristics by group assignment are shown in **Table 1**; the groups were quite similar in accordance with major characteristics with the exception of gender and cancer type. Differences in insurance type and employment status were also present.

MISSING DATA/DATA ENTRY ERRORS

Five percent of surveys entered were checked at random for data entry errors; these checks were performed by study personnel who did not perform the initial data entry and demonstrated a detected error rate of <1%. A total of 448 surveys (258 baseline, 190 post-program) were collected. The number of surveys with complete data for specific outcomes ranged from 427 to 448, indicating that missing data within available surveys was minimal.

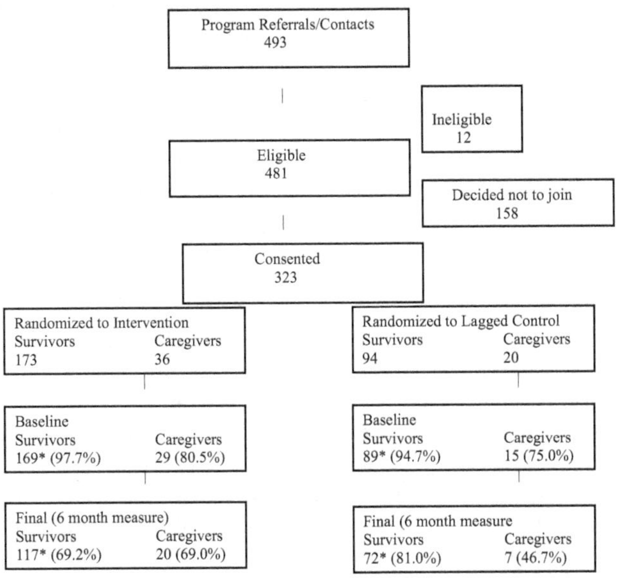

* Subjects included in repeated measures outcome analysis

FIGURE 1 | Study participation.

OUTCOME MEASURES

Baseline, final values measured at 6-month post-program, and change (%) values over time observed among participants in the intervention as compared to the control group are shown in **Table 2.** Statistically significant change over time among participants in the intervention was observed in the following outcomes: provider communication, depression, energy, sleep, and stress. Where change was observed in the controls, they were smaller among most outcomes.

EFFECT SIZES

Effect sizes calculated by Cohen's *d* are shown in **Table 3** for the intervention, control, and the difference in degree of change between the two groups. A beneficial effect was observed over time among participants in the intervention for many outcomes, consistent with the results in **Table 2.** For example, medium effect sizes (0.5–0.75) were shown for provider communication, depression, energy, sleep, and stress. In contrast, small effect sizes (0.16–0.35) or no effects were observed in the control for these same outcomes.

When the effect size for the difference in change in the intervention group relative to the change in the control was evaluated, a small effect was observed in regard to provider communication (0.23), sleep (−0.20), and very small effect for stress-related problems (−0.17).

In addition to the results shown in **Tables 2** and **3**, we also examined the role of interaction between age, time since diagnosis, and outcomes of interest and did not detect possible effect modification (data not shown).

Table 2 | Baseline, final, change, and % change between 6-month outcome measures, by intervention vs. control.

	Intervention ($n = 169$)				Lagged control ($n = 89$)			
6-month outcome	**Baseline value mean (SE)**	**Final value mean (SE)**	**Change mean (SE)**	**Change (%)**	**Base-line value mean (SE)**	**Final value mean (SE)**	**Change mean (SE)**	**Change (%)**
Days active	3.0 (0.2)	3.0 (0.2)	0.1 (0.2)	1.7	2.9 (0.2)	2.8 (0.3)	−0.1 (0.3)	−4.3
Minutes active	143.4 (12.3)	192 (27.3)	48.7 (28.2)	34.0	124.4 (17.0)	155.1 (35.0)	30.6 (36.5)	24.6
Self-efficacy	70.2 (1.7)	72.4 (2.0)	2.3 (1.9)	3.2	73.6 (2.3)	77.7 (2.6)	4.0 (2.5)	5.5
Provider communication	3.1 (0.1)	3.7 (0.1)	0.5** (0.1)	16.7	3.5 (0.1)	3.8 (0.1)	0.3 (0.1)*	7.4
Depression	8.5 (0.4)	6.9 (0.5)	1.62** (0.5)	−19.1	7.8 (0.6)	7.2 (0.6)	−0.7 (0.6)	−8.5
Health status	2.7 (0.1)	2.7 (0.1)	0.0 (0.1)	0.4	2.7 (0.1)	2.6 (0.1)	−0.1 (0.1)	−2.2
Energy	2.2 (0.1)	2.5 (0.1)	0.3** (0.1)	13.8	2.1 (0.1)	2.4 (0.1)	0.3 (0.1)*	12.9
Pain	3.2 (0.2)	3.0 (0.2)	−0.3 (0.2)	−8.0	3.5 (0.3)	3.7 (0.3)	0.2 (0.3)	5.9
Sleep problems	5.3 (0.2)	4.0 (0.3)	−1.3** (0.2)	−24.9	5.6 (0.3)	4.9 (0.3)	−0.7 (0.3)*	−12.7
Stress problems	5.1 (0.2)	4.1 (0.2)	−1.0** (0.22)	−19.1	5.4 (0.3)	4.8 (0.3)	−0.6 (0.3)*	−10.3

**Statistically significant change between baseline and final measures; $p<0.05$.*

***Statistically significant change between baseline and final measures; $p < 0.001$; repeated measures analysis.*

Table 3 | Effect sizes (Cohen's *d*) in 6-month outcomes, by intervention vs. control and change between groups.

Outcome	Effect size in intervention group (*n* = 169)	Effect size observed in control group (*n* = 89)	Effect size of difference in change between intervention and control
Days active	0.03	−0.05	0.06
Minutes active	*0.25	0.12	0.06
Self-efficacy	0.17	*0.23	0.08
Health status	0.02	−0.08	0.08
Provider communication	**0.75	*0.29	*0.23
Depression	**−0.50	*−0.16	*−0.18
Energy	**0.51	*0.35	0.03
Pain	−0.17	0.11	*−0.19
Sleep problems	**−0.72	*−0.31	*−0.20
Stress problems	**0.63	*−0.28	*−0.17

**Borderline/small effect (0.2).*
***Medium effect (0.5).*

DISCUSSION

These outcome analyses of the adapted version of the Stanford CDSMP for cancer survivors indicate demonstrable beneficial effects in many outcomes (**Tables 2** and **3**); further, no outcomes worsened following participation in the intervention when we evaluated the group-level comparisons. The outcomes that improved with the CTS program (e.g., provider communication, depression, sleep problems, and stress-related problems; see **Table 3**) are particularly salient to the challenges faced by cancer survivors. For example, fragmented and poorly coordinated systems of care make provider communication an important skill for the cancer survivor. Sleep, depression, and pain are commonly reported symptoms as described in the previously cited IOM report, and it is notable that a non-medical, relatively inexpensive and brief educational intervention delivered in the community setting had positive impact on these common yet potentially serious issues.

Improvement over time between the baseline and 6-month measure was also observed in three domains among the controls, although generally to a lesser degree than those in the intervention (see **Table 2**). For example, we observed a 19.1% mean difference depression scores measured by the PHQ-8 over time in the intervention group in contrast to only 8.5% decline in the controls over time. Further, the difference over time was statistically significant in the intervention but not in the control group. This difference in the magnitude of effect over time observed in the intervention vs. control groups is illustrated by comparing effect size. Effect sizes take into account the size of measurement error in the data but do not rely on sample size or statistical significance for their interpretation; therefore, they are meaningful when evaluating the relative impact of an intervention. In the case of depression, for example, the effect size in the intervention group over time was a medium/large effect (−0.50) vs. a small effect (−0.16) in controls (**Table 3**). Similarly, striking differences in effect size among the intervention vs. control groups were observed for pain (−0.17 vs. 0.11), suggesting a net small/medium benefit since the trend in the controls was to worsen over time. Although sample size does not directly impact the calculation of effect size, the finding of effect size differences is considered meaningful when observed in larger, well-designed studies such as reported here.

The heterogeneous nature of our study population in this intentionally pragmatic design allows us to estimate the benefits of the program in the real world by examining effect sizes (i.e., effectiveness). However, it also dampens the ability to detect statistically significant differences because by design, it does not use carefully constructed homogeneous study populations to minimize variation as in efficacy trials. The ability to demonstrate statistical significance in an effectiveness evaluation is strongly influenced by the number of persons in relevant subgroups where the intervention may be more or less efficacious; however, these subgroups are not necessarily known to the researchers or able to be detected in the real-world setting of the evaluation. The fact that we that we did not see statistically significant difference between the change over time in the intervention vs. control is likely a consequence of the heterogeneous nature of our real-world study population; but the difference in effect sizes represents the impact of the intervention by measuring the magnitude of this difference observed over time in the two groups and highlights the external validity of our findings.

Other studies of the CDSMP have similarly evaluated effect size to evaluate the impact of the program. A 2008 Cochrane Collaboration review (11) of self-management education interventions demonstrated effect sizes observed in multiple reports of other populations similar to or smaller than those observed in the current study. For example, of the 17 randomized trials of lay-led self-management programs in this review demonstrated effect sizes for pain of 0.10 (current study 0.11) and depression of 0.16 (current study 0.18).

Although we did not observe an effect with self-efficacy as observed in other trials (ranging from 0.30 to 0.40), we did observe an improvement in provider communication (0.23). Cancer survivors in the post-treatment period neither have the frequency nor regularity of health system interaction as with other chronic conditions such as asthma and diabetes and therefore may not have had ample opportunity to use their self-management skills, which could be the cause of the neutral scores on this domain. However, the improvement observed in provider communication is a related and similarly important skill for this population. Provider communication is a necessary component of the Chronic Care Model, which promotes collaboration between patients and providers in partnership to achieve improved outcomes (5). This is especially important in survivors who may experience both late and long-term side effects from treatment that can change over time, and may require ongoing vigilance and care.

Another observation from our study could be explored in future research is our observation of improvement over time in the control group, which although was to a lesser degree, was statistically significant in three constructs (energy, sleep, and stress). Other researchers have suggested that positive adjustment or post-traumatic growth over time following a stressful event such as cancer can occur (19–21). Thus, one possible explanation for this finding is that survivors have accepted a "new normal" and therefore the increase over a time is a reflection of this perception. Additionally, there may be some endogenous aspects to a survivor's improvement that could be capitalized upon in future iterations of the program.

Limitations of this study are that we may not have quantitatively measured all the outcomes of relevance in this population. For example, we did not directly measure social support or the unique benefits among caregivers such as family communication. Additionally, while the majority of respondents completed the final measure, we were unable to measure final outcomes in all respondents. However, we utilized repeated measures analysis to utilize data from all respondents regardless of completion to minimize this potential source of bias. Additionally, we chose to include survivors in the post-treatment stage only to support the unmet need for transition support. Although it is reasonable to expect that similar benefits would be observed in survivors at other points in the continuum, additional evaluations with survivors at other time points should be conducted.

A recent review of 16 self-management programs that have been utilized with a variety of cancer survivor populations promotes the use of the Chronic Care Model and particularly support for self-management in addressing needs across the continuum from diagnosis to survivorship (22). Aspects of self-management highlighted in this review as beneficial for survivors are also highly visible "active ingredients" in the CTS program and include: goal setting, realistic action plans, partnering with providers, and identifying aspects of health and healthcare that patients can self-manage with confidence. Although the attention to self-management interventions in this population is increasing, this review concludes that there is an urgent need for the translation of these interventions into practice, particularly in the post-treatment period. The authors suggest that interventions at this point in time can be especially helpful in easing transition to less regular contact with oncologists and dealing with the psychosocial and functional challenges into survivorship.

Contemporary views of effectiveness have evolved to suggest that it is influenced not only by efficacy, but reach of the program as well as implementation with fidelity (23). Our enrollment of over 300 cancer survivors and caregivers to this effectiveness study and the diversity of the study population according to cancer type, time since diagnosis, age, and other characteristics as shown in **Table 1** suggests that this program can reach and appeal to the general cancer population. By partnering with a community agency with state-wide reach for delivery of the original CDSMP Program with certified facilitators and extensive experience in delivering the program, we were further able to deliver the new adapted version in keeping with the principles of original program method. When taken in sum, these outcome and implementation data demonstrate that survivors who participate in the CTS program experience a small but measurable net gain over time in important survivorship domains in comparison to those who receive no intervention, and that the program can fill an important gap in meeting the ongoing need for management of post-diagnosis issues in this growing segment of the U.S. population.

The implementation of self-management support is particularly challenging in the cancer environment for a number of reasons including the use of multiple specialty care providers from diagnoses through to treatment and survivorship, lack of an evidence base to guide follow-up surveillance and decision making, complex late and long-term side effects requiring detailed patient history and records, and limited oncology system capacity. While the delivery of self-management programs to date has been driven by innovations in primary care, a recent emerging trend in support of needed system and policy change for cancer survivors is the establishment of patient-centered medical homes (PCMH) in the oncology setting (24). Future research is needed to support policy change to ensure that patients receive self-management support that is tailored to their cancer needs across oncology and a variety of other settings, driven by patient needs and preferences. Additional research is also needed to understand which outcomes are most relevant in this population toward demonstrating cost-effectiveness that can inform needed system and policy change.

Decreased emergency room visits and hospitalizations are of relevance to cost in other chronic illness populations (14), but outcomes such as overuse of care/screening may be even more important for cancer survivors. Patterns of care outcomes are difficult to track in with multiple payor systems, but policy changes to support the collection and analysis where possible in Medicaid/Medicare or other single-payor systems should be pursued to further evaluate outcomes from self-management support for cancer survivors. The CTS has enormous potential to be widely disseminated by tapping into existing channels in the community and among providers that have already been established with the CDSMP Program; however, the successful implementation of self-management interventions such as the CTS is reliant upon buy-in by oncology providers, survivors, and the healthcare system to recognize benefits such as those observed in the current report. As evidence continues to mount on the effectiveness of the CDSMP in other chronic disease populations (25, 26), and models of survivorship care continue to develop, policy and system support for self-management as a vital and viable component in successful transition to survivorship is needed.

ACKNOWLEDGMENTS

This publication was supported by the Centers for Disease Control and Prevention (CDC) and the National Cancer Institute through the Cancer Prevention and Control Research Network, a network within the CDC's Prevention Research Centers Program (University of Colorado, U48DP001938; Texas A&M University, U48DP001924). The contents of this article are solely the responsibility of the authors and do not necessarily represent the official views of the CDC or NCI. Additionally, we thank Stanford Patient Education Research Center for program development and technical assistance and the Consortium for Older Adult Wellness in Colorado for program dissemination.

REFERENCES

1. American Cancer Society. *Cancer Facts and Figures 2012.* Atlanta: ACS (2012).
2. Hewitt M, Greenfield S, Stovall E. *From Cancer Patient to Cancer Survivor: Lost in Transition.* The National Academies Press (2005).
3. Stull VB, Snyder DC, Demark-Wahnefried W. Lifestyle interventions in cancer survivors: designing programs that meet the needs of this vulnerable and growing population. *J Nutr* (2007) **137**(1 Suppl):243S–8S.

4. Patnaik JL, Byers T, Diguiseppi C, Denberg TD, Dabelea D. The influence of comorbidities on overall survival among older women diagnosed with breast cancer. *J Natl Cancer Inst* (2011) **103**(14):1101–11. doi:10.1093/jnci/djr188
5. Wager EH. Chronic disease management: what will it take to improve car for chronic illness? *Eff Clin Pract* (1998) **1**(1):2–4.
6. Lorig KR, Holman H. Self-management education: history, definition, outcomes, and mechanisms. *Ann Behav Med* (2003) **26**(1):1–7. doi:10.1023/A:1021718304633
7. Nolte S, Elsworth GR, Sinclair AJ, Osborne RJ. The extent and breadth of benefits from participating in chronic disease self-management course: a national patient-reported outcomes survey. *Patient Educ Couns* (2007) **65**(3):351–60. doi:10.1016/j.pec.2006.08.016
8. Brady TJ, Murphy L, O'Colmain BJ, Beauchesne D, Daniels B, Greenberg M, et al. A meta-analysis of health status, health behaviors, and health care utilization outcomes of the chronic disease self-management program. *Prev Chronic Dis* (2013) **10**:1201–12. doi:10.5888/pcd10.120112
9. Bandura A. *Self-Efficacy: The Exercise of Control*. New York: W.J. Freeman (1997).
10. Risendal B, Dwyer A, Seidel R, Lorig K, Katzenmeyer C, Coombs L, et al. Adaptation of the chronic disease self-management program for cancer survivors: feasibility, acceptability, and lessons for implementation. *J Cancer Educ* (2014) 29:762–71. doi:10.1007/s13187-014-0652-8
11. Foster C, Wright D, Hill J, Hopkinson J, Roffe L. Psychosocial implications of living 5 years or more following a cancer diagnosis: a systematic review of the research evidence. *Eur J Cancer* (2009) **18**(3):223–47. doi:10.1111/j.1365-2354.2008.01001.x
12. Foster C, Fenlon D. Recovery and self-management following a cancer diagnosis. *Br J Cancer* (2011) **105**:S21–8. doi:10.1038/bjc.2011.419
13. Lorig K, Stewart A, Ritter P, González V, Laurent D, Lynch J. *Outcome Measures for Health Education and other Health Care Interventions*. Thousand Oaks CA: Sage Publications (2012).
14. Ory MG, Ahn S, Jiang L, Smith ML, Ritter PL, Whitelaw N, et al. Successes of a national study of the chronic disease self-management program: meeting the triple aim of health care reform. *Med Care* (2013) **51**(11):992–8. doi:10.1097/MLR.0b013e3182a95dd1
15. Kulinski KP, Boutaugh M, Smith ML, Ory MG, Lorig K. Setting the stage: measure selection, coordination, and data collection for a national self-management initiative. *Front Public Health* (2015) **2**:206. doi:10.3389/fpubh.2014.00206
16. Kroenke K, Spitzer RL, Williams JB. The PHQ-9: validity of a brief depression severity measure. *J Gen Intern Med* (2001) **16**:606–13. doi:10.1046/j.1525-1497.2001.016009606.x
17. Fairclough D. *Design and Analysis of Quality of Life Studies in Clinical Trials*. 2nd ed. London, UK: Chapman and Hall, CRC Press (2012).
18. Rosnow RL, Rosenthal R. Computing contrasts, effect sizes, and counternulls on other people's published data: general procedures for research consumers. *Pyschol Methods* (1996) **1**:331–40. doi:10.1037/1082-989X.1.4.331
19. Cordova MJ, Andrykowski MA. Responses to cancer diagnosis and treatment: posttraumatic stress and posttraumatic growth. *Semin Clin Neuropsychiatry* (2003) **8**(4):286–96.
20. Barskova T, Oesterreich R. Post-traumatic growth in people living with a serious medical condition and its relations to physical and mental health: a systematic review. *Disabil Rehabil* (2009) **31**(21):1709–33. doi:10.1080/09638280902738441
21. Bellizzi KM, Smith AW, Reeve BB, Alfano CM, Bernstein L, Meeske K, et al. Posttraumatic growth and health-related quality of life in a racially diverse cohort of breast cancer survivors. *J Health Psychol* (2010) **15**(4):615–26. doi:10.1177/1359105309356364
22. McCorkle R, Ercolano E, Lazenby M, Schulman-Green D, Schilling LS, Lorig K, et al. Self-management: enabling and empowering patients living with cancer as a chronic illness. *CA Cancer J Clin* (2011) **61**(1):50–82. doi:10.3322/caac.20093
23. Glasgow RE, Lictenstein E, Marcus AC. Re-thinking the efficacy to effectiveness transition. *Am J Public Health* (2003) **93**(8):1261–7. doi:10.2105/AJPH.93.8.1261
24. Sprandio J. Oncology patient-centered medical home. *J Oncol Pract* (2012) **8**(3S):47s–9s. doi:10.1200/JOP.2012.000590
25. Ory MG, Ahn S, Jiang L, Lorig K, Ritter P, Laurent DD, et al. National Study of Chronic Disease Self-Management: six-month outcome findings. *J Aging Health* (2013) **25**(7):1258–74. doi:10.1177/0898264313502531
26. Ory MG, Smith ML, Patton K, Lorig K, Zenker W, Whitelaw N. Self-management at the tipping point: reaching 100,000 Americans with evidence-based programs. *J Am Geriatr Soc* (2013) **61**(5):821–3. doi:10.1111/jgs.12239

18

Fall prevention in community settings: Results from implementing *Stepping On* in three states

Marcia G. Ory[1]*, Matthew Lee Smith[2], Luohua Jiang[3,5], Robin Lee[4], Shuai Chen[5], Ashley D. Wilson[1], Judy A. Stevens[4] and Erin M. Parker[4]

[1] Department of Health Promotion and Community Health Sciences, Texas A&M Health Science Center, College Station, TX, USA
[2] Department of Health Promotion and Behavior, The University of Georgia College of Public Health, Athens, GA, USA
[3] Department of Epidemiology, University of California, Irvine, CA, USA
[4] National Center for Injury Prevention and Control, Centers for Disease Control and Prevention, Atlanta, GA, USA
[5] Department of Statistics, Texas A&M University, College Station, TX, USA

Edited by:
Michal Grivna, United Arab Emirates University, United Arab Emirates

Reviewed by:
Wilma Alvarado-Little, AlvaradoLittle Consulting LLC, USA
Katherine Henrietta Leith, University of South Carolina, USA

***Correspondence:**
Marcia G. Ory, Department of Health Promotion and Community Health Sciences, Texas A&M Health Science Center, 1266, College Station, TX 77843–1266, USA
e-mail: mory@sph.tamhsc.edu

Stepping On is a community-based intervention that has been shown in a randomized controlled trial to reduce fall risk. The Wisconsin Institute for Healthy Aging adapted *Stepping On* for use in the United States and developed a training infrastructure to enable dissemination. The purpose of this study is to: (1) describe the personal characteristics of *Stepping On* participants; (2) quantify participants' functional and self-reported health status at enrollment, and (3) measure changes in participants' functional and self-reported health status after completing the program. Both survey and observed functional status [timed up and go (TUG) test] data were collected between September 2011 and December 2013 for 366 participants enrolled in 32 *Stepping On* programs delivered in Colorado, New York, and Oregon. Paired *t*-tests and general estimating equations models adjusted for socio-demographic factors were performed to assess changes over the program period. Among the 266 participants with pre–post survey data, the average participant age was 78.7 (SD $\pm$ 8.0) years. Most participants were female (83.4%), white (96.9%), and in good health (49.4%). The TUG test scores decreased significantly ($p < 0.001$) for all 254 participants with pre–post data. The change was most noticeable among high risk participants where TUG time decreased from 17.6 to 14.4 s. The adjusted odds ratio of feeling confident about keeping from falling was more than three times greater after completing *Stepping On*. Further, the adjusted odds ratios of reporting "no difficulty" for getting out of a straight back chair increased by 89%. Intended for older adults who have fallen in the past or are afraid of falling, *Stepping On* has the potential to reduce the frequency and burden of older adult falls.

Keywords: fall prevention, evidence-based program, *Stepping On*, older adult

INTRODUCTION

Although older adults fall more frequently than younger people, falls are not a normal part of aging (1). Over the past three decades, researchers have identified the major modifiable fall risk factors as well as effective fall interventions (2–4). Some interventions shown to be effective in randomized control trials have been translated into programs and implemented in community settings. One such program is *Stepping On*, which was developed in Australia (5) and later adapted for use in the United States by the Wisconsin Institute for Healthy Aging (WIHA). The WIHA now provides training for *Stepping On* leaders as well as an implementation manual and evaluation plan (6, 7).

Stepping On is a group program proven to reduce falls and build confidence in ambulatory older adults who have fallen previously or are afraid of falling (8). A randomized trial of *Stepping On* found that participants' risk of falling was approximately 30% lower than those who did not receive the intervention (5). Stevens (2014) noted that a recent analysis also found that *Stepping On* showed a positive return on investment of 59% (J. Stevens, CDC, personal communication. 8/1/2014).

As described in the WIHA Implementation Manual (6), the program is delivered by a trained leader and a peer leader, who apply adult education and social learning principles to teach older adults about fall risk factors and strategies to reduce their fall risk. The traditional program consists of a group of 10–14 participants attending a 2 hour session held once a week for seven consecutive weeks. Content is provided by the program leaders and by invited health professional "guest experts." During the program, older adults learn how to improve their balance and strength, increase their safety at home and in the community, and the importance of vision assessment and medication reviews.

In 2011, the Centers for Disease Control and Prevention (CDC) launched a 5-year project funding State Departments of Health to implement *Stepping On* in selected communities in Oregon, Colorado, and New York. This was part of a larger project in which the CDC funded these states to reduce falls and fall-related injuries by engaging fall prevention coalitions, healthcare organizations, and other partners to implement evidence-based fall prevention programs in clinical and community settings. *Stepping On* is intended for older adults with moderate fall risk, such as an older adult who fell in the past year or is afraid of falling. Additional information about CDC's fall prevention initiative can be found elsewhere (9).

This manuscript describes the results of implementing *Stepping On* during the first 2 years of the project. The purposes were to: (1) describe the personal characteristics and session attendance of *Stepping On* participants; (2) quantify participants' functional and self-reported health status at enrollment, and (3) measure changes in participants' functional and self-reported health status after completing the program.

MATERIALS AND METHODS

PROGRAM PLANNING AND PARTICIPANT RECRUITMENT

The WIHA offered training for master trainers who, in turn, trained local group facilitators. State program leads (i.e., designated contacts at the State Departments of Health) recommended facilitators who were part of local public health or aging services delivery systems. Following the *Implementation Guide* (6), state program leads and facilitators worked together to identify appropriate sites for *Stepping On* programs.

Program participants were recruited through a variety of channels, including distributing flyers, conducting informational presentations, making personal contact in places where older adults congregated such as senior centers, recreation centers, or senior housing or retirement homes, as well as through contacts with their health care providers and television, newspaper, and radio advertisements.

Stepping On staff used a standardized admission form and screening questions to identify appropriate participants. To be eligible, a participant needed to be 60 years of age or older, live independently in the community, and be able to walk without the help of another person or with an assistive device (e.g., walker, scooter). Although some information about chronic illnesses was obtained during the screening process, information on the number and type of chronic conditions was not systematically collected as part of the evaluation survey.

In preparation for program delivery, each state conducted training sessions for *Stepping On* program leaders. The program was delivered in multiple settings, including healthcare organizations, senior housing or assisted living facilities, faith-based organizations, recreational facilities, and senior centers. Additional information about program preparation, implementation, and evaluation can be found in the *Stepping On Implementation Guide* (6).

DATA COLLECTION

Data were collected from multiple sources. Attendance was recorded at each session and these records were used to describe participant retention over the 7 week program. Program completion was defined as attending five of the seven sessions. A 20-question self-administered questionnaire was used to collect data at the initial *Stepping On* session (enrollment or baseline survey) and at the last session (program completion or post-intervention survey). Each survey took about 15 minutes to complete and assistance was provided to participants who needed help filling out the forms. Survey questions included participant characteristics (e.g., age group, gender, race, ethnicity), general health status (excellent, very good, good, fair, and poor), and whether the participant had been referred to the program by a healthcare provider. Also measured were satisfaction with their current physical activity level (very, mostly, somewhat, or not at all satisfied) and confidence in their ability to keep themselves from falling (five-point scale ranging from strongly agree to strongly disagree). Self-reported functional ability was assessed by the reported level of difficulty in performing various activities (e.g., climbing one flight of stairs) on a four-point scale ranging from (1) no difficulty to (4) unable to do (10).

The *Timed Up and Go* (TUG) test was used to measure functional status at the first and last *Stepping On* sessions. This test has been widely used to assess functional mobility and predict fall risk (11, 12) and has been validated among community-dwelling older adults (13). The test measures the time in seconds for a participant to "stand up from a standard arm chair, walk at [his or her] typical or normal pace to a line on the floor 3 m away, turn, return, and sit down again" (14). Participants who completed the TUG in <12 s were classified as having low fall risk and those who took 12 or more seconds were classified as high risk (15).

The Texas A&M University Institutional Review Board granted approval to analyze secondary data on program participants and outcomes collected using survey instruments and functional assessments.

STATISTICAL ANALYSES

To identify potential biases from loss to follow-up, we used the chi-square test to compare participant characteristics, number of sessions attended, and TUG results from participants who completed both the baseline and post-intervention surveys to those who only completed the baseline survey (were lost to follow-up). Two-tailed paired t-tests were used to compare participant's TUG results at the start and end of the program. General estimating equation (GEE) models using a logit link function were used to compare self-reported health status, satisfaction with activity levels, confidence in not falling, and self-reported functional status indicators at the start and end of the program. GEE models are longitudinal data models that use all available data in model estimation (i.e., do not require paired data) and can account for the correlation among repeated measures from the same participant. Each GEE model controlled for age group, gender, race, and program location. All models were run using SAS version 9.3 (SAS Institute Inc., Cary, NC, USA).

RESULTS

PROGRAM IMPLEMENTATION AND PARTICIPANT CHARACTERISTICS

Between September 1, 2011 and December 31, 2013, the three states hosted four *Stepping On* training sessions. There were 64 leaders trained and 32, 7-week *Stepping On* programs delivered. Four hundred nineteen participants aged 60 years and older enrolled and 336 participants (80.2%) completed the enrollment or baseline survey. Of these, 274 (81.5%) participants attended five or more sessions and 138 (41.1%) attended all seven sessions.

Table 1 | Characteristics of *Stepping On* participants.

	All enrolled participants[a]	Participants who completed both the baseline enrollment and post-intervention surveys	Participants who completed only the baseline enrollment survey		
	$N=336$	$n=266$	$n=70$		
	N (%)	*N* (%)	*N* (%)	X^2	*p*
Program location				0.90	0.639
Oregon	60 (17.9)	45 (16.9)	15 (21.4)		
Colorado	91 (27.1)	74 (27.8)	17 (24.3)		
New York	185 (55.1)	147 (55.3)	38 (54.3)		
Age group				0.58	0.749
60–69	53 (15.8)	44 (16.5)	9 (12.9)		
70–79	119 (35.4)	93 (35.0)	26 (37.1)		
80+	164 (48.8)	129 (48.5)	35 (50.0)		
Gender				0.01	0.914
Female	279 (83.3)	221 (83.4)	58 (82.9)		
Male	56 (16.7)	44 (16.6)	12 (17.1)		
Missing	1	1	0		
Race				2.61	0.106
White	316 (96.0)	253 (96.9)	63 (92.7)		
Non-white	13 (4.0)	8 (3.1)	5 (7.4)		
Missing	7	5	2		
Ethnicity (Hispanic/Latino)				2.07	0.151
Hispanic	7 (2.1)	4 (1.5)	3 (4.4)		
Non-Hispanic	322 (97.9)	256 (98.5)	66 (95.7)		
Missing	7	6	1		
General health status				3.09	0.214
Excellent or Very Good	114 (34.1)	96 (36.2)	18 (26.1)		
Good	168 (50.3)	131 (49.4)	37 (53.6)		
Fair/Poor	52 (15.6)	38 (14.3)	14 (20.3)		
Missing	2	1	1		
Referred to program by healthcare provider	22 (6.7)	19 (7.2)	3 (4.6)	0.57	0.452
Missing	8	3	5		
Timed up and go (tug) time at enrollment				0.78	0.378
Low risk (enrollment TUG <12 s)	165 (50.3%)	135 (51.5%)	30 (45.5%)		
High risk (enrollment TUG ≥ 12 s)	163 (49.7%)	127 (48.5%)	36 (54.6%)		
Missing	8	4	4		
Participants who completed 70%+ of sessions	274 (81.6%)	252 (94.7%)	22 (31.4%)	147.60	<0.001

[a] *Enrolled participants include all persons 60 years and older who filled out the baseline survey on the first day of the program (336/419 Stepping On participants). Individual survey questions may have had missing data.*

As indicated in **Table 1**, of the 336 participants who completed the baseline survey, 60 (17.9%) attended programs in Oregon, 91 (27.1%) in Colorado, and 185 (55.1%) in New York (**Table 1**). The age distribution was similar among participants in each state. The mean age was 78.7 (SD ± 8.0) years. Overall, the majority of people who enrolled were female (83.3%), white (96.0%), and non-Hispanic (97.9%). The majority of participants reported good (50.3%) or excellent to very good health (34.1%). Only 22 (6.7%) participants were referred to *Stepping On* by a healthcare provider.

There were 266 (63.5%) participants who completed both the baseline and post-intervention surveys; 70 completed only the baseline survey and were considered drop outs. Among the 266 participants with pre-post survey data, the average participant age was 78.7 (SD ± 8.0) years. Most participants were female (83.4%), white (96.9%), and in at least good health (85.6%). The majority of the participants with baseline and post-intervention surveys (94.7%) completed 70% of the seven session program. There were no statistically significant differences between those who completed both surveys (the analytical sample) and those who only completed the baseline survey except in terms of class completion (**Table 1**).

PARTICIPANT FUNCTIONAL PERFORMANCE

Of 336 participants with baseline data, 254 (75.6%) completed the TUG test at both baseline and post-intervention (**Table 2**). Of these, 123 (48.4%) were classified as high risk. After completing *Stepping On*, overall TUG scores significantly decreased 2.1 s (SD ± 3.1). The change was greatest among high risk participants whose TUG scores decreased an average of 3.2 s (SD ± 3.9).

SELF-REPORTED HEALTH AND FUNCTIONAL OUTCOMES

Table 3 compares self-reported health and functional outcomes at baseline enrollment and post-intervention. Odds ratios were adjusted for gender, age, race, and state. The adjusted odds ratio (aOR) of reporting excellent or very good health status increased by 56% (aOR = 1.56, 95% CI 1.22–2.00). The odds of being very or mostly satisfied with their physical activity levels increased significantly (aOR = 1.74, 95% CI 1.36–2.23) as did their confidence that a fall could be avoided (aOR = 4.60, 95% CI 2.94–7.22). Three of the five items assessing functional status indicated improvement (**Table 3**). Participants were more likely to report no difficulty in walking one block (aOR = 1.36, 95% CI 1.09, 1.69); getting out of a straight backed chair (aOR = 1.89, 95% CI 1.43–2.50); and climbing one flight of stairs (aOR = 1.42, 95% CI 1.11–1.82). Controlling for the number of sessions attended did not substantially affect our results (data not shown).

Table 2 | Changes in *Stepping On* participants' timed up and go (TUG) times in seconds from baseline to post-intervention[a].

Changes in timed up and go (TUG) times (in seconds)	Baseline TUG		Post-intervention TUG		Change in TUG from baseline to post-intervention[b]		
	N	Mean (±SD)	*N*	Mean (±SD)	*N*	Mean (±SD)	*p*-value
TUG times for all participants	254	13.5 (±5.7)	254	11.4 (±4.7)	254	−2.1 (±3.1)	<0.001
High risk (enrollment TUG time ≥12 s)	123	17.6 (±5.6)	123	14.4 (±4.9)	123	−3.2 (±3.9)	<0.001
Low risk (enrollment TUG time < 12 s)	131	9.6 (±1.4)	131	8.6 (±1.8)	131	−1.0 (±1.5)	<0.001

SD, standard deviation.

[a]While 329 participants completed the TUG at enrollment, this table highlights the 254 participants who completed the TUG at both baseline and post-intervention.

[b]Paired t-tests with an alpha of 0.05 were used to compare changes in participant's TUG time between baseline and post-intervention. A reduction in time indicates a positive functional improvement.

Table 3 | Changes in *Stepping On* participants' self-reported health and functional outcomes from baseline to post-intervention[a].

Self-reported health and functional outcome measures	Baseline (*N* = 266)[b]	Post-intervention (*N* = 266)[b]	Adjusted change from baseline to post-intervention[c]	
	N (%)	*N* (%)	Odds ratios from logistic models	*p*-value
Health status, satisfaction, and confidence				
Excellent or very good health status	96 (36.2%)	123 (46.8%)	1.56 (1.22, 2.00)	<0.001
Very/mostly satisfied with physical activity levels	123 (46.8%)	155 (59.4%)	1.74 (1.36, 2.23)	<0.001
Feel confident not falling (strongly agree or agree)	180 (69.8%)	237 (91.2%)	4.60 (2.94, 7.22)	<0.001
Self-reported functional status				
No difficulty in walking across room	195 (75.0%)	204 (79.4%)	1.23 (0.95, 1.59)	0.121
No difficulty in walking one block	144 (55.8%)	161 (62.4%)	1.36 (1.09, 1.69)	0.007
No difficulty in stooping, crouching, kneeling	59 (23.0%)	66(25.8%)	1.12 (0.86, 1.46)	0.403
No difficulty in getting out of a straight back chair	154 (59.7%)	189 (73.3%)	1.89 (1.43, 2.50)	<0.001
No difficulty in climbing one flight of stairs	102 (40.2%)	125 (48.6%)	1.42 (1.11, 1.82)	0.006

[a]Data are reported for the n = 266 participants who completed both the baseline and post-intervention surveys.

[b]The sample size is slightly smaller than 266 for some health outcomes due to missing data on individual outcome measures. The amount of missing data ranges from 0 to 5% for different outcomes.

[c]Adjusted odds ratios from GEE logistic regression modeling the probability of response = 1 at an alpha of 0.05. All models account for repeated measures from the same participant and are adjusted for gender, age, race, and program location. An odds ratio >1 represents a positive improvement in self-reported health.

DISCUSSION

This study examined 2 years of evaluation data collected from older adults aged 60 years and older who participated in the *Stepping On* community-based fall prevention program. We observed improvements in both the observed and self-reported functional abilities of program participants. Comparing data collected at baseline enrollment and program completion, *Stepping On* was associated with significant improvements in TUG scores and in self-reported measures of health status, satisfaction with their physical activity levels, and fall-related confidence. This suggests that *Stepping On* contributes to functional improvements and may also contribute to participants' general sense of well-being. The largest improvement was seen in feeling confident that falls could be avoided, which increased from approximately 70% at enrollment to over 90% after completion of the *Stepping On* program. Given that fear of falling is a fall risk factor (16–19), reduced fear coupled with increased functional ability is important components of an effective fall prevention program.

Recruitment and retention of participants is a concern for most fall prevention programs. While the race and ethnicity of *Stepping On* participants reflected the population from which they were recruited, there was a low percentage of male participants. There were limited numbers of referrals from health care providers, which suggest the need for better linkages between clinical and community approaches to fall prevention (20). Involvement of health care professionals can be critical for motivating older patients at risk of falling to enroll in and complete evidence-based fall prevention programs.

In regards to participant retention, we observed some attrition; however, the majority of the 366 enrolled participants (81.5%) completed at least 70% of the sessions. *Stepping On* runs only 7 weeks, so program attrition may be less of a problem than for longer running programs. For example, the fall prevention program, Tai Chi Moving for Better Balance (TCMBB), requires two 1 hour sessions over the course of 12 weeks (21). For TCMBB, only about half of the participants completed at least 70% of the program sessions (22). It also may have helped that *Stepping On* includes a social component, a break halfway through the 2 hour session, when participants can mingle and share refreshments. Further, it is possible that using the TUG test may have helped retain participants. While no data were systematically collected on participants like or dislike of the TUG test, multiple participants told their leaders that they enjoyed receiving their TUG times. The importance of timely performance feedback has been documented previously as a motivating factor for program participation (23).

LIMITATIONS

This study has a number of limitations that must be acknowledged. Participants were self-selected and this may limit the generalizability of the results to the broader older adult population in those communities. As we did not collect data on co-morbid conditions, we could not determine if our participants were similar to the broader population of older adults who were fearful of falling or had experienced prior falls. Similarly, we were unable to assess the extent to which co-morbid conditions were related to our study outcomes.

In order to minimize the reporting burden on the program implementation staff, we used a limited number of self-reported outcomes and one timed functional assessment (i.e., the TUG test). Although there was training provided for conducting the TUG (24), including available step-by-step online videos, this training was limited. Therefore, results may not be comparable to standardized TUG tests administered by trained professionals and some misclassification of a participant's fall risk may have occurred. While participants reported improvements in self-reported functional ability and demonstrated better TUG scores, we do not know if there was a reduction in falls. Data about falls were not collected because of anticipated problems with recall bias.

Although we did not assess fidelity directly, we believe that program fidelity was maintained by training and certifying group facilitators and using the detailed *Implementation Guide* that emphasized the importance of program fidelity.

CONCLUSION

Stepping On was previously shown to be effective at reducing fall risk in a randomized controlled trial. Intended for older adults who have fallen in the past or are afraid of falling, *Stepping On* applies adult education and social learning principles to teach older adults strategies that they can use to reduce their risk of falling. *Stepping On* participants practice balance and strength exercises, learn how to increase their safety at home and in the community, and learn about the importance of vision assessment and medication reviews. This study confirms that the program provides positive benefits and reduces fall risk factors among participants when implemented in multiple community-based settings in three states.

ACKNOWLEDGMENTS

We thank the Colorado, New York, and Oregon State Injury Prevention Centers for coordinating The *Stepping On* programs and collecting the study data and Margaret Kaniewski and Heidi Ehrenreich with the Centers for Disease Control and Prevention for their programmatic support and critical review of the manuscript. This research was supported in part by the Centers for Disease Control and Prevention, Prevention Research Centers Special Initiative Project, with funding from the National Center for Injury Prevention and Control for the State Fall Prevention Program under 5U48DP001924, and the Research Participation Program at the Centers for Disease Control and Prevention administered by the Oak Ridge Institute for Science and Education through an interagency agreement between the U.S. Department of Energy and CDC. The findings and conclusions in this report are those of the authors and do not necessarily represent the official position of the Centers for Disease Control and Prevention.

REFERENCES

1. Stevens J, Noonan R, Rubenstein L. Older adult fall prevention: perceptions, beliefs, and behaviors. *Am J Lifestyle Med* (2010) **4**(1):16–20. doi:10.1177/1559827609348350
2. Tinetti M, Baker D, Garrett P, Gottschalk M, Koch M, Horwitz R. Yale FICSIT: risk factor abatement strategy for fall prevention. *J Am Geriatr Soc* (1993) **41**(3):315–20.
3. Rubenstein LZ. Falls in older people: epidemiology, risk factors and strategies for prevention. *Age Aging* (2006) **35**(Suppl 2):ii37–41. doi:10.1093/ageing/afl084

4. Stevens JA, Baldwin GT, Ballesteros MF, Noonan RK, Sleet DA. An older adult falls research agenda from a public health perspective. *Clin Geriatr Med* (2010) **26**(4):767–79. doi:10.1016/j.cger.2010.06.006
5. Clemson L, Cumming RG, Kendig H, Swann M, Heard R, Taylor K. The effectiveness of a community-based program for reducing the incidence of falls in the elderly: a randomized trial. *J Am Geriatr Soc* (2004) **52**(9):1487–94. doi:10.1111/j.1532-5415.2004.52411.x
6. Wisconsin Institute for Healthy Aging. *Stepping on an Implementation Guide: How to Prepare for, Implement, and Evaluate Stepping on in Community Settings.* Centers for Disease Control and Prevention (2012). Available from: https://wihealthyaging.org/_data/files/SO_materials/Stepping-On-Manual_10-17-2013.pdf.
7. Mahoney JE. "Stepping On": stepping over the chasm from research to practice. *Front Public Health* (2015) **2**:148. doi:10.3389/fpubh.2014.00148
8. Stevens JA. *A CDC Compendium of Effective Fall Interventions: What Works for Community-Dwelling Older Adults.* Atlanta, GA: Centers for Disease Control and Prevention. National Center for Injury Prevention and Control. Division of Unintentional Injury Prevention (2010).
9. Kaniewski M, Stevens JA, Parker EM, Lee R. An introduction to the Centers for Disease Control and Prevention's efforts to prevent older adult falls. *Front Public Health* (2015) **2**:119. doi:10.3389/fpubh.2014.00119
10. Wallace RB, Herzog AR. Overview of the health measures in the health and retirement study. *J Hum Resour* (1995) **30**:S84–107. doi:10.2307/146279
11. Hutton I, Gamble G, McLean G, Butcher H, Gow P, Dalbeth N. Obstacles to action in arthritis: a community case-control study. *Int J Rheum Dis* (2009) **12**(2):107–17. doi:10.1111/j.1756-185X.2009.01392.x
12. Shumway-Cook A, Brauer S, Woollacott M. Predicting the probability for falls in community-dwelling older adults using the timed up & go test. *Phys Ther* (2000) **80**(9):896–903.
13. Bohannon RW. Reference values for the timed up and go test: a descriptive meta-analysis. *J Geriatr Phys Ther* (2006) **29**(2):64–8. doi:10.1519/00139143-200608000-00004
14. Podsiadlo D, Richardson S. The timed "up & go": a test of basic functional mobility for frail elderly persons. *J Am Geriatr Soc* (1991) **39**(2):142–8.
15. Bischoff HA, Stahelin HB, Monsch AU, Iversen MD, Weyh A, von Dechend M, et al. Identifying a cut-off point for normal mobility: a comparison of the timed 'up and go' test in community-dwelling and institutionalised elderly women. *Age Ageing* (2003) **32**(3):315–20. doi:10.1093/ageing/32.3.315
16. Tennstedt S, Howland J, Lachman M, Peterson E, Kasten L, Jette A. A randomized, controlled trial of a group intervention to reduce fear of falling and associated activity restriction in older adults. *J Gerontol B Psychol Sci Soc Sci* (1998) **53**(6):384–92. doi:10.1093/geronb/53B.6.P384
17. Tinetti ME, Baker DI, McAvay G, Claus EB, Garrett P, Gottschalk M, et al. A multifactorial intervention to reduce the risk of falling among elderly people living in the community. *N Engl J Med* (1994) **331**(13):821–7. doi:10.1056/NEJM199409293311301
18. Tinetti ME, Richman D, Powell L. Falls efficacy as a measure of fear of falling. *J Gerontol* (1990) **45**(6):239–43. doi:10.1093/geronj/45.6.P239
19. Vellas BJ, Wayne SJ, Romero LJ, Baumgartner RN, Garry PJ. Fear of falling and restriction of mobility in elderly fallers. *Age Ageing* (1997) **26**(3):189–93. doi:10.1093/ageing/26.3.189
20. Stevens JA, Phelan EA. Development of STEADI: a fall prevention resource for health care providers. Health Promot Pract [Internet]. (2012); [1-10 pp.]. Available from: http://www.ncbi.nlm.nih.gov/pubmed/23159993
21. National Center for Injury Prevention and Control. *Tai chi: Moving for Better Balance a Guide for Program Implementation.* (2011). p. 1–146. Available from: http://api.ning.com/files/lpWX79eu*NgqhrxYqum3lrPOm6Dp4GRQCK9J1qwtJylSBPaJ2W38NVNJNcBqszLkRplWB9ee-lwV4PIN-hUoPujtn*zU9vRw/TCManual_Compiled__v19.pdf
22. Ory MG, Smith ML, Parker EM, Jiang L, Chen S, Wilson AD, et al. Fall prevention in community settings: results from implementing Tai Chi: Moving for Better Balance in three states. *Front Public Health* (2015) **2**:258. doi:10.3389/fpubh.2014.00258
23. American College of Sports Medicine. *ACSM's Guidelines for Exercise Testing and Prescription.* 9 ed. Baltimore, MD: Lippincott Williams & Wilkins (2013). 480 p.
24. Centers for Disease Control and Prevention (CDC). STEADI (Stopping Elderly Accidents, Deaths & Injuries) Tool Kit for Health Care Providers Atlanta, GA, (2014). Available from: http://www.cdc.gov/homeandrecreationalsafety/Falls/steadi/index.html?s_cid=tw_injdir154.

19

Chronic Disease Self-Management Program in the workplace: Opportunities for health improvement

Matthew Lee Smith[1]*, Mark G. Wilson[1], David M. DeJoy[1], Heather Padilla[1], Heather Zuercher[1], Phaedra Corso[2], Robert Vandenberg[3], Kate Lorig[4] and Marcia G. Ory[5]

[1] *Workplace Health Group, Department of Health Promotion and Behavior, College of Public Health, The University of Georgia, Athens, GA, USA*
[2] *Department of Health Policy and Management, College of Public Health, The University of Georgia, Athens, GA, USA*
[3] *Department of Management, Terry College of Business, The University of Georgia, Athens, GA, USA*
[4] *Stanford Patient Education Research Center, Department of Medicine, Stanford School of Medicine, Palo Alto, CA, USA*
[5] *Department of Health Promotion and Community Health Sciences, Texas A&M Health Science Center School of Public Health, College Station, TX, USA*

Edited by:
Harshad Thakur, Tata Institute of Social Sciences, India

Reviewed by:
Xiaoyun Liu, Peking University, China
Nilesh Chandrakant Gawde, Tata Institute of Social Sciences, India

****Correspondence:***
Matthew Lee Smith, Department of Health Promotion and Behavior, College of Public Health, The University of Georgia, 330 River Road, 315 Ramsey Center, Athens, GA 30602, USA
e-mail: health@uga.edu

Disease management is becoming increasingly important in workplace health promotion given the aging workforce, rising chronic disease prevalence, and needs to maintain a productive and competitive American workforce. Despite the widespread availability of the Chronic Disease Self-Management Program (CDSMP), and its known health-related benefits, program adoption remains low in workplace settings. The primary purpose of this study is to compare personal and delivery characteristics of adults who attended CDSMP in the workplace relative to other settings (e.g., senior centers, healthcare organizations, residential facilities). This study also contrasts characteristics of CDSMP workplace participants to those of the greater United States workforce and provides recommendations for translating CDSMP for use in workplace settings. Data were analyzed from 25,664 adults collected during a national dissemination of CDSMP. Only states and territories that conducted workshops in workplace settings were included in analyses ($n = 13$ states and Puerto Rico). Chi-squared tests and t-tests were used to compare CDSMP participant characteristics by delivery site type. CDSMP workplace participant characteristics were then compared to reports from the United States Bureau of Labor Statistics. Of the 25,664 CDSMP participants in this study, 1.7% ($n = 435$) participated in workshops hosted in worksite settings. Compared to CDSMP participants in non-workplace settings, workplace setting participants were significantly younger and had fewer chronic conditions. Differences were also observed based on chronic disease types. On average, CDSMP workshops in workplace settings had smaller class sizes and workplace setting participants attended more workshop sessions. CDSMP participants in workplace settings were substantially older and a larger proportion were female than the general United States workforce. Findings indicate opportunities to translate CDSMP for use in the workplace to reach new target audiences.

Keywords: chronic disease self-management, evidence-based program, workplace wellness, evaluation, translational research

INTRODUCTION

Chronic diseases are multi-dimensional and affect all aspects of people's lives, especially work (1, 2). People with chronic diseases are constantly required to make decisions that affect their health, which have ramifications for work performance and employability. It has been reported that, depending on the chronic condition involved, between 22 and 49% of employees experience difficulties meeting physical work demands, while between 27 and 58% have problems meeting psychosocial work requirements (3). These problems can lead to job loss or premature departure from the workforce.

To complicate matters, the American workforce is aging. The Bureau of Labor Statistics (BLS) predicts that between 2006 and 2016, the number of workers aged 65–74 years will increase by 83%, and those aged 75 and older will increase by 84% (4). Many of these older workers will have one or more chronic diseases; 77% of older adults currently have two or more comorbidities (5). Recognizing the growing prevalence of obesity and other cardiovascular risk factors (e.g., hypertension, hypercholesterolemia, diabetes) and related chronic conditions among working-aged Americans (6), interventions are needed to arm middle-aged and older employees with skills and strategies to manage their diseases and associated symptoms.

Disease management is increasingly recognized as an important component of workplace health promotion given our aging workforce, the prevalence of chronic conditions, and the importance of maintaining a productive and competitive American workforce (7–11). Currently, most workplace-based disease management programs are offered by health insurance providers and operate largely independent of other on-site health promotion activities (2). Mounting evidence supports the effectiveness and growing importance of disease management programing in workplace settings (12–15). Unfortunately, workplace-delivered disease management activities may have limited reach because they are expensive and require medically trained providers/facilitators (2). These activities may also have narrow scopes (i.e., focus on one specific disease or condition).

Stanford's Chronic Disease Self-Management Program (CDSMP) is among the most widely disseminated and researched evidence-based programs (16, 17) and is extremely effective in helping individuals better manage their chronic disease and related complications (18–20). Developed based on over 20 years of research at Stanford University, CDSMP is currently offered in over 30 countries and a variety of languages[1]. Traditionally delivered through the aging services network, this robust program has been delivered in a wide variety of community settings (e.g., senior centers, healthcare organizations, residential facilities, faith-based organizations, and tribal centers). CDSMP has the advantages of being inexpensive and easily disseminated. It is not disease or condition specific and can be delivered effectively by lay leaders with minimal training using a train-the-trainer model.

To date, CDSMP has not been widely implemented by workplace settings or incorporated into workplace health promotion programing (21). In part, low-implementation rates in workplace settings may be a consequence of CDSMP being primarily delivered through the aging services network, which predominately targets older adults, many of whom may no longer in the workforce. Additionally, the standard CDSMP structure and format (i.e., 2.5 h sessions, once a week for six consecutive weeks) may not appear amenable to widespread implementation in work organizations. For these reasons, it is important to investigate characteristics of CDSMP uptake in workplace settings and explore opportunities for reaching and better serving the American workforce.

Using data from the first 100,000 participants collected during a 2-year national dissemination of CDSMP, the primary purpose of this study was to compare personal and delivery characteristics of adults who attended CDSMP in the workplace relative to other settings (e.g., senior centers, healthcare organizations, residential facilities). To contextualize CDSMP implementation in workplace settings, this study also contrasts characteristics of CDSMP workplace participants relative to those of the greater United States workforce. Building upon these findings, we highlight potential opportunities for translating CDSMP for use in workplace settings to overcome traditional barriers, reach new customer markets, and improve work performance indicators while maintaining the program's well-documented effectiveness.

MATERIALS AND METHODS

PROGRAM DESCRIPTION

The CDSMP has been introduced and disseminated in the United States as a method to empower patients with self-management skills to deal with their chronic conditions (22). Drawing upon social learning theory (23), CDSMP is an evidence-based, peer-led intervention consisting of six highly participative classes held for 2.5 h each, once a week, for six consecutive weeks (22). CDSMP has resulted in improved healthcare and health (18, 20), while potentially saving healthcare costs (19).

DATA SOURCE AND STUDY POPULATION

Cross-sectional data for this study were obtained from a nationwide delivery of CDSMP as part of the American Recovery and Reinvestment Act of 2009 (i.e., Recovery Act) *Communities Putting Prevention to Work: Chronic Disease Self-Management Program* initiative (16). The United States Administration on Aging led this initiative in collaboration with the Centers for Disease Control and Prevention (CDC) and the Centers for Medicare and Medicaid Services to support the delivery of CDSMP in 45 states, Puerto Rico, and the District of Columbia (17). This initiative was originally designed to have 50,000 Americans complete at least 4 out of 6 CDSMP sessions between 2010 and 2012 and to embed CDSMP delivery structures into statewide systems (16).

For this study, data were analyzed from 25,664 participants who attended CDSMP workshops in 13 states and 1 territory that delivered the program in workplace settings (i.e., to reduce threats for systematic bias associated with state-specific delivery infrastructures or preferences) and had no missing data for variables of interest. We also utilized 2012 BLS data from the United States Department of Labor to compare CDSMP participant characteristics to those of the larger American workforce[2].

MEASURES

The primary variable of interest in this study was whether or not CDSMP participants attended program workshops in workplace settings. Data from states that did not deliver one or more CDSMP workshops were omitted from study analyses. Among included states, workshop delivery site type was dichotomized into worksite settings and non-worksite settings. Non-worksite settings included senior centers, area agencies on aging (AAA), healthcare organizations, residential facilities, community or multipurpose centers, faith-based organizations, educational institutions, and tribal centers. Other workshop-level variables of interest included the number of participants enrolled in the workshop (i.e., continuous number ranging from 1 to 20 individuals) and the number of workshop sessions attended (i.e., "successful completion" is defined as attending 4 or more of the 6 possible sessions) (20).

Participant characteristics of interest in this study included age (i.e., measured continuously in years as well as categories consistent with those reported by the United States Department of Labor), sex, ethnicity, and race. Rural–urban commuting area codes based on participants' ZIP were used to categorize participants' residence (metro vs. non-metro). The number and type of self-reported chronic conditions was also recorded (i.e., arthritis, cancer, depression, diabetes, heart disease, hypertension, lung disease, stroke, osteoporosis, and other chronic conditions).

ANALYSES

To compare the characteristics of the participants who attended CDSMP workshops in workplace settings and those who participated in other settings, we used chi-square tests for categorical variables and independent-sample t-tests for continuous variables. Only data for the following states and territories were included in analyses: Alabama, Arizona, Florida, Hawaii, Maine,

[1] http://patienteducation.stanford.edu/programs/cdsmp.html

[2] http://www.bls.gov/data/#employment

Maryland, Massachusetts, Missouri, New Jersey, North Carolina, Oregon, Puerto Rico, Virginia, and Wisconsin. Statistical analyses for this descriptive study were performed using SPSS (version 21).

RESULTS

CDSMP PARTICIPATION IN WORKPLACE SETTINGS

Of the 25,664 participants who attended CDSMP workshops in these 13 states and 1 territory, 435 (1.70%) did so at a workplace setting. As seen in **Table 1**, the average age of workplace setting participants was 61.12 (±14.69) years. The majority of workplace setting participants was under age 65 years (58.6%), female (80.9%), non-Hispanic (96.1%), and white (61.6%). Over 63% reported living in metro areas. On average, workplace setting participants self-reported having 2.29 (±1.50) chronic conditions, with 41.4% reporting 3 or more coexisting conditions. The most frequently reported chronic conditions were hypertension (43.9%), arthritis (40.0%), diabetes (28.0%), and depression (22.5%). Almost 35% of participants reported some other chronic condition. On average, CDSMP workshop held in workplace settings had 10.82 (±3.89) participants. On average, these participants attended 4.84 (±1.46) of the 6 workshop sessions, with 85.1% successfully completing the workshop.

Compared to CDSMP participants in non-workplace settings, workplace setting participants were significantly younger and had fewer chronic conditions. A significantly smaller proportion of workplace setting participants had arthritis, hypertension, stroke, whereas a significantly larger proportion of these participants had other chronic condition types. A significantly larger proportion of participants in workplace settings were non-Hispanic and non-white, although a significantly larger proportion of non-workplace setting participants were African American. On average, CDSMP workshops in workplace settings had significantly fewer participants, and participants in workplace settings attended significantly more workshop sessions.

Compared to 2012 estimates from the United States Department of Labor, a larger proportion of CDSMP participants in workplace settings were over age 50 years, female, non-Hispanic, and non-white.

DISCUSSION

Findings from this descriptive study indicate that CDSMP adoption is low in the workplace, with merely 1.7% of participants in this sample attending workshops in workplace settings. Over 66% of workplace setting participants had two or more chronic conditions, which indicates the need for a widely available, high-quality disease self-management intervention. While significantly smaller proportions of workplace setting participants had arthritis, hypertension, and stroke relative to non-workplace setting participants (conditions more prevalent in the older adult population), it is interesting that rates of self-reported chronic conditions among workplace setting participants were generally comparable to rates among non-workplace setting participants. This aligns with previous reports indicating the American workforce is developing chronic conditions and accruing more comorbidities during their extended time on the job before their delayed retirement (24).

Compared to non-workplace setting participants in this study, workplace setting participants were significantly younger (i.e., on average 6.7 years younger); however, they were substantially older than the American workforce (i.e., 5.2% of the 2012 workforce aged 65 and older compared to 51.4% of CDSMP workplace setting participants). Further, when compared to the American workforce, males and Hispanics were underrepresented in CDSMP workplace settings. This finding highlights potential opportunities to expand program reach to new target audiences. When CDSMP was delivered in workplace settings, a significantly larger proportion of participants successfully completed the workshop relative to those in non-workplace settings (i.e., 85.1% compared to 78.1%). Clearly there is potential to expand CDSMP reach and adoption among the American workforce.

OPPORTUNITIES TO TRANSLATE CDSMP FOR USE IN THE WORKPLACE

Agencies such as the CDC are promoting coordinated approaches to workplace health that encompass interventions to address the multi-factorial influences of health risk and employee wellness (25). Aligned with CDC's goal of increasing the number of science-based initiatives in worksites (26), implementing and evaluating CDSMP in workplace settings is a viable strategy to improve employee health using a proven evidence-based intervention. Even though there is considerable need in worksite health promotion for efficacious disease management programs, CDSMP has not been tested in a format conducive for broad-based worksite dissemination. If CDSMP were appropriately tailored to the needs of middle-aged and older workers and delivered through workplace settings, this translated version would have potential to reduce healthcare utilization and boost work productivity and retention. This combination of benefits coupled with relatively low-delivery costs and scalability should be attractive to almost all employers and employer groups (i.e., leverage for making "a business case" to adopt CDSMP). Further, this model has potential to be extremely cost-effective and yield substantial returns on investment.

UNIQUE NATURE OF WORKSITES

Although there is considerable potential for offering CDSMP in workplaces, in order to maximize program effectiveness, it needs to be translated to accommodate the unique nature of worksite settings. Generally speaking, the typical worker is paid a certain amount of money, to work a defined period of time, to accomplish specific tasks or outcomes that will benefit the organization's goals and enable them to support themselves and their families. Organizations, in turn, are focused on maximizing the outcomes and minimizing the costs to achieve those outcomes, most of which are driven by the people, environment, and materials needed to produce the product or outcome. So, both the worker and organization have a strong economic incentive, time constraints, and interrelated goals and/or outcomes that are restricted by the environment in which they operate. These factors vary from organization to organization and job to job. As a result, any intervention implemented in worksites must be tailored to these unique characteristics. For CDSMP to be effective in worksite settings, it must be cost-effective, not too disruptive of work schedules, and achieve varying work-related outcomes (both individual and organizational). And, most importantly, it must do so within the constraints of the workplace environment.

Table 1 | National sample characteristics by CDSMP delivery site type.

	U.S. Workforce Statistics (2012)[a]	Total CDSMP participants (n=25,664)	Worksite setting (n=435)	Non-worksite setting (n=25,229)	χ^2 or t	P
Age	–	67.70 (±14.35)	61.12 (±14.69)	67.82 (±14.31)	9.67	<0.001
Under 50	66.8%	11.2%	20.0%	11.0%	108.82	<0.001
50–64	28.0%	23.9%	38.6%	23.7%		
6574	4.2%	30.2%	20.0%	30.4%		
75+	1.0%	34.7%	21.4%	35.0%		
Sex						
Male	53.0%	21.2%	19.1%	21.2%	1.14	0.286
Female	47.0%	78.8%	80.9%	78.8%		
Hispanic ethnicity						
No	–	89.0%	96.1%	88.9%	22.70	<0.001
Yes	15.4%	11.0%	3.9%	11.1%		
Race						
White	80.5%	66.7%	61.6%	66.8%	85.66	<0.001
African American	11.2%	20.9%	14.0%	21.0%		
Asian/Pacific Islander	5.5%	4.7%	12.9%	4.5%		
American Indian/Alaska naive	–	1.0%	2.1%	0.9%		
Other multiple races	–	6.8%	9.4%	6.7%		
Number of chronic conditions	–	2.50 (±1.65)	2.29 (±1.50)	2.50 (±1.65)	2.90	0.004
0	–	9.2%	9.2%	9.2%	3.94	0.268
1	–	21.4%	24.6%	21.3%		
2	–	23.9%	24.8%	23.9%		
3+	–	45.5%	41.4%	45.6%		
Participant residence						
Metro	–	78.5%	63.4%	78.7%	59.01	<0.001
Non-metro	–	21.5%	36.6%	21.3%		
Number of participant enrolled in workshop	–	12.59 (±4.03)	10.82 (±3.89)	12.62 (±4.03)	9.23	<0.001
Number of sessions attended	–	4.53 (±1.63)	4.84 (±1.46)	4.53 (±1.63)	−4.48	<0.001
Successful completion: no	–	21.8%	14.9%	21.8%	12.16	<0.001
Successful completion: yes	–	78.2%	85.1%	78.1%		
Disease prevalence						
Arthritis	–	47.1%	40.0%	47.2%	8.99	0.003
Cancer	–	10.9%	12.0%	10.9%	0.49	0.486
Depression	–	23.1%	22.5%	23.1%	0.09	0.770
Diabetes	–	32.1%	28.0%	32.1%	3.29	0.070
Heart disease	–	18.6%	16.6%	18.6%	1.18	0.277
Hypertension	–	48.7%	43.9%	48.8%	4.12	0.042
Lung disease	–	19.1%	16.1%	19.1%	2.51	0.113
Stroke	–	5.4%	3.2%	5.4%	4.12	0.042
Osteoporosis	–	14.6%	12.2%	14.7%	2.10	0.148
Other	–	30.3%	34.7%	30.2%	4.07	0.044

[a] *Unadjusted estimates of employed persons (U.S. Bureau of Labor Statistics; http://www.bls.gov/data/#employment).*

–, Workforce data not available for comparison purposes.

CDSMP TRANSLATION

As with any translation, it is imperative to maintain the program's integrity, which assures that the original intervention effects will be achieved. This could be accomplished by keeping the content, program duration, and number of contact hours constant, but modifying the session length (and thereby increasing the number of sessions) and incorporating worksite-specific strategies. This translation should also include efforts to complement existing workshop content to include topics, skills, and examples more relevant to working-aged individuals. It would afford researchers and evaluators an opportunity to introduce and assess new outcomes measures related to work performance and productivity. Such modifications may overcome barriers to workplace adoption as well as foster more universal cross-industry appeal in small rural jobsites and Fortune 500 companies alike. In the event that a workplace-based CDSMP were created, the new intervention would need to be standardized (as with any evidence-based program), with careful attention given to implementation manuals, fidelity standards, leader training (i.e., new and/or "bridge" trainings for T-trainers, master trainers, lay leaders), workshop materials, and evaluation tools and protocol.

Translation benefits

A key advantage of offering CDSMP to working adults would be that the program could reach younger individuals and those who are earlier in the time course of their chronic conditions, thereby reducing the likelihood of costly and debilitating complications. A workplace-based CDSMP has the potential to reach large numbers of working adults, which is not occurring through current workplace disease management delivery models or traditional CDSMP delivery channels.

Although delivered in workplace settings, a workplace-based CDSMP would benefit from ongoing collaboration with the aging services network and local community-based organizations to ensure long-term program sustainability. Further, a workplace-based CDSMP would readily complement other existing on-site health promotion initiatives that target healthy lifestyle behaviors and healthy decision-making.

LIMITATIONS

As with any study, there were limitations that should be addressed. Because of the grand scale nature of this national initiative, only self-report sociodemographics and administrative records were collected. No outcome data were obtained. Of the 45 states and 2 territories involved in this study, only 13 states and Puerto Rico offered workshops in workplace settings, thus, only data from these areas were included in study analyses to reduce possible bias when making comparisons. However, because 2012 BLS data contained data from all states and territories, comparisons with CDSMP participant data were less than ideal. Further, BLS data only contained a few variables to which CDSMP participant data could be compared (e.g., no information about rurality or disease diagnoses). This limited these authors' ability to fully realize the aims of this study.

CONCLUSION

This study provides a unique glimpse into the under-explored realm of CDSMP delivered in workplace settings. Findings suggest considerable opportunities for translating CDSMP for use in workplace settings to overcome traditional barriers, reach new target audiences, and improve work performance indicators while maintaining the program's effectiveness. While the recommendations put forth in this paper are those of the authors, additional workplace-based CDSMP translation efforts are inevitable.

ACKNOWLEDGMENTS

The American Recovery and Reinvestment Act of 2009 (i.e., Recovery Act) Communities Putting Prevention to Work: Chronic Disease Self-Management Program initiative, led by the United States Administration on Aging in collaboration with the Centers for Disease Control and Prevention and the Centers for Medicare and Medicaid Services, allotted $32.5 million to support the translation of the Stanford program in 45 States, Puerto Rico, and the District of Columbia. The National Council on Aging served as the Technical Assistance Resource Center for this initiative and collected de-identified data on program participation.

Research reported in this publication was supported by the National Heart, Lung, And Blood Institute of the National Institutes of Health under Award Number R01HL122330. The content is solely the responsibility of the authors and does not necessarily represent the official views of the National Institutes of Health.

REFERENCES

1. Detaille SI, van der Gulden JWJ, Engels JA, Heerkens YF, van Dijk FJ. Using intervention mapping (IM) to develop a self-management programme for employees with a chronic disease in the Netherlands. *BMC Public Health* (2010) **10**:353. doi:10.1186/1471-2458-10-353
2. Richling DE. Disease management for employed populations. 2nd ed. In: Pronk NP, editor. *ACSM's Worksite Health Handbook: A Guide to Building Healthy and Productive Companies.* Champaign, IL: Human Kinetics (2009). p. 286–95.
3. Lerner D, Allaire S, Reisine S. Work disability resulting from chronic health conditions. *J Occup Environ Med* (2005) **47**(3):253–64. doi:10.1097/01.jom.0000150206.04540.e7
4. Bureau of Labor Statistics. *Older Workers [Internet].* (2008). Available from: http://www.bls.gov/spotlight/2008/older_workers/
5. Agency for Health Research and Quality. *Medical Expenditure Panel Survey Household Component: 2010 Full Year Consolidated Data File.* Rockville, MD (2010). Available from: http://meps.ahrq.gov/data_stats/download_data_files_detail.jsp?cboPufNumber=HC-138
6. Bhattacharya J, Choudhry K, Lakdawalla D. Chronic disease and severe disability among working-age populations. *Med Care* (2008) **46**(1):92–100. doi:10.1097/MLR.0b013e3181484335
7. Goetzel RZ, Pei X, Tabrizi MJ, Henke RM, Kowlessar N, Nelson CF, et al. Ten modifiable health risk factors are linked to more than one-fifth of employer-employee health care spending. *Health Aff* (2012) **31**(11):2474–84. doi:10.1377/hlthaff.2011.0819
8. Special Committee on Health, Productivity, and Disability Management. Healthy workforce/healthy economy: The role of health, productivity, and disability management in addressing the nation's health care crisis. *J Occup Environ Med* (2009) **51**(1):114–9. doi:10.1097/JOM.0b013e318195dad2
9. Collins JJ, Baase CM, Sharda CE, Ozminkowski RJ, Nicholson S, Billotti GM, et al. The assessment of chronic health conditions on work performance, absence, and total economic impact for employers. *J Occup Environ Med* (2005) **47**(6):547–57. doi:10.1097/01.jom.0000166864.58664.29
10. Hoffman C, Rice D, Sung H-Y. Persons with chronic conditions. Their prevalence and costs. *J Am Med Assoc* (1996) **276**(18):1473–9. doi:10.1001/jama.276.18.1473
11. Hwang W, Weller W, Ireys H, Anderson G. Out-of-pocket medical spending for care of chronic conditions. *Health Aff* (2001) **20**(6):267–78. doi:10.1377/hlthaff.20.6.267
12. Nyman JA, Abraham JM, Jeffery MM, Barleen NA. The effectiveness of a health promotion program after 3 years: evidence from the University of Minnesota. *Med Care* (2012) **50**(9):772–8. doi:10.1097/MLR.0b013e31825a8b1f
13. Caloyeras JP, Liu H, Exum E, Broderick M, Mattke S. Managing manifest diseases, but not health risks, saved PepsiCo money over seven years. *Health Aff* (2014) **33**(1):124–31. doi:10.1377/hlthaff.2013.0625
14. Varekamp I, Verbeek JH, van Dijk FJH. How can we help employees with chronic diseases to stay at work? A review of interventions aimed at job retention and based on an empowerment perspective. *Int Arch Occup Environ Health* (2006) **80**(2):87–97. doi:10.1007/s00420-006-0112-9
15. Pelletier K. A review and analysis of the clinical and cost-effectiveness studies of comprehensive health promotion and disease management programs at the

worksite: update VI 2000-2004. *J Occup Environ Med* (2005) **47**(10):1051–8. doi:10.1097/01.jom.0000174303.85442.bf

16. Ory MG, Smith ML, Patton K, Lorig K, Zenker W, Whitelaw N. Self-management at the tipping point: Reaching 100,000 Americans with evidence-based programs. *J Am Geriatr Soc* (2013) **61**(5):821–3. doi:10.1111/jgs.12239
17. ARRA. *Communities Putting Prevention to Work: Chronic Disease Self-Management Program [Internet]*. US Department of Health and Human Services, Administration on Aging (2012). Available from: https://www.cfda.gov/index?s=program&mode=form&tab=core&id=04e3dca0a3218583cc472c28f5d26644
18. Ory M, Ahn S, Jiang L, Lorig K, Ritter P, Laurent D, et al. National study of chronic disease self-management. *J Aging Health* (2013) **25**(7):1258–74. doi:10.1177/0898264313502531
19. Ahn S, Basu R, Smith ML, Jiang L, Lorig K, Whitelaw N, et al. The impact of chronic disease self-management programs: healthcare savings through a community-based intervention. *BMC Public Health* (2013) **13**:1141. doi:10.1186/1471-2458-13-1141
20. Ory MG, Ahn S, Jiang L, Smith ML, Ritter PL, Whitelaw N, et al. Successes of a national study of the chronic disease self-management program: meeting the triple aim of health care reform. *Med Care* (2013) **51**(11):992–8. doi:10.1097/MLR.0b013e3182a95dd1
21. Smith ML, Ory MG, Ahn S, Kulinski KP, Jiang L, Horel S, et al. National dissemination of chronic disease self-management education programs: an incremental examination of delivery characteristics. *Front Public Health* (2015) **2**:227. doi:10.3389/fpubh.2014.00227
22. Lorig K, Holman H, Sobel D, Laurent D. *Living a Healthy Life with Chronic Conditions.* 3rd ed. Boulder, CO: Bull Publishing Company (2006).
23. Bandura A. Social cognitive theory of self-regulation. *Organ Behav Hum Decis Process* (1991) **50**(2):248–87. doi:10.1016/0749-5978(91)90022-L
24. Sliverstein M. Meeting the challenges of an aging workforce. *Am J Ind Med* (2008) **51**:269–80. doi:10.1002/ajim.20569
25. Centers for Disease Control and Prevention [Internet]. *Workplace Health Model* (2013). Available from: http://www.cdc.gov/workplacehealthpromotion/model/index.html
26. Centers for Disease Control and Prevention [Internet]. *About Work@Health* (2014). Available from: http://www.cdc.gov/workathealth/about.html

20

The conversion of a practice-based lifestyle enhancement program into a formalized, testable program: From Texercise *Classic* to Texercise *Select*

Marcia G. Ory[1]*, Matthew Lee Smith[2], Doris Howell[1], Alyson Zollinger[1], Cindy Quinn[1], Suzanne M. Swierc[3] and Alan B. Stevens[4]

[1] *Department of Health Promotion and Community Health Sciences, Texas A&M Health Science Center School of Public Health, College Station, TX, USA*
[2] *Department of Health Promotion and Behavior, College of Public Health, The University of Georgia, Athens, GA, USA*
[3] *Big Brothers Big Sisters of South Texas, San Antonio, TX, USA*
[4] *Baylor Scott & White Health, Temple, TX, USA*

Edited by:
Sanjay P. Zodpey, Public Health Foundation of India, India

Reviewed by:
Mary Altpeter, University of North Carolina at Chapel Hill, USA
Robert Otto Valdez, University of New Mexico, USA

Correspondence:
Marcia G. Ory, Department of Health Promotion and Community Health Sciences, School of Public Health, Texas A&M Health Science Center, TAMU 1266, College Station, TX 77843, USA
e-mail: mory@sph.tamhsc.edu

Little is known about the structure, content, and benefits of practice-based or grass roots health programs that have been widely delivered by a variety of community organizations and stakeholders. This perspective will document the natural history of Texercise *Classic*, a state-endorsed but previously untested lifestyle health promotion program. It will: (1) discuss Texercise *Classic's* participant reach and adoption over time; (2) describe the rationale and processes employed to formalize Texercise *Classic* into a more structured program known as Texercise *Select*; (3) outline the essential elements and activities included in Texercise *Select* and contrast them with those included in Texercise *Classic*; and (4) highlight key components for uniform facilitator training. The discussion will reflect upon the evolution of Texercise, compare and contrast the benefits and challenges of each program, and review the "next steps" for Texercise *Select*. In contrasting Texercise *Classic* and *Select*, it is important to understand the benefits and challenges of both programs. Preliminary results indicate that Texercise *Select* is effective, yet its ability to sustain the same reach as Texercise *Classic* remains unknown and an area for future study.

Keywords: translational research, program implementation, program evaluation, older adults, physical activity

INTRODUCTION

With greater recognition of the value of health promotion for adults across the life-course (1), a multitude of programs now exist to improve health and wellness among older adults (2, 3). These programs recognize that older adults are able and willing to engage in health promotion programs and can derive substantial health benefit from those programs (4). There have been two programmatic streams to meet the needs of the rapidly growing population of older adults: (1) practice-based or grass roots programs promoted by community-based organizations; and (2) research-tested programs developed and tested in academic research centers.

Included in the first programmatic stream, health promotion/disease prevention programs have traditionally been delivered by non-academic community-based practitioners with the generic goals of maintaining or improving health (5–8). Because these programs are delivered in real-world settings, they have a greater potential for large population reach and long-term sustainability; however, they are typically unstructured and hence not easily replicable or testable. Further, even when based on "best practices," such programs may have minimal attention to behavioral change theories and little to no formal evaluation to document intervention effectiveness or characterize essential program elements (9–12).

A second programmatic stream involves the recent nation-wide movement toward the widespread dissemination of evidence-based programs (EBPs) for older adults that were developed and tested by academics in controlled settings. This movement reflects the assumption that EBPs are preferable because they are "assumedly" more efficient and cost-effective than programs that are not theoretically based and rigorously evaluated (13). With the initiation of the Administration on Aging (AoA) Evidence-based Disease Prevention Initiative (14, 15), substantial knowledge has been gained about the nature and effectiveness of EBPs for older adults, especially those related to fall prevention, chronic disease self-management, and specific lifestyle behaviors such as physical activity or healthy nutrition (16–18).

Less is known, however, about the structure, content, and benefits of grass roots health programs that have been delivered by a variety of community organizations across vast geographic distances (i.e., regional or state-wide health promotion campaigns or community walking programs). Further, little attention has been given to understand how these programs might contribute to practice-based evidence. Given the recent emphasis on administrative policies within the Administration on Community Living (ACL), which give funding preference to EBPs (19), it is especially important to understand how these long-standing, community-based health promotion programs have functioned in the past and how they might be adapted to permit formal evaluation and be eligible for governmental funding streams.

This perspective article presents a case study of Texercise, a community-based health promotion movement established in 1999 to help Texans ages 45 and older live healthier lives. Based on a historical review of existing Texercise materials, supplemented by information provided by key Texercise staff, this article will examine the processes employed to structure the original Texercise program (referred to as Texercise *Classic*) so that it could be formally evaluated. Specifically, this article will: (1) document the natural history of Texercise *Classic*, including its programmatic reach and adoption across Texas over the past decade and a half; (2) describe the rationale and processes employed to formalize Texercise *Classic* into a more structured program known as Texercise *Select*; (3) outline the essential elements and activities included in Texercise *Select* and contrast them with those included in Texercise *Classic*; and (4) highlight key components for uniform facilitator training. The discussion will reflect upon the evolution of Texercise, the comparisons across the two program types, and the "Next Steps" for Texercise *Select*.

NATURAL HISTORY

Texercise *Classic* emerged from a vision by the state public health and aging services leadership to help the growing number of Texans age well. We highlight some salient events in the development and evolution of Texercise. Starting as a state-wide public health campaign in the late 1990s, this grass roots program was officially launched in 2002 as part of the Governor's Challenge Walk for Wellness. Under the Governor's Office, Texercise was envisioned as a state-wide health promotion program to encourage individuals and communities to adopt healthy lifestyle habits such as physical activity and good nutrition. In 2005, strong endorsement was received from the Governor's Office through Executive Order (20), which stated that "The Department of Aging and Disability Services, Department of State Health Services, Governor's Advisory Council on Physical Fitness, and other appropriate state and community organizations shall continue to promote and expand the internationally recognized Texercise program as a means to ensure healthy lifestyles in older Texans." In 2006, under the auspices of the Texas Department of Aging and Disability Services (DADS), Texercise became more formalized with the creation of a 12-week face-to-face fitness program, with the tag line "*Fit for the Health of It!*", and the identification of community-based volunteers or "program champions" to promote Texercise. In 2009, with input from experts such as Dr. Kenneth Cooper from the internationally known Cooper Clinic (21), the 12-week program and materials were updated to include attention to both physical activity and nutrition. The basis for the nutritional content was the existing information sheets developed by nutrition experts at DADS. We also utilized some standard nutrition items that other EBPs employ as well, such as the USDA my plate, and had all materials reviewed by a nutrition expert at the Texas A&M Health Science Center School of Public Health.

Thanks to the collaboration between DADS and its partners, what has become known as Texercise *Classic* is available free-of-charge and includes resources and incentives such as pedometers, resistance bands, pledge sheets, and 12-week daily fitness and nutrition logs distributed to participants during the program. Using a lay-leader facilitator model, Texercise *Classic* has been delivered through a variety of settings including worksites, senior centers, faith-based organizations, and long-term care facilities.

Texercise *Classic* has reached more than 15,000 Texans starting with 794 participants in 2006 and growing to 3,400 participants in 2012. Further, since 2003, over 160,000 Texercise handbooks (available at www.texercise.com) about how to initiate an exercise program have been distributed to individuals wanting to exercise on their own (22). Despite its widespread reach across Texas and national recognition (e.g., the International Council on Active Aging Industry Innovator Award; President's Council on Fitness, Sports, and Nutrition Community Leadership Award; and the Texas Cardiovascular Health Promotions Award), Texercise *Classic* had never been formally evaluated.

In 2012, a contract was awarded to the Texas A&M Health Science Center in collaboration with Baylor Scott & White Health to review and evaluate the program. The primary aims of this contract were to formalize the processes and procedures (including materials and facilitator training) and collect more detailed information from participants with the hopes of establishing a rigorous, scientific evidence base for this program. This evaluation has generated a new phase of activity.

FORMALIZATION PROCESSES AND PROCEDURES

PROCESS OVERVIEW

We identified in the beginning stages of the evaluation project that the loosely structured nature of the existing Texercise *Classic* program would make program evaluation difficult. Initially, Texercise *Classic* was designed as a participant-driven grass roots program in which participants, in collaboration with group leaders, decide upon the nature and amount of group exercises. While this strategy offered substantial choice, the lack of uniformity between workshops offered made it difficult to examine effectiveness and generalize to all Texercise programs. The Texas A&M research team and DADS staff jointly decided to utilize existing program materials and activities to create a more formally designed program. As indicated in **Table 1**, the resulting "structured" program is known as Texercise *Select*. Texercise *Select* is implemented in 12 weeks, which includes 2 weeks for participant recruitment and 10 weeks of 1.5-hour sessions conducted twice a week. Utilizing evidence-based skills and tools, each session incorporates interactive educational discussions, interactive activities related to physical activity and/or nutrition topics, and 30–45 minutes of actual exercise.

ESSENTIAL INTERVENTION ELEMENTS

Pulling from foundational concepts in evidence-based health and wellness programs (23–26), the research team developed the "structured" Texercise *Select* program, manual, and training that operationalized essential intervention elements and processes. To accomplish this task, the research team reviewed the literature as well as comparable EBPs. This review enabled the team to identify key exercise and behavior change elements that would work best in the Texercise context (e.g., ideal session length, ideal class duration, and types of effective exercises). Drawing on social cognitive learning principles (27), the entire program was designed heavily around the concept of self-efficacy with a goal of having participants take a more active role in their health through health choices and behaviors. The underlying programmatic intent was to increase self-efficacy and behavioral skills so that participants would continue to engage in healthy aging activities after the program ended.

Table 1 | Texercise *Select* topics, objectives, and resources by week.

Week	Sessions and topics	Objectives
1 & 2	None: participant recruitment	
3	Session 1: Ready, Set, Get Active: Launching an Active Lifestyle	Describe the 11 principles of physical activity success Identify their personal exercise levels Understand the importance of a warm-up and cool-down Set realistic goals related to physical activity
	Session 2: Ready, Set, Eat Healthy! Healthy Eating for a Healthy Lifestyle	Understand the benefits of healthy eating as well as the nutritional components of a healthy diet Make an achievable and realistic nutrition goal Describe the purpose of a nutrition log
4	Session 3: Ready, Set, Get Moving! Getting & Staying Physically Active	Recognize the essential components of being and staying physically active Practice endurance, strength, balance, and stretching exercises safely and correctly Create an action plan
	Session 4: Ready, Set, Eat Healthy! Eating a Balanced and Healthy Diet	Recognize the essential components of a balanced and healthy diet Practice new exercises safely and correctly Select and incorporate five sources of fruits and vegetables into their diets
5	Session 5: Ready, Set, Hydrate! Hydration for Health	Explain the basis and requirements of proper hydration Practice previous exercises safely and correctly Identify barriers and apply problem-solve skills when action planning
	Session 6: Ready, Set, Eat Proper Portions! Establishing a Sense of Portion Control	Understand healthy portion sizes for most types of foods Practice new exercises safely and correctly Identify ways to eat sensible portions
6	Session 7: Ready, Set, Go Endurance! A Focus on Endurance	Identify ways to safely increase endurance Practice exercises safely and correctly Evaluate previous action plan and apply strategies to overcome challenges with personal action plans
	Session 8: Ready, Set, Decode Food Labels! Understanding Food Labels	Explain the fundamental components of a food label Practice new exercises safely and correctly Evaluate dietary logs and action plans and apply strategies to overcome challenges
7	Session 9: Ready, Set, Prevent Injury! Injury Prevention for Better Health & Safety	Identify and apply injury prevention methods before, during, and after physical activity Practice safe and correct exercises Evaluate previous action plans and apply strategies to overcome challenges
	Session 10: Ready, Set, Cook Healthy! Cooking Healthy for Improved Nutrition	Identify and apply healthy cooking modifications to maximize nutritional intake Practice new exercises safely and correctly Recognize challenges and apply strategies to improve dietary behaviors
8	Session 11: Ready, Set, Get Strength Training	Understand and apply the fundamentals of strength training introduced in class Practice exercises safely and correctly Evaluate previous action plans and challenges Identify and apply strategies to overcome challenges with personal action plans
	Session 12: Ready, Set, Eat Out Healthy: Eat Healthy When Dining Out	Identify and apply strategies to make healthy choices when eating outside the home Practice exercises safely and correctly Create a healthy meal or menu
9	Session 13: Ready, Set, Don't Stress! Stress Management & Mental Health	Recognize and discuss healthy behaviors that reduce stress Practice exercises safely and correctly Evaluate previous actions plans
	Session 14: Ready, Set, Prevent Chronic Illness! Healthy Preventive Behaviors	Identify and select strategies to overcome challenges with action plans/goals Recognize and discuss healthy behaviors Practice exercises safely and correctly Identify ways to prevent and better manage chronic illnesses

(Continued)

Table 1 | Continued

Week	Sessions and topics	Objectives
10	Session 15: Ready, Set, Keep Fitness Fun! Keeping Fitness Fun	Practice exercises safely and correctly Identify ways to make long-term fitness enjoyable Identify and select strategies to overcome challenges with action plans/goals
	Session 16: Ready, Set, Eat Healthy! Eating Healthy During the Holidays	Identify healthy eating alternatives during the holidays Practice exercises (safely and correctly) Recognize unhealthy eating habits
11	Session 17: Ready, Set, Stay Committed! Staying Committed to Fitness & Review	Practice exercises safely and effectively Apply the two-step approach to creating an action plan Identify and apply strategies to overcome challenges Identify and apply safe ways to stay physically active (review)
	Session 18: Ready, Set, Stay Nutritious! Keeping Nutrition a Lifestyle & Review	Identify and apply ways to stay committed to nutritional goals and healthy eating Practice new exercises safely and correctly Identify and apply skills maintaining a healthy lifestyle
12	Session 19: Ready, Set, GO! Moving Forward Successfully	Identify and apply ways to stay physically active and eat nutritiously Practice exercises safely and correctly Identify and apply strategies to overcome barriers of physical activity and healthy eating
	Session 20: Ready, Set, CELEBRATE!	Identify and apply ways to stay committed to physical activity nutritional goals and healthy eating Demonstrate exercises safely and correctly

Texercise *Select* sessions were organized around a "Ready, Set, Go, Stay" rubric developed by our our Texas A&M program designers to help participants know what they needed to do to initiate healthier behaviors, engage in those behaviors, and to make them part of their everyday routines. Typically, each session has a physical activity and nutrition educational component, with the exception of the weekly session that focused more generally on managing emotional issues and general lifestyle behaviors. Using handout materials that had already been developed by experts for Texercise *Classic* (22), the course activities were intended to help participants apply strategies for enhancing healthy lifestyle behaviors. For example, group brainstroming was utilized to help participants identify solutions to common barriers. Class instructors also taught participants the essence of action planning – identifying, setting, and implementing realistic goals.

Although the program was structured (e.g., class length, discussion topics, and types of exercise specified), it was designed to be highly participatory and interactive with participants learning to actively engage in behavior change principles such as goal setting, problem solving, tracking behaviors, and providing support to fellow class participants. In addition to a peer-to-peer learning approach, Texercise *Select* was built around a lay-leader model, which has proven highly successful in the delivery of other EBPs for older adults (17, 28–30). This is consistent with the new exercise guidelines for older adults that stress the importance of risk management in the delivery of physical activity programs (25, 26, 31). Formal training sessions (i.e., a 6-hour group training) were hosted by the research team to provide lay-leaders (known in Texercise *Select* as facilitators) with information about how to safely introduce exercises. These training sessions were supplemented with course material that included screening questions and safety tips for participants (32).

Given the high probability of behavioral relapse in achieving one's desired lifestyle behavioral goals (24), the curriculum was designed for 10 weeks to increase the likelihood that behaviors would be adopted and become habit through ongoing reinforcement. It included attention to explicit strategies for helping participants stay committed. This involved hands-on practice of different behavioral skills (e.g., goal setting) combined with discussion about ways to overcome barriers and meet physical activity and healthy eating goals. Additionally, participants were encouraged to incorporate more walking into their daily routines and use the Texercise workout DVD at least 1 day each week outside of class (reinforced by program facilitators at the conclusion of each session).

COMPARISON OF TEXERCISE *CLASSIC* AND *SELECT*

Table 2 compares the elements of Texercise *Classic* with those of Texercise *Select.* When compared to Texercise *Classic,* Texercise *Select* has some similarities and many substantial differences. We draw upon Schulz and colleague's (33) taxonomy of interventions to describe some of the most prominent similarities and differences. When Texercise *Classic* was first designed, less was known about best practices for exercise training for older adults, and the program concepts were more implicitly related to best practices (rather than explicitly related to best practices). In contrast, Texercise *Select* was designed by individuals with formal training in exercise science and behavioral science as related to older adults. As such, this version of the program has benefited from an emerging science and practice base in both of these disciplines (26). Additionally, when creating Texercise *Select,* the developers drew upon the RE-AIM and other public health frameworks (34–36), for understanding the importance of key implementation and dissemination elements such as maximizing population reach, adoption, implementation, and sustainability.

Table 2 | Comparison of features in Texercise *Classic* and *Select*.

	Texercise *Classic*	Texercise *Select*
THEORETICAL UNDERPINNINGS		
Built around best practices for exercise training	Not explicit, but implicit through endorsement of Dr. Kenneth Cooper	Yes, using ACSM for older adult guidelines
Built upon best practices for behavioral change	Actual theoretical basis not clearly stated	Social cognitive theory (self-efficacy and other behavior change principles) RE-AIM framework Diffusion of innovation
PROGRAM STRUCTURE, APPROACH, AND POPULATION TARGET		
Total program duration	12 weeks of chosen exercise/activity	12 weeks: 2 weeks of recruitment plus 10 weeks, 2×/week of actual sessions equals 20 sessions total
Number of weeks of active intervention	12 weeks of chosen exercise	10 weeks, 2×/week of actual classes equals 20 sessions total
Amount of time per class	Variable	Structured – 90 minutes
Sensitivity to participant characteristics	Can be lay lead, leaders can be representative of the participants Participants do not need to be cognitively able to understand possible educational components Spanish materials are available	Can be lay led, leaders can be representative of the participants Participants must be cognitively able to understand the educational component including action planning Not yet translated to Spanish
PROGRAM DESIGN		
Intervention manual	General guidance with class instructors are only given the Texercise pink packet that includes: Promotional DVD Texercise handbook Pledge sheets Incentives (pedometers, t-shirts, etc.) and have access to the online resources	Structured manual for program facilitators with detailed session outlines
Adaptability	All aspects can be adapted, except involving some sort of PA Anyone can make an adaptation to the program including sites and class leaders Adaptations can be made at any time	Exercises can be adapted to participant level of PA Field coordinators/class facilitators cannot make adaptation to essential features of the program
PROGRAM CONTENT		
Attention to physical activity and nutrition	Possibility with the fact sheets Not necessary or monitored to see if the info provided to participants is factual	Built into the program First session of the week deals with a physical activity topic Second session of the week deals with a nutrition topic
Use of information sheets	Optional	Integrated into class curriculum
Opportunity for engaging in in-class exercises	Yes	Yes
Recommended exercises	Variable	Drawn from prescribed list with goal of 30–45 minutes of exercise per session that must include flexibility, strength, balance, and endurance
Opportunity for interactive class discussions on goal setting and problem solving	Due to the variability of the classes this is unknown Goal setting and problem solving are not specifically addressed in the classic class	Utilizes action planning and brainstorming Physical activity and dietary logs are kept through the first half of the sessions Uses incentives for behavior change Tracking and monitoring behavior (logs) Teaches problems solving Provides skill building (i.e., learning exercises) Provides social support
TRAINING AND EVALUATION		
Training of instructors	Variable	Structured – 1 day 6 hour training
Pre-post assessment	None	Part of curriculum
Fidelity monitoring	None	On-site class fidelity checklist Post class survey for participants

Although both programs are viewed as 12-week programs (with 10 weeks of active programing), the structure varies across the two programs, which makes the actual program duration and class time likely to vary as well. Texercise *Classic* and *Select* both provide time for participants to engage in group exercises and demonstrate some sensitivity to individual participant's needs, preferences, and level of physical functioning. One primary difference relates to program flexibility in that Texercise *Classic* operates under general guidance in contrast to Texercise *Select* that has a detailed implementation manual, which limits any adaptation to essential program characteristics or general program flow. Given the flexibility in structure and lack of detailed facilitator manual, it is assumed that Texercise *Classic* attends less consistently to both physical activity and nutrition aspects of healthy living. Texercise *Classic* was also assumed less likely to utilize the information sheets, demonstrate specific exercises, and promote interactive class discussions about goal setting and problem solving. However, the extent to which this is true is unknown because Texercise *Classic* has never been formally evaluated. Finally, the two programs differ in instructor training, evaluation, and fidelity monitoring with only Texercise *Select* including a pre- and post-assessments and a fidelity checklist as part of the program. While Texercise *Select* was evaluated as part of a research study, it should be noted that the capacity for on-site fidelity check monitoring in grand scale dissemination efforts may be limited.

TEXERCISE FACILITATOR TRAINING

When developing Texercise *Select*, the research team decided to utilize the term "facilitator" for program "lay" or "peer" leaders who are typically community volunteers versus health professionals. This decision was intended to emphasize that facilitators are not experts; rather, their role was to "facilitate" participants' ability to influence their health and functioning by presenting them with the concepts and exercises included within the program. The facilitator training was seen as essential for maintaining treatment fidelity (37, 38). Total facilitator training time consisted of one 6-hour day, with a structured training manual to which facilitators could refer after training. As specified in the training manual (39), the facilitator training was divided into five main topic blocks, each lasting between 30 minutes and 1.5 hours. Topics were delivered by the Texas A&M trainers through an interactive lecture style, including activities that allowed facilitators to apply presented information and elicit group feedback.

The training included a brief program overview of Texercise *Select* and an introduction to the format of each session in the curriculum. The training provided an opportunity for facilitators to observe and practice selected exercises, as well as to observe and demonstrate their ability to engage in group facilitation roles. During the demonstration session, trainers played the roles of the facilitators during a session and facilitators played the role of participants.

To demonstrate competency to lead a Texercise class, facilitators were assigned a Texercise session and tasked with four activities: (1) identifying the session topic; (2) identifying session materials needed; (3) identifying session activities; and (4) choosing one exercise from each exercise category (i.e., one warm-up, one upper body, and one lower body strength activity) and demonstrating it. Facilitators were then critiqued by trainers and any issues discussed and clarified.

Twenty-nine facilitators were trained during this pilot study. The curriculum was originally developed with two Texas A&M trained facilitators per class in mind. Once the research team began working with organizations to identify implementation sites and facilitators, it became apparent the class would most likely be led by one trained facilitator with assistance from another person who had not gone through the formal A&M training session. Given the pilot nature of this demonstration study, the Texas A&M class trainers were available by telephone and email to provide additional assistance to newly trained facilitators.

SUMMARY OF EVIDENCE-BASED STEPS

We employed several steps in transforming *Texercise Select* into a testable and replicable EBP. These involved: (1) inventorying the current literature to identify foundational concepts in evidence-based health and wellness programs, with special emphasis on strategies for promoting participant's self-efficacy for engaging in physical activity and peer-to-peer learning; (2) evaluating the match between existing programmatic elements and anticipated delivery capacity and structure to ensure program adoptability and maximal population coverage; (3) organizing the sessions around a "ready, set, go, stay" framework for ease of implementation; (4) developing a standardized manual and training protocol; (5) incorporating fidelity checks and quality assurance into the implementation and evaluation processes; and (6) identifying a practical measurement battery to assess pre–post intervention outcomes.

DISCUSSION

As indicated in our brief historical review, the evolution of Texercise mirrors many of the critical steps taken during the development and evaluation of an evidence-based health promotion program. This review also demonstrates the interaction between state-wide policy priorities, community practice, and research. Unlike research-based programs that often struggle for scalability, its state governmental sponsorship made Texercise *Classic* widely available and disseminated through existing community partners and delivery systems even before it was formally evaluated. Further, participation in Texercise *Classic* has grown state-wide for over 15 years, confirming the importance of high level endorsements and community buy-in for achieving long-term program sustainability (40–42). Its relatively low cost and use of volunteer networks have also been probable factors in its successful dissemination (43).

Although there have not been systematic studies, it is likely that Texercise *Classic* gained steam, in part, because it was endorsed by the Governor, codified in executive orders, supported for implementation as part of state services, and stimulated through active encouragement of public–private partnerships. Texercise *Classic* grew from a public health campaign with community-friendly handouts to a face-to-face group program based on best practices and expert opinion. As evolved by science, Texercise *Classic* progressed from an exercise program focused on physical activity to a behaviorally based program including attention to both physical activity and nutrition. Additionally, over time, with the movement toward evidence-based programing with replicable and demonstrated effects, the program was redesigned as Texercise *Select* to include explicit attention to best practices about exercise training and behavioral change found in other successful lifestyle programs that meet the highest tier criteria Evidence-based Disease Prevention and Health Promotion Program (19).

The development of new programs or the formalization of existing programs can expand the evidence base as it pertains to older adult health and wellness. While community-generated programs such as Texercise *Classic* may have already demonstrated success based on their reach and adoption, new policies from federal funders in the U.S. aging services sector are restricting reimbursement to reproducible health promotion programs with proven benefits (16, 19). As such, this case study illustrates the processes and procedures involved in the formalization of this community-generated program to advance its sophistication, replicability, and likelihood of evoking health benefits among its participants. To mirror requirements for EBP status, Texercise *Select* is now characterized by a set of essential features including formal manual and training infrastructure for widespread delivery (44, 45). Thus, the process described in this review represents the first steps toward formalizing Texercise *Select*, which is undergoing systematic evaluation to examine program effectiveness. Looking forward, the RE-AIM framework (46) will be used as a guide for examining strategies for demonstrating Texercise *Select* program effectiveness and public health impact, especially around program implementation, scalability, and sustainability issues.

In contrasting Texercise *Classic* and *Select*, it is important to understand the benefits and challenges of both programs. Texercise *Classic* has demonstrated its widespread appeal and sustainability by continual delivery for more than ten years by volunteer facilitators who do so without external financial support. As indicated in interviews with stakeholders (47), it is a program that has name recognition, is easy to implement, and is well-liked by program facilitators and participants alike. However, its greatest strength – flexibility in the content and type of delivery – is also its greatest potential weakness as an EBP. Such flexibility makes it difficult to replicate consistently, know exactly what program components are being implemented, and measure the extent to which participants are benefiting (or in what ways). Specific outcomes are unknown but are likely to be quite variable and affected by individual delivery settings, facilitators, and participant populations.

Conversely, Texercise *Select* provides structured training for facilitators and a scripted curriculum that, if followed, should result in positive health outcomes similar to those of other evidence-based lifestyle programs. Yet, some existing partners who primarily offer exercise programs might not like (or be able to implement) the reconfigured program with fidelity. For example, some park and recreation programs might easily adapt the exercise training part but not be as comfortable with facilitating the behavioral lifestyle educational aspects.

However, in terms of program impact, Texercise *Select* is likely to be more effective than Texercise *Classic* in changing lifestyle behaviors because of its standardized incorporation of evidence-based behavioral change principles. Yet, it is also unknown whether Texercise *Select* will be as appealing to community organizations and able to sustain the same reach and adoption as Texercise *Classic*. This issue illustrates a potential trade-off often seen when attempting to simultaneously achieve public health reach and effectiveness (48), and remains an area for future study.

The research team was able to redesign Texercise and conduct standardized training within two months. This accelerated timeframe was possible because of the research team's familiarity with EBPs and leader training as well as the insights provided by the original state-based developers of Texercise. Working together, opportunities, challenges, and potential solutions were identified. Texercise has a brand that is already established throughout the state with an existing network of partners. This brand was capitalized upon during the transition from Texercise *Classic* to Texercise *Select*. While a new name was considered for Texercise *Select*, the Texercise name was kept to ensure recognition and consistency. Both programs will continue to be promoted and supported in Texas because DADS sees value in allowing their partners to choose the appropriate program to offer based on their settings and participants.

NEXT STEPS

The purpose of this article was to illustrate the evolution of a grass roots program to become a theoretically derived and research-tested program. The further expansion of Texercise *Select* is dependent, in part, upon demonstrating positive outcomes comparable to those found in similar EBPs for seniors. An initial pilot test of the feasibility of implementation and outcomes was conducted in 2013. Preliminary results are promising (49, 50), with significant pre-post improvements ($P < 0.05$) seen in positive health behaviors (i.e., increased aerobic activity, weekly fruit/vegetable consumption, and daily water consumption) with large effect sizes for physical activity and smaller ones for nutrition behaviors. Additionally, enhanced dissemination of Texercise *Select* requires infrastructure resources such as the widespread availability of standardized training. Toward this end, DADS is updating the training and implementation manual so it will be web-based and easily accessible by community partners and potential facilitators. Although initial outcome results are promising, further study is needed to understand factors associated with the ability of Texercise *Select* to be widely disseminated and sustained over time. Once the results of initial pilot testing from 2013 are fully published, we recommend a state-wide campaign with DADS's current Texercise partners to help spread the word about the benefits of implementing evidence-based programing for seniors and how Texercise *Select* might be broadly disseminated through existing community channels.

ACKNOWLEDGMENTS

We thank study participants, research, and administrative staff. This study was supported by a grant from the Texas Department of Aging and Disability Studies. The research presented was also supported in part through the Community Research Center for Senior Health, a joint partnership between Scott & White Healthcare, Texas A&M Health Science Center, and the Central Texas Aging & Disability Resource Center. The Center is funded through a grant from the National Institute on Aging (Award Number RC4AG038183-01). The contents of this work are solely the responsibility of the authors and do not necessarily represent the official views of DADS or NIH.

REFERENCES

1. Ory MG, Smith ML, Resnick B. Changing behavior throughout the life-course: translating the success of aging research. *Transl Behav Med* (2012) **2**:1–4. doi:10.1007/s13142-012-0129-4
2. Prohaska TR, Anderson LA, Binstock RH. *Public Health for an Aging Society.* Baltimore: JHU Press (2012). 456 p.
3. Haber D. *Health Promotion and Aging: Practical Applications for Health Professionals.* Sixth ed. New York: Springer Publishing Company (2013). 513 p.
4. Ory M, Kinney Hoffman M, Hawkins M, Sanner B, Mockenhaupt R. Challenging aging stereotypes: strategies for creating a more active society. *Am J Prev Med* (2003) **25**(3):164–71. doi:10.1016/S0749-3797(03)00181-8
5. National Prevention Council. *National Prevention Strategy.* Washington, DC: U.S. Department of Health and Human Services, Office of the Surgeon General (2011).
6. National Center for Chronic Disease Prevention and Health Promotion. *Helping People to Live Long and Productive Lives and Enjoy a Good Quality of Life.* Atlanta, GA: Centers for Disease Control and Prevention (2009).
7. Task Force on Community Preventive Services. Recommendations to increase physical activity in communities. *Am J Prev Med* (2002) **22**(4 Suppl):67–72. doi:10.1016/S0749-3797(02)00433-6
8. National Center for Injury Prevention and Control. *Preventing Falls: How to Develop Community-Based Fall Prevention Programs for Older Adults.* Atlanta, GA: Centers for Disease Control and Prevention (2008).
9. Bryant LL, Altpeter M, Whitelaw NA. Evaluation of health promotion programs for older adults: an introduction. *J Appl Gerontol* (2006) **25**(3):197–213. doi:10.1177/0733464806288562
10. Glanz K, Bishop DB. The role of behavioral science theory in development and implementation of public health interventions. *Annu Rev Public Health* (2010) **31**:399–418. doi:10.1146/annurev.publhealth.012809.103604
11. Harris JR, Cheadle A, Hannon PA, Lichiello P, Forehand M, Mahoney E, et al. A framework for disseminating evidence-based health promotion practices. *Prev Chronic Dis* (2012) **9**:E22.
12. Merzel C, D'afflitti J. Reconsidering community-based health promotion: promise, performance, and potential. *Am J Public Health* (2003) **93**(4):557–74. doi:10.2105/AJPH.93.4.557
13. Brownson RC, Fielding JE, Maylahn CM. Evidence-based public health: a fundamental concept for public health practice. *Annu Rev Public Health* (2009) **30**:175–201. doi:10.1146/annurev.publhealth.031308.100134
14. Administration on Aging. *AoA Evidence-Based Prevention Program.* Washington, DC: Department of Health and Human Services (2013).
15. Administration for Community Living. *ARRA – Communities Putting Prevention to Work: Chronic Disease Self-Management Program.* Atlanta, GA: Department of Health and Human Services (2012).
16. National Council on Aging. *Where to Find Evidence-Based Programs.* Washington, DC (2013). Available from: http://www.ncoa.org/improve-health/center-for-healthy-aging/where-to-find-evidence-based.html
17. Ory MG, Smith ML, Wade A, Mounce C, Wilson A, Parrish R. Implementing and disseminating an evidence-based program to Prevent falls in older adults, Texas, 2007-2009. *Prev Chronic Dis* (2010) **7**(6):A130.
18. Ory MG, Ahn S, Jiang L, Smith ML, Ritter PL, Whitelaw N, et al. Successes of a national study of the chronic disease self-management program: meeting the triple aim of health care reform. *Med Care* (2013) **51**(11):992–8. doi:10.1097/MLR.0b013e3182a95dd1
19. Administration on Aging. *Disease Prevention and Health Promotion Services (OAA Title IIID).* Washington, DC: Department of Health and Human Services (2014).
20. Office of the Governor Rick Perry. *Executive Order RP42 – Relating to the Creation of the Aging TexasWell Advisory Committee and Plan.* (2005). Available from: http://governor.state.tx.us/news/executive-order/3687/
21. Cooper KH. *Texans Urged to Follow Kids' Lead; Shed "Fattest" Label.* Texas Department of Aging and Disability Services (2013). Available from: http://www.dads.state.tx.us/texercise/partners/cooper.html
22. Texas Department of Aging and Disability Services. *Texercise: A How-to Handbook for Lifelong Health and Wellness.* (2014). Available from: http://www.dads.state.tx.us/texercise/resources/handbook/english/index.html
23. Ory M, Jordan P, Bazzarre T. The behavior change consortium: setting the stage for a new century of health behavior-change research. *Health Educ Res* (2002) **17**(5):500–11. doi:10.1093/her/17.5.500
24. Ory MG, Smith ML, Mier N, Wernicke MM. The science of sustaining health behavior change: the health maintenance consortium. *Am J Health Behav* (2010) **34**(6):647–59. doi:10.5993/AJHB.34.6.2
25. Cress M, Buchner D, Prohaska T, Rimmer J, Brown M, Macera C, et al. Best practices for physical activity programs and behavior counseling in older adult populations. *Eur Rev Aging Phys Act* (2006) **3**(1):34–42. doi:10.1007/s11556-006-0003-9
26. Chodzko-Zajko W, American College of Sports Medicine. *ACSM's Exercise for Older Adults.* Philadelphia: Lippincott Williams & Wilkins (2013). 256 p.
27. Bandura A. *Social learning theory.* Englewood Cliffs, NJ: Prentice Hall (1977). 247 p.
28. Bodenheimer T, Chen E, Bennett HD. Confronting the growing burden of chronic disease: can the US health care workforce do the job? *Health Aff* (2009) **28**(1):64–74. doi:10.1377/hlthaff.28.1.64
29. Brady TJ, Murphy L, O'Colmain BJ, Beauchesne D, Daniels B, Greenberg M, et al. A meta-analysis of health status, health behaviors, and health care utilization outcomes of the chronic disease self-management program. *Prev Chronic Dis* (2013) **10**:120112. doi:10.5888/pcd10.120112
30. Wilcox S, Dowda M, Griffin SF, Rheaume C, Ory MG, Leviton L, et al. Results of the first year of active for life: translation of 2 evidence-based physical activity programs for older adults into community settings. *Am J Public Health* (2006) **96**(7):1201–9. doi:10.2105/AJPH.2005.074690
31. Ory M, Resnick B, Jordan PJ, Coday M, Riebe D, Garber CE, et al. Screening, safety, and adverse events in physical activity interventions: collaborative experiences from the behavior change consortium. *Annals Behav Med* (2005) **29**(2):20–8. doi:10.1207/s15324796abm2902s_5
32. Program on Healthy Aging. *EASY Exercise and Screening for You.* Texas A&M Health Science Center School of Public Health (2008). Available from: http://easyforyou.info/
33. Schulz R, Czaja SJ, McKay JR, Ory MG, Belle SH. Intervention taxonomy (ITAX): describing essential features of interventions (HMC). *Am J Health Behav* (2010) **34**(6):811–21. doi:10.5993/AJHB.34.6.15
34. Gaglio B, Shoup JA, Glasgow RE. The RE-AIM framework: a systematic review of use over time. *Am J Public Health* (2013) **103**(6):e38–46. doi:10.2105/AJPH.2013.301299
35. Lobb R, Colditz GA. Implementation science and its application to population health. *Annu Rev Public Health* (2013) **34**:235–51. doi:10.1146/annurev-publhealth-031912-114444
36. Brownson RC, Colditz GA, Proctor EK. *Dissemination and Implementation Research in Health: Translating Science to Practice.* New York: Oxford University Press (2012). 560 p.
37. Bellg AJ, Borrelli B, Resnick B, Hecht J, Minicucci DS, Ory M, et al. Enhancing treatment fidelity in health behavior change studies: best practices and recommendations from the NIH behavior change consortium. *Health Psychol* (2004) **23**(5):443–51. doi:10.1037/0278-6133.23.5.443
38. Frank JC, Coviak CP, Healy TC, Belza B, Casado BL. Addressing fidelity in evidence-based health promotion programs for older adults. *J Appl Gerontol* (2008) **27**(1):4–33. doi:10.1177/1090198114543007
39. Texas Department of Aging and Disability Services. *Texercise Training Manual.* Available from: http://www.dads.state.tx.us/texercise/resources/index.html
40. Evashwick C, Ory M. Organizational characteristics of successful innovative health care programs sustained over time. *Fam Community Health* (2003) **26**(3):177–93. doi:10.1097/00003727-200307000-00003
41. Estabrooks PA, Smith-Ray RL, Dzewaltowski DA, Dowdy D, Lattimore D, Rheaume C, et al. Sustainability of evidence-based community-based physical activity programs for older adults: lessons from active for life. *Transl Behav Med* (2011) **1**(2):208–15. doi:10.1007/s13142-011-0039-x
42. Scheirer MA, Dearing JW. An agenda for research on the sustainability of public health programs. *Am J Public Health* (2011) **101**(11):2059–67. doi:10.2105/AJPH.2011.300193
43. Rogers EM. *Diffusion of Innovations.* 5th ed. New York: Free Press (2003). 551 p.
44. Altpeter M, Bryant L, Schneider E, Whitelaw N. Evidence-based health practice: knowing and using what works for older adults. *Home Health Care Serv Q* (2006) **25**(1–2):1–11. doi:10.1300/J027v25n01_01
45. Center for Healthy Aging. *Module 2: What is EBHP?.* Washington, DC: National Council on Aging (2014).

46. Human Nutrition Foods and Exercise. *Reach Effectiveness Adoption Implementation Maintenance.* Blacksburg, VA: Virginia Tech College of Agriculture and Life Sciences (2014).
47. Stevens Ab, Thiel S, Thorud JL, Smith ML, Howell D, Cargill J, et al. Increasing the availability of physical activity programs for older adults: lessons learned from Texercise stakeholders. *J Aging Phys Activ* (in press).
48. National Collaborating Centre for Methods and Tools. *Assessing the Public Health Impact of Health Promotion Initiatives.* Hamilton, ON: McMaster University (2010).
49. Ory MG, Smith ML, Jiang J, Howell D, Chen S, Pulczinski J, et al. Texercise effectiveness: an examination of physical function and quality of life. *J Aging Phys Activ.* (2015) (in press).
50. Smith ML, Ory MG, Jiang L, Howell D, Chen S, Pulczinski J, et al. Texercise select effectiveness: an examination of physical activity and nutrition outcomes. *Transl Behav Med* (2015) (in press).

21

Developing an evidence-based fall prevention curriculum for community health workers

Julie A. St. John[1]*, Tiffany E. Shubert[2], Matthew Lee Smith[3], Cherie A. Rosemond[4], Doris A. Howell[5], Christopher E. Beaudoin[6] and Marcia G. Ory[7]

[1] Department of Public Health, Graduate School of Biomedical Sciences, Texas Tech University Health Sciences Center, Abilene, TX, USA
[2] Division of Geriatrics, School of Medicine, University of North Carolina at Chapel Hill, Chapel Hill, NC, USA
[3] College of Public Health, The University of Georgia, Athens, GA, USA
[4] Center for Health Promotion and Disease Prevention, University of North Carolina at Chapel Hill, Chapel Hill, NC, USA
[5] Program on Healthy Aging, Texas A&M Health Science Center School of Public Health, College Station, TX, USA
[6] Department of Communication, Texas A&M University, College Station, TX, USA
[7] Department of Health Promotion and Community Health Sciences, Texas A&M Health Science Center School of Public Health, College Station, TX, USA

Edited by:
Sanjay P. Zodpey, Public Health Foundation of India, India

Reviewed by:
Milka Dancevic Gojkovic, Public Health Institute of Federation of Bosnia and Herzegovina, Bosnia and Herzegovina
Shridhar Murlidharrao Kadam, Public Health Foundation of India, India

***Correspondence:**
Julie A. St. John, Department of Public Health, Graduate School of Biomedical Sciences, Texas Tech University Health Sciences Center, 1718 Pine Street, Abilene, TX 79601-3044, USA
e-mail: julie.st-john@ttuhsc.edu

This perspective paper describes processes in the development of an evidence-based fall prevention curriculum for community health workers/promotores (CHW/P) that highlights the development of the curriculum and addresses: (1) the need and rationale for involving CHW/P in fall prevention; (2) involvement of CHW/P and content experts in the curriculum development; (3) best practices utilized in the curriculum development and training implementation; and (4) next steps for dissemination and utilization of the CHW/P fall prevention curriculum. The project team of CHW/P and content experts developed, pilot tested, and revised bilingual in-person training modules about fall prevention among older adults. The curriculum incorporated the following major themes: (1) fall risk factors and strategies to reduce/prevent falls; (2) communication strategies to reduce risk of falling and strategies for developing fall prevention plans; and (3) health behavior change theories utilized to prevent and reduce falls. Three separate fall prevention modules were developed for CHW/P and CHW/P Instructors to be used during in-person trainings. Module development incorporated a five-step process: (1) conduct informal focus groups with CHW/P to inform content development; (2) develop three in-person modules in English and Spanish with input from content experts; (3) pilot-test the modules with CHW/P; (4) refine and finalize modules based on pilot-test feedback; and (5) submit modules for approval of continuing education units. This project contributes to the existing evidence-based literature by examining the role of CHW/P in fall prevention among older adults. By including evidence-based communication strategies such as message tailoring, the curriculum design allows CHW/P to personalize the information for individuals, which can result in an effective dissemination of a curriculum that is evidence-based and culturally appropriate.

Keywords: community health workers, promotores, curriculum development, training, fall prevention, older adults

INTRODUCTION

"I've fallen and I can't get up," was a phrase made popular by LifeCall in 1989. This commercial was a dramatized version of an older adult's fall. However, this situation is the reality for numerous older adults in the United States. Falls are a threat to the lives, independence, and health of adults – especially those aged 65 and older. Every 18 s an older adult visits an emergency department as a result a fall, and every 35 min an older adult dies due to injuries from such a fall (1–7).

Other significant consequences are associated with falls. For example, one in three adults aged 65 and older fall each year, costing the U.S. healthcare system more than $30 billion dollars annually (1). This problem is even more significant due to the rapidly expanding aging population (8). In light of the rate of falls among older adults, physical and fiscal costs, severity of falls, and population growth among adults ages 65 and older, researchers are investigating how to effectively prevent and reduce falls among older adults.

Research has demonstrated that a large proportion of falls among community-dwelling older adults are preventable (9, 10). Numerous documented strategies address fall prevention among older adults – community programing, primary care practice guidelines, and integration of physical therapists into models of care (11). Despite the growth of evidence-based fall prevention programs and the emergence of state-wide fall prevention policy efforts, there continues to be a gap in community adoption of fall prevention interventions among underserved, rural, minority, and low-income populations (12). Literature is lacking regarding: (1) the reasons why fall prevention policies and programs are or are not adopted and spread in community settings; (2) the most efficient practices for creating a trained workforce for delivering interventions; (3) the best strategies for reaching out to underserved populations in terms of recruitment, geographic, and needs-based challenges; and (4) how to connect community and clinical care settings (12). A lack of infrastructure for disseminating and implementing interventions to community-based programs has contributed significantly to this gap.

The Policies, Programs, and Partners for Fall Prevention (PPPFP) study incorporated multi-level intervention strategies to develop several dissemination approaches (13). This paper focuses on a training Community Health Workers/Promotores (CHW/P) to deliver fall prevention messages to older adults. CHW/P are described as frontline public health workers, serving as liaisons between health and social services and the community. They facilitate access and improve the quality and cultural competence of service delivery by utilizing a wide array of skill sets (14–17). CHW/P are trusted members of the target community, work for pay or as volunteers, and typically share ethnicity, language, socioeconomic status, and life experiences with the community members served. As such, CHW/P can communicate with other members of the healthcare system to ensure that community members' care is sensitive to cultural and community issues. Research has demonstrated the effectiveness of CHW/P among targeted Hispanic populations in achieving positive health outcomes through health education, case management, service coordination, and referrals (18–31). Specifically, CHW/P are effective due to their cultural similarity and understanding of the population they serve, as well as the subsequent trust clients have in them. These CHW/P characteristics are largely due to their residing in the same communities. Further, studies have demonstrated the effectiveness of CHW/P in providing social support to help Hispanics adopt behavior change (24–30).

One of the greatest challenges in effective fall prevention is ensuring the population at risk actually receives recommended interventions. CHW/P can serve as liaisons for older adults at risk for falling, making sure they are referred to accessible services and helping make sure interventions at the community or healthcare level are supported to maximize program adherence. The literature supports CHW/P as a conduit to increase fall prevention awareness, but there is a gap in fall prevention training for CHW/P. This perspective paper will describe the development and implementation of the fall prevention curriculum for CHW/P with a focus on: (1) making the case for developing evidence-based CHW fall prevention training; and (2) explaining programmatic activity, including informal focus groups, module development, pilot testing, curriculum refinement, continuing education units (CEUs) approval, and next steps in dissemination.

MAKING THE CASE FOR DEVELOPING AN EVIDENCE-BASED CHW FALL PREVENTION TRAINING

A preparatory national scan of CHW/P curriculum, trainings, and resources about fall prevention among older adults was conducted in October–December 2011, revealing a lack of a comprehensive fall prevention curricula specifically designed for CHW/P. The scan included searches conducted on web-based search engines and phone calls and emails to CHW/P organizations, networks, associations, state CHW program offices, employers, and academic institutions. No curricula on fall prevention for older adults specifically for CHW/P were located. A wider search revealed an evidence-based curriculum to train nurse assistants in fall prevention in home health settings, which has been available since 2007. Based on the best practice strategies discussed in detail in the following section, along with fall prevention strategies, we developed a series of CHW/P curriculum entitled, "How can CHW/Promotores help older adults stay safe from falls and related injuries?" The curriculum was developed by the study team from October 2012 to May 2013 and piloted in McAllen, Texas, on June 4–5, 2013, in English and Spanish with 49 CHW/P. Revisions were made from July 2013 to December 2013, and the revised curriculum was deployed nationally in face to face and virtual formats in April 2014. This project was approved by the Institutional Review Board at Texas A&M University.

EMPLOYMENT OF BEST PRACTICE APPROACHES

To effectively develop and train CHW/P, we employed three best practices: (1) utilization of CHW/P to deliver health education messages; (2) adult learning theory; and (3) tailored messaging. Studies have demonstrated CHW/P are effective in delivering health education to community residents due to shared ethnicity, language, socioeconomic status, and life experiences with the community members they serve (18–31). The project team included CHW/P throughout the development of processes to train and engage CHW/P to deliver fall prevention health education messages. Specifically, CHW/P identified the needs of their communities, reviewed the training materials, and identified gaps in information and service.

Second, an adult learner-centered training approach that considers characteristics of the target audience was utilized. CHW/P are typically between the ages of 20 and 65, have lower educational attainment with reading and math skills ranging between 4th and 8th grade levels, and are non-native English speakers. Adult learner-centered educational strategies engage learners in problem-based learning and teaching. Rather than a "lecture," learner-centered approaches engage learners in hands-on, interactive activities based upon discussion and skill-building exercises (32–35).

Third, tailored messaging was incorporated into the CHW/P fall prevention curriculum. Message tailoring deploys information and change strategies to reach one specific person based on the individual characteristics (36, 37). Tailoring differs from targeting of general audiences and segmenting of subgroups by customizing (or personalizing) educational approaches and messages to the individual. CHW/P were trained to employ tailoring to effectively educate clients. Instead of providing general education to their overall audience – or more refined education to certain subgroups within that overall audience – CHW/P made assessments about and delivered education based on the characteristics of individuals in their constituency, including culture, language, health literacy, education, gender, age, and pertinent experiences, beliefs, and attitudes. Tailoring-based approaches acknowledge how individuals differentially use, learn, and benefit from varied educational and messaging approaches. The purpose of developing training with integrated tailored messaging taught via adult learning strategies was to support CHW/P to utilize their strengths to ensure optimization of fall prevention interventions.

EXPLAINING PROGRAMMATIC ACTIVITY

INFORMAL FOCUS GROUPS TO IDENTIFY NEED

The lead partner was a Texas Department of State Health Services (DSHS) Certified CHW/P Training Center. The curriculum incorporated the eight competencies recognized by the Texas DSHS CHW/P Training and Certification Program: (1) communication; (2) teaching; (3) advocacy; (4) interpersonal skills; (5) service coordination; (6) capacity building; (7) organization; and (8) knowledge-based skills. Texas certifies CHW/P and requires a minimum of 20 CEUs (i.e., 10 DSHS-certified and 10 non-certified CEUs) every 2 years for recertification. To maximize adoption, the project team developed the curriculum in English and Spanish and met DSHS requirements for CEUs for CHW/P in Texas. **Figure 1** depicts the five-step training development module process, which is discussed in detail in the ensuing paragraphs.

Prior to material development, the project team conducted informal conversations with CHW/P about fall prevention (Step 1). These conversations identified potential gaps in knowledge to inform curriculum development and identify cultural influences and attitudes critical for message tailoring. This procedure ensured the training modules integrated input from the CHW/P and created a framework to integrate characteristics unique to CHW/P (e.g., culture, language, and gender) to best tailor messages.

MODULE DEVELOPMENT

The feedback from the informal focus groups and input by content experts in healthy aging, fall prevention, health messaging, and CHW/P training contributed to developing and refining tailoring-based training modules in English and Spanish. The curriculum was developed for any CHW/P instructor (whether

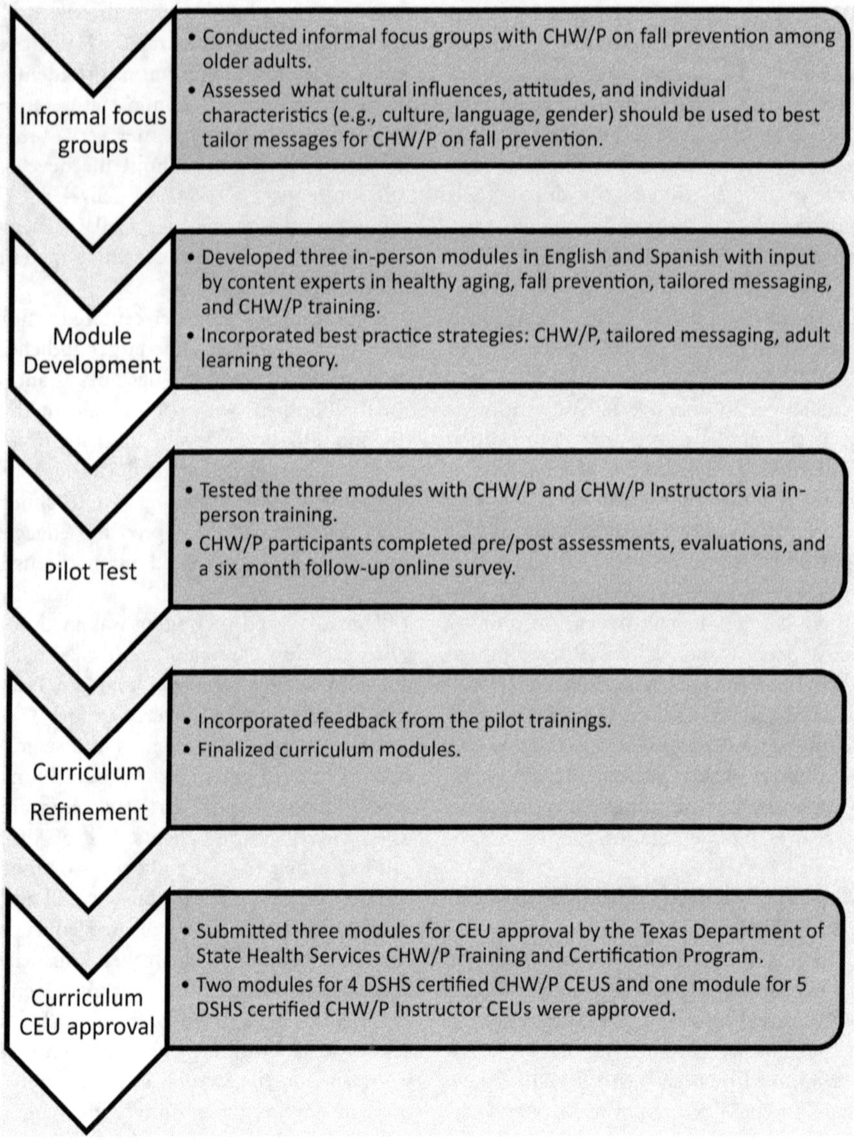

FIGURE 1 | Process of CHW/P fall prevention training module development.

DSHS-certified or not) and those with varying knowledge about fall prevention (whether a novice or expert). The intent was for any CHW/P to use the curriculum and training guide to train other CHW/P about fall prevention among older adults. Specific objectives included:

- Explain that falls are not a normal part of aging and the majority of falls are preventable.
- Articulate why preventing and reducing falls and related injuries among older people is especially important.
- Increase awareness about risk factors for falling inside and outside the home.
- Develop and augment observation, reporting, and communication skills to improve communication with older adults and their families around fall prevention.
- Describe ways to help prevent or manage falls in older adults.
- Develop fall prevention plans.
- Explain and discuss different approaches to changing health behaviors.
- Apply behavior change strategies to fall prevention and reduction.
- Teach health behavior change strategies to CHW/P and older adults.

As shown in **Table 1**, the three in-person training modules addressed the following topics: (1) fall risk factors and strategies to reduce/prevent falls (4 h in length); (2) communication strategies to reduce risk of falling and develop fall prevention plans (4 h in length); and (3) using health behavior change theories to prevent and reduce falls (5 h in length). The first two modules were designed to be completed independently but were linked in theme and content. The third module focuses on equipping CHW/P Instructors to apply health behavior theory to fall prevention and reinforces fall risk factors and strategies to prevent falls and related injuries.

Course materials included: an introduction for trainers, facilitator's guides, participant handouts, case studies, pre/post-assessments, and evaluations. Pre/post-assessments measured knowledge and confidence related to fall prevention and communication strategies. The evaluations gathered participant demographic information and satisfaction with the training. The curriculum incorporated teaching methods focusing on increasing self-awareness and skill building through practical application, including case scenarios, role play, group work, and interactive presentations. Refer to **Table 1** for detailed content.

PILOT TESTING

After developing the modules, each module was pilot tested with a group of CHW/P and CHW/P Instructors (i.e., 44 participants for Module 1; 41 for Module 2; and 18 for Module 3). CHW/P and CHW/P Instructors were recruited via emails and word-of-mouth. Two DSHS-certified, experienced, bilingual, and bicultural CHW/P Instructors conducted the in-person trainings in English and Spanish – with all materials provided in both languages. The pilot included evaluation and assessment onsite after completion of each training module and an online survey deployed 6 months after training to assess knowledge and implementation in their roles as CHW/P.

CURRICULUM REFINEMENT

The team refined the curriculum based on feedback from the pilot test. Specific feedback and revisions to the final curriculum included:

(1) Standardized wording for CHW/P and fall prevention terminology.
(2) Refined case studies.
(3) Added detailed physical activity exercises.
(4) Added a handout on local, state, and national resources; a glossary of terms; and a fall-related Frequently Asked Questions (FAQ) handout.

CONTINUING EDUCATION UNITS APPROVAL

The final step of the curriculum development process included submitting the three modules in English and Spanish for CEU approval by the Texas DSHS CHW/P Training and Certification Program. Each of the three models was approved. Information regarding the CEU approval process can be found at http://www.dshs.state.tx.us/mch/chw.shtm; information regarding the CHW/P fall prevention modules may be found at http://nchwtc.tamhsc.edu/.

NEXT STEPS IN DISSEMINATION

The curriculum was converted into an online format for broader dissemination (http://nchwtc.tamhsc.edu/fall-prevention-curriculum). The online formats include two courses:

1. *CHW/P Course*: Preparing CHWs/Promotores to prevent and reduce falls among older.
2. *CHW/P Instructor Course*: Helping older adults change their health behaviors to prevent falls and related injuries: health behavior change theories.

For the online format, CHW/P complete pre/post-assessments, an evaluation, and a 6-month follow-up survey. The goal of this approach is to create a feasible and sustainable training method that minimizes resources while maximizing dissemination – particularly in rural and remote communities that have CHW/P but do not have local CHW/P training programs. This strategy is designed to support implementation sustainability because CHW/P who received training from the fall prevention modules can continue to revisit these modules at no incurred cost in their future health outreach, education, and promotion strategies.

DISCUSSION

This perspective paper describes the development of a fall prevention curriculum for CHW/P. Given the access of CHW/P to at-risk older adults and their effectiveness to educate and promote behavior change, CHW/P are logical partners in promoting fall prevention strategies. However, to date, little has been attempted to engage CHW/P in fall prevention interventions, despite the scope of the problem. More specifically, there has not been another evidence-based curriculum on fall prevention among older adults specifically designed for CHW/P.

Table 1 | Contents of CHW/P fall prevention training modules.

Fall prevention: curriculum for community health workers/promotores How can CHW/promotores help older adults stay safe from falls and related injuries?			
Session title	**Content outline**	**Target audience**	**Session length**
Session 1: ways to prevent falls and related injuries in older adults	1. Statistics on falls among older adults a. Why talk about fall prevention? b. Goals of the session c. The facts on falls 1) U.S. falls statistics 2) Local falls statistics 2. Common risk factors for falling a. Individual risk factors 1) Physical mobility 2) Medications 3) Transitioning home from hospital 4) Fear of falling 5) Traumatic brain injury (TBI) 6) Cognitive impairment a. Environmental risk factors 1) Home safety 2) Safety factors outside the home 3. How to identify and address risk factors a. Assessments 1) Home fall prevention assessment for older adults 2) Check your risk for falling – self assessment b. Communication strategies Closed and open-ended questions 4. How to prevent and reduce falls a. Prevention tips 1) Regular exercise program 2) Have healthcare provider review medications 3) Have vision checked 4) Make home safer b. Putting information into action 1) Case studies & role play 2) Identification of resources	CHW/P	4 h/4 CEUs
Session 2: learning skills to reduce falls and related injuries	1. Risk factors for falls a. Individual risk factors 1) Physical mobility 2) Medications 3) Transitioning home from hospital 4) Fear of falling 5) Traumatic brain injury (TBI) 6) Cognitive impairment b. Environmental risk factors 1) Home safety 2) Safety factors outside the home 2. Enhance communication skills to tailor messages and ask open-ended questions a. Strategies to communicate effectively about falls prevention 1) Closed and open-ended questions 2) Observe, record, and report 3) Communicating with older adults a) What to do if an older adult falls b) How to get up from a fall	CHW/P	4 h/4 CEUs

(Continued)

Table 1 | Continued

Session title	Content outline	Target audience	Session length
	4) Communicating with care givers 5) Communicating with health professionals b. Tailored messaging 1) Assessment a) Stage of behavioral change of the individual b) Personal characteristics of the individual 2) Message creation and delivery a) Analyze falls prevention strategies b) Identify characteristics c) Develop relevant messages 3. Apply communication skills to case scenarios and identify risk factors to reduce risk of falling a. Case studies b. Role play 4. Develop and implement a fall prevention plan a. Role play b. Interview an older adult 5. Identify resources for fall prevention a. Group and individual activities		
Session 3: helping older adults change their health behaviors to prevent falls and related injuries: health behavior change theories	1. Theories of health behavior change a. Why talk about behavior change b. Health belief model 1) Constructs a) Perceived susceptibility b) Perceived severity c) Perceived benefits d) Perceived barriers e) Perceived self-efficacy f) Cues to action 2) Scenarios c. Trans-theoretical model 1) Stages of change a) Pre-contemplation b) Contemplation c) Preparation d) Action e) Maintenance 2) Processes of change 3) Scenarios d. Theory of reasoned action/theory of planned behavior 1) Constructs a) Attitude b) Norm c) Intention d) Perceived behavioral control 2) Scenarios 2. Fall prevention risk factors a. Individual risk factors 1) Physical mobility 2) Medications 3) Transitioning home from hospital 4) Fear of falling	CHW/P instructors	5 h/5 CEUs

(Continued)

Table 1 | Continued

Session title	Content outline	Target audience	Session length
	5) Traumatic brain injury (TBI) 6) Cognitive impairment b. Environmental risk factors 1) Home safety 2) Safety factors outside the home 3. Strategies for managing falls a. Regular exercise program b. Have healthcare provider review meds c. Have vision checked d. Make home safer 4. Tailored communication a. Communication approaches 1) General messaging 2) Targeted messaging 3) Segmented messaging 4) Tailored messaging b. Reasons to tailor messages c. Research on tailoring d. Steps in tailoring 1) Analyze a health problem 2) Identify pertinent characteristics 3) Develop pertinent messaging e. Key fall prevention messages 5. Application of behavior change concepts to fall prevention and reduction a. Review game b. Case studies 6. Skills to work with older adults/CHW/P to implement behavioral changes to prevent falls a. Interviews with older adults b. Practice assessments		

Numerous studies have highlighted the utilization of CHW/P and their effectiveness in helping their target populations achieve positive health outcomes through health education, promotion, and outreach (17–31). CHW/P are effective in these roles due to their cultural similarity and understanding of the population they serve and the subsequent trust that residents have in them (17–31). Specifically, CHW/P-led educational interventions have led to increased participant self-efficacy, knowledge, and adoption of preventive behaviors (38–43). Further, studies have demonstrated the effectiveness of CHW/P in providing social support to help participants adopt behavior change (38–40). One intent of this project was to build on the literature that has demonstrated the effectiveness of CHW/P in educational interventions to improve knowledge and adoption of behavior changes by the target population to include fall prevention education and promotion for older adults, which previously was a gap in the literature, given the significant burden and cost of falls by older adults in the U.S.

An innovative aspect of the study was to actively engage CHW/P in all stages of the curriculum development, which included pilot testing, refining, and implementation. The curricula utilized best practice strategies of CHW/P, adult learning theory, and tailored messaging, as well as evidence-based fall prevention strategies. The structured engagement of CHW/P during the development process had many benefits. First, the included messages, content, and format of the curricula were relevant, acceptable, and comprehendible for the CHW/P and CHW/P Instructors. Second, the messages, content, and format were appropriate for older adults who would be reached by the fall prevention activities. Third, by vetting the modules among the intended community, the goal of widespread adoption, dissemination, and sustainability was more realistic and obtainable. A potential limitation of the CHW/P curriculum on fall prevention among older adults is that the impact of the curriculum on reducing falls and injuries caused by falls by older adults could depend on the actual implementation of the curriculum – relying on the capacity of CHW/P programs, trainers, and employers – rather than on the actual curriculum. The project team anticipated this limitation and attempted to address this potential limitation through detailed instructions, tools, and resources within the curriculum and through providing additional technical assistance upon request to CHW/P, CHW/P instructors or trainers, and CHW/P employers on how to utilize and implement the curriculum with CHW/P and older adults.

The future directions of this project as a translated curriculum in an online format has great potential to broaden its reach and further disseminate the modules – particularly in rural areas where CHW/P training programs are scarce and communities have a greater population of older adults. Key will be to assess the ease of use, esthetics, and platform selected for online content to ensure CHW/P can successfully access and complete the online modules and revisit resources and training materials. Careful and strategic selection of partners for promoting and supporting this internet-based curricula can substantially impact uptake and utilization. The project team members will rely on existing partners and collaborators to broadly disseminate the self-paced, online training modules available for CHW/P and CHW/P Instructors in English or Spanish.

CONCLUSION

This perspective paper describes the process of evaluating the CHW/P training curriculums, identifying a gap in the curriculum, and then the process of developing a CHW/P curriculum that specifically targets management of fall prevention. The goal of the curriculum is to equip and mobilize CHW/P so they can play a key role in joining other public health professionals in the fight to prevent and reduce injuries among older adults due to falling. In other areas, CHW/Ps have proven effective in helping individuals adopt preventive behaviors through educational interventions (38–43). The curriculum development was the first step in determining if a similar model could be used for fall prevention. The process we undertook validated that CHW/Ps had a need for this type of curriculum, were interested in the curriculum, and could improve their knowledge by participating in the curriculum. Engaging CHW/P remains especially vital in that CHW/P have a unique opportunity to reach out to older adults who may otherwise be neglected and have an increased risk for falling.

ACKNOWLEDGMENTS

The authors would like to acknowledge the funder of this project – the Centers for Disease Control Prevention Research Centers. The research was supported with funding support from the Centers for Disease Control and Prevention under Cooperative Agreement Number 1U48 DP001924 with the Texas A&M Health Science Center School of Rural Public Health Center for Community Health Development and Cooperative Agreement Number U48-DP001944 with the University of North Carolina at Chapel Hill Prevention Research Center. The funding for the fall prevention CHW/P curriculum was provided by the Centers for Disease Control and Prevention Special Interest Project 12-058. The findings and conclusions in article are those of the author(s) and do not necessarily represent the official position of the Centers for Disease Control and Prevention. The authors would also like to thank the CHW/P who provided input into the curriculum development and participated in the pilot-test and to acknowledge the following CHW/P and instructors for their contribution in the development modules: Denise Adame, Aracely Garibay, Lupita Garza, Leticia Gutierrez, Dinorah Martinez, and Paula Saldaña. The authors also want to express their appreciation to Stephanie Bomberger and Katharine Nimmons who provided administrative support during this project.

REFERENCES

1. Stevens JA, Corso PS, Finkelstein EA, Miller TR. The costs of fatal and nonfatal falls among older adults. *Inj Prev* (2006) **12**:290–5. doi:10.1136/ip.2005.011015
2. Alexander BH, Rivara FP, Wolf ME. The cost and frequency of hospitalization for fall–related injuries in older adults. *Am J Public Health* (1992) **82**(7):1020–3. doi:10.2105/AJPH.82.7.1020
3. Stevens JA, Dellinger AM. Motor vehicle and fall related deaths among older Americans 1990–98: sex, race, and ethnic disparities. *Inj Prev* (2002) **8**:272–5. doi:10.1136/ip.8.4.272
4. Jager TE, Weiss HB, Coben JH, Pepe PE. Traumatic brain injuries evaluated in U.S. emergency departments, 1992–1994. *Acad Emerg Med* (2000) **7**(2):134–40. doi:10.1111/j.1553-2712.2000.tb00515.x
5. Faul M, Xu L, Wald MM, Coronado VG. *Traumatic Brain Injury in the United States: Emergency Department Visits, Hospitalizations, and Deaths.* Atlanta, GA: Centers for Disease Control and Prevention, National Center for Injury Prevention and Control (2010).
6. Thomas KE, Stevens JA, Sarmiento K, Wald MM. Fall-related traumatic brain injury deaths and hospitalizations among older adults – United States, 2005. *J Safety Res* (2008) **39**(3):269–72. doi:10.1016/j.jsr.2008.05.001
7. Scott JC. Osteoporosis and hip fractures. *Rheum Dis Clin North Am* (1990) **16**(3):717–40.
8. U.S. Department of Health and Human Services Health Resources and Services Administration on Aging. *Aging Statistics.* (2014). Available from: http://www.aoa.gov/AoARoot/Aging_Statistics/index.aspx
9. Gillespie LD, Robertson MC, Gillespie WH, Sherrington C, Gates S, Clemson LM, et al. Interventions for preventing falls in older people living in the community. *Cochrane Database Syst Rev* (2012) **9**:CD007146.
10. Moyer VA. Prevention of falls in community-dwelling older adults: U.S. Preventive Services Task Force Recommendation Statement. *Ann Intern Med* (2012) **157**(3):197–204. doi:10.7326/0003-4819-157-8-201210160-00533
11. Michael YL, Lin JS, Whitlock EP, Gold R, Fu R, O'Connor E, et al. *Interventions to Prevent Falls in Older Adults: An Updated Systematic Review.* Rockville, MD: Agency for Healthcare Research and Quality (US) (2010). Available from: http://www.ncbi.nlm.nih.gov/books/NBK51683/
12. Noonan RK, Sleet DA, Stevens JA. Closing the gap: a research agenda to accelerate the adoption and effective use of proven older adult fall prevention strategies. *J Safety Res* (2011) **42**(6):427–30. doi:10.1016/j.jsr.2010.12.002
13. Kaniewski M, Stevens JA, Parker EM, Lee R. An introduction to the Centers for Disease Control and Prevention's efforts to prevent older adult falls. *Front Public Health* (2015) **2**:119. doi:10.3389/fpubh.2014.00119
14. U.S. Department of Health and Human Services Health Resources and Services Administration Bureau of Health Professions. *Community Health Worker National Workforce Study.* (2007). Available from: http://bhpr.hrsa.gov/healthworkforce.chw/
15. American Public Health Association. *Community Health Worker Section.* (2013). Available from: http://www.apha.org/membergroups/sections/aphasections/chw/
16. Texas Department of State Health Services and health and Human Services Commission. *Report to the Texas Legislature, as Required by H.B. 2610, 82nd* Legislature, Regular Session. (2012). Available from: http://www.dshs.state.tx.us/mch/chw.shtm
17. Viswanathan M, Kraschnewski J, Nishikawa B, Morgan LC, Thieda P, Honeycutt A, et al. Outcomes of community health worker interventions. *Evidence Report/Technology Assessment, Number 181, Agency for Healthcare Research and Quality.* (2009). Available from: http://www.ahrq.gov/downloads/pub/evidence/pdf/comhealthwork/comhwork.pdf
18. Staten LK, Scheu LL, Bronson D, Peña V, Elenas J. Pasos Adelante: the effectiveness of a community-based chronic disease prevention program. *Prev Chronic Disease* (2005) **2**(1):A18.
19. Crowe JL, Keifer MC, Salazar MK. Striving to provide opportunities for farm worker community participation in research. *J Agric Saf Health* (2008) **14**(2):205–19. doi:10.13031/2013.24351
20. Larkey LK, Gonzalez JA, Mar LE, Glantz N. Latina recruitment for cancer prevention education via community based participatory research strategies. *Contemp Clin Trials* (2009) **30**(1):47–54. doi:10.1016/j.cct.2008.08.003

21. Ramos IN, May M, Ramos KS. Environmental health training of promotoras in colonias along the Texas-Mexico border. *Am J Public Health* (2001) **91**(4):568–70. doi:10.2105/AJPH.91.4.568
22. Levine DM, Becker DM, Bone LR. Narrowing the gap in health status of minority populations: a community-academic medical center partnership. *Am J Prev Med* (1992) **8**(5):319–23.
23. Witmer A, Seifer SD, Finocchio L, Leslie J, O'Neil EH. Community health workers: integral members of the health care work force. *Am J Public Health* (1995) **85**(8 Pt 1):1055–8. doi:10.2105/AJPH.85.8_Pt_1.1055
24. Balcázar H, Alvarado M, Cantu F, Pedregon V, Fulwood R. A promotora de salud model for addressing cardiovascular disease risk factors in the US-Mexico border region. *Prev Chronic Dis* (2009) **6**(1):A02.
25. Baquero B, Ayala GX, Arredondo EM, Campbell NR, Slymen DJ, Gallo L, et al. Secretos de la Buena Vida: processes of dietary change via a tailored nutrition communication intervention for Latinas. *Health Educ Res* (2009) **24**(5):855–66. doi:10.1093/her/cyp022
26. Elder JP, Ayala GX, Slymen DJ, Arredondo EM, Campbell NR. Evaluating psychosocial and behavioral mechanisms of change in a tailored communication intervention. *Health Edu Behav* (2009) **36**(2):366–80. doi:10.1177/1090198107308373
27. Heisler M, Spencer M, Forman J, Robinson C, Shultz C, Palmisano G, et al. Participants' assessments of the effects of a community health worker intervention on their diabetes self-management and interactions with healthcare providers. *Am J Prev Med* (2009) **37**(6 Suppl 1):S270–9. doi:10.1016/j.amepre.2009.08.016
28. McCloskey J. Promotores as partners in a community-based diabetes intervention program targeting Hispanics. *Fam Community Health* (2009) **32**(1):48–57. doi:10.1097/01.FCH.0000342816.87767.e6
29. Medina A, Balcazar H, Hollen ML, Nkhoma A, Mas FS. Promotores de Salud: educating Hispanic communities on heart-healthy living. *Am J Health Edu* (2007) **38**(4):194–202. doi:10.1080/19325037.2007.10598970
30. Postma J, Karr C, Kieckhefer G. Community health workers and environmental interventions for children with asthma: a systematic review. *J Asthma* (2009) **46**(6):564–76. doi:10.1080/02770900902912638
31. Deitrick LM, Paxton HD, Rivera A, Gertner EJ, Biery N, Letcher AS, et al. Understanding the role of the promotora in a Latino diabetes education program. *Qual Health Res* (2010) **20**(3):386–99. doi:10.1177/1049732309354281
32. Yannacci J, Roberts K, Ganju V. *Principles from Adult Learning Theory, Evidence-Based Teaching, and Visual Marketing: What are the Implications for Toolkit Development?*. Center for Mental Health Quality and Accountability, NRI, Inc. (2006). Available from: http://ebp.networkofcare.org/uploads/Adult_Learning_Thoery_2497281.pdf
33. Green ML, Ellis PJ. Impact of an evidence-based medicine curriculum based on adult learning theory. *J Gen Intern Med* (1997) **12**(12):742–50. doi:10.1046/j.1525-1497.1997.07159.x
34. Neame RLB, Powis DA. Toward independent learning: curricular design for assisting students to learn how to learn. *J Med Educ* (1991) **56**:886–93.
35. Comings JP, Soricone L, Santos M. *An Evidence-Based Adult Education Program Model Appropriate for Research. NSCALL Occasional Paper.* Cambridge, MA: National Center for the Study of Adult Learning and Literacy (2006). Available from: http://www.nscall.net/fileadmin/resources/research/op_comings4.pdf
36. Kreuter MW, Farrell D, Olevitch L, Brennan L. *Tailored Health Messages: Customizing Communication with Computer Technology.* Mahwah, NJ: Lawrence Erlbaum (1999).
37. Foerster SB, Kizer KW, Disogra LK, Bal DG, Krieg BF, Bunch KL. California's "5 a day – for better health!" campaign: an innovative population-based effort to effect large-scale dietary change. *Am J Prev Med* (1995) **11**(2):124–31.
38. Hansen LK, Feigl P, Modiano MR, Lopez JA, Sluder SE, Moinpour CM, et al. An educational program to increase cervical and breast cancer screening in Hispanic women. *Cancer Nurs* (2005) **28**(1):47–53. doi:10.1097/00002820-200501000-00007
39. Larkey L. Las Mujeres Saludables: reaching Latinas for breast, cervical and colorectal cancer. *J Community Health* (2006) **31**(1):69–77. doi:10.1007/s10900-005-8190-2
40. Livaudais JC, Coronado GD, Espinoza N, Islas I, Ibarra G, Thompson B. Educating Hispanic women about breast cancer prevention: evaluation of a home-based promotora-led intervention. *J Womens Health (Larchmt)* (2010) **19**(11):2049–56. doi:10.1089/jwh.2009.1733
41. Luque JS, Mason M, Reyes-Garcia C, Hinojosa A, Meade CD. Salud es Vida: development of a cervical cancer education curriculum for promotora outreach with Latina farmworkers in rural southern Georgia. *Am J Public Health* (2010) **101**(12):2233–5. doi:10.2105/AJPH.2011.300324
42. Moralzes EA, Rao SP, Livaudais JC, Thompson B. Improving knowledge and screening for colorectal cancer among Hispanics: overcoming barriers through a promotora-led home-based educational intervention. *J Cancer Edu* (2012) **27**:533–9. doi:10.1007/s13187-012-0357-9
43. O'Brien MJ, Halbert CH, Bixby R, Pimentel S, Shea JA. Community health worker intervention to decrease cervical cancer disparities in Hispanic women. *J Gen Intern Med* (2010) **25**(11):1186–92. doi:10.1007/s11606-010-1434-6

22

Translation of the Otago Exercise Program for adoption and implementation in the United States

Tiffany E. Shubert[1]*, Matthew Lee Smith[2], Marcia G. Ory[3], Cristine B. Clarke[1], Stephanie A. Bomberger[4], Ellen Roberts[5] and Jan Busby-Whitehead[5]

[1] Center for Aging and Health, University of North Carolina, School of Medicine, Chapel Hill, NC, USA
[2] College of Public Health, The University of Georgia, Athens, GA, USA
[3] Department of Health Promotion and Community Health Sciences, Texas A&M School of Public Health, College Station, TX, USA
[4] University of North Carolina Center for Health Promotion and Disease Prevention, Chapel Hill, NC, USA
[5] Division of Geriatrics, University of North Carolina, School of Medicine, Chapel Hill, NC, USA

Edited by:
Sanjay P. Zodpey, Public Health Foundation of India, India

Reviewed by:
Xiaoguang Ma, University of South Carolina, USA
Nilesh Chandrakant Gawde, Tata Institute of Social Sciences, India

***Correspondence:**
Tiffany E. Shubert, Center for Aging and Health, University of North Carolina, School of Medicine, Old Clinic, Campus Box 7550, Chapel Hill, NC 27599-7550, USA
e-mail: tshubert@med.unc.edu

Background: The Otago Exercise Program (OEP) is an evidence-based fall prevention program developed, evaluated, and disseminated in New Zealand. The program was designed for delivery in the home by physical therapists (PTs). It was not known if American PTs would require additional training and resources to adopt the OEP. This article describes the process of translating the OEP for dissemination in the US. Processes included reviewing and piloting the New Zealand training materials to identify implementation challenges, updating training materials to be consistent with American physical therapy practices, piloting the updated training materials in an online format, and determining if the online format reached the target PT audience.

Methods – Process Activities: The New Zealand manual was reviewed by expert American PTs and a training webinar was piloted with 56 American PTs. Feedback suggested that the program itself was understood by PTs, but training materials required modification related to documentation and reimbursement policies. Additional content was developed and integrated into an online training module. The online training was piloted and then deemed adequate by seven PT subject matter experts. The online training was launched in March 2013. Demographic and practice data were collected to characterize the PTs attending the online training as well as perceived barriers and facilitators to implementation ($n = 522$). Perceived facilitators include the effectiveness of the OEP to facilitate adoption, but the lack of agency support, billing and reimbursement challenges pose a significant barrier to OEP implementation.

Conclusion: The OEP required additional information to facilitate adoption by American PTs. Online training that specifically targets PTs appears to effectively reach the target audience and be well received by participants. More research is required to determine the impact of online training on a PT's adoption and implementation of this material into their practice.

Keywords: fall prevention, health promotion, physical therapy, balance, aging, policy

INTRODUCTION

Older adult falls are a significant public health problem (1). The reasons why older adults fall are complex and typically a result of multiple, interacting risk factors unique to the individual as they interact with their physical environment (2). The most common risk factors for falling are leg muscle weakness, difficulty walking, polypharmacy (too much or the wrong type of medications), cognitive impairment, vision impairment, and challenges within the environment (3). Of greatest concern are the falls experienced by those aged 75 and over. It is estimated that 50% of adults in this age group fall annually (4). These falls result in the greatest number of visits to healthcare providers and significant morbidity and mortality (5).

Given the extensive and complex nature of falls among older adults, interventions to prevent falls and related injuries have been studied for over two decades. Several fall prevention programs have been developed, tested, and proven effective to reduce falls among community-dwelling older adults (6). To facilitate the dissemination and implementation of these programs, the Centers for Disease Control and Prevention (CDC) published "Compendium of Effective Fall Interventions: What Works for Community-Dwelling Older Adults" in 2008 (7), with a second edition in 2010 (6). The second edition of the Compendium lists 22 interventions that have effectively reduced the rate of falls or fall-related injury. Each intervention includes a summary of the outcomes, program setting, target audience, content (key elements, frequency, and duration), and delivery system (who is qualified to deliver, level of training required). Of the 22 interventions, only three have incorporated and expanded the key elements into an implementation manual and training system to ensure program delivery with fidelity across community (Tai Chi: Moving For Better Balance and Stepping On) (8, 9) and home-based (the Otago Exercise Program – OEP) settings (10).

These three programs target older adults with the physical and mental abilities to live in non-institutional settings. Tai Chi is most appropriate for those older adults with the greatest mobility skills (11), Stepping On is for those older adults who are transitioning to be less mobile (12), and the OEP is the most effective for those older adults who are the least mobile and at the highest risk of falling (6). The OEP target audience may have limited mobility and access to group exercise settings, which differs from the other two programs in that it was designed to be delivered in the home (10).

The OEP was developed and evaluated in New Zealand in the late 1990s and proven effective in randomized controlled trials at reducing falls in high-risk older adults by 35% (13, 14). Due to the complex medical conditions inherent in the target audience, the OEP was delivered by healthcare professionals. The creators of the New Zealand OEP deemed that physical therapists (PTs), who receive extensive training in musculoskeletal rehabilitation, should at a minimum supervise, and ideally implement, the OEP (10). PTs have the training and expertise to evaluate an individual's risk of falling; identify additional medical risk factors such as orthostatic hypotension, polypharmacy, arrhythmia; refer to other healthcare providers to manage risk; and prescribe and progress an older adult through a fall prevention program (15).

The OEP is an innovative model of low frequency of physical therapy sessions over a long duration. The original program was delivered in six visits over a year. The first four visits are in the first 2 months of the program (i.e., the initial visit, a visit a week later, then a visit 2 weeks later, then 4 weeks later); then follow-up visits are conducted at 6 and 12 months with monthly "check-in" phone calls between (13, 16). This type of model sets the stage for the patient engagement and ownership of their exercise program. The program only works if the patient does the exercises. The OEP achieves that goal with over 35% of participants stating they perform the exercises three times a week 1 year after the start of the program (13).

Given the robust results of the OEP, and the above average adherence and compliance rates, the CDC selected the OEP as one of three evidence-based fall prevention programs for dissemination in the United States. The implementation and dissemination materials for the OEP were developed in New Zealand. These materials offered a concise summary of the research supporting the OEP and step-by-step instructions about how the program was prescribed (10). However, the New Zealand manual did not account for policies and practices unique to the American healthcare system, nor did it provide any guidance about how to integrate the OEP into the workflow of a PT. It was not known if American PTs would require additional training and resources to adopt the OEP and implement it as intended.

The purpose of this article is to describe the process of translating the OEP for dissemination in the United States. Processes included reviewing and piloting the New Zealand OEP training materials with PTs to identify implementation challenges, updating the OEP training materials to be more consistent with American physical therapy practices, piloting the updated training materials in an online format, and then determining if the online format reached the target audience of PTs who work with frail older adults.

METHODS – PROCESS ACTIVITIES

TRANSLATION OF THE OTAGO EXERCISE PROGRAM FOR DISSEMINATION IN THE UNITED STATES

The OEP was developed and tested for dissemination and implementation in a country with a nationalized healthcare system. A manual to describe the implementation process was published in 2003 by the program developers (10). Before dissemination in the United States, it was deemed necessary to review all training materials and make modifications to support adoption and implementation by an American audience. Part of translation plan developed by the American team responsible for translating the OEP was to create and integrate a centralized system to offer education and training to PTs.

The following plan was deployed to review and revise the OEP manual and training materials for dissemination in the United States:

1. PTs with expertise in fall prevention and implementation of the OEP were to review the materials and identify any revisions necessary to support program adoptions
2. Pilot a real-time webinar based on the revised manual for American audiences amongst a small group of PTs from three states – Oregon, Colorado, and New York that were participating in the Centers for Disease Control Fall Prevention Pilot Project
3. Identify "lessons learned" from Otago implementation based on feedback from the webinars
4. Revise training materials based on lessons learned
5. Develop an online training program for broad dissemination in the United States
6. Pilot training with a small group of practicing PTs for feedback
7. Revise and deploy online training
8. Determine if online training was reaching the target audience of PTs most likely to adopt and implement the OEP in their practice settings.

REVISIONS SPECIFIC TO AMERICAN PTs

Expert PTs (T. Shea and T. Shubert) who had extensive knowledge of the OEP implementation both in the United States and in New Zealand worked with one of the OEP program developers (C. Robertson) to review the Otago Exercise Programme Manual (10). Revisions were made to the original manual. A United States version of the OEP Manual was released and made available in early 2012 (http://www.med.unc.edu/aging/cgec/exercise-program). The content of this manual was presented in a 1-hour training webinar offered four times in 2012 to 56 PTs. The 56 PTs who attended had been recruited by their respective State Division of Public Health Units (OR, CO, NY) to participate in a project to implement the OEP as part of the Fall Prevention Pilot Project. Attendance at the webinars was the first step in that process, and they were recruited via personal invitation from their state partners.

The training webinars were designed to pilot the material. Throughout the course of each webinar, therapists were encouraged to ask questions either by telephone or using the online chat function. We anticipated that many of the questions would be about how to actually prescribe the program; however, questions and discussions were more about implementation differences between New Zealand and America and how to address these differences. The following themes were identified as common challenges to implementation throughout the webinars:

1. The theory and implementation of evidence-based health promotion programs were not common knowledge for PTs.
2. In the original OEP research studies, subjects were at risk of falls but not actually seeing a PT for a diagnosed impairment. In order for Medicare to reimburse a PT for an episode of care, there needs to be a diagnosed impairment that requires "skilled and necessary" physical therapy (17).
3. Subjects in the original OEP research scored at risk of falls. This criterion was used for PTs to implement the OEP as part of the plan of care. Given that patients required skilled therapy, they were often weak and required a dose of physical therapy before starting the OEP. This dose of physical therapy was necessary to improve their strength and mobility so that they would be able to participate at the appropriate frequency and duration.
4. The OEP exercises were not unique to physical therapy, but the low frequency of PT visits and long duration of the OEP was deemed be an innovative practice model. Typical courses of physical therapy follow a model for 2–3 times a week for a period of 4–8 weeks. There was concern from therapists that the OEP model with its low frequency and long duration would be considered outside of the acceptable course of therapy. Being outside of normative values may result in a "red flag" to be audited by Medicare.
5. The OEP offered an opportunity to standardize practice around fall prevention. The literature demonstrates significant variations in clinical care around falls. Standardizing practice was appealing to some PTs and distasteful to others (18, 19).
6. The OEP was delivered in the home; however, the policies for billing and reimbursement for Physical Therapy under Medicare Part A (Home Health) make it virtually impossible to implement Otago over a year period.
7. A new model of PT delivery of care, which has emerged, allows for delivering physical therapy in the home but billing under Medicare Part B (outpatient). Though this model allows for greater opportunity to deliver the OEP over the year-long period, the paperwork burden on the PT was still sizeable.
8. Webinars and online training were deemed as an acceptable mode of training by PTs.

Given the feedback from the webinars, the content from the New Zealand manual was deemed appropriate for teaching therapists exercise program specifics. However, they believed that implementation in the United States would require additional information about how to integrate the program into the workflow, given documentation, billing, and reimbursement requirements. It was also identified that therapists would benefit from additional background about the theory behind evidence-based programs and the research behind the OEP.

The feedback from the PTs was then incorporated into the training manual. The PTs who attended the webinar agreed that the content of the OEP did not need to be presented in a face-to-face setting because much of the actual program was common to both PT practice and education. It was deemed that an online medium would be acceptable to disseminate the training to PTs in the United States.

DEVELOPMENT OF ONLINE TRAINING PROGRAM

The online curriculum was an adaption of the webinar and developed by the same authors. The curriculum incorporated "adult learning theory" using video, interactive assignments, and required posting to external discussion boards (**Figure 1**). The online

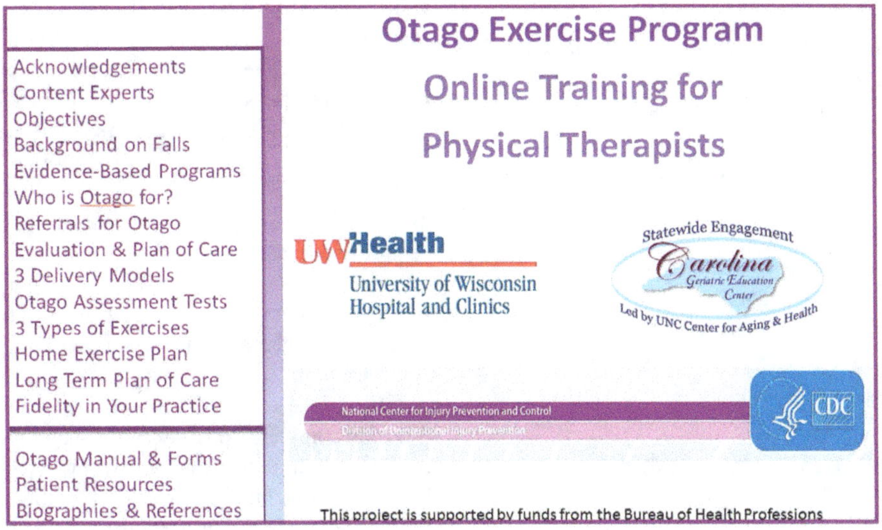
Acknowledgements
Content Experts
Objectives
Background on Falls
Evidence-Based Programs
Who is Otago for?
Referrals for Otago
Evaluation & Plan of Care
3 Delivery Models
Otago Assessment Tests
3 Types of Exercises
Home Exercise Plan
Long Term Plan of Care
Fidelity in Your Practice
Otago Manual & Forms
Patient Resources
Biographies & References
Otago Exercise Program
Online Training for
Physical Therapists
UWHealth
University of Wisconsin
Hospital and Clinics
Statewide Engagement
Carolina
Geriatric Education Center
Led by UNC Center for Aging & Health
National Center for Injury Prevention and Control
CDC
This project is supported by funds from the Bureau of Health Professions

FIGURE 1 | Otago online training program and activities.

version was developed into a power point and piloted by seven subject matter expert (SME) PTs – three knowledgeable about the OEP and four without prior experience of the OEP. All clinicians had at least 5 years of clinical experience.

The SMEs were invited to review the content from a select group of PTs who had received advanced certification in geriatrics, and who had contacted the researchers independent of the online training to learn more about the efforts to implement the OEP.

The SMEs were instructed to complete the course including outside assignments, quizzes, and a final exam. The SMEs then evaluated the following with open-ended questions (**Table 1**): (1) Course logistics – was it easy to find, navigate, complete? (2) Course content – was the information interesting, helpful, presented with fidelity to the original program? (3) Clinical usability/feasibility – could they apply this in their clinical setting? (4) Research – was it presented in a meaningful way? The responses were summarized and reviewed by course creators and independent external consultant.

Table 1 | Otago online pilot evaluation open-ended questions.

Logistics
1. Describe how you found the course navigation to be. Was it easy to get around?
2. Were the directions clear to access phConnect?
3. How well did the quizzes cover the content in your opinion?
4. What was your opinion on the usefulness of the case studies presented in the videos?
5. How realistic did the case studies feel to you?
6. How easy was it to post questions on PH Connect?

Content
1. Tell me three things you remember from the content?
2. Was there anything that felt incompletely explained?
3. Was there anything that seemed too elementary?
4. ....or too advanced?

Your motivation
1. How different does the Otago Exercise Program feel from your customary PT practice?
2. How likely are you to use some of what you learned in the online course?
3. How motivated do you feel as a result of this experience to start using the Otago Exercise Program with your patients?

Research
1. How convincing did you find the research we presented?
2. Is the push toward using evidenced-based programs in PT more important to you now than it was at the beginning of the course?

Fidelity
1. How strictly do you think PTs have to stick to the Otago Exercise Program?

What unanswered questions do you still have regarding
1. The assessment tests
2. Billing for Otago
3. Choosing the exercises
4. On the Otago schedule and continuum?

The SMEs reported that the course was acceptable and engaging. The training was deemed adequate in length (2–3 h) and appropriately priced ($25). The curriculum was easy to navigate. The content was acceptable and clinically relevant. The exercise videos and case studies were well received; however, clinicians with several years of experience (>5) felt that the video cases were too contrived and not realistic.

Subject matter experts listed the following additional concerns:

1. "The OEP is appropriate for clinical use, but I have concerns about billing, reimbursement, and program fidelity" (four SMEs made this statement)
2. "The OEP may be challenging to implement and deliver for therapists who are not in-home Part B providers" (two SMEs).

DEPLOYMENT OF ONLINE TRAINING PROGRAM

The feedback from the SMEs was collated and revisions to the course were made. The course was deployed in March 2013. The course was advertised via the University of North Carolina at Chapel Hill's School of Medicine website, national listserv for PTs, and word-of-mouth. Key partners such as the American Physical Therapy Association and CDC informed various groups interested in balance and fall prevention. The online training program continues to be advertised through monthly postings on national listservs for PTs, quarterly webinars for the National Falls Free Coalition, and at national and international meetings and conferences.

To minimize cost barriers, the course was priced at $25. Upon completion of the course, the registrants received 2 Continuing Education Units (CEUs). Many states require PTs to attend and report a minimum amount of continuing competence training annually to renew their license. These courses are often expensive. We felt offering low-cost CEUs would add an additional incentive to therapists interested in completing the training.

Participants enrolled in the course via the Area Health Education Center Connect website. The course was described as a 3-hour experience, which could be started and stopped at any time. After registration, participants completed a demographic form including key characteristics about their clinical practice (e.g., number of years in practice, percent of caseload over the age of 65), a pre-assessment of confidence in skills, and a baseline test about falls knowledge. The course had three other mini-quizzes embedded into the content throughout the course: (1) knowledge assessment of standardized protocols for functional tests; (2) an assessment of ability to evaluate functional tests and prescribe appropriate exercises from the OEP; and (3) an evaluation to assess the mastery of the concept of fidelity. Participants were not allowed to proceed to the next course section until they had demonstrated mastery of the content per the quiz score. Upon completion of the course, but before participants were awarded CEUs, they had to pass a final exam of 10 questions with a minimum score of 80% and complete a post-assessment about confidence in skills; an intention to implement survey that included items about perceived barriers and facilitators; and an evaluation of the course presentation and content. All participants received a follow-up survey via email 6 weeks after completing the course to assess level of program implementation. All participant data were collected with tools embedded in the training. Data were exported, de-identified, cleaned, and analyzed at 6 and 13 months post deployment.

RESULTS

It was unknown if the PTs who registered for the course would be the target audience for adoption. The goal was for PTs who worked primarily with older adults to complete the course. It was also unknown if the perceived facilitators and barriers by a larger audience would be consistent with the pilot results from the webinars. To ensure that the target audience was actually reached, frequencies for trainee demographics and perceived facilitators and barriers were calculated using data of the first 552 PTs enrolled in the course.

CHARACTERISTICS OF ONLINE OEP TRAINEES

The characteristics of all the OEP trainees who completed the training in the first 11 months of deployment are described in **Table 2**. During that time frame, 552 PTs, physical therapy assistants, and students enrolled in physical therapy programs enrolled in the course, and 398 completed the training. **Table 3** describes the characteristics of the trainees practice settings. Of the 398, 30% were not in practice. These individuals were either students, researchers, or from other professions. The remaining 279 were predominately therapists with significant experience in geriatrics (211 had over 8 years of experience working with older adults) and worked primarily in geriatric settings (75% of sample stated more than 75% of their caseload was over the age of 65).

Table 2 | Demographics of therapists who completed the online program (*N* = 398).

	% Sample
Age	
20–29	23
30–39	21
40–49	20
50–59	29
60+	7
Gender	
Male	25
Female	75
Race	
White	89
African-American	1
Asian	5
Native American	1
Other	4
Practice setting	
Rural	30
Suburban/urban	66
Other	4
Patient care	
Full time	45
Part time	25
Not in practice	30

PERCEIVED FACILITATORS AND BARRIERS TO PROGRAM IMPLEMENTATION (TABLE 4)

Trainees were instructed to "Please estimate the degree to which each of the following items will *facilitate* your ability to implement Otago," and were given a list of 11 potential facilitators. Facilitators ranged from administrative support (i.e., would supervisors pay for copying of materials and help support documentation) to payor policies (i.e., what were the local Medicare polices toward longer duration of treatments with low frequencies) to compliance issues (i.e., would patients actually do the exercises on their own?). Trainees were also asked to "Please estimate the degree to which each of the following items will be a *barrier* to your ability to implement Otago," and were given a list of 14 barriers. Barriers ranged from getting weights for patients to co-pays to paperwork issues. **Table 5** lists the top three perceived facilitators and the top 3 perceived barriers.

DISCUSSION

This study described the process of translating a research-based intervention developed in a country with nationalized healthcare for use in clinical practice within the United States. This article described the process of translating the OEP to facilitate adoption

Table 3 | Characteristics of therapist practice (*N* = 279).

	%
Years in practice	
≤3	14
4–7	10
≥8	76
Years working with older adults	
≤3	14
4–7	16
≥8	70
Average # visits/week	
0–9	17
10–19	27
20–39	46
>40	90
% of caseload age 65 or older?	
<25%	4
25–49%	6
50–74%	15
>75%	75
Experience with evidence-based health promotion programs (EBHP)	
Ever referred?	
Yes	36
No	61
I do not know	3
Which program? (Select all that apply)	
Matter of balance (*n* = 25)	9
Stepping on (*n* = 15)	5
Tai Chi (*n* = 75)	27
Other (*n* = 21)	8

Table 4 | List of facilitators and barriers.

Facilitators	Barriers
I have active support from my Agency's administration	My agency does not have reimbursement or billing policies in place
I have an internal "champion" or key leader who is supportive of Otago	Current Medicare reimbursement practices do not support delivery of the program
My agency has enough staff member, skills, resources to support the work and phone calls	Poor patient compliance
My agency is/will be able to modify reimbursement and billing practices to fit Otago guidelines	My agency is not set up keep patients on caseload over an extended period of time
The program is low cost and does not need substantial resources to continue	My agency does not have a system for follow-up phone calls
The research data helped convince my Agency of the value	It is difficult to get weights for patients
The research data helped convince referral partners (physicians, accountable care organizations) of value	Patients will not continue with a different Part B provider
The research data and program structure helped convince me of the value	Patients unable or do not want to pay co-pays
My patients like the program	Medicare C payors will not cover Otago
The program is supported by community and state-based fall coalitions	No way to transition patient from home health to Part B
I am able to bill as a Part B provider	Agency does not have enough trained staff members, skills, resources to support the work
Other facilitators (please specify)	Agency leadership does not support the work.
	Turnover among therapists implementing Otago
	Other barriers (please specify)

Table 5 | Top three facilitators and top three barriers.

	Not at all	Somewhat	A lot
Facilitators			
I have active support from my Agency's administration	23	95	155
The program is low cost and does not need substantial resources to continue	18	119	131
The research data helped convince my Agency of the value	19	118	130
Barriers			
My agency is not set up to keep patients on caseload over an extended period of time	66	127	65
Patients unable or do not want to pay co-pays	38	160	59
My agency does not have a system for follow-up phone calls	94	114	50

in the United States. Inherent in this process was identifying the barriers to adoption presented by implementing a program developed in a different healthcare system as well as identifying and implementing solutions to these barriers. In addition to translating the intervention materials, this process included the development of an efficient and effective system to disseminate training to PTs. A secondary purpose of this project was to determine if online training was an acceptable and feasible mechanism to reach our target audience of PTs.

The process of translating an intervention developed and tested in another county was innovative, and our experience indicates that it may be challenging to overcome barriers imposed by implementing programs under different healthcare systems. Two unanticipated challenges unique to the American healthcare system became apparent during the translation process: (1) reimbursement issues and (2) current policies regarding frequency and duration of physical therapy treatment.

Significant changes in Medicare Home Health Payment Policies were implemented during the time period of 2010–2013 (20, 21). When the OEP was first selected by the CDC to disseminate, it was assumed that PTs in the home health setting would be able to deliver Otago as intended and be reimbursed for their services. However, in October 2011, CMS released "The Final Rule" for implementation in 2012 (20, 21). The "Final Rule" significantly changed reimbursement for home health rehabilitation services with the goal of assuring equal access to services and reduce financial gaming. In essence, the final rule limited an episode of home health to no more than 60 days (it can be extended but with much paperwork) and reimbursed therapists at lower rates as more therapy was utilized. The 60-day limitation, in conjunction with an increase in acuity of home health patients and a 3–8% reduction in reimbursements depending on the patient's acuity, effectively made it impossible for home health therapists to deliver Otago with fidelity.

Alternative models proposed by the American translation team leveraged PTs that treat patients in outpatient settings and have the ability to keep their patients on caseload for a longer period of time; however, this poses a significant challenge to the fidelity of the program. Innovative models that have therapists work with patients in the home, but bill as an outpatient have been investigated and demonstrate promise. However, this model for delivering therapy is relatively new and does not have widespread penetration.

Despite the popularity of evidence-based programs among public health professionals serving older adult populations (22), clinicians such as PTs are often not familiar with such evidence-based programs. The concept of fidelity, or delivering a program as intended, was not familiar to the majority of learners. More than 64% of those who took the training had never referred or incorporated an evidence-based health promotion program into their treatment plan. Many therapists felt that a standardized program was not flexible enough to meet the needs of their patients. The gaps identified through the work with the SMEs and the pilot testing with the PTs indicated that OEP content would be easy to convey to PTs, but the implementation of the program with fidelity would prove to be a challenge.

In recognition of these challenges, the online training was revised to include several case studies to demonstrate different implementation models including a home health to outpatient and an outpatient only case. Additionally, we believe the online model afforded several advantages over the traditional face-to-face model: (1) cost-effectiveness – participants were charged $25 to attend versus a face-to-face course, which is typically $100–200; (2) reach – in the first 9 months of deployment, we had participants from all 50 states take the training; (3) community – participants were invited to other opportunities to support their work; and (4) convenience – participants could start and stop the training whenever they liked.

In the first 9 months, the online training appears to be an effective mechanism to target PTs who work primarily with aging patients. The program itself was advertised through a word-of-mouth, website, and a few physical therapy-based listserv. The "early adopters" who completed the program were those who would be considered "senior" therapists (in practice 8 or more years) and spent the majority of their clinical practice time working with older adults. This supports that our target audience was reached. One concerning item was that only 13% of the sample were categorized as "new" therapists (3 years or less of clinical practice). The low number of new graduates may reflect the demographics within the greater practice setting and that the majority of PTs in geriatrics are older and more seasoned (23).

The perceived barriers and facilitators to program implementation provided significant insights about the challenges of the OEP adoption and implementation. At the end of the online training, therapists were asked to rate the extent an item was considered to be a facilitator or a barrier to implementation. The top facilitator was support from Agency administration. Therapists who implement the OEP without agency support are responsible for procuring weights, copying home exercise program handouts, and ensuring all paperwork is completed correctly and in a timely manner. One therapist estimated the personal cost of implementing the OEP at about $50/patient. Agencies that supported the OEP created systems to procure ankle weights for patients to use as part of the exercise program and ensured that all photocopying costs were absorbed by the agency as opposed to the therapist. Agency support is critical for program success, and more efforts should be made toward demonstrating the value of the OEP at the agency level.

Barriers included system-based challenges to maintaining a patient on caseload, concerns about costs to the patients in the form of co-pays, and the inability to perform follow-up phone calls. Interestingly, the therapists who completed the training did not perceive the billing and reimbursement challenges to be a barrier to program implementation. This may be because the therapists were being asked to rate these items immediately upon completing the online training and before actually implementing the program.

CONCLUSION

The implementation of standardized fall prevention programs into physical therapy practice is not as simple or as straightforward as anticipated. PTs are well versed in the content of the OEP but were not familiar with the frequency, duration, and standardization of the program. In general, PTs appreciated the effectiveness of the program, but there are challenges inherent to reimbursement for providing the OEP with fidelity to appropriate patients. Online training appears to be an effective way to disseminate the OEP to PTs who work with older adults; however, we anticipate that additional support and resources will be necessary for PTs to implement the OEP with fidelity to impact the nature of falls.

ACKNOWLEDGMENTS

This work was supported in part by the Bureau of Health Professions (BHPr), Health Resources and Services Administration (HRSA), Department of Health and Human Services (DHHS) under grant #UB4HP19053, Carolina Geriatric Education Center. This information, content, and conclusions are those of the author and should not be construed as the official position or policy of, nor should any endorsements be inferred by the BHPr, HRSA, DHHS, or the U.S. Government. The Centers for Disease Control Prevention Research Center at Texas A&M Health Science Center, School of Rural Public Health Center for Community Health Development also provided funding support from the Centers for Disease Control and Prevention Cooperative Agreement Number 1U48 DP001924, and the Centers for Disease Control Prevention Research Center at the University of North Carolina, Chapel Hill Prevention Research Center, supported by Cooperative Agreement Number U48-DP001944. The findings and conclusions in this paper are those of the author(s) and do not necessarily represent the official position of the Centers for Disease Control and Prevention.

REFERENCES

1. Stevens J. *Falls Among Older Adults: An Overview* (2013) [cited 2013 August 5]. Available from: http://www.cdc.gov/HomeandRecreationalSafety/Falls/adultfalls.html
2. Tinetti ME, Kumar C. The patient who falls: "It's always a trade-off". *JAMA* (2010) **303**:258–66. doi:10.1001/jama.2009.2024
3. *Prevention of Falls in Older Persons AGS/BGS Clinical Practice Guidelines* (2010) [cited 2012 October 15]. Available from: http://www.medcats.com/FALLS/frameset.htm
4. CDC. *Self-Reported Falls and Fall-Related Injuries Among Persons Aged >65 Years – United States, 2006* (2008) [cited 2014 June 1]. Available from: http://www.cdc.gov/mmwr/preview/mmwrhtml/mm5709a1.htm

5. Stevens J. *The Cost of Falls Among Older Adults* (2012) [cited 2012 December 1]. Available from: http://www.cdc.gov/HomeandRecreationalSafety/Falls/fallcost.html
6. Stevens J. *A CDC Compendium of Effective Fall Inteventions: What Works for Community-Dwelling Older Adults.* 2nd ed. Atlanta, GA: Centers for Disease Control and Prevention, National Center for Injury Prevention and Control (2010).
7. Stevens J. *Preventing Falls: What Works a CDC Compendium of Effective Community Based Interventions from Around the World.* Atlanta, GA: National Center for Injury Prevention and Control (2008).
8. Li F, Harmer P, Glasgow RB, Mack K, Sleet D, Fisher KJ, et al. Tai Chi: moving for better balance – development of a community-based falls prevention program. *Am J Public Health* (2008) **98**(7):1195–8.
9. Clemson L, Cumming RG, Kendig H, Swann M, Heard R, Taylor K. The effectiveness of a community-based program for reducing the incidence of falls in the elderly: a randomized trial. *J Am Geriatr Soc* (2004) **52**:1487–94. doi:10.1111/j.1532-5415.2004.52411.x
10. Campbell AJ, Robertson MC. *Otago Exercise Programme to Prevent Falls in Older People: A Home-Based, Individually Tailored Strength and Balance Retraining Program.* Otago, NZ: Accident Compensation Corporation (2003).
11. Cho J, Smith ML, Shubert TE, Jiang L, Ahn S, Ory MG. Gait speed among older participants enrolled in an evidence-based fall risk reduction program: a subgroup analysis. *Front Public Health* (2015) **3**:26. doi:10.3389/fpubh.2015.00026
12. Ory MG, Smith ML, Jiang L, Lee R, Chen S, Wilson AD, et al. Fall prevention in community settings: results from implementing Stepping On in three states. *Front Public Health* (2015) **2**:232. doi:10.3389/fpubh.2014.00232.
13. Campbell AJ, Robertson MC, Gardner MM, Norton RN, Buchner DM. Falls prevention over 2 years: a randomized controlled trial in women 80 years and older. *Age Ageing* (1999) **28**:513–8. doi:10.1093/ageing/28.6.513
14. Thomas S, Mackintosh S, Halbert J. Does the "Otago Exercise Programme" reduce mortality and falls in older adults? A systematic review and meta-analysis. *Age Ageing* (2010) **39**:681–7. doi:10.1093/ageing/afq102
15. American Physical Therapy Association. Guide to physical therapist practice. Second edition. American Physical Therapy Association. *Phys Ther* (2001) **81**:9–746.
16. Campbell AJ, Robertson MC, Gardner MM, Norton RN, Tilyard MW, Buchner DM. Randomised controlled trial of a general practice programme of home based exercise to prevent falls in elderly women. *BMJ* (1997) **315**:1065–9. doi:10.1136/bmj.315.7115.1065
17. CMS. *Medicare Benefit Policy Manual 002 – Chapter 15 Covered Medical and Other Health Services.* Baltimore, MD: Centers for Medicare & Medicaid Services (2014).
18. Mahoney JE, Shea TA, Przybelski R, Jaros L, Gangnon R, Cech S, et al. Kenosha county falls prevention study: a randomized, controlled trial of an intermediate-intensity, community-based multifactorial falls intervention. *J Am Geriatr Soc* (2007) **55**:489–98. doi:10.1111/j.1532-5415.2007.01144.x
19. Mangione KK, Lopopolo RB, Neff NP, Craik RL, Palombaro KM. Interventions used by physical therapists in home care for people after hip fracture. *Phys Ther* (2008) **88**(2):199–210. doi:10.2522/ptj.20070023
20. APTA. *Highlights of the 2012 Physician Fee Schedule Rule.* Alexandria, VA: American Physical Therapy Association (2012).
21. APTA. *Highlights of the 2014 Physician Fee Schedule Rule.* Alexandria, VA: American Physical Therapy Association (2014).
22. NCOA. *Evidence-Based Health Promotion Programs for Older Adults: Key Factors and Strategies Contributing to Program Sustainability.* Washington, DC: NCOA (2012).
23. APTA. *APTA Physical Therapist Member Demographic Profile.* Alexandria, VA: American Physical Therapy Association (2013).

Gait speed among older participants enrolled in an evidence-based fall risk reduction program: A subgroup analysis

***Jinmyoung Cho*[1,2]*, ***Matthew Lee Smith*[3,2], ***Tiffany E. Shubert*[4], ***Luohua Jiang*[5,6], ***SangNam Ahn*[7,2] and ***Marcia G. Ory*[2]

[1] *Center for Applied Health Research, Baylor Scott & White Health, Temple, TX, USA*
[2] *Department of Health Promotion and Community Health Science, Texas A&M Health Science Center School of Public Health, College Station, TX, USA*
[3] *Department of Health Promotion and Behavior, The University of Georgia, Athens, GA, USA*
[4] *School of Medicine, University of North Carolina, Chapel Hill, NC, USA*
[5] *Department of Epidemiology, School of Medicine, University of California, Irvine, CA, USA*
[6] *Department of Epidemiology and Biostatistics, Texas A&M Health Science Center School of Public Health, College Station, TX, USA*
[7] *Division of Health Systems Management and Policy, The University of Memphis, Memphis, TN, USA*

Edited by:
Sanjay P. Zodpey, Public Health Foundation of India, India

Reviewed by:
Cheryll Diann Lesneski, The University of North Carolina at Chapel Hill, USA
Preeti Negandhi, Indian Institute of Public Health Delhi, India

Correspondence:
Jinmyoung Cho, Department of Health Promotion and Community Health Science, Texas A&M Health Science Center, School of Public Health, Center for Applied Health Research, Baylor Scott and White Health, MS-01-501, 2401 S 31st Street, Temple, TX 76508, USA
e-mail: jcho@sw.org, jinmyoung.cho@sph.tamhsc.edu

Background: Functional decline is a primary risk factor for institutionalization and mortality among older adults. Although community-based fall risk reduction programs have been widely disseminated, little is known about their impact on gait speed, a key indicator of functional performance. Changes in functional performance between baseline and post-intervention were examined by means of timed up and go (TUG), a standardized functional assessment test administered to participants enrolled in A Matter of Balance/Volunteer Lay Leader (AMOB/VLL) model, an evidence-based fall risk reduction program.

Methods: This study included 71 participants enrolled in an AMOB/VLL program in the Brazos Valley and South Plain regions of Texas. Paired *t*-tests were employed to assess program effects on gait speed at baseline and post-intervention for all participants and by subgroups of age, sex, living status, delivery sites, and self-rated health. The Bonferroni correction was applied to adjust inflated Type I error rate associated with performing multiple *t*-tests, for which *p*-values <0.0042 (i.e., 0.5/12 comparisons) were deemed statistically significant.

Results: Overall, gait speed of enrolled participants improved from baseline to post-intervention ($t = 3.22$, $p = 0.002$). Significant changes in TUG scores were observed among participants who lived with others ($t = 4.45$, $p < 0.001$), rated their health as excellent, very good, or good ($t = 3.05$, $p = 0.003$), and attended program workshops at senior centers ($t = 3.52$, $p = 0.003$).

Conclusion: Findings suggest community-based fall risk reduction programs can improve gait speed for older adults. More translational research is needed to understand factors related to the effectiveness of fall risk reduction programs in various populations and settings.

Keywords: older adults, A Matter of Balance/Volunteer Lay Leader model, timed up and go

FALLS AMONG OLDER ADULTS

Falls among older adults are a serious public health problem in America (1). Approximately one-fourth of older adults aged 80 years and older experience at least two falls per year (2–4). As the risk of falling increases with advanced age, dramatic escalations in fall-related morbidity, hospitalization, institutionalization, and mortality can be expected to accompany the aging of the population (5). Direct annual medical care costs related to falls have been estimated at almost $20 billion and are projected to increase sharply in the coming decades (6, 7).

Various demographic, functional, and health factors are known to increase the risk for falling among older adults (8). These factors include age (2, 4), being female (9, 10), a prior history of falls (2, 4), gait and mobility deficits (2, 4, 9, 11), and poor self-reported health status (9, 10). In addition to personal characteristics, particular attention has been paid to the environmental circumstances surrounding falls, such neighborhood environments or program delivery settings (12).

Fall-prevention programs and integration of prevention services have been shown to decrease fall recurrence (13) and reduce health-care costs (14). However, literature about the effectiveness of evidence-based fall-prevention programs for improving objectively measured functional performance has been limited for programs delivered in the community by lay facilitators.

Given its ease of use and standardization, gait speed, often called "timed up and go (TUG)," has been frequently used to assess functional performance as an outcome measurement for effective interventions (15, 16). Many studies have demonstrated a strong relationship between gait speed and fall-related risk, health and functional status, institutionalization, and mortality among older adults (17–19). To address the existing research gaps, the overall goal of this study was to examine improvement in functional performance among older participants enrolled in A Matter of Balance/Volunteer Lay Leader (AMOB/VLL) model, an evidence-based fall risk reduction program.

A MATTER OF BALANCE/VOLUNTEER LAY LEADER FALL RISK REDUCTION PROGRAM

A Matter of Balance (AMOB), established at the Roybal Center for Enhancement of Late-Life Function at Boston University, is an evidence-based program to reduce risk of falls among older adults (20). The effectiveness of the AMOB program was originally tested through a randomized clinical trial, which showed positive improvements in physical activity and mobility control (21). Derived from the original program, the AMOB/VLL model has been adapted for widespread community dissemination in various health and aging sectors (22, 23). Delivered by trained lay-led facilitators in 38 states, it is presented in 2-h sessions for 8 weeks. One hour is taught by a physical therapist. This hour focuses on the role of exercise in fall prevention. It is not meant to be a standalone session, but rather an introduction for older adults to build upon. At the end of AMOB, participants are more likely to exercise and intended activity (21). Each session includes specific goals for older adults to reduce the risk of falling and continue remaining active and independent (24). The major goals of the program are as follows: to make participants perceive control, to increase their confidence, and to learn falls are controllable. The design of intervention targets behavior change and emphasizes building fall self-efficacy and setting goals for increasing physical activity through lectures, group discussions, various problem-solving and role-playing activities, exercise and assertiveness training, and individual assignments (24).

Since 2006, a well-established infrastructure has facilitated the delivery of the intervention to older adults in Texas (24). The network for aging services arranged a signed agreement with the Texas Association of Area Agencies on Aging (AAA) for implementation of the AMOB/VLL program in many AAA regions. The program targets low-income older minority adults and their caregivers and focuses on reaching a diverse population in a large geographic area. Residential facilities, health-care institutions, public health departments, faith-based organizations, business sectors, and local government were included as partners with the Texas AAA sites to build fall-prevention capacity (24, 25).

PURPOSE OF STUDY

Although community-based health promotion programs result in for improvement in falls efficacy, overall health status, and increased physical activities (11, 26), less is known about their impact on physical performance (i.e., TUG) among older participants. The purposes of this study were to (a) assess the changes in physical performance measured by the TUG test from baseline to post-intervention and (b) compare the improvement in physical performance by personal characteristics and delivery sites. A conceptual model for this study is shown in **Figure 1**. This model depicts the fall risk reduction program as an intervention that can have positive effects on changes in physical performance. If participation in AMOB results in improved efficacy as well as improved physical performance, physical therapists may want to include AMOB as a program for appropriate patients. To better understand who may benefit

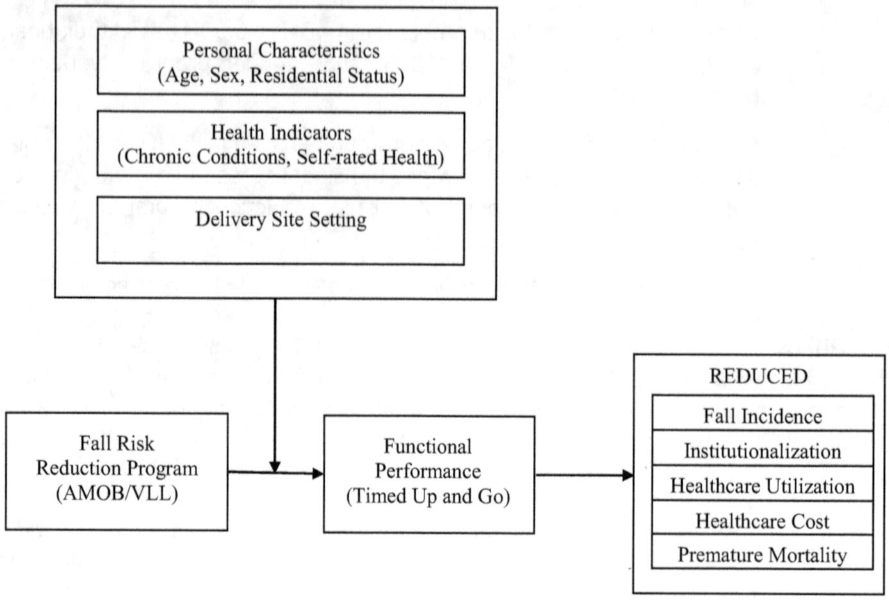

FIGURE 1 | Conceptual model.

the most from this program, personal characteristics and delivery sites act as moderators between the fall risk reduction program (as illustrated by the AMOB/VLL model) and physical performance as measured by the TUG test. In turn, the TUG measurements are associated with long-term improvements in reduced health-care use and costs as well as enhanced health and well-being.

METHODS

PROCEDURES AND PARTICIPANTS

A total of 301 participants enrolled in the Texas AMOB/VLL fall risk reduction program between September 2007 and April 2009 in two regional AAAs: Brazos Valley and South Plain. Although functional assessment was optional in the statewide AAA delivery of the AMOB/VLL program, assessments were conducted in some classes that taught these two regions. Workshop leaders were trained in assessment procedures and performed assessments in eight of the AMOB/VLL classes, which served as the basis for this study. A total of 171 participants who attended classes in these two regions but who were not assessed using the TUG were excluded; thus, 76 participants completed the TUG test at baseline and post-intervention, whereas 54 participants did not complete the test at both times. Boxplots were used to screen for outliers for TUG scores from both baseline and post-intervention. Results indicated the presence of three outliers, who were then omitted. An additional two cases reporting an "other" ethnic group were excluded to maximize racial and ethnic homogeneity of participants for this study. As a result, only non-Hispanic White participants were included in this study. **Figure 2** shows the recruitment flow diagram, indicating that 71 participants were included in study analyses.

MEASURES

Timed up and go test

The TUG test, introduced in 1991 by Podsiadlo and Richardson (27), has been used extensively for over a decade to predict fall risk and to examine functional mobility among older adults (26, 28). It assesses the time in seconds that participants required to "rise from a standard arm chair, walk at your typical or normal pace to a line on the floor 3 meters away, turn, return, and sit down again" (p. 64) (27). This test was validated to test physical functioning and mobility among community-dwelling older adults (26) and showed high predictive validity with the Berg Balance Scale (27). Those who completed the TUG tasks in more than 14 s also showed lower scores on the Berg Balance Scale, which was associated with higher risk for institutionalization (26).

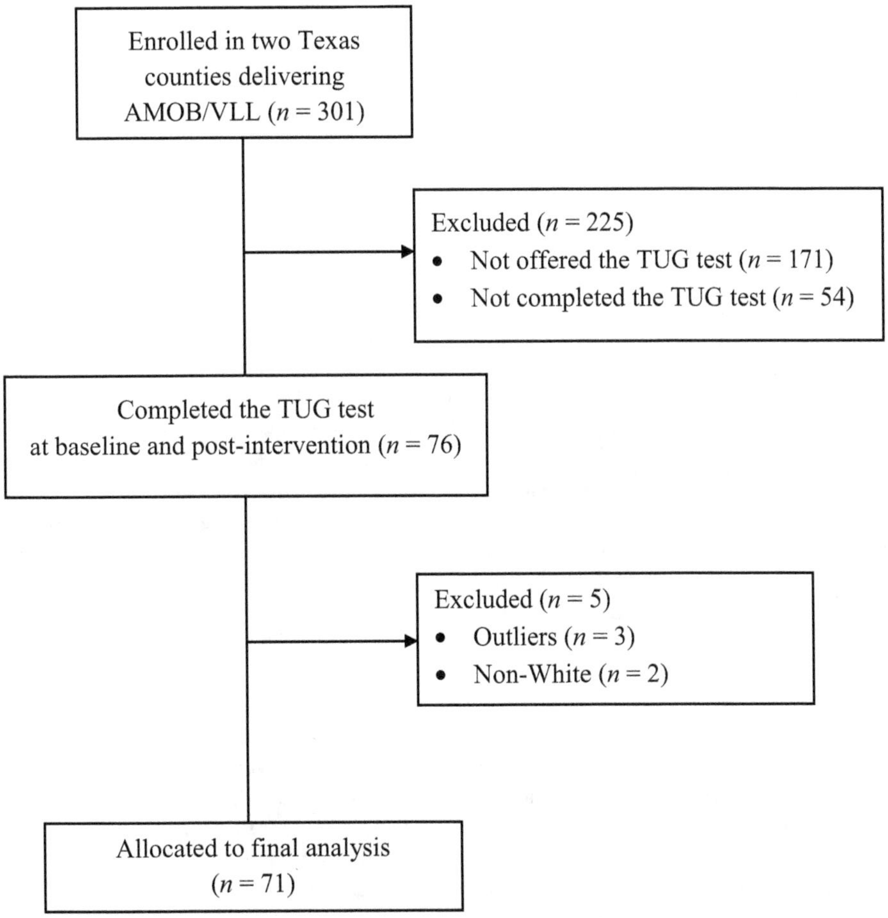

FIGURE 2 | Diagram for study participants inclusion.

Personal characteristics

Age was coded as a continuous variable based on a participant's birth date and ranged from 56 to 95. The age was then categorized into three groups for the purpose of the study: young-old (up to 69 years), mid-old (from 70 to 79 years), and old-old (80 years and older). *Sex* was scored 0 if the participant was male and 1 if the participant was female. *Living status* was scored 1 if participants lived with others and 0 if they lived alone. *Self-rated health* was included. Self-rated health, a single item measuring in which participants rate current status of their overall health, has been widely used as a significant predictor of physical and psychological health such as mortality or functionality among various populations (29–32). Many studies have shown that the single item is a reliable and valid measure reflecting objective health status (e.g., cardio-cerebral vascular diseases, visual impairment) (32–34). At baseline, participants were also asked to self-report their perceived health status: "Would you say that in general your health is poor, fair, good, very good, or excellent?" For comparisons of self-rated health, the responses were divided into two categories (i.e., poor/fair vs. good/very good/excellent).

Delivery sites

To compare outcomes at the various settings in which the AMOB/VLL program was conducted in the Brazos Valley and South Plain regions, delivery site types were obtained from administrative data. Delivery site categories included senior centers, community centers, faith-based organizations, residential facilities, and other Parks Department facilities. For comparisons of delivery sites, five sites were categorized into three groups: senior centers and community centers, residential facilities, and others.

Table 1 | Characteristic of the study participants.

Characteristics	Frequency (%)
Age, mean (SD) (range: 56–95)	77.8 (9.3)
Sex	
Male	13 (19.4)
Female	54 (80.6)
Residential status	
Living alone	29 (43.9)
Living with others	37 (56.1)
Self-rated health	
Excellent	5 (7.7)
Very good	17 (26.2)
Good	27 (41.5)
Fair	15 (23.1)
Poor	1 (1.5)
Numbers of chronic condition	
None	11 (15.5)
1–2	44 (61.9)
3+	16 (22.5)
Delivery sites	
Senior centers	15 (21.1)
Community centers	2 (2.8)
Residential facilities	37 (52.1)
Faith-based organizations	9 (12.7)
Other-parks department facilities	8 (11.3)

Different numbers of missing cases were observed for each variable. Missing cases were excluded from calculations and analyses.

Data analysis

The paired t-test was employed to compare mean TUG scores for all participants pre- and post-intervention. Statistical significance was examined at the level of 0.05 for this test. Then, a series of paired t-tests were employed to compare the TUG scores by subgroups: age groups, sex, residential status, delivery sites, and self-rated health. Bonferroni's correction was applied for subgroup (12 groups) comparisons to adjust the inflated Type I error rate associated with performing multiple t-tests, for which p-values <0.0042 (i.e., 0.5/12 comparisons) were deemed statistically significant. Statistical analyses were conducted with SPSS statistical software (version 20.0). As an indicator of practical significance, Cohen's d standardized effect sizes were calculated to compare intervention effects from baseline to post-intervention within each group.

RESULTS

SAMPLE CHARACTERISTICS

Table 1 summarizes characteristics of study participants. The average age of the study participants was 77.8 (SD = 9.3) years old. The majority of participants was female (80.6%), and more than half the participants lived with others (56.1%). Over three quarters of the participants rated their health good, very good, or excellent (75.4%). Most participants had at least one chronic health problem (84.4%). Within the two regional AAAs, the AMOB/VLL program was implemented in residential facilities (52.1%), senior centers (21.1%), faith-based organizations (12.7%), other Parks Department facilities (11.3%), and community centers (2.8%).

CHANGES IN TIMED UP AND GO TEST

Before the paired t-test for the TUG score was conducted, the TUG scores at baseline and post-intervention were observed. Almost a third of participants (28.2%) at baseline and 22.5% of participants at post-intervention performed slower than 14 s, which represents a critical value on the TUG test. **Table 2** presents results of the paired t-tests for TUG scores among all AMOB/VLL program participants and by subgroups from baseline to post-intervention. Among all participants, the average TUG score at baseline was 12.89 (SD = 5.08) and changed to 11.95 (SD = 4.30) at post-intervention ($t = 3.22$, $p = 0.002$). When comparing TUG score changes by subgroup, three significant improvements were found. First, participants who lived with others showed significant changes in TUG scores from baseline ($M = 12.61$, SD = 5.92) to post-intervention ($M = 11.32$, SD = 5.04), $t = 4.45$, $p < 0.001$. The effect size (Cohen's d) was 0.23. Second, participants who attended the AMOB/VLL program at senior centers or community centers showed statistically significant improvement in TUG scores from 14.96 (SD = 7.20) at baseline to 13.30 (SD = 6.21) at post-intervention, $t = 3.52$, $p = 0.003$. Cohen's d was 0.25. Third, those who perceived their health good, very good, or excellent showed significant improvement in TUG scores: 12.77 (SD = 5.41)

Table 2 | Average TUG scores in pre- and post-test by groups.

	Pre (SD)	Post (SD)	*t*-Value	*p*	Cohen's *d*
Total participants	12.89 (5.08)	11.95 (4.30)	3.22	0.002	0.25
Age groups					
Young-old ($n=14$)	9.74 (2.21)	8.89 (2.06)	2.60	0.018	0.40
Mid-old ($n=16$)	11.67 (3.43)	10.83 (2.80)	2.25	0.040	0.27
Old-old ($n=34$)	14.85 (6.06)	13.82 (5.00)	2.20	0.035	0.19
Sex					
Male ($n=13$)	12.41 (4.00)	11.53 (3.59)	1.33	0.208	0.23
Female ($n=54$)	12.95 (5.45)	12.08 (4.62)	2.77	0.008	0.17
Living status					
Living alone ($n=29$)	12.93 (4.05)	12.66 (3.44)	0.52	0.605	0.07
Living with others ($n=37$)	12.61 (5.92)	11.32 (5.04)	4.45	<0.001	0.23
Delivery sites					
Senior/community centers ($n=15$)	14.96 (7.20)	13.30 (6.21)	3.52	0.003	0.25
Residential facilities ($n=38$)	13.58 (4.51)	12.79 (3.69)	1.56	0.128	0.19
Others ($n=19$)	9.90 (2.27)	9.24 (2.02)	2.54	0.020	0.31
Self-rated health groups					
Excellent/VG/good ($n=57$)	12.77 (5.41)	11.87 (4.56)	3.05	0.003	0.18
Fair/poor ($n=11$)	13.08 (2.78)	11.86 (3.36)	1.25	0.240	0.40

Different numbers of missing cases were observed for each variable. Missing cases were excluded from calculations and analyses.

at baseline and 11.87 (SD = 4.56) at post-intervention, $t=3.05$, $p=0.003$. The effect size was 0.18.

DISCUSSION

The primary objective in this study was to examine changes in functional performance between baseline and post-intervention among participants enrolled in the Texas AMOB/VLL fall risk reduction program. Several important findings emerged from this study. First, the average score for all participants' walking speed assessed with the standardized TUG test improved from baseline to post-intervention. These findings demonstrate that this fall risk reduction program can improve gait speed among old participants in addition to its previously reported benefits for falls efficacy and fear of falling (22). Second, subgroup comparisons showed significant improvements among those who rated their health more positively, lived with others, and attended program workshops in senior centers or community centers. These findings reveal that improvement in functional performance (i.e., TUG) may be directly associated with participating in a fall risk reduction program for these subgroups.

The most significant aspect of this study was the incorporation of an objectively measured functional assessment to compare participant improvement based on self-reported measures. Because most measures from evidence-based programs have been based on self-reported information, such as health-related quality of life, number of falls, and number of chronic conditions within the previous week or month, a couple of other researchers noted that self-reported measures might produce recall bias as a data collection limitation (23, 35, 36). Using a standardized functional assessment test (i.e., TUG) can contribute to the validation of previous findings that reported improvements in the ability to perform important social and role functions (23, 36).

Findings of the current study also highlight the importance of physical health, social, and environmental correlates to enhance the effectiveness of the evidence-based program. First, the analyses revealed that better perception of health was associated with significant improvement on the TUG test. It is obvious that those who perceived their health to be of better status showed significant improvement because these individuals may be more likely to have fewer chronic conditions and may be less influenced by daily activity limitations. However, the largest standardized Cohen's effect size (Cohen's $d=0.40$) was notably observed among participants who self-reported their health to be fair/poor despite the lack of statistical significance of the TUG score change. In other words, those with worse health status may show larger changes in functional assessments because they have greater opportunity for improvement, whereas those healthier participants who score high at baseline have little room for improvement (36). This finding points to the need for future research to increase understanding of the functional improvements of individuals of different health status levels and detect underlying statistical effects, such as regression to the mean.

Second, the significant improvement in gait speed based on residential status emphasizes the importance of social correlates on the effectiveness of the evidence-based program. Results showed significant improvement in functional performance from baseline to post-intervention among participants who live with others. This finding is consistent with previous studies that has shown the significant relationship between physical activities and support from family or friends (37, 38). Living with others is likely to prevent older adults from social isolation, which has been identified as a barrier to physical activity (38). This finding may also indicate that participants who lived with others had social support mechanisms that may have encouraged them to attend more AMOB/VLL program sessions (i.e., received more intervention dose) and engage in recommended physical activities outside class time.

Third, findings of this study suggest delivery settings in which evidence-based programs that are implemented can enhance physical performance among old participants. Participants who attended workshops in senior centers or community centers showed significant improvement in TUG scores from baseline to post-intervention, which may highlight an environmental benefit for delivering evidence-based programs to older adults in these group settings. This finding may be associated with the notion that these participants were healthier upon program enrollment or that the location of the delivery site was more accessible, which increased their attendance (i.e., intervention does) and led to significant improvement.

In an attempt to disseminate widely fall-prevention programs, the Texas AAA sites have continued to build fall-prevention capacity by partnering with the public health network and others to establish programs in various settings, such as residential facilities, faith-based organizations, workplace setting, health-care institutions, public health departments, and governmental facilities (25). Although other studies have identified differences in program outcomes by delivery site types (35), further investigation is warranted to understand the influence of delivery site on functional assessment measures among lay-led fall-prevention programs.

LIMITATIONS AND IMPLICATIONS

The findings of this study showed significant TUG score changes associated with this fall risk reduction program; however, a few notable limitations were associated with this study. First, this study included only 71 study participants. The small sample size may limit generalization of our findings to other populations. Second, as stated in the procedures and participant section, older minority adults were excluded from this study because too few participated for meaningful analyses. Although Texas is a geographically large and demographically diverse state, the two minority group cases were intentionally excluded to yield a homogeneous sample of participants. If enough minorities had been available for meaningful comparisons, we may find ethnic difference in functional performance among more diverse groups of participants. Finally, if objective method of rating current health status (e.g., biomarkers) was used in the fall risk reduction program instead of self-rated health, the result may provide an association between health status and functional capacity among old participants.

The findings from the current study have considerable implications for future research on translational studies. Although this study provides an important view of the use of TUG tests in a community-based fall risk reduction program, additional research is needed to link functional assessment scores to the actual fall experience, subsequent health-care use, and the availability of supportive environments illustrated in our conceptual model of fall risk behaviors, interventions, and long-term outcomes. First, the capacity for objective functional measurement among community-dwelling older adults should be built into evidence-based fall-prevention programs. For example, instructor manuals for lay leaders should include a training session about objective functional measurement. Such provider training is important for maintaining measurement necessary for research assessment. In recognition of the importance of objective measurements for purposes of both research and programing, this type of training has been built into CDC's State Fall Prevention Program (39). Furthermore, future studies should focus on participants' degree of disability to examine more comprehensively the effectiveness of evidence-based fall risk reduction programs in different populations. Considering the extent of the disability or investigating the difference in physical performance between fallers and non-fallers may suggest detailed strategies to promote physical activity for older adults with various baseline functional levels. Also, more translational research is needed to understand potential modifiable and non-modifiable correlates related to effectiveness of fall risk reduction programs on functional performance within various populations and settings.

ACKNOWLEDGMENTS

A Matter of Balance/Voluntary Lay Leader (AMOB/VLL) is a major program activity in the Aging Texas Well's Texas Healthy Lifestyles Initiative. Statewide implementation is supported by the Department of Aging and Disability Services and administered through the Texas Association of Area Agencies on Aging. The evaluation is conducted by the Texas A&M Health Science Center School of Public Health. We recognize faculty support from The Center for Community Health Development, which is a member of the Prevention Research Centers Program, supported by the Centers for Disease Control and Prevention cooperative agreement number 5U48 DP000045. The findings and conclusions in this article are those of the author(s) and do not necessarily represent the official position of Department of Aging and Disability Services or the Centers for Disease Control and Prevention.

REFERENCES

1. Sleet DA, Moffett DB, Stevens J. CDC's research portfolio in older adult fall prevention: a review of progress, 1985-2005, and future research directions. *J Safety Res* (2008) **39**:259–67. doi:10.1016/j.jsr.2008.05.003
2. Rubenstein LZ. Falls in older people: epidemiology, risk factors and strategies for prevention. *Age Ageing* (2006) **35**:37–41. doi:10.1093/ageing/afl084
3. Tinetti M. Preventing falls in elderly persons. *N Engl J Med* (2003) **348**:42–9. doi:10.1056/NEJMcp020719
4. American Geriatrics Society, British Geriatrics Society, American Academy Of Orthopaedic Surgeons Panel on Falls Prevention. Guideline for the prevention of falls in older persons. *J Am Geriatr Soc* (2001) **49**:664–72. doi:10.1046/j.1532-5415.2001.49115.x
5. Persad CC, Cook S, Giordani B. Assessing falls in the elderly: should we use simple screening tests or a comprehensive fall risk evaluation? *Eur J Phys Rehabil Med* (2010) **46**:249–59.
6. Stevens JA, Corso PS, Finkelstein EA, Miller TR. The costs of fatal and non-fatal falls among older adults. *Inj Prev* (2006) **12**:290–5. doi:10.1136/ip.2005.011015
7. Roudsari BS, Ebel BE, Corso PS, Molinari NA, Koepsell TD. The acute medical care costs of fall-related injuries among the U.S. older adults. *Injury* (2005) **36**:1316–22. doi:10.1016/j.injury.2005.05.024
8. Ullmann G, Williams HG, Plass CF. Dissemination of an evidence-based program to reduce fear of falling, south Carolina, 2006-2009. *Prev Chronic Dis* (2012) **9**:E103.
9. Kato R, Takagi C, Sakurai N, Hoshi T. Risk factors for falls and survival after falling in elderly people in a community. *Nihon Koshu Eisei Zasshi* (2012) **59**:305–14.
10. Muraki S, Akune T, Ishimoto Y, Nagata K, Yoshida M, Tanaka S, et al. Risk factors for falls in a longitudinal population-based cohort study of Japanese men

and women: the ROAD study. *Bone* (2013) **52**:516–23. doi:10.1016/j.bone.2012.10.020

11. Viccaro LJ, Perera S, Studenski SA. Is timed up and go better than gait speed in predicting health, function, and falls in older adults? *J Am Geriatr Soc* (2011) **59**:887–92. doi:10.1111/j.1532-5415.2011.03336.x
12. Landy DC, Mintzer MJ, Silva AK, Dearwater SR, Schulman CI. Hispanic ethnicity and fatal fall risk: do age, gender, and community modify the relationship? *J Surg Res* (2012) **175**:113–7. doi:10.1016/j.jss.2011.02.035
13. Tinetti ME. Prevention of falls and fall injuries in elderly persons: a research agenda. *Prev Med* (1994) **23**:756–62. doi:10.1006/pmed.1994.1130
14. Rizzo J, Baker D, McAvay G, Tinetti M. The cost-effectiveness of a multifactorial targeted prevention program for falls among community elderly persons. *Med Care* (1996) **34**:954–69. doi:10.1097/00005650-199609000-00007
15. Cesari M, Kritchevsky SB, Newman AB, Simonsick EM, Harris TB, Penninx BW, et al. Added value of physical performance measures in predicting adverse health-related events: results from the health, aging and body composition study. *J Am Geriatr Soc* (2009) **57**:251–9. doi:10.1111/j.1532-5415.2008.02126.x
16. Abellan van Kan G, Rolland Y, Andrieu S, Bauer J, Beauchet O, Bonnefoy M, et al. Gait speed at usual pace as a predictor of adverse outcomes in community-dwelling older people an international academy on nutrition and aging (IANA) task force. *J Nutr Health Aging* (2009) **13**:881–9. doi:10.1007/s12603-009-0246-z
17. Beauchet O, Fantino B, Allali G, Muir SW, Montero-Odasso M, Annweiler C. Timed up and go test and risk of falls in older adults: a systematic review. *J Nutr Health Aging* (2011) **15**:933–8. doi:10.1007/s12603-011-0062-0
18. Studenski S, Perera S, Patel K, Rosano C, Faulkner K, Inzitari M, et al. Gait speed and survival in older adults. *JAMA* (2011) **305**:50–8. doi:10.1001/jama.2010.1923
19. Huang WW, Perera S, VanSwearingen J, Studenski S. Performance measures predict onset of activity of daily living difficulty in community-dwelling older adults. *J Am Geriatr Soc* (2010) **58**:844–52. doi:10.1111/j.1532-5415.2010.02820.x
20. Lachman M, Weaver S, Bandura M, Elliott E, Lewkowicz C. Improving memory and control beliefs through cognitive restructuring and self-generated strategies. *J Gerontol* (1992) **47**:293–9. doi:10.1093/geronj/47.5.P293
21. Tennstedt S, Howland J, Lachman M, Peterson E, Kasten L, Jette A. A randomized, controlled trial of a group intervention to reduce fear of falling and associated activity restriction in older adults. *J Gerontol B Psychol Sci Soc Sci* (1998) **53**:384–92. doi:10.1093/geronb/53B.6.P384
22. Healy TC, Peng C, Haynes MS, McMahon EM, Botler JL, Gross L. The feasibility and effectiveness of translating A Matter of Balance into a Volunteer Lay Leader model. *J Appl Gerontol* (2008) **27**:34–51. doi:10.1177/0733464807308620
23. Smith ML, Ahn SN, Sharkey JR, Horel S, Mier N, Ory MG. Successful falls prevention programming for older adults in Texas: rural-urban variations. *J Appl Gerontol* (2012) **31**:3–27. doi:10.1177/0733464810378407
24. Ory MG, Smith ML, Wade AF, Wright JC, Parrish R. Addressing falls in Texas: evidence-based fall prevention programming for older adults. *Tex Public Health J* (2010) **62**:15–20.
25. Cho J, Smith ML, Ahn S, Kim K, Appiah B, Ory MG. Effects of an evidence-based falls risk-reduction program on physical activity and falls efficacy among oldest-old adults. *Front Public Health* (2015) **2**:182. doi:10.3389/fpubh.2014.00182
26. Shumway-Cook A, Brauer S, Woollacott M. Predicting the probability for falls in community-dwelling older adults using the timed up & go test. *Phys Ther* (2000) **80**:896–903.
27. Podsiadlo D, Richardson S. The timed up and go – a test of basic functional mobility for frail elderly persons. *J Am Geriatr Soc* (1991) **39**:142–8.
28. Hutton I, Gamble G, McLean G, Butcher H, Gow P, Dalbeth N. Obstacles to action in arthritis: a community case-control study. *Int J Rheum Dis* (2009) **12**:107–17. doi:10.1111/j.1756-185X.2009.01392.x
29. Benjamins MR, Hummer RA, Eberstein IW, Nam CB. Self-reported health and adult mortality risk: an analysis of cause-specific mortality. *Soc Sci Med* (2004) **59**:1297–306. doi:10.1016/j.socscimed.2003.01.001
30. Idler EL, Angel RJ. Self-rated health and mortality in the NHANES-I epidemiologic follow-up study. *Am J Public Health* (1990) **80**:446–52. doi:10.2105/AJPH.80.4.446
31. Appels A, Bosma H, Grabauskas V, Gostautas A, Sturmans F. Self-rated health and mortality in a Lithuanian and a Dutch population. *Soc Sci Med* (1996) **42**:681–9. doi:10.1016/0277-9536(95)00195-6
32. Murata C, Kondo T, Tamakoshi K, Yatsuya H, Toyoshima H. Determinants of self-rated health: could health status explain the association between self-rated health and mortality? *Arch Gerontol Geriatr* (2006) **43**:369–80. doi:10.1016/j.archger.2006.01.002
33. Molarius A, Janson S. Self-rated health, chronic diseases, and symptoms among middle-aged and elderly men and women. *J Clin Epidemiol* (2002) **55**:364–70. doi:10.1016/S0895-4356(01)00491-7
34. Wu S, Wang R, Zhao Y, Ma X, Wu M, Yan X, et al. The relationship between self-rated health and objective health status: a population-based study. *BMC Public Health* (2013) **13**:320. doi:10.1186/1471-2458-13-320
35. Smith ML, Ory MG, Belza B, Altpeter M. Personal and delivery site characteristics associated with intervention dosage in an evidence-based fall risk reduction program for older adults. *Transl Behav Med* (2012) **2**:188–98. doi:10.1007/s13142-012-0133-8
36. Smith ML, Jiang L, Ory MG. Falls efficacy among older adults enrolled in an evidence-based program to reduce fall-related risk sustainability of individual benefits over time. *Fam Community Health* (2012) **35**:256–63. doi:10.1097/FCH.0b013e318250bdb8
37. Wilcox S, Der Ananian C, Sharpe PA, Robbins J, Brady T. Correlates of physical activity in persons with arthritis: review and recommendations. *J Phys Act Health* (2005) **2**:230–52.
38. Gordon NF, Gulanick M, Costa F, Fletcher G, Franklin BA, Roth EJ, et al. Physical activity and exercise recommendations for stroke survivors: an American heart association scientific statement from the council on clinical cardiology, subcommittee on exercise, cardiac rehabilitation, and prevention; the council on cardiovascular nursing; the council on nutrition, physical activity, and metabolism; and the stroke council. *Stroke* (2004) **35**:1230–40.
39. Center for Disease Control and Prevention, National Center for Injury Prevention and Control, Stopping Elderly Accidents, Dealths, & Injuries. *STEADI Implementation Guide: For Health Care Providers.* Washington, DC: Center for Disease Control and Prevention (2012).

24

Effects of an evidence-based falls risk-reduction program on physical activity and falls efficacy among oldest-old adults

Jinmyoung Cho[1,2]*, Matthew Lee Smith[3], SangNam Ahn[4], Keonyeop Kim[5], Bernard Appiah[6] and Marcia G. Ory[2]

[1] Center for Applied Health Research, Baylor Scott and White Health, Temple, TX, USA
[2] Department of Health Promotion and Community Health Science, Texas A&M Health Science Center, School of Public Health, College Station, TX, USA
[3] Department of Health Promotion and Behavior, College of Public Health, The University of Georgia, Athens, GA, USA
[4] Division of Health Systems Management and Policy, School of Public Health, The University of Memphis, Memphis, TN, USA
[5] Department of Preventive Medicine, Graduate School of Public Health, Kyungpook National University, Daegu, South Korea
[6] Department of Public Health Studies, Texas A&M Health Science Center, School of Public Health, College Station, TX, USA

Edited by:
Sanjay P. Zodpey, Public Health Foundation of India, India

Reviewed by:
Suresh Narayanrao Ughade, Government Medical College, India
Muni Rubens, Florida International University, USA

***Correspondence:**
Jinmyoung Cho, Center for Applied Health Research, Baylor Scott and White Health, Department of Health Promotion and Community Health Science, Texas A&M Health Science Center, School of Public Health, 2401 S 31st Street, MS-01-501, Temple, TX 76508, USA
e-mail: jinmyoung.cho@sph.tamhsc.edu; jcho@sw.org

Purpose of the study: The current study was designed to examine changes in falls efficacy and physical activities among oldest-old and young-old participants in a falls risk-reduction program called a matter of balance/volunteer lay leader model.

Design and methods: An oldest-old group (aged 85 years and older; $n = 260$) and a young-old group (aged between 65 and 84 years old; $n = 1,139$) in Texas with both baseline and post-intervention measures were included. Changes in Falls Efficacy Scale scores and weekly physical activity levels were examined from baseline to post-intervention. Repeated measures analysis of covariance were employed to assess program effects on falls efficacy.

Results: Results showed significant changes in falls efficacy from baseline to post-intervention, as well as a significant interaction effect between time (baseline and post-intervention) and physical activity on falls efficacy.

Implications: Findings from this study imply the effectiveness of evidence-based programs for increasing falls efficacy in oldest-old participants. Future implications for enhancing physical activities and reducing fear of falling for oldest-old adults are discussed.

Keywords: oldest-old adults, falls efficacy, falls risk-reduction program

INTRODUCTION

The population of oldest-old adults – or those 85 years and older – is one of the fastest growing segments of the American population and is estimated to increase from 5.7 million to 19 million by 2050 (1). Despite growth among this population segment, relatively less attention is given to the oldest-old population compared to people aged younger than 85 years old (2). Attention to health status among oldest-old adults is critical because approximately half of those in this age group experience limitations in functioning, which not only impacts their health and independence (3) but also has societal implications on escalating health care utilization and costs (4, 5).

Substantial research has identified functional and behavioral factors associated with loss of independence among the aging population (6, 7). Less physical activity, for example, is increasingly seen as a major contributor to health deterioration and mortality, even among oldest-old adults (8, 9). Lower levels of physical activity contribute to increased number of medical comorbidities in oldest-old populations (10, 11). In addition, anxiety or fear of falling is related to risk for subsequent falls and limited physical activity among older adults (12, 13). For instance, in a sample of adults aged 70 years and older living in a community, over half had fallen at least once during the previous 6 months or restricted their daily activities or both because of a fear of falling (13).

Heterogeneity exists in levels of physical activity among oldest-old adults, despite the lower overall physical activity levels, suggesting the value in identifying modifiable factors associated with higher activity levels. A sense of efficacy, particularly falls efficacy – "the degree of confidence in performing common daily activities without falling" (14) (p. M141) – has been found as a significant factor for physical activity among older adults. Higher levels of efficacy have been related to faster gait speeds (15, 16) as well as lower levels of fear of falling (17); furthermore, physical activity interventions have shown significant positive effects on physical performance related to efficacy (18–20).

A MATTER OF BALANCE (AMOB) FALLS RISK-REDUCTION PROGRAM

Previous research indicates that falls risks can be ameliorated, especially through increases in physical activities, which are combined with behavioral strategies to help older adults prevent or manage falls (21–25). Behavioral interventions have been identified to improve falls efficacy (12, 26, 27). A matter of balance (AMOB) is an evidence-based program to reduce falls risk among older adults based on cognitive restructuring methods (28). Established at the

Roybal Center for Enhancement of Late-Life Function at Boston University, the original AMOB program was tested through a randomized clinical trial (RCT) (22). The major outcome variables of the program included significant improvements of perceived capacity to manage the risk of falling and confidence in everyday activities without falling. Two primary aims of the AMOB included (a) reducing fear of falling and (b) increasing physical, social, and functional activity (22).

Because the goal of AMOB/volunteer lay leader (VLL) is to build falls efficacy and encourage physical activities, many researchers have examined the effects of AMOB/VLL and found improvement in overall health status, as well as falls efficacy among older adults (29–33). For example, Ory and colleagues (29) found that Texas AMOB/VLL participants showed significant improvements in falls efficacy, physical activity, and normal everyday routines. These results are consistent with other studies that included participants from South Florida and South Carolina (34, 35). Ullmann and colleagues (35) found that South Carolina participants showed greater confidence in managing falls and performing activities of daily living, as well as improvements in functional mobility. In addition to short-term benefits in behavioral outcomes from the program, Smith et al. (36) observed significant yet modest improvements in falls efficacy were maintained 6 months after intervention. Furthermore, improvements in falls efficacy and physical activity have been identified in studies examining the rurality of participants' residence, participant ethnicity, and the influence of class size and session attendance on health outcomes. Rural residents, Hispanic participants, and participants in smaller size classes with higher attendances showed significant improvements in falls efficacy and physical activity compared to their own counterparts (30, 37, 38).

The extant studies documenting improvements associated with AMOB/VLL typically include a full range of older participants (e.g., all those 65 years and older). Scant research has examined benefits in falls efficacy and physical activities uniquely among oldest-old adults (39). A call has been raised to examine those aged 85 years and older as a separate age group (e.g., a forth age) because of the unique nature and challenges faced by those in this subgroup (40–42). Age-related stereotypes about the benefits of health promotion programs for seniors (43), however, might be a barrier to examining physical activities programs among the oldest-old adults (39). Despite current knowledge of the potential effectiveness of behavioral interventions across the life span (43), few studies have focused specifically on examining the joint influence of falls efficacy and physical activities in the oldest-old population.

The purposes of this study were, therefore, to (a) assess the changes in falls efficacy and physical activity from baseline to post-intervention among oldest-old adults and (b) examine the effect of the interaction between improvement of physical activity from baseline to post-intervention on falls efficacy, with a targeted focus on oldest-old participants. A conceptual model for this study is shown in **Figure 1**. This model depicts the AMOB/VLL falls risk-reduction program as a predictor for changes in physical activity and falls efficacy. In addition, improvement of physical activity acts as a moderator between falls efficacy and falls risk-reduction program.

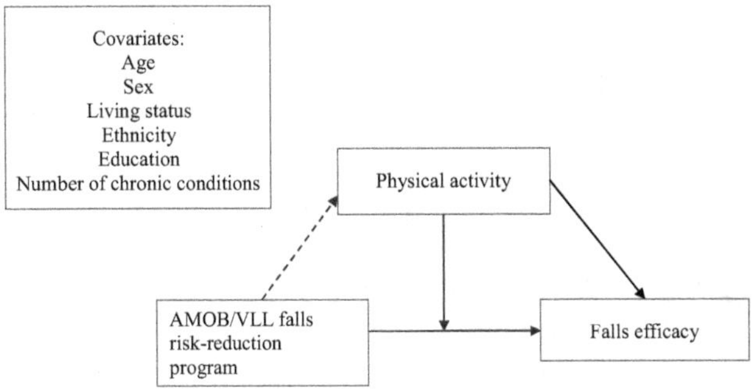

FIGURE 1 | Conceptual model.

MATERIALS AND METHODS

INTERVENTION ELEMENTS

A matter of balance/volunteer lay leader entails a lay leader model and is widely disseminated in the health and aging services sectors (44). The intervention is typically delivered by a pair of trained lay leaders, known as coaches (30, 32, 44). AMOB/VLL was designed to modify fall-related factors, such as behaviors, attitudes, and environmental aspects that increase falling risk among older adults (45). Standardized AMOB/VLL workshops take place at licensed delivery sites and are facilitated by certified coaches to ensure program fidelity (44). As facilitators, these lay leaders use an extensively detailed training manual and two instructional videos (32). The AMOB/VLL intervention consists of eight 2-h sessions either once a week for 8 weeks or twice a week for 4 weeks (30). Early sessions focus on individual behavior and mindsets with an emphasis on decreasing the fear of falling and increasing participants' confidence to prevent falls; later sessions focus on environmental aspects, so leaders assist participants to change their physical surroundings to reduce risk factors for falling and learn exercises to increase balance and strength (30, 46, 47).

Because the intervention processes focus on building fall-related self-efficacy and setting realistic goals for increasing activity, the intervention includes a variety of components, such as lectures, group discussions, mutual problem solving, role-play activities, exercise training, assertiveness training, and home assignments. A standard definition of a "successful" class completion (i.e., attending five or more of the eight sessions) and an ideal class size (i.e., 8–12 older adults) has been established (38).

PARTICIPANTS

As noted in our previous research (31, 37), a total of 3,276 participants enrolled in the Texas AMOB/VLL Falls-Prevention Intervention between September 2007 and April 2009 through local area agencies on aging (AAA) and other community-based organizations. Eighteen AAA regions offered 243 classes during that period. The authors obtained Institutional Review Board (IRB) approval at Texas A&M University to analyze secondary data on program participants and the effectiveness of the program.

PROCEDURES AND INSTRUMENTS

The same instruments were used at baseline and after completion of an intervention. A paper-based questionnaire included 28 items.

The survey items included four different formats (i.e., Likert-type scales, yes/no, closed response, and open ended). Public health and aging research experts who established a common database for evaluation of program effectiveness in a national consortium of studies helped guide the selection of the measures (48). Participants took approximately 15 min to complete the baseline and post-intervention instruments, respectively.

MEASURES

Personal characteristics

Six personal characteristic variables were used: age, sex, race/ethnicity, education, living status, and number of chronic conditions. Age was treated as a continuous variable and was based on a participant's birth date. Sex was scored 1 if the participant is female. Race or ethnicity was scored 0 if the participant is non-Hispanic White, and 1 if non-White. Education was scored 0 if a participant's highest level of education was less than high school graduation, 1 if graduated from high school, and 2 if more than a high school education. Living status was scored 0 if participants lived alone and 1 if they lived with others. The self-reported number of chronic conditions ranged from zero to seven and was considered as a continuous variable.

Falls efficacy scale

Falls efficacy was assessed with the scale developed by Tennstedt et al. (22). The scale consists of five items that measure participants' perceived ability to manage risk of falls or actual falls (22). Participants were asked to rate the following statements: (1) you can find a way to get up if you fall, (2) you can find a way to reduce falls, (3) you can protect yourself if you fall, (4) you can increase your physical strength, and (5) you can become more steady on your feet. Ratings were used with a four-point Likert scale: 1 = not sure at all, 2 = not very sure, 3 = somewhat sure, and 4 = absolutely sure. Cronbach's α was 0.87 for the five items of falls efficacy. Scores ranged from 5 to 20 with higher scores indicating higher levels of managing risk of falls. These falls efficacy scores were collected from participants at baseline and post-intervention.

Physical activity

Physical activity was measured using one item that asked participants to report the number of days they were physically active in the previous 7 days (i.e., scores could range from 0 to 7 days). Participants were given examples of physical activities (e.g., brisk walking, bicycling, vacuuming, gardening, or anything else that causes one to breathe faster); however, the actual physical activities in which the participant engaged were not independently documented. Physical activity was measured at baseline and post-intervention. Furthermore, the change in the number of days from baseline to post-intervention was assessed. Improvement indicates a greater number of days at post-intervention than baseline; no-improvement indicates a same or less number of days at post-intervention when compared with baseline. Based on the change in number of days from baseline to post-intervention, the authors defined two groups for physical activity: improvement (scored 1) and no-improvement (scored 0).

DATA ANALYSIS

Three different analyses were performed. In univariate analyses, frequencies were calculated for personal characteristics, falls efficacy, and physical activity. In bivariate analyses, Pearson's chi-square tests were conducted to examine the goodness of fit for frequency distributions and the independence between categorical participants' characteristics (e.g., sex, living status) (49). Multivariate analyses were also performed to obtain adjusted estimates. SAS (ver. 9.2, 2010) Proc Mixed (50) procedures were used when conducting two repeated measures analysis of covariance (ANCOVA) to calculate the adjusted mean changes in falls efficacy scale scores by physical activity groups (i.e., those who showed improvement vs. those with no-improvement). As far as the measurement of physical activity, many previous studies on the program have showed the intervention effects on physical activities (29–33). When we tested a model including physical activity in this study (not shown in this study), this independent variable showed significant effects on falls efficacy in both age groups after controlling for covariates (i.e., slope $\beta = 0.30$, $p < 0.001$ for oldest-old group; slope $\beta = 0.28$, $p < 0.001$ for young-old group). Assuming significant effects of physical activity on falls efficacy, the physical activity levels were purposively categorized into two groups to see the interaction effect between levels of physical activity (i.e., improvement group vs. no-improvement) and the intervention. In other words, independent variables included time (two time points: baseline and post-intervention) and two levels of physical activity (improvement vs. no-improvement) worked as a moderator. Age, sex, race/ethnicity, education, living status, and number of chronic conditions at baseline were also included as covariates. Many methodological experts of longitudinal studies have advised centering time-varying covariates (51, 52); therefore, we centered age and the number of chronic conditions before conducting advanced analyses. Specifically, we examined whether time (baseline and post-intervention) and two levels of physical activity influence the changes in falls efficacy. In addition, we examined the interaction effect between time (baseline and post-intervention) and physical activity groups (improvement vs. no-improvement) to detect the difference in change of falls efficacy. Covariates and one of the independent variables, time (baseline and post-intervention), were included in the first model. Two levels of physical activity (improvement vs. no-improvement) and interaction term between time (baseline and post-intervention) and physical activity groups were included in the second model.

RESULTS

SAMPLE DESCRIPTION

As shown in **Figure 2**, a total of 3,276 participants enrolled in the Texas AMOB/VLL fall risk-reduction program. About 30% of the total participants ($n = 978$) who were younger than 65 years old were excluded. Among those who met our inclusion criteria ($n = 2{,}298$), 899 participants (39.1%) did not complete post-intervention survey instruments. Only those who completed both baseline and post-intervention assessments ($n = 1{,}399$) were included in this study. Those aged 85 years and older were categorized into the oldest-old group as a target group for this study ($n = 260$); those aged between 65 and 84 years represent young-old group as a comparison age group ($n = 1{,}139$).

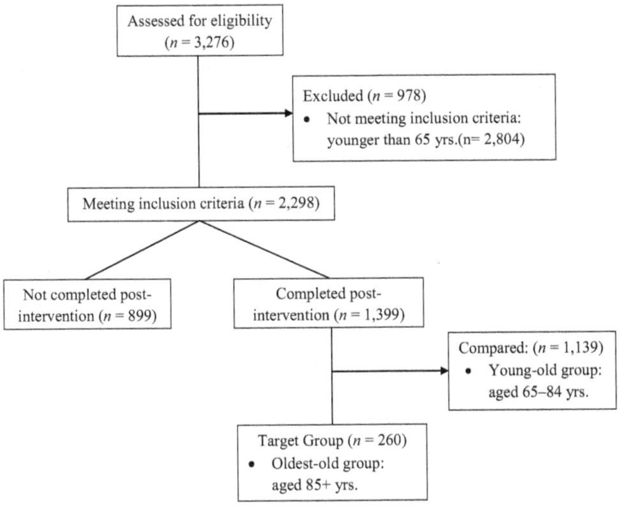

FIGURE 2 | Diagram for participants inclusion. No statistical differences found in sex, age, and the number of chronic conditions. Statistical differences found between those who completed and did not complete post-intervention for African-Americans, Hispanics, and those with less than high school education.

In addition, we examined characteristics associated with program completion. Although no significant differences were apparent by sex, age, or the number of chronic conditions at baseline (not shown in tables), a significant race/ethnicity difference ($p < 0.05$) was identified between those who completed post-intervention (inclusion group; $n = 1,399$) and those who did not complete post-intervention (exclusion group; $n = 899$). African-American participants represented over 25% and Hispanic participants represented 4.6% among those who did not complete the baseline and post-intervention assessment (exclusion group); African-American participants constituted 17.0% and Hispanic participants constituted 7.9% among those who completed the baseline and post-intervention assessment (inclusion group). Furthermore, a significant education difference ($p < 0.05$) occurred. Those who had less than high school graduation constituted 17.6% among those who completed both baseline and post-intervention (inclusion group), but those who had less than high school graduation constituted 26.4% among the exclusion group.

BASELINE CHARACTERISTICS

Table 1 shows study participants' characteristics at baseline for those having both baseline and post-assessment data between oldest-old and young-old group. For the oldest-old group, the mean age was 87.84 (SD = 2.84) years old; 76.4% were female, and 70.2% of the group lived alone. The majority of the group (86.5%) was non-Hispanic White, and about half the group (55.5%) had an education above high school. Over 90% of the group (94.6%) attended five or more workshop sessions. The average number of self-reported chronic conditions was 1.64 (SD = 1.14). Participants in the oldest-old group engaged in physical activities on three or more days on average ($M = 3.55$, SD = 2.56). In addition, their average falls efficacy score was 13.58 (SD = 3.92). For the young-old group, the mean age was 76.43 (SD = 5.24) years old;

Table 1 | Participant characteristics at baseline.

	Oldest-old group (n = 260)	Young-old group (n = 1,139)	F/χ^2
Age[a]	87.84 (±2.84)	76.43 (±5.24)	1,156.67***
Sex			1.59
Male	59 (23.6)	216 (20.0)	
Female	191 (76.4)	863 (80.0)	
Living status			26.53***
Living alone	177 (70.2)	575 (52.4)	
Living with one or more others	75 (29.8)	523 (47.6)	
Ethnicity			21.21***
White not Hispanic	212 (86.5)	775 (72.5)	
African-American	21 (8.6)	202 (18.9)	
Hispanic	12 (4.9)	92 (8.6)	
Education levels			0.21
Less than high school	45 (17.6)	196 (17.6)	
High school graduate	69 (27.0)	285 (25.6)	
More than high school	142 (55.5)	632 (56.8)	
Number of sessions attended			
Less than 5 sessions	14 (5.4)	47 (4.1)	0.78
5–8 sessions	246 (94.6)	1,087 (95.9)	
Number of chronic conditions[a]	1.64 (±1.14)	1.75 (±1.20)	1.58
Ave. days of physically active[a] (0–7)	3.55 (±2.56)	3.46 (±2.29)	0.23
Ave. score of falls efficacy scale[a] (5–20)	13.58 (±3.92)	14.42 (±3.65)	9.37**

[a] *Means (±SD) reported for continuous variables.*
$^{**}p < 0.01$, $^{***}p < 0.001$.

80% were female, and about half of the comparison group (52.4%) lived alone. The majority of the group (72.5%) was non-Hispanic White, and about half the group (56.8%) had an education above high school. Over 90% of the group (95.9%) attended five and more sessions. The average number of chronic conditions was 1.75 (SD = 1.20). Participants in the young-old group engaged in slightly less physical activities ($M = 3.46$, SD = 2.29). Furthermore, the average falls efficacy score of this group was 14.42 (SD = 3.65).

CHANGE IN FALLS EFFICACY

Table 2 presents the results of repeated measures ANCOVA in the oldest-old group and the young-old group. Two models were compared for each group in **Table 2**. For the oldest-old group, time was statistically significant for change of falls efficacy from baseline to post-intervention in Model 1. In other words, the mean scores of falls efficacy scores significantly increased from baseline to post-intervention (slope: $\beta = 1.98$, $p < 0.001$). In addition, improvement of days of physical activities and the interaction term between time (baseline and post-intervention) and physical activities were included in Model 2. Both physical improvement and the interaction term were significant (slopes: $\beta = 1.32$, $p < 0.05$,

Table 2 | Models for changes in falls efficacy among oldest-old group and young-old group.

Predictors	Oldest-old group ($n = 190$)		Young-old group ($n = 1{,}015$)	
	Model 1	**Model 2**	**Model 1**	**Model 2**
Intercept	15.50	14.98	11.96	12.40
Covariates				
Age	−0.17 (0.07)*	−0.16 (0.07)*	−0.01 (0.01)***	−0.07 (0.01)***
Sex (female = 1)	−0.99 (0.51)	−0.93 (0.51)	−0.62 (0.22)**	−0.57 (0.51)*
Living status (living alone = 0)	−0.68 (0.48)	−0.63 (0.49)	0.16 (0.17)	0.19 (0.18)
Ethnicity (White not Hispanic = 1)	−0.78 (0.69)	−0.66 (0.69)	0.24 (0.22)	0.08 (0.24)
Education (less than HS = 1)	0.33 (0.29)	0.29 (0.29)	0.28 (0.12)*	0.34 (0.14)*
Number of chronic condition	−0.25 (0.19)	−0.22 (0.19)	−0.52 (0.07)***	−0.52 (0.08)***
Time (baseline = 0)	1.98 (0.30)***	1.33 (0.39)***	2.03 (0.12)***	1.71 (0.16)***
Improvement of physically active (Improved = 1)		1.32 (0.52)*		1.05 (0.42)*
Time*improvement of physically active		1.43 (0.58)*		0.73 (0.25)**
AIC (Akaike's information criteria)	1818.3	1814.6	9640.2	8359.1

Figures shown in the table are metric coefficients and standard errors (in parentheses).
$^*p < 0.05$, $^{**}p < 0.01$, $^{***}p < 0.001$.

$\beta = 1.43$, $p < 0.05$, respectively). These results indicate that the mean score of falls efficacy in improvement group was higher than in the no-improvement group and mean scores of falls efficacy in both improvement group and no-improvement group at baseline were different from those at post-intervention.

Similar results of changes in falls efficacy were found in the young-old group. Time was statistically significant for change of falls efficacy from baseline to post-intervention in Model 1 (slope: $\beta = 2.03$, $p < 0.001$); both physical improvement and the interaction term were statistically significant (slopes: $\beta = 1.05$, $p < 0.05$, $\beta = 0.73$, $p < 0.01$, respectively) in Model 2.

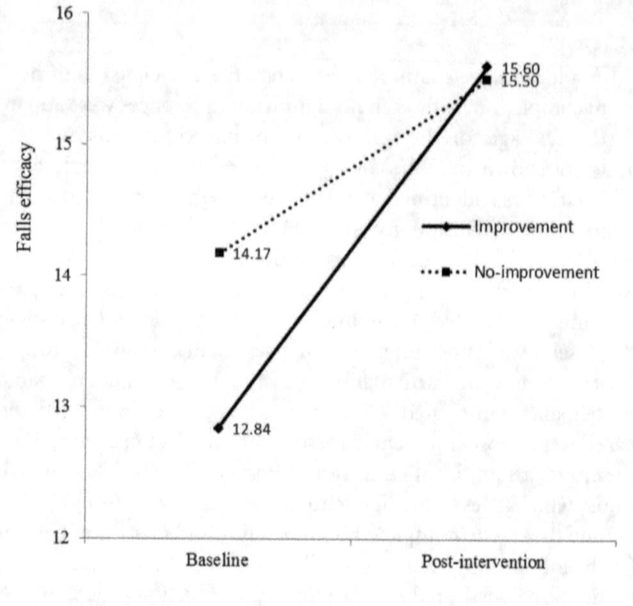

FIGURE 3 | Falls efficacy at baseline and post-intervention by physical activity groups (improvement vs. no-improvement) in oldest-old group.

RELATIONSHIP BETWEEN IMPROVEMENT OF PHYSICAL ACTIVITIES AND FALLS EFFICACY

As shown in Model 2 (**Table 2**), the interaction term between time (baseline and post-intervention) and physical activity had significant effects on falls efficacy in both oldest-old and young-old groups. This indicates mean scores of falls efficacy in both improvement group and no-improvement group at baseline were different from those at post-intervention. To examine interactions, methodologists have advised plotting the figure (53). As shown in **Figure 3** for oldest-old group, the improvement group in physical activity had lower score of falls efficacy at baseline than the no-improvement group, but after they participated in the AMOB/VLL program, their falls efficacy score improved greater than the participants in the no-improvement group. In other words, the improvement in falls efficacy was associated with increased physical activity as well as program participation among oldest-old participants. The young-old group also showed same trends; the improvement group in physical activity had lower score of falls efficacy at baseline, but their score improved greater than the participants in the no-improvement group (**Figure 4**).

DISCUSSION

Many previous studies have assessed falls efficacy and physical activities among participants in the AMOB/VLL program and shown the effectiveness of the program. Most studies, however, did not differentiate oldest-old participants from general old adults. Specification of age group may contribute to a closer look at the effectiveness of evidence-based program in falls efficacy and physical activities. The aim of this study was to examine physical and psychological benefits among oldest-old adults enrolled in the Texas AMOB/VLL falls risk-reduction program. First, this study contributes to understanding of falls efficacy among oldest-old adults by extending the evidence base of the AMOB/VLL falls risk-reduction program. Our findings confirm the increased falls efficacy among oldest-old adults in Texas similar to that reported

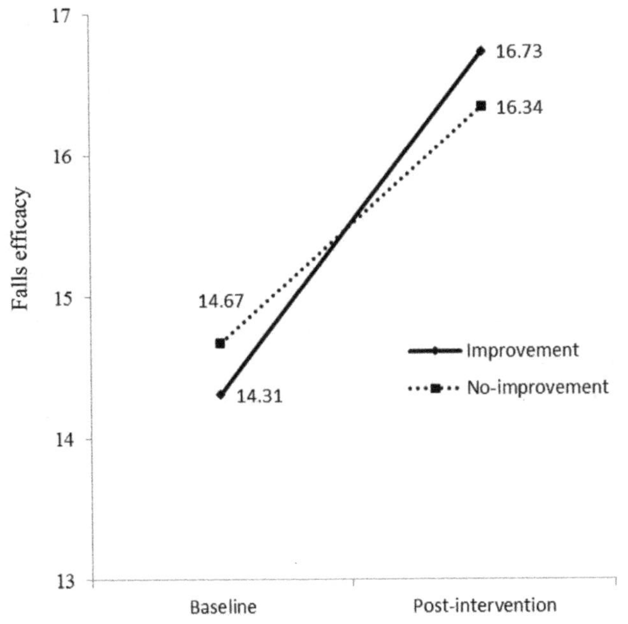

FIGURE 4 | Falls efficacy at baseline and post-intervention by physical activity groups (improvement vs. no-improvement) in young-old group.

previously for the general population of older adults (29, 31, 38, 44) From baseline to post-intervention, oldest-old participants who enrolled in the AMOB/VLL intervention showed significant improvement in falls efficacy as shown in the young-old group. This finding indicates that entry into the program may have a significant effect on changes in confidence of managing falls-related risks from baseline to post-intervention. A few studies showed that the effect of psychological variables is attenuated for those over 75 years old (54, 55). Our results, however, indicate that older adults, especially those aged 85 years and older, can improve their own self-beliefs related to risks of falling through intervention (56, 57).

Second, this study suggests a mechanism for overcoming psychological barriers. Our results suggest that increased physical activities contributed to improving falls efficacy among oldest-old adults enrolled in an evidence-based falls risk-reduction program. From baseline to post-intervention, as noted above, participants showed significant improvement in falls efficacy; however, 44% of participants who enrolled in the intervention showed significant improvement in days of physical activities in the improvement group while 56% of participants indicated decline or same days of physical activities in the no-improvement group. At baseline, the falls efficacy scores of the improvement group ($M = 12.84$, $SD = 4.78$) were lower than those of the no-improvement group ($M = 14.17$, $SD = 4.35$). There was a significant difference between the two falls efficacy scores, $t(306) = 2.57$, $p < 0.01$. This indicates that the AMOB/VLL intervention contributed to differential improvement in the falls efficacy between the two groups. At post-interventions, falls efficacy scores of the improvement group and no-improvement group were 15.60 ($SD = 4.71$) and 15.50 ($SD = 4.18$), respectively. There was no significant difference between the two falls efficacy scores at post-intervention, $t(305) = 0.198$, $p = 0.579$.

This finding provides another significant benefit of evidence-based programs in improving the quality of life among oldest-old population. Most studies related to the effectiveness or benefits of evidence-based program have focused on separate health-related outcomes, such as health behaviors, self-efficacy, or falling or injury rates (29, 58, 59). The results of this study, however, provide critical evidence suggesting that the AMOB/VLL program can positively affect psychological beliefs (i.e., falls efficacy), as well as physical activities among oldest-old participants at the same time. One possible explanation of the synergy/doubled/combined effect of physical and psychological improvement from the falls risk-reduction program may be that oldest-old adults had more barriers for physical activities than younger counterparts. Through a systemic review of physical activity in oldest-old adults, Baert and colleagues (60) have reported many different types of barriers, such as physical impairment (61), weakness of physical strength (62), being too tired (59), fear of injury or pain (63), or the belief that older people cannot change (64). Our oldest-old participants enrolled in the AMOB/VLL intervention may, however, overcome those barriers. In particular, the group that improved their physical activities may enhance ability or strategy of prevention of falls risks and this, in turn, contribute to improve falls efficacy.

LIMITATIONS

Some limitations were related to this study, despite noteworthy findings. First, the study variables collected at baseline and post-intervention were self-reported. We should consider the possibility of recall bias because participants were asked to recall occurrences within the previous week or month (31). Second, the participants in this study were recruited from only one geographic region of the United States (i.e., Texas). Participants from more demographically diverse states of United States or other countries might demonstrate different patterns in the change in falls efficacy. More studies from other states and in diverse settings could contribute to generalization of the results. Third, participants were not randomly assigned into the intervention, nor were a true comparison group included in the study design (i.e., older adults who did not receive the AMOB/VLL intervention). With translational research studies, the main objective is to replicate outcomes previously obtained in more controlled intervention designs across different groups. Hence, such translational studies are often not designed as RCTs (65); nevertheless, our use of a one group design in this study limits our ability to definitively confirm the presence of significant intervention effects between baseline and post-intervention on falls efficacy and physical activity. As such, we recommended that future studies include both intervention and comparison groups to detect true intervention effects (e.g., RCT by specified age groups). Admittedly, self-selection bias may be another limitation for this study because participants chose to enroll in the AMOB/VLL program. However, our findings are similar to those reported in other studies in which no treatment comparison group was used (22, 44).

Fourth, the single item used to measure physical activity asked participants to report the number of days they were physically active in the previous 7 days. We were limited in our ability to perform more complex analyses with this variable or weight specific physical activities. In addition, because this variable simply asks the number of days physically active, not the number of minutes, the ability to detect change is less because the item is not very sensitive to change. Thus, we elected to measure changes in physical activity from baseline to post-intervention as "improved/not improved." We acknowledge that this decision may be influenced by a potential ceiling effect among those who were physically active upon entering the program. This may have accounted for fewer significant improvements in physical activity to be observed at post-intervention. If a more specified scale (e.g., measuring duration such as minutes per activity) or more specific items related to falling (exercise vs. daily living) were used, the effectiveness of fall-reduction programs may become more pronounced. Fifth, 899 participants who did not complete post-intervention assessments were excluded from study analyses. The target group of this study was participants aged 85 years and older; thus, we believe a majority of missing data from participants aged from 65 to 84 years did not strongly impact our intervention findings. Nevertheless, strategies are needed to raise participant retention and assessment response rate, which can reduce a selection bias in future implementation efforts. Sixth, **Figures 3** and **4** show that intervention effects influenced changes in falls efficacy levels differently for physical activity groups, regardless of age groups. Because baseline levels of falls efficacy were substantially lower in the improvement group compared to the no-improvement group, the effect on improvement group participants would be expected to be larger than the no-improvement group participants. Again, a ceiling effect may account for the less change in falls efficacy for the no-improvement group relative to the improvement group. Levels of falls efficacy at post-intervention were similar in both groups. Because, regardless of age, participants in this study showed significant improvements after the intervention, we acknowledge there may be other extraneous effects that were not captured in this study. Future researchers may elect to collect a more encompassing set of measures to assess the complex factors associated with falls efficacy improvement among participants. Finally, only a short-term assessment of this intervention program was conducted (e.g., at 8 weeks post-intervention initiation). The study outcomes may be more robust if participants were studied for 6 months or 1 year (66).

IMPLICATIONS FOR RESEARCH

The findings from this study have considerable implications for future research on aging studies. Most notably, the inclusion of the young-old group in this study emphasizes the magnitude of intervention benefits for the oldest-old population. Although it is expected that younger seniors may benefit from the intervention more than their older counterparts, findings of this study indicate both groups' improvement in physical activity was associated with improvements in falls efficacy. Moreover, oldest-old participants showed larger rate of improvement when compared to the younger-old participants. Future studies should focus on participants aged 85 years and older to examine what characteristics are associated with the effectiveness of evidence-based programs, such as AMOB/VLL. Detailed examination of whether physical activities from the AMOB/VLL could influence cognitive function/mood, remove barriers for physical activities, or improve those with specific conditions, such as dementia, are foci for future research. This study examined an interaction effect between physical activity and time (from baseline to post-intervention) on falls efficacy among oldest-old adults. As a couple of differences between those included and excluded were identified (i.e., education and ethnicity) and additional interaction effects were not investigated in this study, we acknowledge there may have been other factors that influenced program participation and falls efficacy among these participants. More specifically, future studies should explore confounding effects among participant samples with diverse racial/ethnic backgrounds (e.g., African-American, Hispanic) and differing education levels (e.g., 17.6% did not complete high school) to assess their influences on intervention effects.

IMPLICATIONS FOR PRACTITIONERS AND POLICY MAKERS

The results of this study suggest that more practical and policy applications are needed, especially for oldest-old population. Although the oldest-old group (i.e., over 85 years old) will form a large proportion of global population in the next couple of decades (1, 39), few studies have been conducted on the effectiveness of evidence-based programs for oldest-old population compared to younger groups (i.e., younger than 85 years old) (67). In contrast to misconceptions and age-related stereotypes (39), the results of this study suggest that systematic strategies must be employed to develop falls risk-reduction programs for oldest-old adults. We recommend that falls risk-reduction programs be developed or modified, specifically targeting different age groups (e.g., younger than 85 years old vs. 85 years old and over) and different levels of physical activities. This may allow oldest-old adults to gain a more powerful intervention effect and to enhance their physical activities and falls prevention and, in turn, may contribute to reducing medical expenses for falls; furthermore, staff from nursing homes or senior centers as well as health professionals could be trained to develop appropriate ways to make environments more physical activity friendly for oldest-old residents in long-term care facilities.

To summarize, findings from the present study are unique in that they show simultaneous physical and psychological benefits of AMOB/VLL among oldest-old participants. This study re-emphasizes the critical effectiveness of an evidence-based fall risk-reduction program on oldest-old participants by increasing their levels of physical activity and falls efficacy. Identifying characteristics of oldest-old participants who benefit from this intervention has the potential to enhance its effectiveness and inform the development of systematic strategies to encourage enrollment and participation among oldest-old adults.

ACKNOWLEDGMENTS

A matter of balance/voluntary lay leader (AMOB/VLL) is a major program activity in the Aging Texas Well's Texas Healthy Lifestyles Initiative. State-wide implementation is supported by the Department of Aging and Disability Services and administered through the Texas Association of Area Agencies on Aging. The evaluation is conducted by the Texas A&M Health Science Center, School of Public Health. We recognize faculty support from The Center for Community Health Development, which is a member of the

Prevention Research Centers Program, supported by the Centers for Disease Control and Prevention cooperative agreement number 5U48 DP000045. The findings and conclusions in this article are those of the author(s) and do not necessarily represent the official position of Department of Aging and Disability Services or the Centers for Disease Control and Prevention.

REFERENCES

1. Federal Interagency Forum on Aging-Related Statistics. *Older Americans 2010: Key Indicators of Well-Being.* Washington, DC: U.S. Government Printing Office (2010).
2. Zhao J, Barclay S, Farquhar M, Kinmonth AL, Brayne C, Fleming J. The oldest old in the last year of life: population-based findings from Cambridge city over-75s cohort study participants aged 85 and older at death. *J Am Geriatr Soc* (2010) **58**:1–11. doi:10.1111/j.1532-5415.2009.02622.x
3. Edlund BJ, Lufkin SR, Franklin B. Long-term care planning for baby boomers: addressing an uncertain future. *Online J Issues Nurs* (2003) **8**(2):3.
4. Strunk BC, Ginsburg PB, Banker MI. The effect of population aging on future hospital demand. *Health Aff (Millwood)* (2006) **25**:w141–9. doi:10.1377/hlthaff.25.w141
5. Yeaworth RC. Long-term care and insurance. *J Gerontol Nurs* (2002) **28**:45–51. doi:10.3928/0098-9134-20021101-10
6. Boyle PA, Buchman AS, Wilson RS, Bienias JL, Bennett DA. Physical activity is associated with incident disability in community-based older persons. *J Am Geriatr Soc* (2007) **55**:195–201. doi:10.1111/j.1532-5415.2007.01038.x
7. Paterson DH, Warburton DE. Physical activity and functional limitations in older adults: a systematic review related to Canada's physical activity guidelines. *Int J Behav Nutr Phys Act* (2010) **7**:38. doi:10.1186/1479-5868-7-38
8. Fernández-Ballesteros R, Zamarrón MD, Díez-Nicolás J, Lopez-Bravo MD, Molina MA, Schettini R. Mortality and refusal in the longitudinal 90+ project. *Arch Gerontol Geriatr* (2011) **53**:e203–8. doi:10.1016/j.archger.2010.09.007
9. Loland N. Exercise, health, and aging. *J Aging Phys Act* (2004) **12**:170–84.
10. Bijnen FC, Feskens EJ, Caspersen CJ, Mosterd WL, Kromhout D. Age, period, and cohort effects on physical activity among elderly men during 10 years of follow-up: the Zutphen Elderly Study. *J Gerontol A Biol Sci Med Sci* (1998) **53**:M235–41. doi:10.1093/gerona/53A.3.M235
11. von Bonsdorff MB, Rantanen T. Progression of functional limitations in relation to physical activity: a life course approach. *Eur Rev Aging Phys Act* (2011) **8**:23–30. doi:10.1007/s11556-010-0070-9
12. Friedman SM, Munoz B, West SK, Rubin GS, Fried LP. Falls and fear of falling: which comes first? A longitudinal prediction model suggests strategies for primary and secondary prevention. *J Am Geriatr Soc* (2002) **50**:1329–35. doi:10.1046/j.1532-5415.2002.50352.x
13. van Haastregt JC, Zijlstra GA, van Rossum E, van Eijk JT, Kempen GI. Feelings of anxiety and symptoms of depression in community-living older persons who avoid activity for fear of falling. *Am J Geriatr Psychiatry* (2008) **16**(3):186–93. doi:10.1097/JGP.0b013e3181591c1e
14. Tinetti ME, Williams CS. The effect of falls and fall injuries on functioning in community-dwelling older persons. *J Gerontol A Biol Sci Med Sci* (1998) **53**:M112–9. doi:10.1093/gerona/53A.2.M112
15. Rosengren KS, McAuley E, Mihalko SL. Gait adjustments in older adults: activity and efficacy influences. *Psychol Aging* (1998) **13**:375–86. doi:10.1037//0882-7974.13.3.375
16. Tinetti ME, Richman D, Powell L. Falls efficacy as a measure of fear of falling. *J Gerontol* (1990) **45**:239–43. doi:10.1093/geronj/45.6.P239
17. McAuley E, Mihalko SL, Rosengren KS. Self-efficacy and balance correlates of fear of falling in the elderly. *J Phys Act* (1997) **5**:329–40.
18. Kwon MS. Effects of a fall prevention program on physical fitness and psychological functions in community dwelling elders. *J Korean Acad Nurs* (2011) **41**:165–74. doi:10.4040/jkan.2011.41.2.165
19. Li FZ, Fisher KJ, Harmer P, McAuley E. Falls self-efficacy as a mediator of fear of falling in an exercise intervention for older adults. *J Gerontol A Biol Sci Med Sci* (2005) **60**:34–40. doi:10.1093/geronb/53B.1.P43
20. McAuley E, Katula J, Mihalko SL, Blissmer B, Duncan TE, Pena M, et al. Mode of physical activity and self-efficacy in older adults: a latent growth curve analysis. *J Gerontol B Psychol Sci Soc Sci* (1999) **54**:283–92. doi:10.1093/geronb/54B.5.P283
21. Clemson L, Cumming RG, Kendig H, Swann M, Heard R, Taylor K. The effectiveness of a community-based program for reducing the incidence of falls in the elderly: a randomized trial. *J Am Geriatr Soc* (2004) **52**:1487–94. doi:10.1111/j.1532-5415.2004.52411.x
22. Tennstedt S, Howland J, Lachman M, Peterson E, Kasten L, Jette A. A randomized, controlled trial of a group intervention to reduce fear of falling and associated activity restriction in older adults. *J Gerontol B Psychol Sci Soc Sci* (1998) **53**:384–92. doi:10.1093/geronb/53B.6.P384
23. Tennstedt S, Lawrence R, Kasten L. An intervention to reduce fear of falling and enhance activity: who is most likely to benefit? *Educ Gerontol* (2001) **27**:227–40. doi:10.1080/036012701750194969
24. Tinetti ME. Prevention of falls and fall injuries in elderly persons: a research agenda. *Prev Med* (1994) **23**:756–62. doi:10.1006/pmed.1994.1130
25. Tinetti ME. Clinical practice: preventing falls in elderly persons. *N Engl J Med* (2003) **348**:42–9. doi:10.1056/NEJMcp020719
26. Cumming RG, Salkeld G, Thomas M, Szonyi G. Prospective study of the impact of fear of falling on activities of daily living, SF-36 scores, and nursing home admission. *J Gerontol* (2000) **55**:M299–305. doi:10.1093/gerona/55.5.M299
27. Lachman ME, Howland J, Tennstedt S, Jette A, Assmann S, Peterson EW. Fear of falling and activity restriction: the survey of activities and fear of falling in the elderly (SAFE). *J Gerontol B Psychol Sci Soc Sci* (1998) **53**:43–50. doi:10.1093/geronb/53B.1.P43
28. Lachman ME, Weaver SL, Bandura M, Elliott E, Lewkowicz C. Improving memory and control beliefs through cognitive restructuring and self-generated strategies. *J Gerontol* (1992) **47**:293–9. doi:10.1093/geronj/47.5.P293
29. Ory MG, Smith ML, Wade AF, Wright JC, Parrish R. Addressing falls in Texas: evidence-based fall prevention programming for older adults. *Tex Public Health Assoc J* (2010) **62**:15–20.
30. Smith ML, Ahn S, Sharkey JR, Horel S, Mier N, Ory MG. Successful falls prevention programming for older adults in Texas: rural-urban variations. *J Appl Gerontol* (2012) **31**(1):3–27. doi:10.1177/0733464810378407
31. Smith ML, Ory MG, Larsen R. Older women in a state-wide, evidence-based falls prevention program: who enrolls and what benefits are obtained? *Womens Health Issues* (2010) **20**:427–34. doi:10.1016/j.whi.2010.07.003
32. Smith ML, Ory MG, Ahn S, Bazzarre TL, Resnick B. Older adult's participation in a community-based falls prevention exercise program: relationships between the EASY tool, program attendance, and health outcomes. *Gerontologist* (2011) **51**:809–21. doi:10.1093/geront/gnr084
33. Smith ML, Quinn C, Gipson R, Wilson AD, Ory MG. Serving rural communities for falls prevention: the dissemination of *a matter of balance* in the Brazos valley region of Texas. *Tex Public Health Assoc J* (2011) **63**:54–8.
34. Batra A, Melchior M, Seff L, Frederick N, Palmer RC. Evaluation of a community-based falls prevention program in South Florida, 2008–2009. *Prev Chronic Dis* (2012) **9**:110057. doi:10.5888/pcd9.110057
35. Ullmann G, Williams HG, Plass CF. Dissemination of an evidence-based program to reduce fear of falling, South Carolina, 2006–2009. *Prev Chronic Dis* (2012) **9**:110093. doi:10.5888/pcd9.110093
36. Smith ML, Jiang L, Ory MG. Falls efficacy among older adults enrolled in an evidence-based program to reduce fall-related risk: sustainability of individual benefits over time. *Fam Community Health* (2012) **35**(3):256–63. doi:10.1097/FCH.0b013e318250bdb8
37. Smith ML, Ahn S, Mier N, Jiang L, Ory MG. An evidence-based program to reduce fall-related risk among older adults: a comparison of program efficacy by ethnicity. *Californian J Health Promot* (2012) **10**(1):28–44.
38. Smith ML, Hochhalter AK, Cheng Y, Wang S, Ory MG. Programmatic influences on outcomes of an evidence-based falls program for older adults: a translational assessment. *Transl Behav Med* (2011) **1**(3):384–93. doi:10.1007/s13142-011-0058-7
39. Ling CH, Taekema D, de Craen AJ, Gussekloo J, Westendorp RG, Maier AB. Handgrip strength and mortality in the oldest old population: the Leiden 85-plus study. *Can Med Assoc J* (2010) **182**:43. doi:10.1503/cmaj.091278
40. Baltes PB. On the incomplete architecture of human ontogeny: selection, optimization, and compensation as foundation of developmental theory. *Am Psychol* (1997) **52**:366–380. doi:10.1037/0003-066X.52.4.366
41. Baltes PB, Smith J. A systemic-holistic view of psychological functioning in very old age: introduction to a collection of articles from the Berlin aging study. *Psychol Aging* (1997) **12**(3):395–409. doi:10.1037/0882-7974.12.3.395

42. Smith J. Stress and aging: theoretical and empirical challenges for interdisciplinary research. *Neurobiol Aging* (2003) **24**:S77–S80. doi:10.1016/S0197-4580(03)00049-6
43. Ory MG, Hoffman MK, Hawkins M, Sanner B, Mockenhaupt R. Challenging aging stereotypes: strategies for creating a more active society. *Am J Prev Med* (2003) **25**:164–71. doi:10.1016/S0749-3797(03)00181-8
44. Healy TC, Peng C, Haynes MS, McMahon EM, Botler JL, Gross L. The feasibility and effectiveness of translating a matter of balance into a volunteer lay leader model. *J Appl Gerontol* (2008) **27**:34–51. doi:10.1177/0733464807308620
45. Partnership for Healthy Aging. *A Matter of Balance Volunteer Lay Leader Model* (2011). Retrieved from http://www.ncoa.org/improve-health/center-for-healthy-aging/content-library/Matter-of-Balance-6-30-2011.pdf
46. Graafmans WC, Ooms ME, Hofstee HMA, Bezemer PD, Bouter LM, Lips P. Falls in the elderly: a prospective study of risk factors and risk profiles. *Am J Epidemiol* (1996) **143**(11):1129–36. doi:10.1093/oxfordjournals.aje.a008690
47. Stevens JA, Dellinger AM. Motor vehicle and fall related deaths among older Americans 1990-98: sex, race, and ethnic disparities. *Inj Prev* (2002) **8**(4):272–5. doi:10.1136/ip.8.4.272
48. National Council on the Aging. *Conducting Evidence-Based Programs in Senior Centers* (2008). Retrieved from http://www.ncoa.org/improve-health/center-for-healthy-aging/content-library/Conducting_EBPs_in_Senior_Centers-FL8-08.pdf
49. Chernoff H, Lehmann EL. The use of maximum likelihood estimates in x^2 tests for goodness of fit. *Ann Math Stat* (1954) **25**:579–86. doi:10.1214/aoms/1177728726
50. Littell RC, Milliken GA, Stroup WW, Wolfinger RD, Schabenberger O. *SAS for Mixed Models.* 2nd ed. Cary, NC: SAS Institute, Inc (2006).
51. Horney J, Osgood D, Marshall I. Criminal careers in the short-term: intra-individual variability in crime and its relation to local life circumstances. *Am Sociol Rev* (1995) **60**:655–73. doi:10.2307/2096316
52. Raudenbush SW, Bryk AS. *Hierarchical Linear Models: Applications and Data Analysis Methods.* 2nd ed. Thousand Oaks, CA: Sage (2002).
53. Frazier P, Tix A, Barron K. Testing moderator and mediator effects in counseling psychology research. *J Couns Psychol* (2004) **51**:115–34. doi:10.1037/0022-0167.51.1.115
54. Fleming J, Brayne C. Mental and physical factors in relation to falls amongst very old people – prospective follow-up of over 90-year olds in the CC75C study. *Poster Session Presented at the Meeting of the Congress of the International Psychogeriatric Association,* Stockholm (2005).
55. Rapp MA, Gerstorf D, Helmchen H, Smith J. Depression predicts mortality in the young old, but not in the oldest old: results from the Berlin aging study. *Am J Geriatr Psychiatry* (2008) **16**:844–52. doi:10.1097/JGP.0b013e31818254eb
56. Kraaij V, Garnefski N, Maes S. The joint effects of stress, coping and coping resources on depressive symptoms in the elderly. *Anxiety Stress Coping* (2002) **15**:163–77. doi:10.1080/10615800290028468
57. Penrod J, Gueldner S, Poon L. Managing multiple chronic health conditions in everyday life. In: Poon L, Gueldner S, Sprouse B, editors. *Successful Aging and Adaptation with Chronic Diseases.* New York, NY: Springer (2002). p. 181–208.
58. Glasgow RE, Ory MG, Klesges LM, Cifuentes M, Fernald DH, Green LA. Practical and relevant self-report measures of health behaviors for primary care settings. *Ann Fam Med* (2005) **3**:73–81. doi:10.1370/afm.261
59. Wilcox S, Bopp M, Oberrecht L, Kammermann SK, McElmurray CT. Psychosocial and perceived environmental correlates of physical activity in rural and older African American and White women. *J Gerontol B Psychol Sci Soc Sci* (2003) **58**:329–37. doi:10.1093/geronb/58.6.P329
60. Baert V, Gorus E, Mets T, Geerts C, Bautmans I. Motivators and barriers for physical activity in the oldest old: a systematic review. *Aging Res Rev* (2011) **10**:464–74. doi:10.1016/j.arr.2011.04.001
61. Newson RS, Kemps EB. Factors that promote and prevent exercise engagement in older adults. *J Aging Health* (2007) **19**:470–81. doi:10.1177/0898264307300169
62. Forkan R, Pumper B, Smyth N, Wirkkala H, Ciol MA, Shumway-Cook A. Exercise adherence following physical therapy intervention in older adults with impaired balance. *Phys Ther* (2006) **86**:401–10.
63. Heesch KC, Brown DR, Blanton CJ. Perceived barriers to exercise and stage of exercise adoption in older women of different racial/ethnic groups. *Women Health* (2000) **30**:61–76. doi:10.1300/J013v30n04_05
64. Dye CJ, Wilcox S. Beliefs of low-income and rural older women regarding physical activity: you have to want to make your life better. *Women Health* (2006) **43**:115–34. doi:10.1300/J013v43n01_07
65. Wilcox S, Dowda M, Leviton LC, Bartlett-Prescott J, Bazzarre T, Campbell-Voytal K, et al. Active for Life®: results from the translation of two physical activity programs. *Am J Prev Med* (2008) **35**:340–51. doi:10.1016/j.amepre.2008.07.001
66. Müller-Riemenschneider F, Reinhold T, Nocon M, Willich SN. Long-term effectiveness of interventions promoting physical activity: a systemic review. *Prev Med* (2008) **47**:354–68. doi:10.1016/j.ypmed.2008.07.006
67. He W, Muenchrath MN. *U.S. Census Bureau, American Community Survey Reports, ACS-17, 90+ in the United States: 2006–2008.* Washington, DC: U.S. Government Printing Office (2011).

25

Translation of *Fit & Strong!* for middle-aged and older adults: Examining implementation and effectiveness of a lay-led model in Central Texas

Marcia G. Ory [1], Shinduk Lee [1], Alyson Zollinger [1], Kiran Bhurtyal [2], Luohua Jiang [3] and Matthew Lee Smith [4]*

[1] Department of Health Promotion and Community Health Sciences, Texas A&M Health Science Center, School of Public Health, College Station, TX, USA
[2] Office of Surveillance, Evaluation, and Research, Texas Department of State Health Services, Austin, TX, USA
[3] Department of Epidemiology and Biostatistics, Texas A&M Health Science Center, School of Public Health, College Station, TX, USA
[4] Department of Health Promotion and Behavior, College of Public Health, The University of Georgia, Athens, GA, USA

Edited by:
Kerry Stephen Kuehl, Oregon Health & Science University, USA

Reviewed by:
Cheryl Lynn Addy, University of South Carolina, USA
Charles D. Treser, University of Washington School of Public Health, USA

****Correspondence:***
Matthew Lee Smith, Department of Health Promotion and Behavior, College of Public Health, The University of Georgia, 330 River Road, 315 Ramsey Center, Athens, GA 30602, USA
e-mail: health@uga.edu

The *Fit & Strong!* program is an evidence-based, multi-component program promoting physical activity among older adults, particularly those suffering from lower-extremity osteoarthritis. The primary purpose of the study is to examine if the *Fit & Strong!* program translated into a lay-leader model can produce comparable outcomes to the original program taught by physical therapists and/or certified exercise instructors. A single-group, pre–post study design was employed, and data were collected at the baseline ($n = 136$ participants) and the intervention conclusion ($n = 71$) with both baseline and post-intervention data. The measurements included socio-demographic information, health- and behavior-related information, and health-related quality of life. Various statistical tests were used for the program impact analysis and examination of the association between participant characteristics and program completion. As in the original study, there were statistically significant ($p < 0.05$) improvements in self-efficacy for exercise, aerobic capacity, joint stiffness, level of energy, and amount and intensity of physical activities. The odds of completing the program were significantly lower for the participants from rural areas and those having multiple chronic conditions. Successful adaptation of the *Fit & Strong!* program to a lay-leader model can increase the likelihood of program dissemination by broadening the selection pool of instructors and, hence, reducing the potential issue of resource limitation. However, high program attrition rates (54.1%) emphasize the importance of adopting evidence-based strategies for improving the retention of the participants from rural areas and those with multiple chronic conditions.

Keywords: evidence-based program, aging, exercise, implementation research

INTRODUCTION

In recent years, there has been growing interest in evidence-based disease prevention programs that help middle-aged and older adults improve their health and quality of life through self-management strategies. This greater attention has resulted, in part, from an emerging recognition that adults of all ages including older adults can benefit from health promotion programs (1, 2) and a larger appreciation of the value of evidence-based approaches (3–5). Many of these programs incorporate elements to increase physical activity among participants (6–8) because of the importance of mobility for sustained independent living (9, 10). *Fit & Strong!* is an example of one such multi-component physical activity program that combines guided aerobic, strength, and flexibility training with health education (7, 11). Previously tested in a randomized clinical trial, *Fit & Strong!* has demonstrated efficacy to improve participants': (1) self-efficacy (SE), or confidence, for exercise; (2) physical activity adherence; (3) aerobic capacity; and (4) lower-extremity joint pain and stiffness (7, 11).

After a series of successful efficacy trials, the program developers have proactively partnered with multiple agencies to disseminate *Fit & Strong!* to more diverse populations and settings (12). While originally developed for older adults with lower-extremity osteoarthritis, it is now being marketed more broadly as an evidence-based physical activity/behavioral change program that can be delivered to sedentary, older adults through aging services, and public health networks (13, 14).

Despite the potential advantages of widely disseminating *Fit & Strong!* in community settings, some challenges were anticipated in the actual delivery through the aging services network in Central Texas. One identified translational research problem was resource limitation related to the inadequate availability of trained instructors (15, 16). Prior to its translation in Central Texas, eligible instructors for *Fit & Strong!* were limited to physical therapists (PTs) and certified exercise instructors (CEIs) as a means to ensure safety and effectiveness in conducting the program (7, 11, 17). However, this narrow pool of eligible instructors limits possibilities for grand-scale uptake and dissemination. Therefore, in collaboration with the program developers, efforts were taken to modify the instructor criteria and expand the types of instructors deemed appropriate to deliver the *Fit & Strong!* program.

Given the growth of other evidence-based programs delivered using train-the-trainer, lay-leader models through a variety of aging, public health, and health care organizations, questions arose about whether *Fit & Strong!* might similarly be translated to a lay-led model and, thus, broaden the selection pool of instructors and minimize the anticipated resource limitation problem. Of primary concern was whether instructors trained in other evidence-based programs, without exercise training experience, could safely deliver *Fit & Strong!* to seniors with non-specific chronic conditions while maintaining program effectiveness. In response to such questions, this study examined the adaptation of *Fit & Strong!* to a lay-leader model in Central Texas using a quasi-experimental study design. The specific purposes of this study were to: (1) describe the characteristics of participants enrolled in the translated *Fit & Strong!* program; (2) examine factors associated with program attendance; and (3) assess changes in health-related outcomes among participants.

MATERIALS AND METHODS

FIT & STRONG! INTERVENTION

The *Fit & Strong!* program is a multi-component physical activity and behavioral change program that is structured around two key components: (1) participation in group-facilitated (or guided) physical activity; and (2) group-based health education/problem-solving. Over an 8-week period, individuals participate in 24 total sessions, meeting 3 days each week for 90-min each session. Each session begins with 60-min of structured physical activity, which is then followed by a 30-min group-based discussion/problem-solving period (7, 11, 17).

The physical activity component includes: (1) warm-up exercises (5–10 min); (2) low-impact aerobic conditioning (e.g., walking and step aerobics) where participants begin with 10 min of activity and gradually work up to 30 min by the end of the program; (3) strength exercises (primarily lower-extremity) using ankle weights and resistance bands (15–20 min); and (4) cool-down and flexibility exercises (5–10 min) (7, 11, 17). During the group-based discussion/problem-solving component, instructors lead participants in discussions of various health-related topics relying on a program curriculum guide. These interactive sessions are intended to help participants make healthy changes that sustain long-term healthy lifestyle management (e.g., improved arthritis symptom management and physical activity engagement). Toward the end of the program, participants are also encouraged to create an individualized physical activity plan to enable and promote continued physical activity after the 8-week program concludes (7, 11, 17).

ADAPTATION OF THE *FIT & STRONG!* PROGRAM

The proposed adaptation of *Fit & Strong!* in Central Texas involved two modifications: (1) a shift in the required instructor qualification from exercise-experts (i.e., PTs or CEIs) to lay-leaders; and (2) a modification in the training protocol. In response to a shortage of qualified instructors in the targeted communities, especially in the rural sites, program implementers at the Texas A&M Program on Healthy Aging collaborated with the original program developers at the University of Illinois – Chicago to modify the existing qualification requirement for instructors and allow lay individuals to lead *Fit & Strong!* classes. For lay individuals to be qualified to lead *Fit & Strong!* classes, the lay-leaders needed to meet the following criteria: (1) be certified in another evidence-based class (e.g., *A Matter of Balance*, *Chronic Disease Self-Management Program*, or *Diabetes Self-Management Program*) and have experience and comfort leading group classes, if not already a PT or a CEI; (2) participate in the full instructor and supplemental lay-leader trainings conducted by the Master Trainers; and (3) adhere to fidelity standards by following the training manual in conducting the program (18, 19).

Recruitment efforts for lay-leaders consisted of collaboration with community stakeholders who were instrumental in: (1) referring and identifying qualified/capable individuals; and (2) disseminating information (e.g., flyers and emails) about the lay-leader training.

Training for the original *Fit & Strong!* program was conducted by *Fit & Strong!* staff, Master, and T-Trainers (e.g., the most experienced trainers who are able to train and certify Master trainers). Lay individuals as well as CEIs completed the mandatory instructor training, which lasted 8 h (in 1 day) and covered: (1) program background & development; (2) importance of fidelity; (3) roles/responsibilities of instructors in relation to other *Fit & Strong!* team members (e.g., developers); (4) *Fit & Strong!* exercise components (description and demonstration of various types of exercises used throughout the program); (5) *Fit & Strong!* group discussion/problem-solving component (including role plays, facilitator management roles); and (6) data collection, evaluation, and fidelity responsibilities of instructors (18, 19). Lay individuals then completed an additional day of training (half-day, 4 h) tailored to lay-leaders that emphasized basic exercise principles and safety as they applied to the *Fit & Strong!* program.

IMPLEMENTATION AND FIDELITY OF THE TRANSLATED *FIT & STRONG!* PROGRAM

During the implementation of the adapted *Fit & Strong!* program in Central Texas, the Texas A&M *Fit & Strong!* evaluation team along with program developers engaged in best practice quality assurance strategies to assure that the adapted program would be delivered with fidelity (20). This included: (1) fidelity assessments (using a specified fidelity checklist) through observations at the delivery sites; (2) setting up a mechanism for frequent communication with the lay-leaders; and (3) conducting process evaluations of program implementation and participant experiences. The program evaluations assessed participants in terms of: (a) attendance; (b) experiences with the program and instructors; and (c) program impact. Evaluations also included instructors' experiences and assessment of the program (instructor manual, group discussion, and exercise components) as well as the effectiveness of the instructor training. The fidelity assessments and program evaluations provided further guidance and support for instructors in conducting classes more effectively and correctly. These quality assurance strategies helped reinforce adherence to the curricula material presented through the original program manuals.

PROGRAM SETTING AND DELIVERY

Five intervention sites were selected from Central Texas, and 12 different *Fit & Strong!* classes were offered across the various sites from September 2012 through June 2013. Site selection was based on three interrelated criteria: (1) community support for hosting *Fit & Strong!* classes (community "buy-in" was seen as a critical factor for both recruitment and sustainability), (2) facility availability for *Fit & Strong!* classes, and (3) the presence of a sufficient number of older adults who could benefit from *Fit & Strong!* and who were interested in participating in the program. The number of participants in each class ranged from 16 to 25, which roughly paralleled the recommended 20–25 participant maximum ideal (21). Institutional review board approval was obtained at Texas A&M University.

Local senior centers, community centers, and health resource centers served as host agencies for the delivery of the *Fit & Strong!* classes. These host agencies also assisted with program promotion and participant recruitment. For example, a couple of agencies hosted promotional meetings for the program as well as voluntarily conducted on-site program enrollment while coordinating these efforts with Texas A&M program implementers. Many of these agencies expressed appreciation for the offering of a new program at their sites and, thus, were more willing to volunteer their services to assist with promotion and recruitment endeavors.

PARTICIPANTS

Study participants included adults aged 47–94 years who enrolled in *Fit & Strong!* in rural and urban counties in Central Texas between 2012 and 2013. All middle-aged and older adults residing in the area were eligible to enroll in the program; however, only those who had never previously participated in a *Fit & Strong!* class and attended the first or second class session and also completed a baseline survey were included in the study analyses ($n = 136$). As previously mentioned, participants were recruited by host agency members as well as Texas A&M program implementers. Participants were recruited through various sources, including print materials (e.g., program guides, brochures/flyers, and newspaper postings), community resources (e.g., senior clubs/classes and promotional meetings), family or friends (word of mouth), and health care providers. The majority of participants were recruited through print materials (43.4%) and family or friends (28.7%).

MEASURES

Data sources included a baseline survey at the beginning (first and second sessions of each class), a post-test survey at the end of the 8-week program (final week), and an attendance log. Demographic data that was drawn from the baseline survey included age, gender, race/ethnicity, education, marital status, employment status, and annual household income. Several outcome measures were extracted and analyzed based upon these baseline and post-test surveys. Primary outcomes included: (1) SE for exercise and (2) level of physical activity related to aerobic capacity, flexibility, and strength. Secondary outcomes included: (1) self-rated health status; (2) joint pain and stiffness; and (3) level of energy (fatigue). Paralleling assessment protocols being utilized by the original program developers in their program dissemination phase (22), the measurement battery was designed to be administered to older adults in community settings. The surveys were designed to be completed on average in <20 min. Program staff was available during data collection to assist older adults when filling out the forms, as needed.

Self-efficacy for exercise

Self-efficacy for exercise was measured using four items. The items asked how confident participants are in performing different types of exercise (e.g., strength and flexibility), performing vigorous exercises, and performing exercise despite pain or symptoms. Each item is based on a 10-point scale ranging from "not at all confident" (score = 1) to "totally confident" (score = 10). The score for SE for exercise was the mean of the four items. Higher SE scores indicated *higher self-efficacy*. The scale value was set to "missing" if more than one item was missing (23); based on the criteria, seven total *missing* cases were omitted from the analyses. If only one item was missing, the mean of the remaining three items was used. Internal reliability was high for this composite scale (Cronbach's $\alpha = 0.96$).

Aerobic capacity, flexibility, and strength

A slight adaptation of the rapid assessment of physical activity (RAPA) was used to measure the amount and intensity of participants' physical activity (24). The adapted RAPA consisted of eight items, and each item had a "yes" and "no" option. The first six items, which measured the intensity and frequency of physical activity were used to assess *aerobic capacity*.

The six items were: (1) I rarely or never do any physical activity; (2) I do some light or moderate physical activities but not every week; (3) I do some light physical activity every week; (4) I do moderate physical activity every week; (5) I do 30 min or more per day of moderate physical activity, five or more days per week; and (6) I do 20 min or more per day of vigorous physical activities, three or more days per week. Each of the six items reflected a specific level of aerobic capacity. For example, affirmative response to the item "(1)" represents "*sedentary*" and was scored 1; affirmative response to the item "(2)" represents "*under-active*" and was scored 2; affirmative response to the item "(3)" represents "*under-active regular – light activities*" and was scored 3; affirmative response to the item "(4)" represents "*under-active regular*" and was scored 4; and affirmative response to items "(5)" and/or "(6)" represents "*active*" and was scored 5. The highest score among the six items was selected for the aerobic capacity score (25). The remaining two items assessed *strength* and *flexibility*, and affirmative response to each item was scored 1. The strength and flexibility items were summed for descriptive purposes. The summed scale ranged from 0 to 2 (0 = none, 1 = either, and 2 = both).

Self-rated health

A single item was used to assess self-rated health (26), which has been identified as an outstanding predictor of future health (27). This item was a five-point scale with lower values indicating worse *health* (poor = 1) and higher values indicating *better health* (excellent = 5).

Joint pain and stiffness

The Western Ontario and McMasters University Osteoarthritis Index (WOMAC) was used to measure lower-extremity pain and stiffness (28). The adopted WOMAC consisted of seven items: five pain and two stiffness items. All seven items were in a five-point Likert scale structure ranging from "none" (score = 0) to "extreme" (score = 4). Scores for each section were summed to produce composite scales for pain and stiffness. The pain-scale ranged from 0 to 20 with higher values indicating *greater pain*; and the stiffness-scale ranged from 0 to 8 with higher values indicating *greater stiffness.* Internal reliabilities were high for both composite scales (Cronbach's α = 0.89 for pain; 0.86 for stiffness) (29).

Level of energy and fatigue

The level of energy and fatigue was measured using five items (30). Each item was a six-point scale ranging from "none of the time" (score = 0) to "all of the time" (score = 5). Some scores were recoded to have an equal direction of answers among the five items (i.e., higher scores indicate *worse health*). The mean of the five items was used as the composite scale for the level of energy and fatigue. The scale ranged from 0 to 5 with higher values indicating a *lower level of energy* and a *greater level of fatigue.* Internal reliability was high for this composite scale (Cronbach's α = 0.90).

Successful class completion

Attendance was tracked via attendance logs for each session, and the attendance data were used to calculate the attendance and completion rates. "Completion" was defined as attending at least 18 out of the 24 total *Fit & Strong!* sessions per class offering.

RECRUITMENT FLOW

The recruitment flow from initial program enrollment is presented in **Figure 1** as a consort type diagram. This figure begins with all "participant enrollees" and concludes with eligible participants with linked baseline and post-test data who were treated as the analytic sample for outcome analyses. This flow documents reasons for exclusion (e.g., those who took the class previously were not part of the analytical survey) and those lost to follow-up at the end of the program.

A total of 234 participants were enrolled in the program. Among this initial group, 181 (77.4%) individuals were potentially eligible for the outcomes study, 21 (9.0%) individuals did not meet study criteria (e.g., to be considered active, participants needed to attend either the first or second training session), and 32 (13.7%) individuals were repeaters (previous *Fit & Strong!* participants). Among the 181 potentially eligible participants, however, only 136 (75.1%) completed the baseline survey and were, therefore, eligible to be part of the initial participant comparison analyses. Only 71 participants (39.2%) of the 136 eligible participants completed *both* pre and post-test surveys and served as "impact study participants."

DATA ANALYSIS

Characteristics of those who completed both baseline and post-test surveys (matched surveys) were compared to the other participants (non-matched surveys; those who only completed a baseline survey) using χ^2 tests for categorical variables and two-sample t-tests for continuous variables. Next, association between participant characteristics and program completion status for the analytical sample was identified using logistic regression with odd ratios. The impact of *Fit & Strong!* was then evaluated by comparing the outcome measures using various methods (paired-t-test for continuous scales, Wilcoxon Signed Rank Test for ordinal scales, and McNemar test for two-level categorical scales).

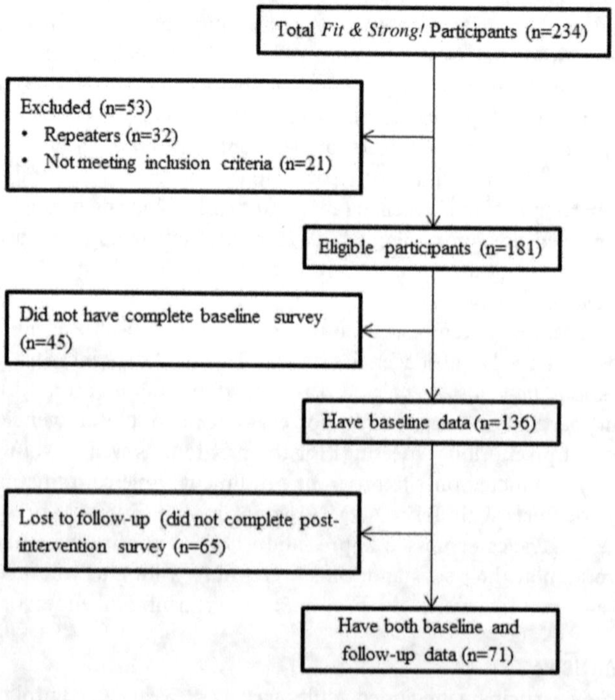

FIGURE 1 | Recruitment flow diagram for *Fit & Strong!* participants.

RESULTS

OBJECTIVE 1: STUDY CHARACTERISTICS

As shown in **Table 1**, the average age of eligible *Fit & Strong!* participants (including all enrollees with baseline surveys) was 73.02 (SD = 9.16) years (49.3% were age 75 and older, and 35.0% were between the ages of 65 and 74). The majority of participants were female (80.2%) and were of non-Hispanic White ethnicity (82.8%). Over 75% had more than a high school degree, and 62.2% were married. Among the four chronic conditions reported (diabetes, hypertension, heart disease, and respiratory problems), hypertension was most frequently reported among the participants (47.3%). Of the 136 eligible participants who completed the baseline survey, 33.8% were from rural counties and 66.2% were from an urban county.

Compared to eligible participants omitted from the impact study because of lack of matched data (completed baseline and post-tests) ($n = 65$), a significantly larger proportion of impact study participants ($n = 71$) were female (87.9 vs. 72.3%, $p = 0.025$). On average, SE at baseline for impact study participants ($p = 0.033$) was significantly higher relative to eligible participants omitted from the impact study; whereas, average self-rated health ($p = 0.028$) at baseline for participants included in the impact study was significantly higher than participants who were not included in the impact study. There were no significant differences by other socio-demographic characteristics and baseline levels of physical activity and illness symptomatology.

OBJECTIVE 2: CLASS COMPLETION

As shown in **Table 1**, the average number of classes attended for all eligible participants who completed baseline surveys was

Table 1 | Baseline characteristics of eligible participants by data availability (i.e., presence of both baseline and post-test surveys).

Baseline characteristics	Categories	Eligible participants with baseline survey ($n=136$)[a]	Eligible participants excluded from the impact study ($n=65$)[b]	Impact study participants ($n=71$)[c]	p-value*
Age	<75	68 (50.7%)	29 (44.6%)	39 (56.5%)	0.168
	≥75	66 (49.3%)	36 (55.4%)	30 (43.5%)	
	Mean (SD)	73.02 (±9.16)	74.25 (±9.82)	71.87 (±8.39)	0.134
Gender	Male	26 (19.8%)	18 (27.7%)	8 (12.1%)	0.025
	Female	105 (80.2%)	47 (72.3%)	58 (87.9%)	
Race/ethnicity	White (not Hispanic origin)	106 (82.8%)	52 (85.2%)	54 (80.6%)	0.486
	Non-White	22 (17.2%)	9 (14.8%)	13 (19.4%)	
Education	≤High school graduate	30 (23.3%)	17 (26.6%)	13 (20.0%)	0.378
	>High school graduate	99 (76.7%)	47 (73.4%)	52 (80.0%)	
Marital status	Married	84 (62.2%)	38 (58.5%)	46 (65.7%)	0.385
	Not married	51 (37.8%)	27 (41.5%)	24 (34.3%)	
Site	Rural	46 (33.8%)	19 (29.2%)	27 (38.0%)	0.279
	Urban	90 (66.2%)	46 (70.8%)	44 (62.0%)	
Reported number of chronic conditions[d]	Mean (SD)[e]	0.83 (±0.82)	0.94 (±0.90)	0.73 (±0.74)	0.168
	Median	1	1	1	
	Mode	0	1	0	
Chronic conditions	Diabetes	18 (13.5%)	11 (17.5%)	7 (10.0%)	0.209
	Hypertension	61 (46.6%)	28 (44.4%)	33 (48.5%)	0.640
	Heart disease	23 (17.3%)	13 (20.6%)	10 (14.3%)	0.334
	Respiratory problems	11 (8.3%)	7 (11.1%)	4 (5.8%)	0.270
Self-efficacy	Mean (SD)[e]	6.95 (±2.44)	6.48 (±2.47)	7.39 (±2.34)	0.033
RAPA (aerobic capacity)	Mean (SD)[e]	3.86 (±1.11)	3.86 (±1.12)	3.85 (±1.11)	0.991
RAPA (strength/flexibility)	None	73 (60.3%)	35 (60.3%)	38 (60.3%)	0.395
	Either	33 (27.3%)	18 (31.0%)	15 (23.8%)	
	Both	15 (12.4%)	5 (8.6%)	10 (15.9%)	
	Strength	22 (18.0%)	8 (13.6%)	14 (22.2%)	0.214
	Flexibility	44 (35.8%)	22 (37.3%)	22 (34.4%)	0.736
Self-rated health	Mean (SD)[e]	3.30 (±0.82)	3.14 (±0.85)	3.45 (±0.78)	0.028
Joint pain	Mean (SD)[e]	4.06 (±3.60)	4.21 (±3.75)	3.90 (±3.48)	0.636
Joint stiffness	Mean (SD)[e]	2.49 (±1.78)	2.59 (±1.86)	2.40 (±1.71)	0.555
Level of energy	Mean (SD)[e]	2.13 (±0.99)	2.18 (±0.98)	2.07 (±1.00)	0.527
***Fit & Strong!* attendance**					
Completion status	Completed	76 (55.9%)	21 (32.3%)	55 (77.5%)	0.000
	Not completed	60 (44.1%)	44 (67.7%)	16 (22.5%)	
Total number of classes attended (MAX = 24)	Mean (SD)[e]	15.96 (±7.16)	11.40 (±7.58)	20.14 (±3.04)	0.000

[a] n = 136 With a slight variation for each variable.

[b] n = 65 With a slight variation for each variable.

[c] n = 71 With a slight variation for each variable.

[d] Chronic conditions: heart diseases, diabetes, hypertension, and respiratory problems.

[e] SD, standard deviation.

**p-value for statistical analyses (i.e., χ^2 or t-tests) for comparing the enrollees with only baseline surveys and the enrollees with both baseline and follow-up surveys. Eligibility criteria for the baseline analysis, or the initial participant comparison analyses, included: (1) attendance of the first or second class sessions, (2) first-time participants (no previous participation in a Fit & Strong! class); and (3) completion of a baseline survey. Eligibility criteria for the impact study analysis included: (1) fulfillment of the aforementioned baseline analysis criteria, and (2) completion of a post-test survey. Participants who fulfilled the baseline analysis criteria and did not complete a post-test survey were excluded from the impact study analysis.*

approximately 16 (SD = 7.16) out of 24. The program completion rate was 55.9% (i.e., attending 18 or more of the 24 sessions). Significant differences were observed when comparing the completion rate and the number of classes attended between the two groups of eligible participants (impact analysis participants vs. non-impact analysis participants). On average, participants in the impact analysis group attended more sessions (average number of sessions attended = 20.14 vs. 11.40, $p < 0.001$) and had higher completion rates (77.5 vs. 32.3%, $p < 0.001$).

As further seen in **Table 2**, there were a few variables that differentiated the participants who did and did not complete the program. Participants from the rural sites were less likely to complete 18 or more classes than the participants from urban sites (OR = 0.41, $p = 0.015$). Those without any chronic conditions were also more likely to complete the program (OR = 2.34, $p = 0.022$); for every increase in number of chronic conditions, the odds of completing the class drops by 46.4%. There were no significant differences by other socio-demographic characteristics or baseline levels of physical activity, general health status, or illness symptomatology.

OBJECTIVE 3: IMPACT OF *FIT & STRONG!*

According to the results illustrated in **Table 3**, in terms of primary outcomes, there were significant improvements in participants' SE for exercise ($p = 0.020$, $d = 0.30$) and aerobic capacity ($p = 0.022$, $d = 0.34$) from baseline to post-test. In terms of the magnitude of improvement at the individual level, there was an 8.1% improvement in SE for exercise and an 11.9% improvement in aerobic capacity. Furthermore, 54.8% of the sample reported an improvement in confidence to exercise and a 29.8% improvement in aerobic capacity. Additionally, there was a shift in the proportion of participants who met the Surgeon General's recommended physical activity guidelines (31). At baseline, 38.7% of the participants were determined to be "active" according to the Surgeon General's guidelines; whereas, by the end of the program, 59.4% of participants were determined to be "active."

In terms of secondary outcomes, there were significant changes observed for joint stiffness, level of energy, and amount and intensity of physical activities related to strength and flexibility ($p < 0.05$). The effect sizes for all secondary outcomes ranged from 0.05 to 0.59. The strongest effect sizes were observed for strength and flexibility scales ($d = 0.59$), then for the level of energy ($d = 0.33$), and then joint stiffness ($d = 0.31$). At the individual participant level, there was a 19.2% improvement in the degree of joint stiffness and an 11.7% improvement in the level of energy. Furthermore, 17.5% of the participants reported improvements in joint stiffness and 27.0% reported improvements in the level of energy. Over one-third of participants reported improvements in the degree of physical activities related to strength. 35.6% reported improvements in the degree of physical activities related to flexibility, and 48.3% reported improvements in the degree of physical activities related to both strength and flexibility.

Table 2 | Comparison of participant baseline characteristics by their program completion status (i.e., attended at least 18 out of 24 sessions).

	n^a	Program completion	
		Odds ratio	p-value[b]
Age	134 (98.5%)	1.008	0.685
Sex (female)	131 (96.3%)	0.433	0.063
Race/ethnicity (non-Hispanic White)	128 (94.1%)	1.562	0.357
Education (>high school graduate)	129 (94.9%)	1.882	0.147
Marital status (married)	135 (99.3%)	1.089	0.812
Site (urban)	136 (100.0%)	0.407	0.015
Reported number of chronic conditions	131 (96.3%)		
Indicative/binary[c] (≥1)		2.337	0.022
Count[d]		0.536	0.006
Baseline self-efficacy	129 (94.9%)	1.113	0.145
Baseline physical activity (aerobic capacity) (active)	118 (86.8%)	0.724	0.400
Baseline physical activity (strength/flexibility)	121 (89.0%)		0.111
None	73 (60.3%)	0.521	0.301
Either	33 (27.3%)	0.268	0.053
Both (ref)	15 (12.4%)		
Baseline self-rated health	134 (98.5%)	1.309	0.213
Baseline joint pain	124 (91.2%)	0.942	0.234
Baseline joint stiffness	128 (94.1%)	0.933	0.488
Baseline level of energy	129 (94.9%)	0.882	0.487

[a] *Number of cases included in the analysis (maximum possible n = 136).*
[b] *p-value from bivariate logistic regression model.*
[c] *Reported number of chronic conditions (0 = no chronic conditions; 1 = at least one chronic condition).*
[d] *Reported number of chronic conditions (count variable ranging from 0 to 4).*

DISCUSSION

As with many evidence-based programs, the randomized trials often use a higher level of interventionists to provide a best case scenario (32, 33). Alternatively, translated models frequently use lay-leaders to expand dissemination efforts while minimizing costs (34, 35). The same is true of the original *Fit & Strong!* program, which originally used PTs or CEIs as class instructors as a means of minimizing harm to participants (7, 17).

The current study examined a lay-leader model of the *Fit & Strong!* program adapted to overcome common challenges to program implementation such as instructor availability (15, 16). Consistent with other findings showing successful applicability of lay-leaders with a variety of physical activity programs in diverse settings (34, 36–38), we saw many positive outcomes and recommend the implementation of a lay-led model. Our program fidelity observations (data not reported here) indicated that group facilitators with more experience in evidence-based programing tended to adhere more closely to program guidelines than instructors with no or limited prior experience adhering to scripted programs.

Our study resonates with previous literature that shows the value of lay-led programs for seniors, especially those with arthritis, which was the original target group for *Fit & Strong!* classes. Cohen et al. (39) compared a lay-led arthritis self-management course and professional-led arthritis self-management course and identified no significant differences for participant outcomes by leader type (although, it should be noted that the courses compared differed slightly in course content). Similarly, Lorig et al. (40) compared a lay-led and a professional-led arthritis

Table 3 | Baseline and post-test comparisons for assessing the impact of *Fit & Strong!* program.

Outcome	n[a]	Mean (SD)[b]		p-value	Effect size[c]	Improvement (%)	Percentage of improved participants (%)
		Pretest	Post-test				
Primary outcomes							
Self-efficacy for adherence to exercise	62 (87.3%)	7.40 (±2.28)	8.00 (±1.99)	0.020	0.30	8.1	54.8
Aerobic physical activity level[d]	57 (80.3%)	3.85 (±1.11)	4.31 (±1.02)	0.022	0.34	11.9	29.8
Secondary outcomes							
Self-rated health[d]		3.45 (±0.78)	3.49 (±0.73)	0.491	0.08	1.2	11.6
Weight	62 (87.3%)	172.02 (±33.87)	168.66 (±36.64)	0.056	0.25	2.0	14.5
Joint pain	62 (87.3%)	3.89 (±3.50)	3.73 (±3.62)	0.714	0.05	4.1	35.5
Joint stiffness	63 (88.7%)	2.38 (±1.73)	1.94 (±1.48)	0.017	0.31	18.7	17.5
Level of energy	63 (88.7%)	2.06 (±0.98)	1.82 (±0.94)	0.010	0.33	11.9	27.0
Strength[e]	59 (83.1%)	14 (22.2%)[f]	34 (52.3%)[f]	0.002			33.9
Flexibility[e]	59 (83.1%)	22 (34.4%)[f]	42 (65.6%)[f]	0.001			35.6
Strength and flexibility[d]	58 (81.7%)	0.56 (±0.76)	1.19 (±0.85)	0.000	0.59		48.3

[a] *Number of cases included in the analysis (maximum possible n = 71).*
[b] *Mean and standard deviation (SD), unless otherwise indicated.*
[c] *Cohen's d [effect sizes of d ≈ 0.2 (small), d ≈ 0.5 (medium), and d ≥ 0.8 (large)].*
[d] *Wilcoxon's paired sign rank test was used.*
[e] *McNemar test was used (No t-statistic).*
[f] *Frequency and valid percentages.*

self-management course, and both courses showed a significant increase in participant knowledge. Participants in the professional-led courses showed a greater gain in knowledge than those in the lay-led courses; however, participants from the lay-led model showed greater improvement in relaxation practice and higher attendance rates (40). These studies utilizing lay-leaders for physical activity programs confirm the feasibility of using a lay-leader model for increasing the availability and adoption of the *Fit & Strong!* program.

The completion rate for those in the impact study (77.5%) was comparable with that found in other research studies using different time-bound evidence-based programs (41). It is not surprising that those in rural areas vs. those in more urban areas were less likely to complete the program given the previously documented challenges to bringing health services or health promotion programs to rural areas (42, 43). Additionally, the fact that those with one or more comorbidities were less likely to complete classes can be attributed to the challenges reported by those facing multiple chronic conditions (44); although, more research is needed to understand how different conditions might affect completion rates. These findings suggest that additional efforts are needed to attract and retain participants from rural areas and those with multiple chronic conditions.

The current study also examined the impact of lay-led *Fit & Strong!* classes on various outcome measures. Participants showed a significant improvement in their aerobic capacity, joint stiffness, level of energy/fatigue, and SE for exercise. Participants also reported greater participation in exercise types (flexibility, strength, or both) such that more individuals met the Surgeon General's recommendations of including exercises targeting flexibility and strength training. These findings are consistent with those of Hughes and colleagues (7, 11), who reported *Fit & Strong!* participant improvement for exercise efficacy, exercise adherence, joint stiffness, physical functioning, and exercise capacity. Hughes reported a 15.6% reduction in participants' stiffness scores at post-test (7), which is consistent with the 19.2% reduction in stiffness scores for participants in the current study. Other measure comparisons could not be made because the current study used different outcome measures than those used by Hughes.

STUDY LIMITATIONS

There are several limitations to this pilot study that should be noted but are acceptable considering this was the initial investigation of a translated intervention. A major limitation for the generalizability of study findings is the small sample size for the final impact study. Additionally, compared to the original *Fit & Strong!* studies (7, 11), there was a relatively high attrition rate (47.9%) from pre to post-test, as commonly found in more community-oriented exercise programs (45). As documented by local program administrators, this high attrition rate was attributed to "loose program adherence/commitment" as some participants preferred "dropping into classes" (i.e., attend at their leisure) as opposed to fully committing to the 8-week program. Others, especially in the rural areas, had limited transportation and, therefore, had difficulties with program attendance. In the current study, we assessed outcomes only for those with complete data, and thus were not able to assess whether those who lacked complete data might have biased study results. However, when we compared the baseline characteristics of the eligible participants included and excluded from the impact analysis, we only found a few significant differences between those two groups, indicating the potential similarity of the two groups.

This study only included a post-test that was administered during the last week of the program. No follow-up assessments were administered after the last session. The lack of follow-up measurements after the program limited our ability to observe any potential long-term effects of utilizing the lay-led *Fit & Strong!* program. However, this study enabled the primary question to be addressed regarding applicability to a broader population of older adults and also the potential value of a lay-led approach for this program in other communities.

Other study limitations can be attributed to program design and evaluation issues. The participants were self-selected into the program from different delivery sites, creating a potential self-selection, or delivery site bias. Also, participants included in the impact analysis had higher SE and self-rated health than those who were not included in the impact analysis, potentially influencing the program impact analysis. This is not surprising given the literature to date suggesting that older adults with better health are more likely to attend and complete a health promotion program (46–48). Such relationships pose a potential intervention bias, which must be considered when interpreting study results.

Finally, participants from this study differed somewhat from participants for which the program was originally intended. Older adults in various physical capacities, including those who were more sedentary or suffered from "achy joints" were recruited for this iteration. In contrast, participants in the original randomized control trials were originally selected based upon the presence of lower-extremity joint stiffness and pain associated with osteoarthritis and related symptomatology. Consequently, it is not possible to do a direct comparison with the earlier studies by Hughes and colleagues (7, 11, 17) since the extent to which participants in the current study had arthritis and specifically osteoarthritis is unknown. Thus, outcomes for arthritis-related symptomatology may have been attenuated in this more generalized study population.

PROGRAM IMPLICATIONS AND FUTURE RESEARCH DIRECTIONS

An important implication of the study is that the *Fit & Strong!* program may benefit the general older adult population and not just those with lower-extremity osteoarthritis. This may be because a substantial proportion of older adults experience some type of joint pain and/or stiffness, not just specifically in the lower-extremity (49) Furthermore, as indicated from program facilitators, *Fit & Strong!* can benefit sedentary older adults who want a beginning level and less intimidating means to start a physical activity regiment. Thus, this program has universal benefits.

Although it is impossible to draw a definitive conclusion, these findings strongly suggest that the *Fit & Strong!* program can be instructed by lay-leaders with standardized training and continued support from the developers and/or on-site Master Trainers. This is important because the training provides lay-leaders (i.e., those without formal exercise or professional training) with guided instruction and ongoing feedback related to program administration as well as proper techniques for exercise progression. These modifications are essential for conducting the program and are seen as critical in allowing the *Fit & Strong!* program to be disseminated more broadly as a lay-led model.

There is now a growing literature on factors affecting recruitment and strategies for boosting program retention (50). Given the reported attrition levels in attendance from entry into the study till class completion, efforts to retain participants from start to finish should focus on committing and motivating participants to fully complete the program. This is often accomplished during enrollment of participants or during the first session, or orientation, of the program (51). Furthermore, instructors should emphasize to participants early on the benefits gained from full participation and should strive to interact and engage participants during sessions and outside of class where necessary (e.g., follow-up phone calls if a participant misses a class).

This pilot study also highlights the need for additional research. Future research should compare lay-led and professional-led *Fit & Strong!* classes in terms of the magnitude of program impact and program fidelity. Also, lay-led *Fit & Strong!* classes should be evaluated/assessed in other settings to draw a more generalizable conclusion about the utility and effectiveness of varying levels of instructor expertise and training components.

CONCLUSION

Overall, utilizing a lay-led model was successfully adapted from the original *Fit & Strong!* program that relied on professional and experienced leaders (PTs and CEIs). The lay-led *Fit & Strong!* model produced outcomes that are consistent with the previous findings from the original intervention. Specifically, the program showed improvement in participants' SE for exercise, aerobic capacity, engagement in strength, and flexibility exercises, while increasing energy levels and decreasing joint stiffness. The magnitude of program attrition in community-based exercise programs can be large; hence, creative strategies are needed to boost participant retention throughout the entire intervention period.

ACKNOWLEDGMENTS

We acknowledge support of Baylor Scott and White HealthCare, St. Joseph's HealthCare System, and Brazos Valley Area Aging on Aging and are appreciative of the delivery sites and older adults who made this translational research possible. We extend special thanks to Doris Howell, Rachel Foster, and Cindy Quinn who assisted in training.

REFERENCES

1. Ory MG, Resnick B, Smith ML. Changing behavior throughout the life-course: translating the success of aging research. *Trans Behav Med* (2012) **2**(2):159–62. doi:10.1007/s13142-012-0129-4
2. Ory MG, Ahn S, Smith ML, Jiang L, Lorig K, Whitelaw N. National study of chronic disease self-management: age comparison of outcome findings. *Health Educ Behav* (2014) **41**(1 Suppl):34s–42s. doi:10.1177/1090198114543008
3. Jacobs JA, Jones E, Gabella BA, Spring B, Brownson RC. Tools for implementing an evidence-based approach in public health practice. *Prev Chronic Dis* (2012) **9**:110324. doi:10.5888/pcd9.110324
4. Task Force on Community Preventive Services. *Preventive Services: What Works to Promote Health?*. New York, NY: Oxford University Press (2005). 36 p.
5. Brownson RC, Fielding JE, Maylahn CM. Evidence-based public health: a fundamental concept for public health practice. *Annu Rev Public Health* (2009) **30**:175–201. doi:10.1146/annurev.publhealth.031308.100134
6. de Jong ORW, Hopman-Rock M, Tak ECMP, Klazinga NS. An implementation study of two evidence-based exercise and health education programmes

for older adults with osteoarthritis of the knee and hip. *Health Educ Res* (2004) **19**(3):316–25. doi:10.1093/her/cyg028

7. Hughes SL, Seymour RB, Campbell R, Pollak N, Huber G, Sharma L. Impact of the Fit & Strong intervention on older adults with osteoarthritis. *Gerontologist* (2004) **44**(2):217–28. doi:10.1093/geront/44.2.217
8. King AC, Baumann K, O'Sullivan P, Wilcox S, Castro C. Effects of moderate-intensity exercise on physiological, behavioral, and emotional responses to family caregiving: a randomized trial. *J Gerontol A Biol Sci* (2002) **57**(1):M26–36. doi:10.1093/gerona/57.1.M26
9. Thibaud M, Bloch F, Tournoux-Facon C, Breque C, Rigaud AS, Dugue B, et al. Impact of physical activity and sedentary behavior on fall risks in older people: a systematic review and meta-analysis of observational studies. *Eur Rev Aging Phys Activ* (2012) **9**(1):5–15. doi:10.1007/s11556-011-0081-1
10. Landi F, Abbatecola AM, Provinciali M, Corsonello A, Bustacchini S, Manigrasso L, et al. Moving against frailty: does physical activity matter? *Biogerontology* (2010) **11**(5):537–45. doi:10.1007/s10522-010-9296-1
11. Hughes SL, Seymour RB, Campbell RT, Huber G, Pollak N, Sharma L, et al. Long-term impact of Fit & Strong! on older adults with osteoarthritis. *Gerontologist* (2006) **46**(6):807–14. doi:10.1093/geront/46.6.801
12. Hughes SL, Seymour R, Cheryl D, Desai P. *Translation of Fit and Strong!: Focus Group Findings from Providers and Instructors in Two States. 61st* Annual Scientific Meeting; Maryland (US). UK: The Gerontologist (2008). 509 p.
13. Center for Healthy Aging, National Council on Aging. *Title III-D Highest Tier Evidence-Based Disease Prevention & Health Promotion Programs Chart.* (2014). 32 p. Available from: http://www.ncoa.org/improve-health/center-for-healthy-aging/content-library/Title-IIID-Highest-Tier-Evidence-FINAL.pdf
14. Centers for Disease Control and Prevention. *Arthritis: Physical Activity Program.* (2011). Available from: http://www.cdc.gov/arthritis/interventions/physical_activity.htm
15. DerAnanian CA, Desai P, Smith-Ray R, Seymour RB, Hughes SL. Perceived versus actual factors associated with adoption and maintenance of an evidence-based physical activity program. *Trans Behav Med* (2012) **2**(2):209–17. doi:10.1007/s13142-012-0131-x
16. Brownson RC, Ballew P, Dieffenderfer B, Haire-Joshu D, Heath GW, Kreuter MW, et al. Evidence-based interventions to promote physical activity: what contributes to dissemination by state health departments. *Am J Prev Med* (2007) **33**(1S):S66–78. doi:10.1016/j.amepre.2007.03.011
17. Seymour RB, Hughes SL, Campbell RT, Huber GM, Desai P. Comparison of two methods of conducting the Fit and Strong! program. *Arthritis Rheum* (2009) **61**(7):879–84. doi:10.1002/art.24517
18. Hughes S, Seymour R, Huber G, Desai P, Der Ananian C, Kunkel C. *Fit & Strong! Instructor Manual 4th* Version [Booklet]. Chicago, IL: Center for Research on Health and Aging, University of Illinois at Chicago (2009).
19. Hughes S, Huber G, Desai P, Smith-Ray R, Heide D. *Fit & Strong! Instructor Training [Booklet].* Chicago, IL: Center for Research on Health and Aging, University of Illinois at Chicago (2012).
20. Center for Healthy Aging, National Council on Aging. *Module 4: Assuring Program Quality: Fidelity.* (2014). Available from: http://www.ncoa.org/improve-health/center-for-healthy-aging/online-training-modules/module-4-assuring-program.html
21. Institute for Health Research and Policy, School of Public Health, University of Illinois at Chicago. *Resource Requirements.* (2014). Available from: http://www.fitandstrong.org/providers/resource_requirements.html
22. Hughes S, Smith-Ray RL, Shah A, Huber G. Translating Fit and Strong!: Lessons learned and next steps. *Front Public Health* (2015) **2**:131. doi:10.3389/fpubh.2014.00131
23. Stanford Patient Education Research Center. *Chronic Disease Self-Efficacy Scales.* (2014). Available from: http://patienteducation.stanford.edu/research/secd32.html
24. Topolski TD, LoGerfo J, Patrick DL, Williams B, Walwick J, Patrick MB. The rapid assessment of physical activity (RAPA) among older adults. *Prev Chronic Dis* (2006) **3**(4):A118.
25. University of Washington Health Promotion Research Center. *How Physically Active are You? – An Assessment of Level and Intensity of Physical Activity.* (2014). Available from: http://depts.washington.edu/hprc/docs/rapa_03_06.pdf
26. Centers for Disease Control and Prevention. *CDC HRQOL-14 "Healthy Days Measure".* (2011). Available from: http://www.cdc.gov/hrqol/hrqol14_measure.htm#1
27. Stanford Patient Education Research Center, Stanford University School of Medicine. *Chronic Disease Self-Management Program Questionnaire Code Book.* Palo Alto, CA: Stanford University (2007). Available from: http://patienteducation.stanford.edu/research/cdCodeBook.pdf
28. Ackerman I. Western Ontario and McMaster Universities Osteoarthritis index (WOMAC). *Aust J Physiother* (2009) **55**(3):213. doi:10.1016/S0004-9514(09)70088-1
29. Olsen IC, Kvien TK, Uhlig T. Consequences of handling missing data for treatment response in osteoarthritis: a simulation study. *Osteoarthritis Cartilage.* (2012) **20**(8):822–8. doi:10.1016/j.joca.2012.03.005
30. Stanford Patient Education Research Center. *Energy/Fatigue.* Palo Alto, CA (2014). Available from: http://patienteducation.stanford.edu/research/energyfatigue.pdf
31. US Department of Health and Human Services. *2008 Physical Activity Guidelines for Americans.* ODPHP Publication No. U0036 (2008). 76 p. Available from: http://www.health.gov/paguidelines/pdf/paguide.pdf
32. Tennstedt S, Howland J, Lachman M, Peterson E, Kasten L, Jette A. A randomized, controlled trial of a group intervention to reduce fear of falling and associated activity restriction in older adults. *J Gerontol B Psychol Sci Soc Sci* (1998) **53B**(6):384–92. doi:10.1093/geronb/53B.6.P384
33. Clemson L, Cumming RG, Kendig H, Swann M, Heard R, Taylor K. The effectiveness of a community-based program for reducing the incidence of falls in the elderly: a randomized trial. *J Am Geriatr Soc* (2004) **52**(9):1487–94. doi:10.1111/j.1532-5415.2004.52411.x
34. Healy TC, Peng C, Haynes MS, McMahon EM, Botler JL, Gross L. The feasibility and effectiveness of translating a matter of balance into a volunteer lay leader model. *J Appl Gerontol* (2008) **27**(1):34–51. doi:10.1177/0733464807308620
35. Clemson L, Swann M, Mahoney J. *Stepping On: Building Confidence and Reducing Falls in Older Adults.* 3rd ed. Cedar Falls, IA: Freiburg Press Inc (2011).
36. Etkin CD, Prohaska TR, Harris BA, Latham N, Jette A. Feasibility of implementing the strong for life program in community setting. *Gerontologist* (2006) **46**(2):284–92. doi:10.1093/geront/46.2.284
37. Krukowki RA, Lensing S, Love S, Prewitt TE, Adams B, Cornell CE, et al. Training of lay health educators to implement an evidence-based behavioral weight loss intervention in rural senior centers. *Gerontologist* (2013) **53**(1):162–71. doi:10.1093/geront/gns094
38. Werner D, Teufel J, Brown SL. Evaluation of a peer-led, low-intensity physical activity program for older adults. *Am J Health Educ* (2014) **45**(3):133–41. doi:10.1080/19325037.2014.893851
39. Cohen JL, Sauter SH, DeVellis RF, DeVellis BM. Evaluation of arthritis self-management courses led by laypersons and by professionals. *Arthritis Rheum* (1986) **29**(3):388–93. doi:10.1002/art.1780290312
40. Lorig K, Feigenbaum P, Regan C, Ung E, Chastain R, Holman HR. A comparison of lay-taught and professional-taught arthritis self-management courses. *J Rheumatol* (1986) **13**(4):763–7.
41. Woodcock C, Korda H, Erdem E, Pedersen S, Kloc M, Tollefson E. *Administration on aging: Chronic Disease Self-Management Program (CDSMP) Process Evaluation.* Report No.: HHSP233201100492G (2013). 142 p. Available from: http://www.aoa.gov/aoaroot/Program_Results/docs/CDSMPProcessEvaluationReportFINAL062713.pdf
42. DiBartolo MC, McCrone S. Recruitment of rural community-dwelling older adults: barriers, challenges, and strategies. *Aging Ment Health* (2003) **7**(2):75–82. doi:10.1080/1360786031000072295
43. Morgan LL, Fahs PS, Klesh J. Barriers to research participation identified by rural people. *J Agric Saf Health* (2005) **11**(4):407–14. doi:10.13031/2013.19719
44. US Department of Health and Human Services. *US Department of Health and Human Services Inventory of Programs, Activities, and Initiatives Focused on Improving the Health of Individuals with Multiple Chronic Conditions (MCC).* Washington, DC: U.S. Department of Health and Human Services Interagency Workgroup on Multiple Chronic Conditions (2011). 103 p. Available from: http://www.hhs.gov/ash/initiatives/mcc/mcc-inventory-20111018.pdf
45. Dishman R, Sallis J. Determinants and interventions for physical activity and exercise. In: Bouchard C, Shepard R, Stephens T editors. *Physical Activity, Fitness and Health: International Preceding and Consensus Statement.* Champaign, IL: Human Kinetics (1994). p. 214–38.
46. Flegal KE, Kishiyama S, Zajdel D, Haas M, Oken BS. Adherence to yoga and exercise interventions in a 6-month clinical trial. *BMC Complement Altern Med* (2007) **7**:37. doi:10.1186/1472-6882-7-37

47. Dattalo M, Giovannetti ER, Scharfstein D, Boult C, Wegener S, Wolff JL, et al. Who participates in Chronic Disease Self-management (CDSM) programs? Differences between participants and nonparticipants in a population of multimorbid older adults. *Med Care* (2012) **50**(12):1071–5. doi:10.1097/MLR.0b013e318268abe7
48. Biedenweg K, Meischke H, Hammerback K, Williams B, Poe P, Phelan EA. Understanding older adults' motivators and barriers to participating in organized programs supporting exercise behaviors. *J Prim Prev* (2014) **35**(1):1–11. doi:10.1007/s10935-013-0331-2
49. Centers for Disease Prevention and Control. Prevalence of doctor-diagnosed arthritis and arthritis-attributable activity limitation – United States, 2007 – 2009. *MMWR Morb Mortal Wkly Rep* (2010) **59**(39):1261–5. Available from: http://www.cdc.gov/mmwr/pdf/wk/mm5939.pdf
50. Ory MG, Lipman PD, Karlen PL, Gerety MB, Stevens VJ, Singh MAF, et al. Recruitment of older participants in frailty/injury prevention studies. *Prev Sci* (2002) **3**(1):1–21. doi:10.1023/A:1014610325059
51. Jiang L, Smith ML, Chen S, Ahn S, Kulinski KP, Lorig K, et al. The role of Session Zero in successful completion of Chronic Disease Self-Management Program workshops. *Front Public Health* (2015) **2**:205. doi:10.3389/fpubh.2014.00205

Development and evaluation of a fidelity instrument for PEARLS

Laura Farren[1], Mark Snowden[2]*, Lesley Steinman[1] and Maria Monroe-DeVita[3]

[1] Health Promotion Research Center, University of Washington, Seattle, WA, USA
[2] Department of Psychiatry and Behavioral Sciences, Harborview Medical Center, University of Washington, Seattle, WA, USA
[3] Division of Public Behavioral Health and Justice Policy, Department of Psychiatry and Behavioral Sciences, University of Washington, Seattle, WA, USA

Edited by:
Matthew Lee Smith, The University of Georgia, USA

Reviewed by:
Rosemary M. Caron, University of New Hampshire, USA
Samuel D. Towne, University of South Carolina, USA

***Correspondence:**
Mark Snowden, Harborview Medical Center, 325 Ninth Avenue, Room PS-5020, Box 359911, Seattle, WA 98104, USA
e-mail: snowden@uw.edu

Purpose: This manuscript describes the development and the preliminary evaluation of a fidelity instrument for the Program for Encouraging Active and Rewarding Lives (PEARLS), an evidence-based depression care management (DCM) program. The objective of the study was to find an effective, practical, multidimensional approach to measure fidelity of PEARLS programs to the original, research-driven PEARLS protocol in order to inform program implementation at various settings nationwide.

Methods: We conducted key informant interviews with PEARLS stakeholders, and held focus groups with former PEARLS clients, to identify core program components. These components were then ranked using a Q-sort process, and incorporated into a brief instrument. We tested the instrument at two time points with PEARLS counselors, other DCM program counselors, and non-DCM program counselors ($n = 56$) in six states. Known-groups method was used to compare findings from PEARLS programs, other DCM programs, and non-DCM programs. We asked supervisors of the counselors to complete the fidelity instrument on behalf of their counselors to affirm the validity of the results. We examined the association of PEARLS program fidelity with individual client outcomes.

Results: Program for Encouraging Active and Rewarding Lives providers reported the highest fidelity scores compared to DCM program providers and non-DCM program providers. The sample size was too small to yield significant results on the comparison between counselor experience and fidelity. Scores varied between PEARLS counselors and their supervisors. PEARLS program fidelity was not significantly correlated with client outcomes, suggesting that other implementation factors may have influenced the outcomes and/or that the instrument needs refinement.

Conclusion: Our findings suggest that providers may be able to use the instrument to assess PEARLS program fidelity in various settings across the country. However, more rigorous research is needed to evaluate instrument effectiveness.

Keywords: fidelity, implementation, depression, evidence-based, older adults

INTRODUCTION

The Program to Encourage Active and Rewarding Lives (PEARLS) was developed in the late 1990s by the University of Washington Health Promotion Research Center, in collaboration with our local Area Agency on Aging and a network of senior centers. PEARLS is a depression care management (DCM) program using the Chronic Care model (1). PEARLS includes active screening for depression, using a trained depression care manager, a team approach, stepped care, and built-in follow-up. Depression care managers deliver brief, evidence-based interventions and provide education and self-management support, proactive outcome measurement, and tracking using the nine-item Patient Health Questionnaire (PHQ-9). PEARLS is a participant-driven program, aimed at teaching individuals effective skills to manage their lives when they get overwhelmed. Case managers, nurses, social workers, and other front-line staff at community-based aging and social service agencies are trained as PEARLS counselors and work with participants, teaching them problem-solving treatment methods in combination with behavioral activation techniques.

In a randomized controlled trial (RCT), the PEARLS program was shown to significantly improve depression treatment outcomes for frail, socially isolated elders with minor depression and dysthymia when compared to the typical care that these clients received (2). Fifty-four percent of PEARLS clients showed at least a 50% decrease in the 20-item Hopkins Symptoms Checklist (HSCL-20) (3) depression score from baseline to 6-months versus 8% of clients in usual care at the same time interval. Forty-four percent of PEARLS clients showed complete remission from depression after 6-months versus 10% of clients in usual care. Compared to usual care, PEARLS participants also had greater health-related quality-of-life improvements in functional well-being ($p = 0.001$) and emotional well-being ($p = 0.048$). Thirty-four percent of individuals in usual care reported any hospitalization during the first 6 months of treatment compared to only 22% of PEARLS clients, suggesting potential health care cost savings (2). A subsequent RCT (4, 5) demonstrated the effectiveness of PEARLS in treating adults of all ages with epilepsy and major depression.

Currently, PEARLS is offered to older adults and adults with epilepsy in approximately 45 sites across 14 states. As it is disseminated nationally, and implemented in various community settings, fidelity becomes increasingly important. Implementation, as it is described in the RE-AIM framework, "refers to the extent to which a program is delivered as intended" both at the site-level and individual level (6). Fidelity is the adherence of a scientifically developed program to the original, research-based protocol, and is necessary for implementing evidence-based programs (7). The literature around evidence-based program implementation emphasizes the importance of maintaining program fidelity to ensure positive outcomes (8–10). Low program fidelity has been shown to negatively impact outcomes (8, 11). Similarly, high program fidelity has been linked to more positive outcomes across a range of evidence-based practices serving a variety of populations (12–14). Dissemination and implementation models such as the Fixsen Implementation framework (10), the RE-AIM framework (15), and the dissemination framework for evidence-based health promotion practices (16) assume that program adaptation is necessary, expected, and must inform program evolution. However, measuring program adaptations, and how those adaptations relate to client outcomes, is an essential step in determining the extent to which an evidence-based program may be modified, while continuing to remain evidence-based.

MATERIALS AND METHODS

The study was completed in three phases. The first phase involved developing a brief, multidimensional instrument for measuring PEARLS fidelity across sites. The second phase involved conducting a preliminary evaluation of that fidelity instrument. The third phase evaluated the association of PEARLS program fidelity instrument scores with individual client outcomes. This study was approved by the University of Washington Institutional Review Board.

INSTRUMENT DEVELOPMENT

We used purposive convenience sampling to identify study participants with experience in PEARLS program development, training, delivery, and receipt. First, we recruited interview participants. The participants included program developers and researchers, program administrators, and PEARLS counselors. Using qualitative methods, we conducted 30–60 min interviews (MS, LS) with these individuals to identify the core, programmatic components of PEARLS from their perspective. Next, we recruited former PEARLS clients who had completed the program within the previous 12 months, and held focus groups with these individuals to identify the core, programmatic components of PEARLS from their perspective. We provided a $25 incentive to focus group participants. Incentives were not provided to interview participants.

After the interview and focus group participants identified program components, we used Q-sort ranking (17) to prioritize these items: we presented the list of possible items to the interview participants on a spreadsheet, along with ranking chips (four 1s, nine 2s, sixteen 3s, nine 4s, and four 5s). The interview participants ranked the items in order of priority ("5" = most core elements of PEARLS to "1" = least core elements of PEARLS), and only used the ranking chips allotted to create a normal distribution. We calculated the numbers of 1s and 2s ("low" ranking) and 4s and 5s ("high" ranking) for each of the items. We then subtracted the number of high rankings from the number of low rankings to come up with a "high-low" score for each item. Those items that received a high-low score >0 were presented back to the interview and focus group participants to confirm that no items were missing. The participants were asked to then identify any additional items. The research team then created multiple-choice questions from each of the items, with five anchor points and a scale of one to five. The interview participants also reviewed the anchor points, provided feedback, and we modified the anchor points based on that feedback. A copy of the resulting PEARLS Fidelity instrument is provided in Data Sheet 1 in Supplementary Material.

PRELIMINARY EVALUATION

We used known-groups method data analysis (18) to conduct a preliminary evaluation of the reliability and validity of the PEARLS fidelity instrument. We compared PEARLS, other DCM programs, and non-DCM programs across six states (CA, FL, GA, IL, MD, WA). The DCM programs included IMPACT (19) and Healthy IDEAS (20). IMPACT is a primary care-based DCM program that has demonstrated effectiveness with diverse populations in a range of clinical settings. Healthy IDEAS is an evidence-based DCM program that integrates depression awareness and management into existing case management services for older adults. The non-DCM programs included other psychotherapy and case management program models. We collected the following data: PEARLS counselors completed (1) the fidelity instrument at two time points, and (2) a survey about their clinical experience at one time point. Clinical supervisors for the PEARLS programs completed the fidelity instrument on behalf of each counselor that they supervised at one time point. We gave the counselors and supervisors the option of completing the fidelity instrument and clinical experience survey online or with a paper and pencil.

The preliminary analysis involved evaluating mean scores and SDs at the site-level and the individual level using paired t-tests. We compared the mean scores for PEARLS sites against the mean scores for the other DCM programs and the non-DCM programs. We also compared site-level mean scores by experience level. We compared individual-level scores by education level (up to 4 years of college and master's degree), by counselor experience (<1 year, 1–3 years, 4–7 years, and 8 or more years), and by PEARLS-specific experience (<1 year, 1–3 years, and 4 or more years). Instrument validity was assessed using sensitivity and specificity, and we used this information to calculate optimal cut-off scores. We also conducted ROC curve analysis, calculating weighted and unweighted areas under the curve (AUC) as a quantitative method for combining sensitivity and specificity into a single metric. Reliability was evaluated using inter-class coefficients (ICC) between the two survey administration time points.

ASSOCIATION WITH CLIENT OUTCOMES

For this study, we worked with eight community partners in four states around the U.S. (CA, NY, WA, VT) to examine the relationship between PEARLS program fidelity and PEARLS client outcomes. These PEARLS programs were based on aging, social services, and mental health agencies and represent diverse geographic settings (urban, rural, suburban), and racial/ethnic minority communities (including African-Americans, Filipinos, and other Asian immigrant communities). Many of these programs serve persons with limited income (as indicated by their eligibility for Medicaid and other assistance programs with less than a high school or college education. Each PEARLS program included one to five PEARLS counselors. The four WA PEARLS programs work with one clinical supervisor. The four PEARLS programs outside of Seattle have their own clinical supervisor. Each PEARLS program graduates up to 25 clients over a 6-month period. Agencies were selected based on their current implementation of PEARLS for at least 1 year and their participation on regular PEARLS technical assistance conference calls. We obtained memorandums of understanding from each participating PEARLS program.

We assessed PEARLS program fidelity by administering the PEARLS fidelity instrument to PEARLS counselors and clinical supervisors. PEARLS client outcomes were obtained from existing de-identified PEARLS client outcome data from clients of participating PEARLS counselors. All PEARLS counselors at participating PEARLS programs were invited to participate in this study. Each counselor was asked to complete the fidelity instrument at two time points over the course of the study. In addition, each counselor provided basic information about her or his clinical experience and demographics. No identifiable information was collected about the counselor. We also invited clinical supervisors at each participating agency to complete a PEARLS fidelity instrument on each participating counselor. We linked the PEARLS clinical supervisor fidelity instrument data to the PEARLS counselor data using a unique code assigned for study purposes only. Each clinical supervisor also provided basic information about their clinical experience and demographics. No identifiable information was collected about the clinical supervisor.

We obtained de-identified depression outcome data from the PEARLS clients of each participating PEARLS counselor 6-months following the fidelity survey administration. The outcome data include baseline and final overall and item PHQ-9 depression scores, as had been done in our prior research (2, 4, 5) examining outcomes from treating clients with major depression. We also obtained data on client age, gender, race/ethnicity, and language spoken. We worked with each participating PEARLS agency to ensure that appropriate human subjects protections were in place before obtaining client data. We analyzed the relationship between PEARLS program fidelity total and item scores with the mean change in PHQ-9 scores between participants' baseline and final PEARLS session. We used Spearman's rank correlation to measure the degree of association between the PEARLS program fidelity scores and the mean change in PHQ-9. We also dichotomized the total PEARLS fidelity score and looked at whether falling above or below the cut-off predicted significant differences in the mean change in the PHQ-9, using independent t-tests to evaluate this difference. Lastly, we summarized responses to the fidelity instrument to examine what adaptations are being made in PEARLS implementation.

RESULTS

INSTRUMENT DEVELOPMENT

Seventeen informants provided input on the initial development of the PEARLS fidelity instrument. Ten people participated in the interviews to identify key components: four program developers and researchers, three program administrators, and three PEARLS counselors. Seven former PEARLS clients participated in focus groups to identify the core, programmatic components of PEARLS from their perspective.

The interview and focus group participants identified 42 program components, including items related to training, supervision, treatment, and eligibility. Eighteen items received a high-low score during the Q-sort ranking process, suggesting higher priority for inclusion in the fidelity instrument. After these 18 items were presented back to the interview and focus group participants, two additional items were added, resulting in a total of 20 multiple-choice items. Each item had five possible text anchor points (score of "1" = least fidelity to "5" = highest fidelity), with the total possible score ranging from 20 to 100. The interview participants reviewed the anchor points, and provided feedback. We modified the anchor points based on that feedback.

Questions are divided into two sections: Program Design and Program Delivery. The Design section includes questions about how the organization implements PEARLS, including training, clinical supervision, client recruitment and referrals, and eligibility criteria. The Delivery section focuses on how the counselor implements PEARLS with their clients, such as the average number of sessions that are delivered at home or that identify and discuss social activities. A copy of the resulting PEARLS Fidelity instrument is provided in Data Sheet 1 in Supplementary Material.

PRELIMINARY EVALUATION

We used known-groups method data analysis to compare 12 depression programs in six states: six PEARLS programs, four other DCM programs, and two non-DCM programs. Fifty-two PEARLS counselors and seven clinical supervisors provided responses to both the fidelity instrument and the experience survey: 16 respondents from six PEARLS programs, 23 respondents from four DCM programs (one IMPACT program and three Healthy IDEAS programs), and 20 respondents from two non-DCM programs. One practitioner from a DCM site was excluded, due to missing data. Seventy-three percent of the participants completed the fidelity instrument online. It took an average of 14 min to complete. Participants averaged 48 days between the first and second time point for taking the survey.

Individual level (PEARLS)

The range of scores was 40–89 for the PEARLS counselors ($n = 16$). Five counselors attended up to 4 years of college and 10 counselors held Master's degrees. Six practiced as a counselor for <1 year, five practiced for 1–3 years, and five practiced for over 8 years. No counselors practiced from 4–7 years. Seven counselors implemented PEARLS for <1 year, five implemented PEARLS for 1–3 years, and two implemented PEARLS for over 4 years. The sample size was too small to yield significant results on the comparison between education level, experience as a counselor, and experience with implementing the PEARLS program.

Site-level (PEARLS, DCM, non-DCM)

Program for Encouraging Active and Rewarding Lives sites reported the highest fidelity score [Mean (SD) 70 (15.5)] compared to sites delivering other DCM programs [55.2 (19.1)] and non-DCM programs [58.0 (13.0)] ($p < 0.05$). Average item scores were 3.56 (0.77) for PEARLS sites compared to 2.9 (0.8) for other DCM sites and non-DCM sites. PEARLS sites with more years of experience reported higher scores (mean 81, range 74–89) than newer programs (mean 59, range 26–81). PEARLS supervisors ($n = 7$) from three PEARLS programs completed the fidelity instrument. Mean fidelity scores were comparable between the supervisor and counselor for all three programs [83 (9) for supervisors and 82 (7) for counselors, $p = 0.87$ (NS)]. Individual item scores were similar, with an average difference of 0.04 between items. Unweighted scoring yielded an AUC in ROC analyses of 0.77. Weighting the overall score improved ROC scores yielding an AUC of 0.81. Optimal cut-off scores for weighted PEARLS fidelity score is 77, yielding a sensitivity of 77% and specificity of 67% for identifying PEARLS counselors and non-PEARLS counselors, respectively (**Figure 1**). Inter-rater reliability was satisfactory, with an overall ICC of 0.77.

ASSOCIATION WITH CLIENT OUTCOMES

Twenty-six PEARLS counselors and six clinical supervisors completed the PEARLS fidelity instrument. The mean PEARLS fidelity score was 79.75 (8.33), which was similar to the average total score of 70 (15) for PEARLS programs in the preliminary evaluation. In contrast, the PEARLS counselor and PEARLS clinical supervisor scores differed by an average of 12.17 points (8.09), with some counselors reporting lower scores and others reporting higher scores than their clinical supervisor, even within the same agency.

Program for Encouraging Active and Rewarding Lives participant data were obtained for 127 persons with a mean age of 69 years (8.87). 38.2% identified as White, 26% identified as Hispanic (59% as Mexican), 21.1% as Asian (mainly Filipino with some Vietnames and Korean participants), 11.4% as African-American, and as other races. Only 21% (26 clients) provided data on their income, with all but three of these clients reporting very low income as defined by the Federal Poverty Level, Median Income, or Housing and Urban Development criteria depending on the PEARLS program. Almost half (46.7%) of the respondents that provided information on language spoken at home ($n = 96$) reported speaking a language other than English. Half of those reporting who they lived with stated that they currently lived alone. We did not collect data on education. The mean change in PHQ-9 was 8.79 (5.50). There was little correlation between PEARLS program fidelity and participant outcomes. The correlation between the overall fidelity score and mean change in PHQ-9 was −0.069 ($p = 0.444$). Several fidelity items were significantly correlated with the mean change in the PHQ-9, but all suggested weak correlations. The most strongly correlated items were those that involved the administration of the PHQ-9 ($r = 0.231$, $p = 0.009$), the use of problem-solving treatment ($r = 0.227$, $p = 0.010$), and the use of homework in between in-person sessions ($r = 0.227$, $p = 0.010$).

We conducted additional analyses removing outliers-data for those counselors and clinical supervisor pairings that had a difference in total fidelity score that was 13 or greater (higher than the mean difference between counselors and clinical supervisors of 12.17). Eighty-four PEARLS participants and 16 counselors were included in this revised dataset. The mean change in PHQ-9 was slightly higher than in the original group [9.00 (5.25)]. The mean (SD) total PEARLS fidelity score was also higher [83.42 (5.29)].

We dichotomized the full dataset to look at whether falling above or below a cut-off for the PEARLS fidelity total score predicted a difference in the mean change in PHQ-9 score. Using the cut-off of 70 (as identified in the preliminary evaluation described above), there was not a significant difference between mean change in PHQ-9 between those falling above or at 70 [$n = 106$, 9.16 (5.42)] and those falling below 70 [$n = 21$, 6.90 (5.69), $p = 0.086$]. The difference was also not significant when the cut point was set at 80 (the mean total PEARLS fidelity score in this correlation study), with a mean PHQ-9 change of 8.94 (5.38) ($n = 81$) for those at or above the cut point and 8.52 (5.78) ($n = 46$) for those below the cut point.

We summarized the responses to the fidelity instrument in **Table 1**. The table provides a snapshot of how PEARLS programs are implementing PEARLS compared to the original research model. Differences exist for clinical supervision, counselor assessment, client eligibility, and the content and format of PEARLS sessions.

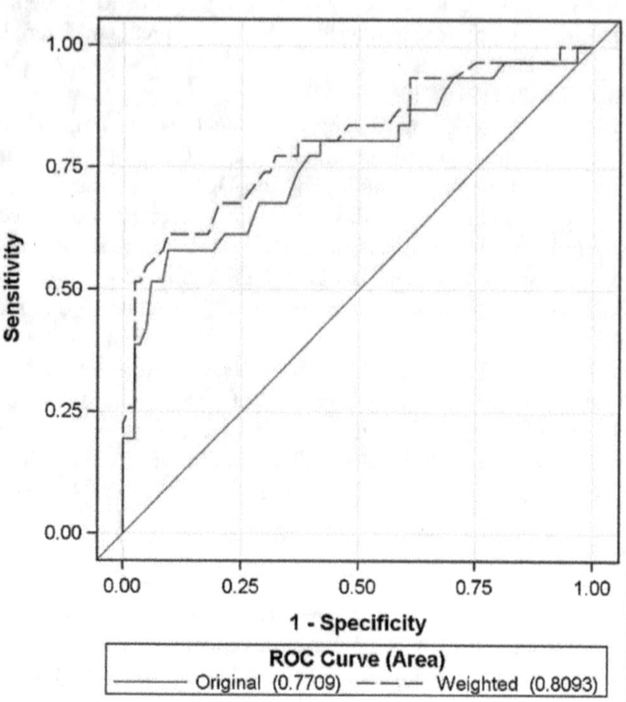

FIGURE 1 | ROC curves for comparisons.

Table 1 | Research to practice: a summary of responses to the PEARLS fidelity instrument as compared to the original PEARLS model.

Original PEARLS model	Practice model
CLINICAL SUPERVISION	
Formal contract with supervisor	89% have formal supervision in place
Bi-monthly supervision	40% meet at least monthly
Each client discussed at each session	Range from "as needed" (16%) to "weekly" (24%)
COUNSELOR ASSESSMENT	
Audiotapes of PEARLS sessions	56% assessed during formal clinical supervision; 28% during job supervision or self-assessment
ELIGIBILITY	
Home-based program	42% deliver PEARLS outside of the home
Older adults (60+)	40% include younger adults (<age 60 years)
PEARLS SESSIONS	
6–8 in-person sessions	71% average ≥6 sessions per client
PHQ-9	80% PHQ-9 at ≥6 sessions
Education about depression using both written and verbal materials	64% counselors use both written and verbal materials
Sessions focus on the present	42% ≤2 sessions focus on the past
Client chooses problems and solutions	42% ≥6 sessions
Homework completed	17% ≥6 sessions, 75% ≥4 sessions
Behavioral activation	46–58% ≥6 sessions
Written PST worksheet	46% ≥6 sessions

DISCUSSION

The PEARLS fidelity instrument is a brief, easy-to-use, low-cost option for PEARLS program staff to assess fidelity during program implementation. The tool takes an average of 14 min to complete, allowing for routine assessments by clinical supervisors and counselors. For example, a PEARLS program may use the fidelity instrument periodically as a way to assess whether a counselor is continuing to maintain fidelity to the original program model, and to identify where adaptations have been made. Clinical supervisors may use the instrument to guide ongoing clinical supervision sessions and activities. Funders of PEARLS programs and agency administrators may be interested in the PEARLS fidelity instrument as a quality assurance tool to guide ongoing implementation.

It is surprising that fidelity to the PEARLS program and client outcomes are not more strongly correlated. Also, the discrepancy between clinical supervisor and counselor ratings suggests that there is variation in how each party completes the instrument, and perhaps in how clinical supervisors are involved in the program. We know, for instance, from PEARLS technical assistance activities that some clinical supervisors are more intimately involved with regularly providing supervision that helps guide counselors in adhering closely to the PEARLS model, while others are brought in less frequently and advise more on co-occurring chronic conditions and medication use than on the PEARLS model. More rigorous research is needed to confirm the effectiveness of the tool (e.g., by comparing the tool to the current gold standard of an in-person, full-day, external evaluation of fidelity) before it is disseminated widely.

Research suggests that translation of evidence-based programs must be completed systematically, both at the site-level and individual level, to assure effectiveness (6). The RE-AIM framework is an important tool that is used by researchers and public health practitioners to inform that dissemination. The framework defines translation across five areas – Reach, Effectiveness, Adoption, Implementation, and Maintenance (6). Assuring the fidelity of a particular program to its original evidence-based design is an important aspect of the implementation phase of dissemination (7–14).

It is important to evaluate PEARLS counselors at the site-level to assure that clients are receiving the best possible treatment. It is also imperative to look at the PEARLS program at the site-level to prove to funding agencies that it is effective (6–14). This is particularly important as many funding sources now require some measure of quality assurance or fidelity for supporting evidence-based programs (e.g., Administration on Aging Title III-D funding for evidence-based disease prevention programing). However, many sites lack adequate funding and staff capacity to conduct in-depth, programmatic assessments; therefore, it is important to develop fidelity tools that are effective, user-friendly, and operate at low-cost.

The PEARLS mean score on the fidelity instrument was lower than expected (70.5 out of a possible 100), and **Table 1** illustrates some of the changes that agencies implementing PEARLS are making. From our work providing technical assistance to PEARLS sites, we believe that a couple of factors may be at play. Many sites have made programmatic changes to address the needs of their staff and the local population, or due to funding and staffing constraints. For instance, while programs would like to meet weekly with their clinical supervisor, they may meet less frequently due to supervisor availability, limited funds to support the supervisor time, and/or smaller PEARLS client caseloads, which make more frequent supervision unnecessary. Another example is the case of programs delivering PEARLS outside the home. This shift has occurred driven by client preferences to meet at places where they are already congregating (e.g., after a nutrition program at a community center) or preferences to meet elsewhere when a spouse or caregiver is at home due to privacy concerns. Some of the changes are to be expected given that the original PEARLS model was based on the research protocol during an RCT. Elements such as having the clinical supervisor review audiotapes of each PEARLS session are not feasible for community-based agencies that do not have the funds, staffing, or resources. Nor is this level of supervision required for the program to be implemented successfully.

Another example is expanding participant eligibility criteria to better align with the multifaceted, complex clients that agencies see every day. Previous research (21) suggested that the strict PEARLS eligibility criteria was screening out more clients than screening them in, frustrating providers who repeatedly refer clients who are ultimately not treated. During our work with PEARLS providers, we have focused their assessment of client eligibility more on client function, whether they are able to attend PEARLS sessions and to do the work during and in between the sessions. In addition, we know that PEARLS programs are making adaptations to fit their local populations. Sites do not use written information with every participant as some are illiterate or have low literacy, or speak a language other than English and materials are interpreted versus translated. In addition, some sites allow younger older adult participants in the program (typically age 50–59 years) as they have no other treatment options, are seen in similar settings, and are as successful as the 60+ population.

These findings also point to the fact that fidelity is only a piece of the implementation of PEARLS. The weak, generally non-significant correlations between fidelity score and client outcomes may suggest that other factors are at play, which impact whether a client improves their depressive symptoms. From our work providing technical assistance to PEARLS programs, we know that at the individual level, motivation, stigma about depression, physical health and management of other comorbidities, informal and formal support, and mobility and function are all factors that influence whether someone successfully participates in PEARLS. At the site-level, other approaches for improving EBP implementation include outcome monitoring, regular and structured supervision, effective organization and climate, rigorous selection and retention of team members, and ongoing consultation and technical assistance (21).

After measuring fidelity, it is important to then provide fidelity feedback to EBP providing agencies so that they can modify their services based on feedback from their fidelity reviews (22). One example of a systematic approach for providing fidelity feedback is from the National Implementing Evidence-Based Practices Project (23). Most of the successfully implementing sites had altered their services based on feedback received during their fidelity reviews, suggesting that the fidelity review process can be effective (22). With PEARLS, we have shared findings from each phase of this fidelity study with participants on our monthly conference calls to provide technical assistance.

The fidelity instrument that we developed in this study may be the most effective way to evaluate effective implementation in various locations and community settings across the country. While independent, observational measures of fidelity are ideal, this instrument provides a practical, user-friendly tool that programs can use internally and at minimal cost for monitoring program quality. Further work is necessary to ascertain the validity of the instrument given the discrepancy between counselor and supervisor ratings and it may need refinement to correlate more strongly with client outcomes.

ACKNOWLEDGMENTS

We thank study participants, research, and administrative staff. This study was supported in part by the CDC Prevention Research Centers (PRC) Program, through cooperative agreement U48 DP000050. Additional PEARLS research funding was provided by the R-18 grant Improving Public Health Practice through Translation Research, #DP001150. The contents of this work are solely the responsibility of the authors and do not necessarily represent the official views of CDC.

REFERENCES

1. Coleman K, Austin BT, Brach C, Wagner EH. Evidence on the chronic care model in the new millennium. *Health Aff* (2009) **28**(1):75–85. doi:10.1377/hlthaff.28.1.75
2. Ciechanowski P, Wagner E, Schmaling K, Schwartz S, Williams B, Diehr P, et al. Community-integrated home-based depression treatment in older adults: a randomized controlled trial. *JAMA* (2004) **291**(13):1569–77. doi:10.1001/jama.291.13.1569
3. Derogatis LR, Lipman RS, Rickels K, Uhlenhuth EH, Covi L. The Hopkins symptom checklist (HSCL): a self-report symptom inventory. *Behav Sci* (1974) **19**(1):1–15. doi:10.1002/bs.3830190102
4. Chaytor N, Ciechanowski P, Miller JW, Fraser R, Russo J, Unutzer J, et al. Long-term outcomes from the PEARLS randomized trial for the treatment of depression in patients with epilepsy. *Epilepsy Behav* (2011) **20**(3):545–9. doi:10.1016/j.yebeh.2011.01.017
5. Ciechanowski P, Chaytor N, Miller J, Fraser R, Russo J, Unutzer J, et al. PEARLS depression treatment for individuals with epilepsy: a randomized controlled trial. *Epilepsy Behav* (2010) **19**(3):225–31. doi:10.1016/j.yebeh.2010.06.003
6. Glasgow RE, Vogt TM, Boles SM. Evaluating the public health impact of health promotion interventions: the RE-AIM framework. *Am J Public Health* (1999) **89**(9):1322–7. doi:10.2105/AJPH.89.9.1322
7. Teague GB, Mueser KT, Rapp CA. Advances in fidelity measurement for mental health services research: four measures. *Psychiatr Serv* (2012) **63**(8):765–71. doi:10.1176/appi.ps.201100430
8. Derzon JH, Sale E, Springer JF, Brounstein P. Estimating intervention effectiveness: synthetic projection of field evaluation results. *J Prim Prev* (2005) **26**(4):321–43. doi:10.1007/s10935-005-5391-5
9. Durlak JA, DuPre EP. Implementation matters: a review of research on the influence of implementation on program outcomes and the factors affecting implementation. *Am J Community Psychol* (2008) **41**(3–4):327–50. doi:10.1007/s10464-008-9165-0
10. Fixsen DL, Naoom SF, Blase KA, Friedman RM, Wallace F. *Implementation Research: A Synthesis of the Literature*. Tampa, FL: The National Implementation Research Network, Louis de la Parte Florida Mental Health Institute, University of South Florida (2005). Contract No.: FMHI Publication #231.
11. Botvin GJ, Baker E, Dusenbury L, Tortu S, Botvin EM. Preventing adolescent drug abuse through a multimodal cognitive-behavioral approach: results of a 3-year study. *J Consult Clin Psychol* (1990) **58**(4):437–46. doi:10.1037/0022-006X.58.4.437
12. Burns T, Catty J, Dash M, Roberts C, Lockwood A, Marshall M. Use of intensive case management to reduce time in hospital in people with severe mental illness: systematic review and meta-regression. *Br Med J* (2007) **335**(7615):336–40. doi:10.1136/bmj.39251.599259.55
13. McGrew JH, Bond GR, Dietzen L, Salyers M. Measuring the fidelity of implementation of a mental health program model. *J Consult Clin Psychol* (1994) **62**(4):670–8. doi:10.1037/0022-006X.62.4.670
14. McHugo GJ, Drake RE, Teague GB, Xie H. Fidelity to assertive community treatment and client outcomes in the New Hampshire dual disorders study. *Psychiatr Serv* (1999) **50**(6):818–24.
15. Glasgow RE, Lichtenstein E, Marcus AC. Why don't we see more translation of health promotion research to practice? Rethinking the efficacy-to-effectiveness transition. *Am J Public Health* (2003) **93**(8):1261–7. doi:10.2105/AJPH.93.8.1261
16. Harris JR, Cheadle A, Hannon PA, Forehand M, Lichiello P, Mahoney E, et al. A framework for disseminating evidence-based health promotion practices. *Prev Chronic Dis* (2012) **9**:E22. doi:10.5888/pcd9.110081
17. Brown SR. Q methodology and qualitative research. *Qual Health Res* (1996) **6**(4):561–7. doi:10.1177/104973239600600408

18. Mowbray CT, Holter MC, Teague GB, Bybee D. Fidelity criteria: development, measurement, and validation. *Am J Eval* (2003) **24**(3):315–40. doi:10.1177/109821400302400303
19. Unutzer J, Katon W, Callahan CM, Williams JW, Hunkeler E, Harpole L, et al. Collaborative care management of late-life depression in the primary care setting – a randomized controlled trial. *JAMA* (2002) **288**(22):2836–45. doi:10.1001/jama.288.22.2836
20. Quijano LM, Stanley MA, Petersen NJ, Casado BL, Steinberg EH, Cully JA, et al. Healthy IDEAS: a depression intervention delivered by community-based case managers serving older adults. *J Appl Gerontol* (2007) **26**(2):139–56. doi:10.1177/0733464807299354
21. Steinman L, Cristofalo M, Snowden M. Implementation of an evidence-based depression care management program (PEARLS): perspectives from staff and former clients. *Prev Chronic Dis* (2012) **9**:E91. doi:10.5888/pcd9.110250
22. Monroe-DeVita M, Morse G, Bond GR. Program fidelity and beyond: multiple strategies and criteria for ensuring quality of assertive community treatment. *Psychiatr Serv* (2012) **63**(8):743–50. doi:10.1176/appi.ps.201100015
23. McHugo GJ, Drake RE, Whitley R, Bond GR, Campbell K, Rapp CA, et al. Fidelity outcomes in the National Implementing Evidence-Based Practices Project. *Psychiatr Serv* (2007) **58**(10):1279–84. doi:10.1176/appi.ps.58.10.1279

National dissemination of multiple evidence-based disease prevention programs: Reach to vulnerable older adults

Samuel D. Towne Jr.[1]*, Matthew Lee Smith[2], SangNam Ahn[1,3], Mary Altpeter[4], Basia Belza[5], Kristie Patton Kulinski[6] and Marcia G. Ory[1]

[1] Department of Health Promotion and Community Health Sciences, Texas A&M Health Science Center School of Public Health, College Station, TX, USA
[2] Department of Health Promotion and Behavior, College of Public Health, The University of Georgia, Athens, GA, USA
[3] Division of Health Systems Management and Policy, School of Public Health, The University of Memphis, Memphis, TN, USA
[4] University of North Carolina at Chapel Hill, Chapel Hill, NC, USA
[5] Biobehavioral Nursing and Health Systems, School of Nursing, University of Washington, Seattle, WA, USA
[6] National Council on Aging, Washington, DC, USA

Edited by:
Sue Ellen Levkoff, University of South Carolina, USA

Reviewed by:
Cheryll Diann Lesneski, UNC-Chapel Hill, USA
Katherine Henrietta Leith, University of South Carolina, USA

***Correspondence:**
Samuel D. Towne Jr., Department of Health Promotion and Community Health Sciences, Texas A&M Health Science Center School of Public Health, College Station, TX 77843-1266, USA
e-mail: towne@sph.tamhsc.edu

Older adults, who are racial/ethnic minorities, report multiple chronic conditions, reside in medically underserved rural areas, or have low incomes carry a high burden of chronic illness but traditionally lack access to disease prevention programs. The Chronic Disease Self-Management Program (CDSMP), A Matter of Balance/Volunteer Lay Leader (AMOB/VLL), and EnhanceFitness (EF) are widely disseminated evidence-based programs (EBP), but the extent to which they are simultaneously delivered in communities to reach vulnerable populations has not been documented. We conducted cross-sectional analyses of three EBP disseminated within 27 states throughout the United States (US) (2006–2009) as part of the Administration on Aging (AoA) Evidence-Based Disease and Disability Prevention Initiative, which received co-funding from the Atlantic Philanthropies. This study measures the extent to which CDSMP, AMOB/VLL, and EF reached vulnerable older adults. It also examines characteristics of communities offering one of these programs relative to those simultaneously offering two or all three programs. Minority/ethnic participants represented 38% for CDSMP, 26% for AMOB/VLL, and 43% for EF. Rural participation was 18% for CDSMP, 17% for AMOB/VLL, and 25% for EF. Those with comorbidities included 63.2% for CDSMP, 58.7% for AMOB/VLL, and 63.6% for EF while approximately one-quarter of participants had incomes under $15,000 for all programs. Rural areas and health professional shortage areas (HPSA) tended to deliver fewer EBP relative to urban areas and non-HPSA. These EBP attract diverse older adult participants. Findings highlight the capability of communities to serve potentially vulnerable older adults by offering multiple EBP. Because each program addresses unique issues facing this older population, further research is needed to better understand how communities can introduce, embed, and sustain multiple EBP to ensure widespread access and utilization, especially to traditionally underserved subgroups.

Keywords: evidence-based programs, community intervention, minority adults, older adults, aging health

INTRODUCTION

The aging of the US population has far reaching effects on the American health care system (1). Chronic disease is becoming endemic among older Americans (2). National statistics indicate most adults aged 65 and older have at least one chronic condition (91%), while nearly three-quarters have two or more chronic conditions (2). Additionally, age-related geriatric conditions are prevalent in this population and have stark public health consequences. Each year, falling affects approximately one-third of older adults in the US (3) contributing to death and serious injuries and costing billions of dollars in healthcare expenses annually (estimated to reach $30 billion by 2020) (4–8). In addition, high blood pressure, high cholesterol, heart disease, arthritis, and diabetes are common among older adults (9), and in many cases comorbidities are also present (10).

Self-management is seen as a critical component of clinical- and community-based health care (11, 12). Although self-management strategies are widely promoted (13), individuals with multiple chronic conditions experience barriers to successful self-care (14). Given that older adults have different chronic diseases, varying comorbidity combinations, and are at differing stages of disease progression, there is need for multiple intervention approaches in any given community.

In concert with public health officials and policy makers' interests to identify effective ways to lessen the impact of chronic disease and other complications among the aging population [e.g., Healthy People 2020 (15)], evidence-based programs (EBP) for older adults have emerged and proliferated in the US (16–20). In recent years, multiple EBP have been disseminated through the US aging services network to address different healthcare concerns experienced by older adults (21). However, there is no "one size fits all" EBP, which highlights the need for communities to introduce multiple programs to meet the various needs of a diverse aging population.

While it is assumed that distinct EBP attract specific types of participants (17, 18) and certain types of participants are more likely to attend EBP at particular types of delivery sites (16), the extent to which EBP attract and retain potentially vulnerable older adults is not fully understood. Older adults deemed vulnerable can include those with comorbid conditions (22), in advanced age, and of racial/ethnic minority status (23–25). Vulnerability can also be defined as older adults residing in areas with limited resources, which include rural areas (26–28), those with limited health care providers, or those with high poverty rates compared to most other areas (29, 30). As such, the purpose of this study was twofold: (1) to measure the extent to which three widely disseminated EBP reached vulnerable older adults and (2) to assess the extent to which delivery areas offered multiple EBP.

MATERIALS AND METHODS

SELECTED EVIDENCE-BASED PROGRAMS

For the purposes of this study, three EBP for older adults were examined. The programs included in this study include: Stanford University's Chronic Disease Self-Management Program (CDSMP), A Matter of Balance/Volunteer Lay Leader (AMOB/VLL), and EnhanceFitness (EF). Each program was selected because of its national dissemination spanning multiple states and well-documented effectiveness for improving health outcomes in community settings.

These EBP have demonstrated their effectiveness in improving health among older adults. CDSMP targets adults with multiple chronic conditions (e.g., teaching self-management skills) and has been shown to be effective at delaying the onset of illness and helping participants improve the management of multiple chronic diseases while reducing hospitalizations (31–34). AMOB/VLL targets older adults, especially those at risk of falling (35) and has been shown to reduce the fear of falling, improve long-term social functioning, and improve long- and short-term mobility in older adults (17, 36–38). EF is a group exercise program (39) that has been shown to improve upper and lower body muscle strength, depression (40), and lower healthcare costs (41).

DATA ANALYSES

We conducted a cross-sectional analysis of three EBP. Participant data and information about program delivery locations were drawn from the National Council on Aging's database of 24 states implementing EBP from 2006 to 2009 as part of the Administration on Aging (AoA) Evidence-Based Disease and Disability Prevention Initiative and 3 states funded by the Atlantic Philanthropies (16). Only data collected between 2006 and 2009 from these initiatives were included in these analyses. These data were linked with the 2013 Area Health Resource File (AHRF) to identify Primary Care Health Professional Shortage Areas (HPSA) and Urban Influence Codes (UIC) (42). HPSA is classified into full-HPSA, partial (only a portion of the county was classified as a HPSA), and a non-HPSA. A HPSA is classified based on geographic area and population size (e.g., primary care physician ratio of less than 3,500 to 1) (43). Rural areas were defined as having a UIC of ≥3 versus urban/metropolitan defined as having a UIC of 1–2. UICs take into consideration the population size and, for rural areas, the relative proximity to metropolitan or micropolitan areas (44). We used ArcGIS version 10.2 for all mapping of data presented in the figures (45). Chi-square tests were used to compare categorical study variables and independent sample *t*-tests were used to assess differences in continuous variables. We used SAS version 9.4 for all statistical analyses (46).

VARIABLES

Vulnerability

Vulnerable adults are the focus of our analysis. Acknowledging that vulnerability can be defined in numerous ways, the operational definition of vulnerability used in this study includes participants meeting one or more of the following criteria: being in advanced age (i.e., age 75 and older), having low income (i.e., self-reporting an annual household income <$15,000), being in a racial/ethnic minority (non-White), having one or more chronic conditions, living in a HPSA (47, 48), living in an area with poverty rates above the median (i.e., based on the percent Federal Poverty Rates in 2008 (14.1%) at the county level according to the 2013 AHRF), or living in a rural area (i.e., counties with UIC ≥3) (49). Only those individuals with one or more chronic conditions were included in our analyses.

Covariates

Sex of the participants who attended the EBP was reported. Income was categorical; however, a missing category for income was included in analyses, as we did not assume this was missing at random.

HANDLING MISSING DATA

As described elsewhere (50), the AoA initiative required only a few participant level variables be collected, including age, sex, living alone status, race/ethnicity, and ZIP Code. Even this limited number of variables was not collected routinely by all state grantees; however, some states chose to routinely collect information related to chronic conditions and income. Missingness (i.e., missing data) was addressed independently according to the analysis performed and variables included. Independently (i.e., only considering each variable's missingness exclusive of other missing variables), our sample size ($n = 48,413$) was gradually reduced when removing missing observations for race ($n = 37,661$), sex ($n = 39,488$), county Federal Information Processing Standard (FIPS) ($n = 36,599$), age ($n = 35,248$), the number of chronic conditions ($n = 22,007$), and income ($n = 22,956$). Dependently, when collectively removing observations for race, sex, county FIPS, and age, our sample size used in univariate and bivariate analysis was 30,185 observations.

RESULTS

REACH INTO VULNERABLE POPULATIONS

Table 1 presents the distribution of participant characteristics in the aggregate and by program type. Of the 30,185 participants enrolled in one of three EBP in this study, the majority participated in CDSMP ($n = 16,612$), followed by AMOB/VLL ($n = 8,391$), and

Table 1 | Distribution of participant characteristics by program.

	CDSMP ($n = 16,612$)		AMOB/VLL ($n = 8,391$)		EF ($n = 5,182$)		Total ($n = 30,185$)	
	n	%	*n*	%	*n*	%	*n*	%
Age group								
<50	1,323[a,b]	8.0	55[b,c]	0.7	135[a,c]	2.6	1,513	5.0
50–64	3,635[a,b]	21.9	656[b,c]	7.8	1,043[a,c]	20.1	5,334	17.7
65–74	5,151[a,b]	31.0	2,120[b,c]	25.3	1,933[a,c]	37.3	9,204	30.5
75 and older	6,503[a,b]	39.2	5,560[b,c]	66.3	2,071[a,c]	34.0	14,134	46.8
Age (mean)	69.6*	77.5*	71.4*	72.1	Age (mean)	69.6*	77.5*	71.4*
	(SD = 13.2)	(SD = 9.1)	(SD = 10.5)	(SD = 12.2)		(SD = 13.2)	(SD = 9.1)	(SD = 10.5)
Race/ethnicity								
White	10,250	61.7	6,270	74.7	3,010	58.1	19,530	64.7
Black or African American	2,136	12.9	581	6.9	987	19.1	3704	12.3
American Indian/Alaska Native	147	0.9	221	2.6	180	3.5	548	1.8
Asian	882	5.3	151	1.8	265	5.1	1,298	4.3
Other	764	4.6	199	2.4	146	2.8	1,109	3.7
Hispanic	2,433	14.7	969	11.6	594	11.5	3,996	13.2
Sex								
Male	3,648	22.0	1,393	16.6	756	14.6	5,797	19.2
Female	12,964	78.0	6,998	83.4	4,426	85.4	24,388	80.8
Number of chronic conditions								
1	4,185	36.6	806	40.9	1,120	37.9	6,111	37.3
2	3,828	33.5	733	37.2	1,048	35.5	5,609	34.3
3	2,379	20.8	332	16.9	544	18.4	3,255	19.9
4	835	7.3	85	4.3	209	7.1	1,129	6.9
5+	217	1.9	14	0.7	33	1.1	264	1.6
Average	2.04* (SD = 1.0)		1.87* (SD = 0.9)		1.98* (SD = 2.0)		2.01 (SD = 1.0)	
Income								
Missing	3,292	47.8	1,498	40.2	1,917	39.8	6,707	43.5
Less than $15,000	1,692	24.6	975	26.2	1,059	22.0	3,726	24.1
$15,000–24,999	820	11.9	479	12.9	742	15.4	2,041	13.2
$25,000–49,999	694	10.07	465	12.48	715	14.84	1,874	12.14
$50,000–75,000	251	3.64	199	5.34	254	5.27	704	4.56
More than $75,000	143	2.07	109	2.93	132	2.74	384	2.49
Rurality								
Rural	2,675	16.10	1,189	14.17	1,437	27.73	5,301	17.56
Urban	13,937	83.90	7,202	85.83	3,745	72.27	24,884	82.44

**Significantly ($p < 0.05$) different by program for select comparisons (i.e., age and the number of chronic conditions).*

[a]Significantly different CDSMP versus EF, within age group.

[b]Significantly different CDSMP versus AMOB/VLL, within age group.

[c]Significantly different AMOB/VLL versus EF, within age group.

EF ($n = 5,182$). On average, participants were aged 72.09 (±12.21) with 46.8% aged 75 and older. The majority of participants were female (80.8%), white (64.7%), and non-Hispanic (87.8%). The mean number of self-reported chronic conditions was 2 (±1.00). Approximately 24% of participants reported household incomes less than $15,000 per year, and 17.6% resided in rural areas.

The average age of participants varied significantly ($p < 0.05$) across program types (i.e., 77.49 for AMOB/VLL, 71.39 for EF, 69.58 for CDSMP) with AMOB/VLL attracting the oldest participants. AMOB/VLL had the highest proportion of participants aged 75 years and older (66.3%) compared to 39.2% for CDSMP and 40.0% for EF. Those with comorbid conditions (i.e., 2 or more chronic conditions) represented 63.4% for CDSMP, 59.1% for AMOB, and 62.1% for EF. The average number of chronic diseases was significantly ($p < 0.05$) different for all comparisons across programs except CDSMP versus EF; CDSMP attracted participants with the most chronic conditions. CDSMP also attracted the largest proportion of Hispanic participants (14.7%). Those residing in rural areas represented 16.0% for CDSMP, 14.2% for AMOB/VLL, and 27.7% for EF. Those reporting incomes less than

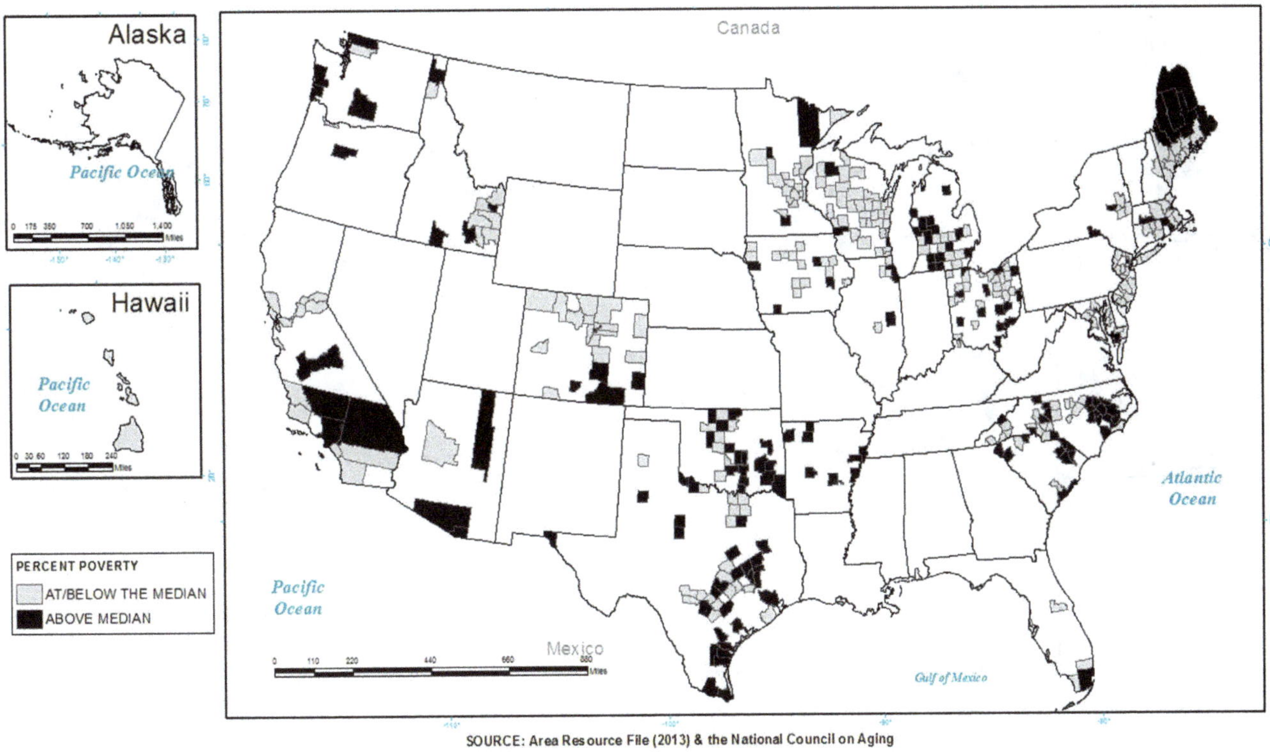

FIGURE 1 | The distribution of areas with a higher poverty rate than the median and a presence of evidence-based programs in 2006–2009.

$15,000 per year were 24.6% CDSMP, 26.2% AMOB/VLL, and 22% EF.

To graphically illustrate the extent to which programs were being delivered in areas classified as vulnerable by poverty rate or health access, a series of three maps highlighting participating states were constructed. **Figure 1** shows where programs were delivered in areas with higher poverty rates than the 2008 median rate. States without shading include those states that were not included in the initiative. Gray shading represents where programs (i.e., CDSMP, AMOB/VLL, EF) were offered in areas equal to or below the 2008 median poverty rate. Black shading represents where programs were offered in areas *higher* than the 2008 median poverty rate. As seen, approximately 49.6% of the participants attended programs in areas with higher poverty rates. A greater proportion of participants in areas with higher poverty rates were served by EF at 58.4%, compared to 52.2% by AMOB/VLL and 45.5% by CDSMP. As can be seen, programs were delivered in high need areas, but the extent varied by state. For example, larger portions of California and North Carolina and smaller proportions of Oklahoma, Maine, and Washington delivered programs in areas with higher poverty.

Figure 2 shows where programs were delivered in areas classified as a HPSA. Gray shading represents where programs (i.e., AMOB/VLL, CDSMP, EF) were offered in a non-HPSA. Black shading represents where programs were offered in a HPSA (full or partial). As presented in the map (**Figure 2**), approximately 88.9% of the participants attended programs in a HPSA. A greater proportion of participants in a HPSA were served by EF at 92.9%, compared to 88.8% by CDSMP and 86.5% by AMOB/VLL. Again, programs were delivered in high need areas, but that the extent varied by state (also seen in **Figure 1**).

Figure 3 depicts the intersection of poverty and HPSA, where black shading represents places where programs were offered in areas classified as both high poverty (above the median percent poverty for 2008 measured at the county) and HPSA (full or partial). As seen, approximately 47.5% of the participants attended programs in areas with both higher poverty rates and that were a HPSA. A greater proportion of participants in these areas were served by EF at 55.7%, compared to 48.6% by AMOB/VLL and 44.3% by CDSMP.

AVAILABILITY OF MULTIPLE EVIDENCE-BASED PROGRAMS

Table 2 presents the distribution of counties that delivered one, two, and three of the EBP included in this study. Overall, 78.8% of counties labeled full-HPSA delivered only one EBP, 18.5% delivered two of the EBP, and 2.6% delivered all three EBP. Approximately 84% of rural counties delivered one of these EBP, and 1.6% delivered all three programs. Nearly 75% of counties within higher poverty areas delivered one EBP versus 2.3% that offered all three EBP.

Table 3 presents the distribution of participants by counties that delivered one, two, and three of the EBP included in this study. Overall, 43.6% of participants attended programs in areas offering only one EBP, 39.6% attended programs offering two of the EBP, and 16.7% attended programs offering all three EBP. Fifty-nine percent of participants in rural counties had only one EBP

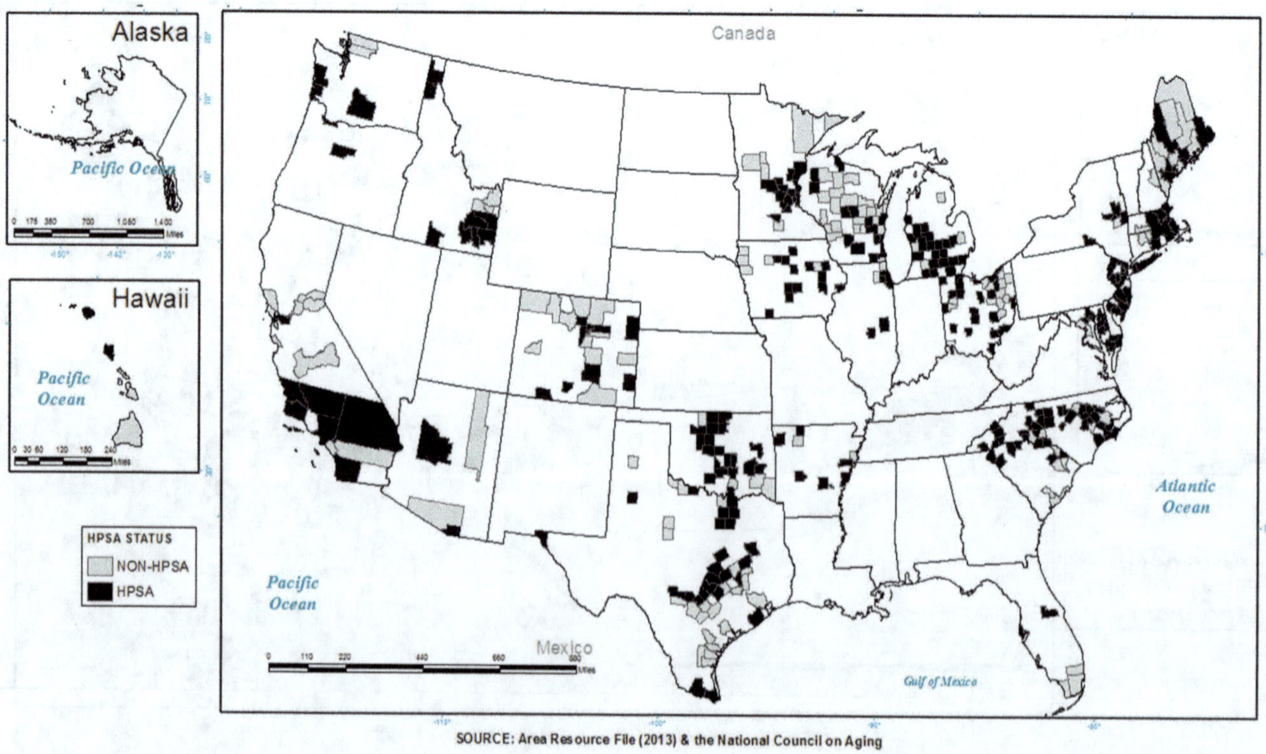

FIGURE 2 | Counties identified as a primary care health professional shortage area (HPSA) with a presence of evidence-based programs.

available to them, and 12.5% had all three programs available in their counties. Approximately 13% of participants within higher poverty areas had all three EBP available in their counties versus 20.8% in areas with lower poverty rates. Among areas that were designated as a full-HPSA, the majority of participants were in areas where one or two EBP were available as compared to 6% in areas where all three EBP were available.

Figure 4 shows the distribution of rural counties that delivered one versus two versus three of the EBP included in this study. As seen, there were very few areas that delivered all three programs (2.3%) and even fewer in rural counties (1.6%), and those that did (i.e., delivered all three programs) were concentrated in just a few states (e.g., AZ, CA, MA, NC, SC, TX).

Table 4 shows the distribution of counties by selected characteristics and programs. Overall, CDSMP was located in the largest number of counties at 419, followed by AMOB/VLL (253), and EF (103). In addition, the majority of counties offering EBP were located in a full or partial-HPSA (see **Table 4**). A higher proportion of the EBP were located in metropolitan areas, as compared to non-metropolitan areas. More counties offering these EBP were also located in lower poverty areas (compared to above the median poverty rate).

DISCUSSION

This study examines the delivery of three EBP delivered to vulnerable individuals (i.e., minority/ethnic individuals, those living in rural or HPSA areas, with low income, and those having one or more chronic conditions or advanced age) within 24 states through the 2006–2009 AoA Evidence-Based Disease and Disability Prevention Initiative and 3 states funded by the Atlantic Philanthropies. The findings reveal that the three EBP reached a substantial percentage of adults who were aged 75 years or older and had incomes below $15,000. The proportion of minority/ethnic participants in each of these three EBP was higher than the current proportion of minority/ethnic adults in US (approximately 22%) in 2012 (51). Additionally, among those with at least one chronic condition, the majority of these participants had comorbid conditions (i.e., two or more chronic conditions) overall and within each program. We note that an overwhelming number of women participated in these programs, which, in part, seems to reflect the larger proportion of women representing the American older adult population. However, this is frequently reported in other national studies of EBP for older adults (16–18, 20). The lower reach to males and ethnic minorities raises questions as to whether the programs lack saliency to specific subpopulations or whether the providers are finding it difficult to find the right strategies to recruit such subpopulations. Further research is needed to explore and examine ways in which nationally coordinated intervention efforts can recruit a greater proportion of diverse populations.

It is not surprising that CDSMP had the largest number of participants, given that all participating states were required to deliver this program, but could add other EBP desired by community partners. The overall distribution of programs (as seen in the figures) illustrates the limited reach within the 27 grantee states during this specific initiative. However, there has been subsequent growth

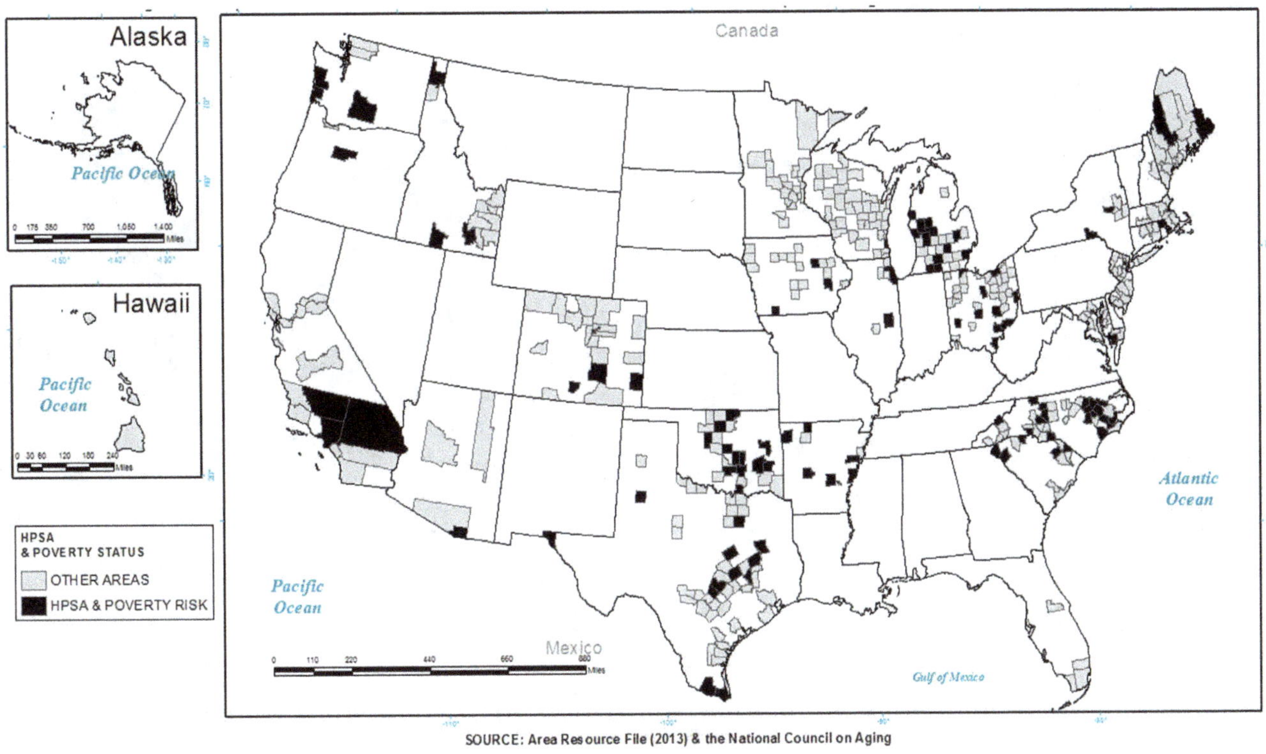

FIGURE 3 | Counties identified as a health professional shortage area, and having higher than the median poverty distribution with the presence of evidence-based programs.

Table 2 | Distribution of counties by availability of multiple evidence-based programs (CDSMP, AMOB/VLL, EF) by health professional shortage area (HPSA), rurality, and poverty status in 2008.

	One program		Two programs		Three programs	
	n	%	*n*	%	*n*	%
HPSA status						
Full-HPSA	183[a]	78.9	43	18.5	6	2.6
Partial-HPSA	159	71.0	57[b]	25.5	8	3.6
Non-HPSA	135[a]	82.8	28[b]	17.2	0	0
Rurality						
Rural	216*	84.4	36*	14.1	4	1.6
Urban	261*	71.9	92	25.3	10	2.8
Poverty rate						
Above median	298*	75.6	85*	21.6	11*	2.8
At/below median	179*	79.6	43*	19.1	3*	1.3
Total	477	77.1	128	20.7	14	2.3

**Significantly ($p < 0.05$) different by characteristic (e.g., rurality).*
[a]Significantly ($p < 0.05$) different non-HPSA versus full-HPSA.
[b]Significantly ($p < 0.05$) different non-HPSA versus partial-HPSA.

Table 3 | Distribution of participants by availability of multiple evidence-based programs (CDSMP, AMOB/VLL, EF) by health professional shortage area (HPSA), rurality, and poverty status in 2008.

	One program		Two programs		Three programs	
	n	%	*n*	%	*n*	%
HPSA status						
Full-HPSA	6,120[a,b]	43.9	6,976[a,b]	50.0	845[b]	6.1
Partial-HPSA	4,477[b,c]	34.7	4,208[b,c]	32.6	4,209[b]	32.6
Non-HPSA	2,577[a,c]	76.9	773[a,c]	23.1	0	0
Rurality						
Rural	3,128*	59.0	1,511*	28.5	662*	12.5
Urban	10,046*	40.4	10,446*	42.0	4,392*	17.7
Poverty rate						
Above median	5,946*	39.7	7,122*	47.6	1,894*	12.7
At/below median	7,228*	47.5	4,835*	31.8	3,160*	20.8
Total	13,174	43.6	11,957	39.6	5,054	16.7

**Significantly ($p < 0.05$) different by characteristic (e.g., rurality).*
[a]Significantly ($p < 0.05$) different non-HPSA versus full-HPSA.
[b]Significantly ($p < 0.05$) different non-HPSA versus partial-HPSA.
[c]Significantly ($p < 0.05$) different partial-HPSA versus full-HPSA.

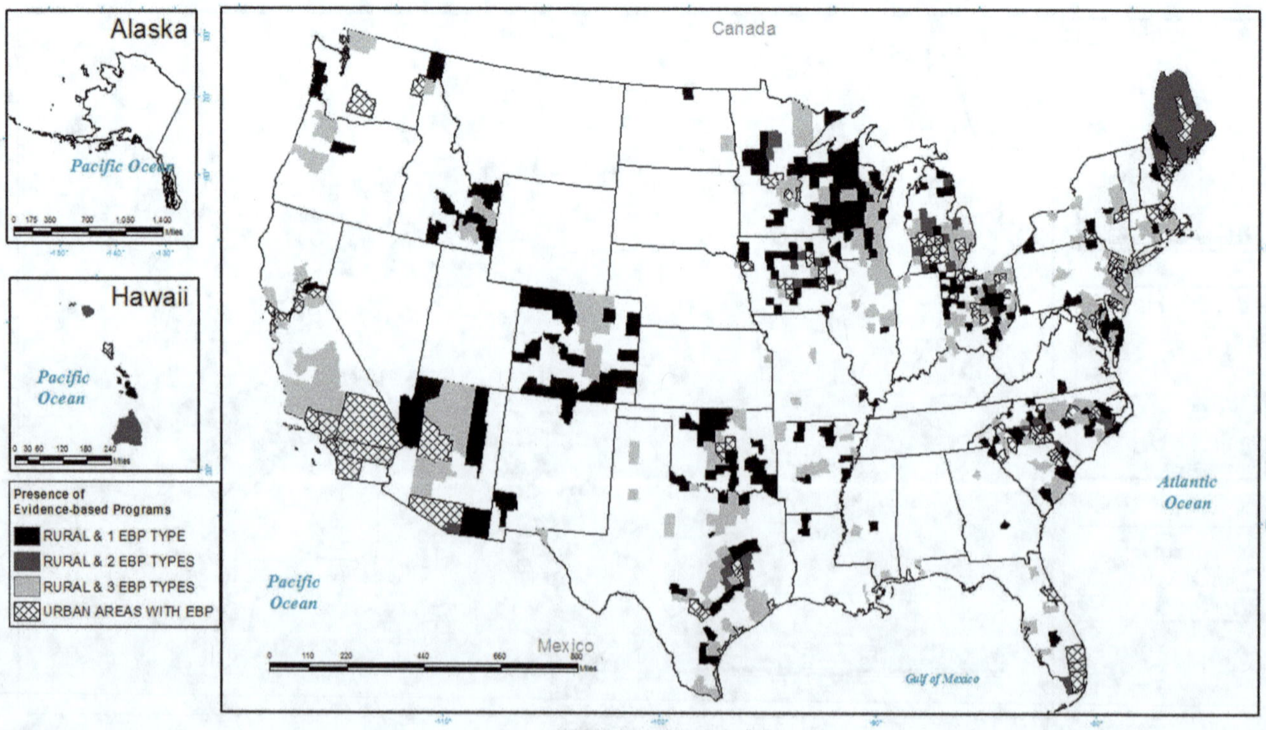

SOURCE: National Council on Aging

FIGURE 4 | Distribution of evidence-based programs (EnhanceFitness, A Matter of Balance/Volunteer Lay Leader Model and the Chronic Disease Self-Management Program) by county and rurality.

in program dissemination and participant reach in recent years. For example, CDSMP was delivered in 27 funded states during the 2006–2009 initiative, but it was delivered in 45 states, the District of Columbia, and Puerto Rico, reaching more than 100,000 older adults from 2010 to 2012 (20). AMOB/VLL was offered in 24 states during 2006–2009, but is now available in over 30 states. Further, EF was delivered in 22 states and is now offered in over 25 states. We recognize that while more states are offering these EBP since the 2006–2009 initiative, there has been variability in their delivery, with some counties increasing their offerings, and others cutting back due to lack of funding.

Having multiple evidence-based interventions available to older adult populations provides an opportunity for better tailoring to the unique needs of seniors with a variety of chronic conditions. Such tailoring may be especially important for the most vulnerable participants (52, 53). Yet, the study data showed that the largest proportion of participants were located in areas where only one program type was offered, regardless of area characteristics. The data also showed that multiple programs are typically less likely to be offered in areas serving the most vulnerable populations (e.g., those living in low income or rural areas and in a HPSA). It was not surprising to find that these areas offered the least number of different programs, as this confirms prior research indicating rural residents have lower access to healthcare services than their urban counterparts (54–56) where there are typically fewer resources and greater distances to providers (57). Drawing from our collective experience implementing and disseminating EBP, we recommend some practical approaches for increasing the delivery of multiple programs in a given area. One approach may include building an infrastructure that can support multiple EBP (58). While the co-ordination of area agency on aging (AAA) funding varies by state (i.e., either centralized or decentralized infrastructure), these EBP may not be capable of reaching certain geographic locations. Moreover, even when communities want to offer these programs, they may not have the program delivery infrastructure to serve the demands in their communities. As such, more research is needed to better understand why states and AAA elect to offer only certain programs, as well as the infrastructure-related challenges associated with EBP delivery (especially as it pertains to multi-program implementation). Further, future research might explore why vulnerable adults only choose to participate in one program despite the potential benefits of participating in multiple programs. Another approach to enhance program delivery capacity could be offering cross-training opportunities for different lay leaders and healthcare professionals so they can lead workshops for multiple programs. Such an approach is being implemented by the Stanford Patient Education Research Center, which offers the suite of chronic disease self-management education programs (Retrieved from http://patienteducation.stanford.edu/training/). Another approach might be to address and solve transportation needs to and from sites offering programs that are often an issue in rural areas.

There were several limitations in the current study. First, this study only examined the three most prevalent EBP being delivered

Table 4 | Distribution of counties by availability of evidence-based programs (CDSMP, AMOB/VLL, EF) by health professional shortage area (HPSA), rurality, and poverty status in 2008.

	CDSMP		AMOB/VLL		EF		CDSMP and AMOB/VLL		CDSMP and EF		AMOB/VLL and EF	
	n	%	*n*	%	*n*	%	*n*	%	*n*	%	*n*	%
HPSA status												
Full-HPSA	165[a]	39.4	90	35.6	32[c]	31.1	37	34.9	12[a]	41.4	12[a]	34.3
Partial-HPSA	149[b]	35.6	97[b]	38.3	51[b, c]	49.5	45[b]	42.5	16[b]	55.2	20[b]	57.1
Non-HPSA	105[a,b]	25.1	66[b]	26.1	20[b]	19.4	24[b]	22.6	1[a,b]	3.5	3[a,b]	8.6
Rurality												
Rural	178*	42.5	81*	32.0	41*	39.8	27*	25.5	8*	27.6	13	37.1
Urban	241*	57.5	172*	68.0	62*	60.2	79*	74.5	21*	72.4	22	62.9
Poverty rate												
Above median	136*	32.5	93*	36.8	45	43.7	31*	29.3	7*	24.1	14	40.0
At/below median	283*	67.5	160*	63.2	58	56.3	75*	70.8	22*	75.9	21	60.0
Total	419		253		103		106		29		35	

**Significantly ($p < 0.05$) different by characteristic (e.g., rurality).*
[a]Significantly ($p < 0.05$) different non-HPSA versus full-HPSA.
[b]Significantly ($p < 0.05$) different non-HPSA versus partial-HPSA.
[c]Significantly ($p < 0.05$) different partial-HPSA versus full-HPSA.

through the AoA Evidence-Based Disease and Disability Prevention Initiative and the Atlantic Philanthropies from 2006 to 2009. While these data are now over 5 years old, no other national database exists; hence, they are particularly powerful for illuminating the two research questions posed in this study. Second, only the three identified programs sponsored by this initiative were included, so that the study does not account for other EBP that might also have been offered by different sponsors. Third, the type of available data and amount of missing data is also a limitation to be acknowledged. In order to reach large numbers of participants being offered EBP through existing community organizations, the amount of required data for this study was limited to a few basic demographic and programmatic factors. Even with this streamlined data collection protocol, there was substantial missing data due to the inability of community providers to systematically collect and release all requested data (e.g., in some healthcare systems providers were not able to release information due to institutional review board restrictions). However, large amounts of missing administrative or programmatic data are not uncommon in evidence-based community interventions (59–62). In addition, analyses that include chronic conditions were limited to data for individuals with one or more chronic conditions. Cases reporting no chronic conditions were omitted because it was impossible to determine whether these cases had no chronic conditions or neglected to respond to these survey items (i.e., missing data). Our analyses do not take into consideration the level of social support among participants; however, future analyses should include this as a possible factor associated with participant outcomes.

Finally, we could not measure the actual penetration among all *possible* participants for these EBP. Future research should examine the extent of reach among those potential participants for these EBP. The cross-sectional nature of the study prevents analysis of trends over time; however, the goal of this study was to measure the overall reach among vulnerable adults, and service delivery characteristics during the initiative period. Future studies should also identify strategies for identifying the dissemination of multiple EBP throughout the US and their interactive impacts on our aging population. At the current time, there is no mechanism for doing so. However, we should look toward a national inventory of EBP for seniors, potentially linked to healthcare utilization outcomes, or community assessments that can track county level changes in health and functioning.

Study findings demonstrate that individually these three EBP have the capacity to appeal to vulnerable populations. Going forward, the challenge is to create an efficient national infrastructure that encourages widespread adoption and bundling of these programs for delivery in underserved populations and areas. Systematical engagement and meaningful involvement of vulnerable populations to fine tune outreach strategies, enhancing linkages with the healthcare system that includes advocating for the importance of evidence-based programing, building marketing strategies and business models, and accelerating adaptation of evidence-based programing are approaches that program administrators, policy makers, and funders can use to continue outreach to vulnerable older adults (63).

New federal initiatives (e.g., Affordable Care Act) (62) are encouraging the aging services network sector to work collaboratively with public health and medical care sectors and other key stakeholders responsible for improving the health and functioning of our rapidly escalating population of older adults with multiple chronic conditions. Growing and sustaining EBP in a diversity of delivery sites that attract a broader range of participants will be critical for achieving a greater population health impact (16).

ACKNOWLEDGMENTS

Administration for Community Living is a primary CDSME workshop funder. Opinions expressed do not necessarily represent official Administration for Community Living policy. The national dissemination of these programs was supported as part of the United States Administration on Aging's Evidence-Based Disease and Disability Prevention program (EBDDP) initiative. In addition to the AoA, this initiative was made possible by partnerships with the Centers for Disease Control and Prevention, Agency for Healthcare Research and Quality (AHRQ), Centers for Medicare and Medicaid Services (CMMS), Health Resources and Services Administration (HRSA), Substance Abuse and Mental Health Services Administration (SAMHSA), and over 30 private foundations. We recognize the support from the AoA with assistance from the National Council on Aging for the evaluation of the EBDDP initiative under co-operative agreement number 90OP0001/01, as well as the Healthy Aging Research Network, funded through the Centers for Disease Control and Prevention's Prevention Research Centers. The findings and conclusions in this article are those of the author(s) and do not necessarily represent the official position of AoA, National Council on Aging, or any other agency. The authors specifically acknowledge the contributions of Nancy Whitelaw, Don Grantt, Wendy Zenker, Kelly Horton, Meghan Thompson, Ashley Wilson, and Linnae Hutchison.

REFERENCES

1. Dall TM, Gallo PD, Chakrabarti R, West T, Semilla AP, Storm MV. An aging population and growing disease burden will require a large and specialized health care workforce by 2025. *Health Aff* (2013) **32**(11):2013–20. doi:10.1377/hlthaff.2013.0714
2. Anderson G. *Chronic Care: Making the Case for Ongoing Care.* Princeton, NJ: Robert Wood Johnson Foundation (2010). Available from: http://www.rwjf.org/content/dam/farm/reports/reports/2010/rwjf54583
3. Yoshida S. *A Global Report on Falls Prevention: Epidemiology of Falls.* World Health Organization (WHO) (2013). Available from: http://www.who.int/ageing/projects/1.Epidemiology%20of%20falls%20in%20older%20age.pdf
4. Carroll NV, Slattum PW, Cox FM. The cost of falls among the community-dwelling elderly. *J Manag Care Pharm* (2005) **11**(4):307–16.
5. Stevens JA, Corso PS, Finkelstein EA, Miller TR. The costs of fatal and non-fatal falls among older adults. *Inj Prev* (2006) **12**(5):290–5. doi:10.1136/ip.2005.011015
6. Roudsari BS, Ebel BE, Corso PS, Molinari NA, Koepsell TD. The acute medical care costs of fall-related injuries among the U.S. older adults. *Injury* (2005) **36**(11):1316–22. doi:10.1016/j.injury.2005.05.024
7. Englander F, Hodson TJ, Terregrossa RA. Economic dimensions of slip and fall injuries. *J Forensic Sci* (1996) **41**(5):733–46.
8. Centers for Disease Control and Prevention. *Falls Among Older Adults: An Overview.* (2014). Available from: http://www.cdc.gov/HomeandRecreationalSafety/Falls/adultfalls.html
9. Centers for Medicare and Medicaid Services. *Chronic Conditions Among Medicare Beneficiaries, Chartbook.* 2012 ed. Baltimore, MD: CMS (2012).
10. Machlin S, Cohen J, Beauregard K. *Health Care Expenses for Adults with Chronic Conditions, 2005.* Rockville, MD: Agency for Healthcare Research and Quality (2008).
11. Wagner EH, Glasgow RE, Davis C, Bonomi AE, Provost L, McCulloch D, et al. Quality improvement in chronic illness care: a collaborative approach. *Jt Comm J Qual Improv* (2001) **27**(2):63–80.
12. Barr VJ, Robinson S, Marin-Link B, Underhill L, Dotts A, Ravensdale D, et al. The expanded chronic care model: an integration of concepts and strategies from population health promotion and the chronic care model. *Hosp Q* (2003) **7**(1):73–82.
13. Bodenheimer T, Lorig K, Holman H, Grumbach K. Patient self-management of chronic disease in primary care. *JAMA* (2002) **288**(19):2469–75. doi:10.1001/jama.288.19.2469
14. Bayliss EA, Steiner JF, Fernald DH, Crane LA, Main DS. Descriptions of barriers to self-care by persons with comorbid chronic diseases. *Ann Fam Med* (2003) **1**(1):15–21. doi:10.1370/afm.4
15. U.S. Department of Health and Human Services. *Healthy People 2020.* (2014). Available from: http://www.healthypeople.gov/2020/default.aspx
16. Smith ML, Belza B, Altpeter M, Ahn S, Dickerson JB, Ory MG. Disseminating an evidence-based disease self-management program for older Americans: implications for diversifying participant reach through delivery site adoption. In: Maddock J, editor. *Public Health: Social and Behavioral Health.* Rijeka, Croatia: InTech (2012).
17. Smith ML, Ory MG, Belza B, Altpeter M. Personal and delivery site characteristics associated with intervention dosage in an evidence-based fall risk reduction program for older adults. *Transl Behav Med* (2012) **2**(2):188–98. doi:10.1007/s13142-012-0133-8
18. Smith ML, Belza B, Braun KL, King S, Palmer RC, Sugihara NS, et al. National reach and dissemination of EnhanceFitness. *Health Behav Policy Rev* (2014) **1**(2):150–60. doi:10.14485/HBPR.1.2.7
19. Ory MG, Smith ML. Exemplifying the evidence-based for health promotion programs across populations and settings. *Family Commun Health* (2012) **35**(3):188–91. doi:10.1097/FCH.0b013e318250bbff
20. Ory MG, Smith ML, Kulinski KP, Lorig K, Zenker W, Whitelaw N. Self-management at the tipping point: reaching 100,000 Americans with evidence-based programs. *J Am Geriatr Soc* (2013) **61**(5):821–3. doi:10.1111/jgs.12239
21. Frank JC, Lau CA. *Empowering Older People to Take More Control of their Health through Evidence-Based Prevention Programs: A Capping Report.* National Council on Aging (2013). Available from: http://www.ncoa.org/improve-health/center-for-healthy-aging/NCOA-Capping-Report_3-26-13_FINAL.pdf
22. Anderson G, Horvath J. The growing burden of chronic disease in America. *Public Health Rep* (2004) **119**(3):263–70.
23. Lasser KE, Himmelstein DU, Woolhandler S. Access to care, health status, and health disparities in the United States and Canada: results of a cross-national population-based survey. *Am J Public Health* (2006) **96**(7):1300–7. doi:10.2105/AJPH.2004.059402
24. Miranda J, Duan N, Sherbourne C, Schoenbaum M, Lagomasino I, Jackson-Triche M, et al. Improving care for minorities: can quality improvement interventions improve care and outcomes for depressed minorities? Results of a randomized, controlled trial. *Health Serv Res* (2003) **38**(2):613–30. doi:10.1111/1475-6773.00136
25. Glover S, Moore CG, Samuels ME, Probst JC. Disparities in access to care among rural working-age adults. *J Rural Health* (2004) **20**(3):193–205. doi:10.1111/j.1748-0361.2004.tb00029.x
26. Gamm L, Hutchison L, Dabney BJ, et al. *Rural Healthy People 2010: A companion document to Healthy People 2010.* College Station, TX: The Texas A&M University System Health Science Center, School of Rural Public Health, Southwest Rural Health Research Center (2003).
27. Norton CH, McManus MA. Background tables on demographic characteristics, health status, and health services utilization. *Health Serv Res* (1989) **23**(6):725–56.
28. Jones CA, Parker TS, Ahearn M, Mishra AK, Variyam JN. *Health Status and Health Care Access of Farm and Rural Populations.* Washington, DC: U.S. Department of Agriculture, Economic Research Service (2009). p. 1–64.
29. Aday LA. *At Risk in America: The Health and Health Care Needs of Vulnerable Populations in the United States.* 2nd ed. San Francisco: Jossey-Bass (2001).
30. Mechanic D, Tanner J. Vulnerable people, groups, and populations: societal view. *Health Aff* (2007) **26**(5):1220–30. doi:10.1377/hlthaff.26.5.1220
31. Lorig KR, Sobel DS, Stewart AL, Brown BW, Bandura A, Ritter P, et al. Evidence suggesting that a chronic disease self-management program can improve health status while reducing hospitalization: a randomized trial. *Med Care* (1999) **37**(1):5–14. doi:10.1097/00005650-199901000-00003
32. Lorig KR, Sobel DS, Ritter PL, Laurent D, Hobbs M. Effect of a self-management program on patients with chronic disease. *Eff Clin Practi* (2001) **4**(6):256–62.
33. Lorig KR, Ritter P, Stewart AL, Sobel DS, Brown BW Jr, Bandura A, et al. Chronic disease self-management program: 2-year health status and health care utilization outcomes. *Med Care* (2001) **39**(11):1217–23. doi:10.1097/00005650-200111000-00008
34. Ory MG, Ahn S, Jiang L, Smith ML, Ritter PL, Whitelaw N, et al. Successes of a national study of the chronic disease self-management program: meeting the triple aim of health care reform. *Med Care* (2013) **51**(11):992–8. doi:10.1097/MLR.0b013e3182a95dd1

35. National Council on Aging. *Center for Healthy Aging: A Matter of Balance.* (2014). Available from: http://www.ncoa.org/improve-health/center-for-healthy-aging/a-matter-of-balance.html
36. Tennstedt S, Howland J, Lachman M, Peterson E, Kasten L, Jette A. A Randomized, controlled trial of a group intervention to reduce fear of falling and associated activity restriction in older adults. *J Gerontol B Psychol Sci Soc Sci* (1998) **53B**(6):384–92. doi:10.1093/geronb/53B.6.P384
37. Healy TC, Peng C, Haynes P, McMahon E, Botler J, Gross L. The feasibility and effectiveness of translating a matter of balance into a volunteer lay leader model. *J Appl Gerontol* (2008) **27**(1):34–51. doi:10.1177/0733464807308620
38. Smith ML, Hochhalter AK, Cheng Y, Wang S, Ory MG. Programmatic influences on outcomes of an evidence-based fall prevention program for older adults: a translational assessment. *Transl Behav Med* (2011) **1**(3):384–93. doi:10.1007/s13142-011-0058-7
39. National Council on Aging. *Center for Healthy Aging. EnhanceFitness.* (2014). Available from: http://www.ncoa.org/improve-health/center-for-healthy-aging/enhance-fi.html
40. Wallace JL, Buchner DM, Grothaus L, Leveille S, Tyll L, LaCroix AZ, et al. Implementation and effectiveness of a community-based health promotion program for older adults. *J Gerontol A Biol Sci Med Sci* (1998) **53A**(4):M301–6. doi:10.1093/gerona/53A.4.M301
41. Ackermann RT, Williams B, Nguyen HQ, Berke EM, Maciejewski ML, LoGerfo JP. Healthcare cost differences with participation in a community-based group physical activity benefit for medicare managed care health plan members. *J Am Geriatr Soc* (2008) **56**:1459–65. doi:10.1111/j.1532-5415.2008.01804.x
42. Area Health Resources Files (ARF). *US Department of Health and Human Services, Health Resources and Services Administration, Bureau of Health Professions.* Rockville, MD (2013).
43. Health Resources and Services Administration. *Health Professional Shortage Areas (HPSAs).* (2014). Available from: http://bhpr.hrsa.gov/shortage/hpsas/designationcriteria/index.html
44. USDA Economic Research Service. *Urban Influence Codes.* (2014). Available from: http://www.ers.usda.gov/data-products/urban-influence-codes.aspx#.U-_DNPldWa8
45. ESRI Inc. *ArcGIS: Release 10.2 by ESRI Inc.* Redlands, CA: Environmental Systems Research Institute. Copyright © 1999–2013.
46. SAS Institute Inc. *SAS 9.4 by SAS Institute Inc.* Cary, NC: Copyright © 2002–2013.
47. Health Resources and Services Administration. *Primary Medical Care HPSA Designation Overview.* (2014). Available from: http://bhpr.hrsa.gov/shortage/hpsas/designationcriteria/primarycarehpsaoverview.html
48. Health Resources and Services Administration. *Primary Medical Care HPSA Designation Criteria: Part 1 – Geographic Areas.* (2014). Available from: http://bhpr.hrsa.gov/shortage/hpsas/designationcriteria/primarycarehpsacriteria.html
49. United States Department of Agriculture Economic Research Service. Available from: http://www.ers.usda.gov/data-products/urban-influence-codes.aspx#.UwahVfldV8E
50. Kulinski KP, Boutaugh M, Smith ML, Ory MG, Lorig K. Setting the stage: measure selection, coordination, and data collection for a national self-management initiative. *Front Public Health* (2015) **2**:206. doi:10.3389/fpubh.2014.00206
51. US Census Bureau. *State and County QuickFacts. USA People Quickfacts.* (2014). Available from: http://quickfacts.census.gov/qfd/states/00000.html
52. Mier N, Ory MG, Toobert D, Smith ML, Osuna D, McKay J, et al. A qualitative case study examining intervention tailoring for minorities. *Am J Health Behav* (2010) **34**(6):822–32.
53. Community Research Center for Senior Health in Partnership. *Toolkit on Evidence-Based Programming for Seniors.* Available from: http://www.evidencetoprograms.com/
54. Council on Graduate Medical Education. *Physician Distribution and Health Care Challenges in Rural and Inner City Areas: Tenth Report to Congress and the Department of Health and Human Services Secretary.* Rockville, MD: Health Resources and Services Administration, US Dept of Health and Human Services (1998).
55. Knapp KK, Paavola FG, Maine LL, Sorofman B, Politzer RM. Availability of primary care providers and pharmacists in the United States. *J Am Pharm Assoc* (1999) **39**(2):127–35.
56. MacDowell M, Glasser M, Fitts M, Nielsen K, Hunsaker M. A national view of rural health workforce issues in the USA. *Rural Remote Health* (2010) **10**(3):1531.
57. Towne SD, Smith ML, Ory MG. Geographic variations in access and utilization of cancer screening services: examining disparities among American Indian and Alaska native elders. *Int J Health Geogr* (2014) **13**:18. doi:10.1186/1476-072X-13-18
58. Scheirer MA. Is sustainability possible? A review and commentary on empirical studies of program sustainability. *Am J Eval* (2005) **26**(3):320–47. doi:10.1177/1098214005278752
59. Edwards KE, Gibson N, Martin J, Mitchell S, Andersson N. Impact of community-based interventions on condom use in the Tłicho region of Northwest Territories, Canada. *BMC Health Serv Res* (2011) **11**(Suppl 2):S9. doi:10.1186/1472-6963-11-S2-S9
60. Mayworm AM, Sharkey JD. Gender-specific mental health outcomes of a community-based delinquency intervention. *J Juv Justice* (2013) **3**(1).
61. Temel S, van Voorst SF, Jack BW, Denktas S, Steegers EA. Evidence-based preconceptional lifestyle interventions. *Epidemiol Rev* (2014) **36**(1):19–30. doi:10.1093/epirev/mxt003
62. *Report to Congress: The Centers for Medicare & Medicaid Services' Evaluation of Community-based Wellness and Prevention Programs under Section 4202 (b) of the Affordable Care Act.* (2014). Available from: http://www.projectenhance.org/Portals/40/Docs/RTC_CommunityBasedWellnessPrograms.pdf
63. Altpeter M, Schneider EC, Whitelaw N. Fostering engagement and independence: opportunities and challenges for an aging society. *Health Educ Behav* (2014) (in press).

28

Fit & Strong! promotes physical activity and well-being in older cancer survivors

Jana Reynolds[1,2]*, **Lorie Thibodeaux**[1,3], **Luohua Jiang**[4], **Kevin Francis**[1] **and Angie Hochhalter**[1]

[1] Baylor Scott & White Health, Temple, TX, USA
[2] Baylor Charles A. Sammons Cancer Center, Baylor University Medical Center at Dallas, Dallas, TX, USA
[3] Seton Medical Center, Austin, TX, USA
[4] School of Rural Public Health, Texas A&M Health Science Center, College Station, TX, USA

Edited by:
Matthew Lee Smith, University of Georgia, USA

Reviewed by:
Emily Joy Nicklett, University of Michigan, USA
Samuel D. Towne, University of South Carolina, USA

***Correspondence:**
Jana Reynolds, Departments of Internal Medicine and Oncology and Hematology, Baylor Charles A. Sammons Cancer Center, Baylor University Medical Center at Dallas, 3410 Worth Street, Dallas, TX 75246, USA
e-mail: jana.reynolds@baylorhealth.edu

Introduction: Physical activity reduces fatigue and depression while improving quality of life in cancer survivors. Exercise is generally considered safe and is recommended to survivors of all ages. Despite the high prevalence of cancer in the elderly, few studies address physical activity interventions targeting this older population. Fit & Strong! is an evidence-based physical activity program shown to improve level of physical activity, exercise-self-efficacy, and mood in older adults with osteoarthritis. This study tests the feasibility and short-term impact of the Fit & Strong! exercise program adapted for older cancer survivors.

Methods: Participants were cancer survivors at least 50 years of age who were not on active treatment with intravenous chemotherapy or radiation. They participated in the 8-week Fit & Strong! program, which included three 90-min sessions per week; 60 min of group physical activity and 30 min of education. Education on osteoarthritis was removed from the Fit & Strong! program and replaced with relevant topics on cancer survivorship issues. Feasibility was measured by the ability to recruit and retain older cancer survivors. Pre and post-intervention surveys evaluated the effect of the intervention on physical activity and quality of life.

Results: The study enrolled 72 cancer survivors to participate in an 8-week exercise program. The mean age of participants was 70. Over two-thirds (68%) of participants completed the program and with a mean attendance rate of 75% (18 of 24 sessions). No safety issues occurred. Improvements from baseline to post-intervention were observed for self-reported minutes of physical activity per week, self-efficacy for aerobic exercise, and symptoms related to depression and anxiety.

Conclusion: This study was successful in recruiting and retaining a population of older cancer survivors to participate in a group exercise program. Significant improvement in level of physical activity and mood suggests this evidence-based physical activity intervention can be adapted to promote health benefits in cancer survivors. Additional studies are necessary to confirm efficacy and assess long-term benefits.

Keywords: evidenced based intervention, older cancer survivors, physical activity, exercise, cancer survivorship

INTRODUCTION

With early cancer detection and greater availability of curative therapy, 64% of cancer survivors in the United States are living five or more years after cancer diagnosis (1, 2). As the number of long-term survivors continues to increase, so has the recognition of negative late and long-term health effects of cancer and cancer treatment (2, 3). It is well documented that once cancer survivors complete their initial treatment, many face persistent fatigue, depression, fear of recurrence, and long-term physical effects of treatment (3–7). Thus, finding ways to combat these long-term health effects in cancer survivors is of paramount importance.

One way to address these long-term effects of cancer and cancer treatment is through increased physical activity. Physical activity in cancer survivors reduces fatigue and depression while improving quality of life (8–12), and at the same time has been shown to be safe in this population (13). It is recommended that cancer survivors of all ages participate in a combination of strength training and moderate aerobic exercise (such as brisk walking) for at least 150 min per week, or to the best of their physical ability. These guidelines are similar to those recommended for the general population (13, 14). Additionally, results from observational studies suggest that participation in physical activity before and/or after diagnoses of certain cancers may serve as a potential preventive measure against recurrence and mortality (4, 15–19).

In the United States, nearly 90% of cancer survivors are aged 50 and older (88%), with persons aged 70 and older accounting for almost half (46%) of all cancer survivors (2). Despite the frequency of cancer in the elderly, the majority of studies targeting physical activity in cancer survivors either exclude or do not achieve high levels of participation from older cancer survivors (20, 21). Given the prevalence of cancer in the older population and lack of evidence-based physical activity programs engaging this population, this study aims to test a group exercise intervention targeting older cancer survivors.

This study chose Fit & Strong!, an evidence-based physical activity program for older adults with osteoarthritis, to adapt to a population of older cancer survivors. The program is a combination of group exercise and education/support. In randomized controlled trials, Fit & Strong! significantly increased participation in physical activity while decreasing levels of anxiety and depression and reducing symptoms of osteoarthritis in adults older than 60 (22–24). We chose to use the Fit & Strong! program because of its relative low cost and ease of reproducibility. Additionally, the program adapts to the abilities of individual participants and thus would be reasonable to implement in a population of older cancer survivors with differing capacities for exercise. The program includes basic education on exercise with the goal of sustainability through a continued home-based program (22–24). Our adaptation replaces the osteoarthritis specific educational curriculum with education addressing important cancer survivorship issues.

The primary aim of the study was to evaluate the feasibility of recruiting and retaining older survivors to participate in an 8-week group exercise intervention and education program. The secondary aim was to test the short-term impact of the Fit & Strong! intervention on self-reported physical activity, self-efficacy for exercise, and quality of life.

MATERIALS AND METHODS

PARTICIPANTS

Participants were eligible for this study if they (1) were 50 years of age or older, (2) had a previous diagnosis of cancer, (3) were not on active cancer treatment such as chemotherapy or radiation, and (4) were self-reported able to engage in light-to-moderate physical activity. Although the intention was to target older cancer survivors (i.e., 65 years of age and up), we chose to allow participants 50 years and older. This age allowance was in recognition that some younger patients with lower functional status, either at baseline or due to cancer or treatment effects, similarly might benefit from the intervention. There was no restriction on type of cancer or years since cancer diagnosis for patient eligibility. Individuals taking oral hormonal or biologic treatments for their cancer were allowed to participate at the discretion of the physician investigator (Jana Reynolds). This study was approved by the Institutional Review Board of Scott & White Healthcare.

RECRUITMENT

Participants were recruited by advertisement put in the local newspaper and flyers placed at senior centers, community cancer survivorship events, and local oncology clinics. The mode of recruitment that generated the most interest in our program, located in rural Central Texas, was newspaper advertisement. Interested individuals contacted the program coordinator and were screened by phone survey to determine whether they met eligibility criteria. Those who met enrollment criteria were invited to participate in the study by enrolling in one of five courses. Participants gave their consent and official enrollment occurred during the first session of each course.

COURSE SETTING

The intervention was offered as an 8-week exercise course with three 90-min sessions per week, for a total of 24 sessions. Approximately 60 min of each session was dedicated to physical activity, and 30 min was dedicated to education. Each course was conducted in a group setting with a goal class size of 8–20 participants. A total of five courses were offered between January 2013 and August 2013. The first course was conducted in a large conference room in a medical office building. Due a higher than anticipated number of participants, the subsequent four courses were offered in a larger aerobics room at a local health center.

SAFETY

All participants were encouraged to consider consulting with a physician prior to beginning of the program. During the eligibility screening phone calls, participants were screened for the presence of specific medical conditions including recent joint surgery or current rehabilitation for joint surgery, known cancer metastases to bone (indicating higher risk of fracture), or history of cardiac disease. Interested participants with these or any other health-related concerns were required to contact their physician to discuss participation prior to enrollment. They were prompted to describe the course as "mild to moderate physical activity that includes walking and light weight lifting," and ask if there were particular types of activities they should avoid. All course instructors were certified in Basic Life Support.

ADAPTATION OF FIT & STRONG! EXERCISE INTERVENTION

Prior to enrolling participants, a license to conduct the Fit & Strong! program was obtained through the Fit & Strong! program office (Institute for Health Research and Policy at the University of Illinois at Chicago). Additionally, our two instructors completed a Fit & Strong! Master Training Program. Fit & Strong! Master Training instruction provided 8 h of education on topics including appropriate types of exercises for older adults and how to implement Fit & Strong! in the community setting. The program supplied instructional manuals for the instructors to follow when facilitating Fit & Strong! courses. In addition to this training, our two instructors held certifications in Chronic Disease Self-Management (Stanford CDSMP). They were experienced in leading group discussion of health behaviors among adults, but our instructors had limited experience leading group exercise activities. At least one of our two trained instructors and one assistant facilitated each 90 min session.

Participants had exercise equipment available as recommended by Fit & Strong! This equipment included resistance bands for arm exercises, 10 pound adjustable ankle weights for leg exercises, and mats for floor-based exercises. Chairs were available for sitting exercises or for those who required modification to their exercise program. Unique to our study, those participating in courses at the local health center had the option to use exercise machines, such as treadmills and stationary bikes, for the aerobics portion of the class.

Fifty to 60 min of each 90-min class session was dedicated to aerobic and strength-training activities. The complete instructor-led exercise routine consisted of a 5- to 15-min warm-up with stretching, 15–20 min of an aerobic activity, 15–20 min of resistance training, and a 5-min cool-down session. Resistance-training exercises followed those recommended in the Fit & Strong! instructor handbook (i.e., leg lifts while seated in a chair). The aerobic component consisted of sustained walking and a low-impact aerobics routine created by our instructors. Each session used this complete exercise routine in the same sequence. Fit & Strong! trained instructors monitored participants and made adaptations of exercises as needed to match participant abilities.

Thirty minutes of each 90-min class session was dedicated to education designed to increase self-efficacy for exercise and exercise adherence (23, 24). The exercise education curriculum was taught by our instructors and a Fit & Strong! manual was provided to each participant for reference during each class. Information on the components of an exercise program and exercise safety was presented (**Table 1**). Participants engaged in group problem-solving activities and set physical activity goals. Two educational sessions specific to osteoarthritis were removed from the original Fit & Strong! curriculum for our program because they were not applicable to all cancer survivors.

Table 1 | Sample course curriculum.

Session	**Fit & Strong! exercise curriculum** **Source: Fit & Strong participant manual (http://www.fitandstrong.org/index.html)**	**Cancer survivorship curriculum** **Source: NCI facing forward: life after cancel treatment (25)**
1	Introduction, consent, and baseline survey	
2	Introduction to Fit & Strong (Ch 1)	Definition of survivorship (preface) and finding a new "Normal" (p. 1)
3	Benefits and barriers of exercise (Ch 2)	Follow-up medical care (pp. 2–5)
4	What to wear (Ch 3)	
5	Pain and exercise modifications (Ch 6)	Creating a wellness plan (pp. 5–11)
6	Warm-up exercises (Ch 7)	Services and community resources (pp. 12–13)
7	Stretching (Ch 8)	Nutrition for cancer survivors[a]
8	Aerobic exercise (Ch 9)	
9		Treatment effects, Part I: fatigue, memory, and concentration (pp. 15–19)
10	Walking (Ch 10)	Treatment effects, Part II: pain and physical changes (pp. 20–31)
11	Strengthening exercise (Ch 11)	
12	Resistance training (Ch 12)	Managing your feelings: stress, depression, anxiety (pp. 37–45)
13	Cool-down exercises (Ch 13)	Finding a meaning (pp. 46–48) and making a difference after Cancer[b]
14	Posture and bone health (Ch 14)	
15	Fall prevention (Ch 15)	Social and work relationships (pp. 49–55)
16	Setting goals (Ch 16)	
17	Other ways to do exercise (Ch17)	Learning to relax: instructor guided relaxation exercise no. 1 (p. 60)
18	Lifestyle changes (Ch 18)	
19	Exercise: a world of options (Ch 19)	Support for caregivers[c]
20	Getting past barriers to exercise (Ch 20)	
21	Diet and exercise (Ch 21)	
22	Stress management (Ch 22)	Learning to relax: instructor guided relaxation exercise no. 2 (pp. 60–61)
23	Maintaining an active lifestyle (Ch 23)	Feedback session on survivorship component
24	Putting it all together (Ch 24) and survey	

Each 90 min session included 60 min of exercise and 30 min of education. A sample schedule for the educational component is listed above. All chapters/page numbers refer to the source listed in heading unless otherwise noted.

[a] *National Cancer Institute: "Eating hints; Before, During, and After Cancer Treatment" pp.44–45 (26).*

[b] *National Cancer Institute: "Facing Forward. Making a difference in cancer" (27).*

[c] *National Cancer Institute: "Facing Forward: when someone you love has completed cancer treatment" (28).*

SURVIVORSHIP EDUCATION COMPONENT OF THE FIT & STRONG! PROGRAM

The adaptation of the Fit & Strong! program tested in this study replaced the original education on osteoarthritis with cancer-related topics. The content for cancer survivorship education came from the National Cancer Institute's *Facing Forward* series along with additional materials from the National Cancer Institute (25–29). Topics included the long-term effects of cancer treatment, self-management of the long-term physical and psychosocial effects of cancer and cancer treatment, nutrition for cancer survivors, support for the caregiver, seeking follow-up medical care, and ways to make a difference after cancer (**Table 1**). Participants were provided copies of the printed materials to reference in class, and if desired, to keep for future reference.

Trained Fit & Strong! instructors incorporated the cancer survivorship materials during the 30 min educational sessions. They presented information from the handouts and then facilitated the group discussion. Clinicians specializing in the cancer care field were invited to teach the cancer-specific curriculum in two to four sessions for each course (Jana Reynolds, Kevin Francis). Participants with cancer-specific questions beyond the scope of the course materials were encouraged to ask their oncologist or health care provider.

OUTCOME MEASURES

The primary aim of feasibility of Fit & Strong! for older cancer survivors was measured by the course completion rate. Participants were considered to have successfully completed the study if they filled out a survey at baseline and course completion, predefined as within 1 week of the 24th (final) session. Instructors documented attendance and calculated the total number of sessions attended by each participant. Self-reported demographics and disease characteristics were obtained at baseline to describe the population and identified potential characteristics of likely participants for similar studies. These data included gender, age, weight, height, ethnicity, race, marital status, employment status, type of cancer, time since treatment completion, and whether one considered if they are living with active cancer (yes/no).

The secondary aim of the study was to test the short-term impact of the intervention on exercise and quality of life. This aim was measured by changes in baseline and post-intervention surveys comparing minutes of physical activity, self-efficacy for exercise, and cancer-related quality of life. The surveys are as follows:

Minutes of physical activity

Participants reported the number of days in the past 7 days and they did moderate to strenuous exercise. They also reported how many minutes, on average, they exercised per day. Physical activity time per week was calculated by multiplying the reported days by the reported minutes, similar to the original Fit & Strong! study (22–24).

Self-efficacy for exercise

Self-efficacy for exercise was measured on a three item scale developed Lorig and colleagues (30). Participants reported their confidence to do frequent aerobic exercise, frequent strengthening exercise, and confidence to participate in exercise without making their symptoms (of chronic disease) worse. This was reported on a 10 point scale of "not at all confident" (score of 1) to "totally confident" (score of 10). A calculation of the mean rating across the three questions determined the score on this measure. This measure showed improvement in exercise-self-efficacy at 2, 6, and 12 months for participants with osteoarthritis in the original Fit & Strong! intervention (22–24).

Cancer-related quality of life

Participants completed the quality of life in adult cancer survivors (QLACS) survey, a 47-item questionnaire with five cancer-specific and seven generic domains. This survey captures issues affecting long-term cancer survivors rather than acute cancer or cancer treatment-related effects. Cancer-related domains of the survey include concerns with appearance, financial problems, distress over recurrence, family-related distress, and benefits of cancer. Generic domains include negative feelings, positive feelings, cognitive problems, physical pain, fatigue, and social avoidance. The scores of each domain and a summary score of the cancer-related (seven items) and generic domains (four items, benefits of cancer not included in the summary score) were reported (31).

At course completion, a course evaluation survey captured the participant's satisfaction with the exercise and cancer-specific portions of the program. It allowed participants to provide suggestions for improvement. The intention of this survey was to provide feedback for future studies.

STATISTICAL ANALYSIS

Participant characteristics at baseline and the study completion rate used descriptive statistics. The impact of the intervention on exercise efficacy, physical activity, and quality of life was assessed using paired t-tests. Significance was defined as $p \leq 0.05$.

RESULTS

Seventy-two (72) cancer survivors participated in one of five courses offered as part of this study, with an average of 14 participants per 8-week course. The mean age of participants was 70.4 (±13.3) years. Forty-nine of the 72 participants completed the course, for a 68% retention rate. The mean number of sessions attended by those who completed the course was 18 out of 24 (75%).

Participant characteristics are illustrated in **Table 2**. The majority of participants were female (82%). The average BMI at baseline was 29.08 (±6.79), with 40% of participants considered obese (BMI 30 or greater). Patients with 18 types of cancer were represented in the study, with the majority (52%) of participants reporting a prior breast cancer diagnosis. Almost half the participants (46%) had been diagnosed and completed cancer treatment at least 5 years prior, with a median time since treatment of 7 years. Though not on active intravenous chemotherapy or radiation per study protocol, six participants (8%) considered themselves to have active cancer during the study.

Participants significantly increased their weekly total minutes of moderate to strenuous exercise from baseline to post-intervention (94.1 vs. 131.5 min, $p = 0.0005$). Their overall

Table 2 | Participant demographics and cancer history.

	N (%)
Age	
<70	37 (52.11)
≥70	34 (47.89)
Sex	
Male	13 (18.06)
Female	59 (81.94)
Race	
White	61 (89.71)
Other	7 (10.29)
Martial Status	
Married	37 (54.41)
Not married	31 (45.59)
Employment Status	
Employed	8 (12.12)
Not employed	58 (87.88)
BMI	
<20	3 (4.41)
20–25	20 (29.41)
25–30	18 (26.47)
30–35	17 (25.00)
35+	10 (14.71)
Type of Cancer	
Breast	37 (52.11)
Colon	5 (7.04)
Prostate	5 (7.04)
Lung	4 (5.63)
Other[a]	20 (28.17)
Time since completion of cancer treatment	
<1 year	14 (20.90)
1–5 years	22 (32.84)
5+ years	31 (46.27)
Participants who consider themselves to have active cancer	
No	66 (91.67)
Yes	6 (8.33)

[a]*Hodgkin's lymphoma, non-Hodgkin's lymphoma, chronic leukemia, multiple myeloma, adenoid cystic cancer, gastrointestinal stromal tumor, bladder, kidney, pancreatic, thyroid, ovarian, uterine, cervical, and vulvar cancer.*

self-efficacy for exercise (i.e., average of the three self-efficacy for exercise items) did not differ from baseline to post-intervention ($p=0.0964$). However, in the measure of self-efficacy for doing for aerobic exercise regularly, participants showed significant improvement in their ratings from baseline to post-intervention ($M_{\text{Baseline}}=7.94$, $M_{\text{Post-intervention}}=8.85$; $p=0.05$) (**Table 3**).

Participants' scores on the generic and cancer-specific subscale of the QLACS survey did not differ from baseline to post-intervention ($p=0.0770$ and $p=0.9303$, respectively). Nonetheless, an improvement in scores on the negative feeling domain (questions related to anxiety and depression) was observed from baseline to post-intervention ($p=0.0198$) (**Table 4**).

In a post-intervention survey of the utility of the course and the cancer-specific education, 79% reported learning something helpful about cancer survivorship that they did not know before starting our course. Sixty-eight percent of participants reported sharing the information on support for caregivers with a friend or a family member. Some enjoyed meeting others with similar experiences and took pleasure in sharing information. All respondents stated that they would recommend the course to another cancer survivor.

One of the survivors thought the survivorship discussions were too emotional. Another reported feeling uncomfortable during voluntary group discussion, preferring more privacy regarding cancer survivorship issues. Some desired a longer exercise course or to be allowed to repeat the course again. Though participants were encouraged to set goals and create a plan for sustained exercise beyond the program, many wanted to continue within the current group setting.

DISCUSSION

Despite the known physical and emotional benefits of exercise in cancer survivors, the majority of studies targeting physical activity in this population either exclude or do not achieve high levels of participation from older cancer survivors (20, 21). Our study was successful in recruiting a population of older cancer survivors with a mean age of 70. The 68% retention rate and 75% session attendance rate is indicative of an intervention individuals were willing to engage in over time. These results support the feasibility of recruiting and retaining older cancer survivors to participate in an 8-week group exercise intervention and education program.

Our study utilized Fit & Strong!, an evidence-based physical activity intervention for older adults with osteoarthritis, as it previously showed long-term physical activity benefits in older adults with a mean age of 73 (23, 24). Hughes and colleagues observed similar retention rate (72%) and attendance (79% of sessions) in their original Fit & Strong! for osteoarthritis study (23). Our study kept the same physical activity content and adapted the educational component of Fit & Strong! by replacing osteoarthritis education with education on common issues facing cancer survivors. No major safety issues were reported.

Participants in our study showed improvement in level of physical activity and mood, supporting the short-term efficacy of Fit & Strong! when adapted to a population of older cancer survivors. Participants successfully increased their self-reported weekly minutes of physical activity from 94.1 minutes at the beginning of the study to 131.5 minutes at the end of the 8-week intervention (**Table 3**). Participants showed significant improvement in the negative feeling domain of the cancer-related quality of life assessment (QLACS), though not in overall quality of life (**Table 4**). The questions in the negative feeling domain address depression and anxiety, which are reported more commonly in cancer survivors and should be a specific measure in future studies (3, 4).

Participants also improved exercise-self-efficacy specific to aerobic activity; however, no changes were observed in overall exercise-self-efficacy (**Table 3**). This is in contrast to the findings of the original Fit & Strong! intervention in which participants

Table 3 | Intervention impact on exercise efficacy and total minutes of physical activity by paired *t*-test.

	Baseline (*n* = 72) Mean (±SD)	Post (*n* = 49) Mean (±SD)	Paired change (*n* = 49) Mean (±SD)	*t*	*p*
1. Confidence to do strength and flexibility exercises 3–4 times a week	8.68 (±1.75)	9.19 (±1.50)	0.45 (±1.86)	1.64	0.1069
2. Confidence to do aerobic exercises 3–4 times a week	7.94 (±2.45)	8.85 (±1.96)	0.69 (±2.37)	2.01	**0.0503**
3. Confidence to exercise without making symptoms (of chronic disease) worse	8.51 (±1.98)	8.60 (±2.20)	0.10 (±2.26)	0.32	0.7511
Overall self-efficacy for exercise (mean of 1–3)	8.39 (±1.73)	8.88 (±1.67)	0.41 (±1.69)	1.70	0.0964
Total minutes of physical activity	94.10 (±87.02)	131.51 (±91.01)	42.22 (±73.80)	3.79	**0.0005**

Bold text indicates statistically significant values ($p \leq 0.05$).

Table 4 | Intervention impact on Quality of Life (QLACS scale) by paired *t*-test.

	Baseline (*n*=72) Mean (±SD)	Post (*n*=49) Mean (±SD)	Paired change (*n*=49) Mean (±SD)	*t*	*p*-value
GENERIC QOL					
Negative feelings[a]	10.18 (±4.40)	9.22 (±3.62)	−1.27 (±3.17)	−2.44	**0.0198**
Positive feelings	10.26 (±4.69)	10.32 (±4.72)	−0.72 (±3.85)	−1.17	0.2509
Cognitive problems	10.47 (±4.02)	10.43 (±3.53)	0.04 (±3.11)	0.10	0.9241
Sexual problems	11.83 (±6.49)	10.29 (±5.55)	−1.59 (±4.81)	−1.78	0.0864
Energy/fatigue	14.81 (±2.81)	14.67 (±4.21)	0.15 (±4.83)	0.21	0.8319
Pain	11.66 (±5.74)	11.00 (±5.52)	−0.54 (±4.95)	−0.69	0.4912
Social avoidance	9.11 (±5.19)	8.57 (±3.73)	0.12 (±3.14)	0.25	0.8049
Generic summary score	77.42 (±24.99)	73.03 (±18.56)	−8.52 (±22.03)	−1.86	0.0770
CANCER-SPECIFIC QOL					
Financial problems	7.00 (±4.75)	6.48 (±4.78)	0.30 (±2.46)	0.80	0.4308
Benefits	19.24 (±6.24)	19.49 (±6.36)	0.51 (±4.38)	0.77	0.4483
Distress-family	9.43 (±5.61)	8.80 (±5.00)	−0.18 (±3.92)	−0.30	0.7621
Appearance	8.80 (±5.70)	8.48 (±4.82)	0.04 (±3.91)	0.08	0.9395
Distress-recurrence	12.79 (±6.33)	12.91 (±6.09)	−0.21 (±3.26)	−0.42	0.6755
Cancer-specific summary score	37.95 (±16.88)	36.89 (±14.81)	−0.12 (±8.87)	−0.09	0.9303

[a] *Questions in the negative feeling domain (1) bothered by mood swings, (2) felt blue or depressed, (3) worried about little things, and (4) felt anxious.*
Bold text indicates statistically significant values ($p \leq 0.05$).

with osteoarthritis showed improvement on the overall exercise-self-efficacy scale at 2, 6, and 12 months (22, 23). One explanation of the variation between the studies is that the self-efficacy scale is more specific to persons with symptoms of osteoarthritis. The item "confidence to do exercise without making symptoms of chronic disease worse" may be more relevant to osteoarthritis pain symptoms rather than a population of cancer survivors with a wide variation of chronic symptoms. A self-efficacy scale examining perceived ability to do exercise without a focus on symptomatology of chronic disease may be more appropriate for cancer survivors.

This study had several limitations. First, this study was not designed to test long-term effects of the intervention on physical activity, self-efficacy, or cancer-related quality of life. Studies of long-term efficacy and sustained benefits will be necessary to establish whether this program is likely to have meaningful impact on outcomes for cancer survivors beyond the 8-week intervention. Second, the study did not measure the effects of the intervention on actual physical health or function; outcomes were limited to self-reported measures. Future studies should consider tests of the intervention effects using direct measures of physical health and function.

Additionally, participants did not meet the 150 minutes of physical activity per week as recommended in the guidelines (13, 14). Though it is reasonable for capable participants to strive to this goal, it may not be necessary to gain benefits of exercise. In a separate study of older cancer survivors, an increase in minutes of physical activity over baseline but to less than a total of 150 minutes per week still showed measurable functional and health-related benefits (32).

Despite the limitations of this study, the majority of the feedback on the program was positive. Most participants indicated that they would recommend a similar course to other survivors. Many participants expressed appreciation for meeting other cancer survivors and sharing experiences. Most participants in our study were female (82%), suggesting this type of group intervention may be of particular interest to females. Almost half of the participants were at least 5 years post-cancer treatment, indicating older cancer survivors are interested in a cancer-related exercise program long after they finish their treatment (**Table 2**). Cancer survivors undergoing therapy were excluded from the protocol for the purpose of keeping baseline characteristics similar and to minimize conflicts between class times and cancer treatment schedules. Given that exercise is safe for most patients while undergoing treatment, it would be reasonable to include them in future programs (20).

Anecdotally, many participants reported a desire to continue the course indefinitely as their primary exercise program. The Fit & Strong! intervention focuses primarily on initiating an exercise routine that could be sustained in one's home after course completion. The original version was not designed to continue in a group setting. Cancer survivors may benefit from an additional adaptation that helps participants find appropriate community-based group exercise programs with social support similar to the Fit & Strong! program. It would also be reasonable to consider monthly maintenance classes open to all graduates to help inspire and refocus exercise goals for long-term sustainability of benefits.

CONCLUSION

Results of this pilot study support the feasibility of implementing an 8-week exercise intervention for older cancer survivors. Short-term efficacy of the Fit & Strong! program was noted from baseline to the end of the 8-week intervention by increases in minutes of physical activity, increased self-efficacy for aerobic exercise, and decreased negative feelings in the quality of life (QLACS) scale. Tests of efficacy and effectiveness over time are needed to determine the utility of this intervention as a program to promote sustained physical activity among older cancer survivors and support long-term health outcomes.

REFERENCES

1. Frieden TR, Jaffe HW, Stephens JW, Thacker SB, Zaza S, Centers for Disease Control and Prevention (CDC). Cancer Survivors – United States, 2007. *MMWR Morb Mortal Wkly Rep* (2011) **60**(9):269–72.
2. American Cancer Society. *Cancer Treatment and Survivorship Facts & Figures 2014 – 2015.* Atlanta: American Cancer Society (2014).
3. Stein KD, Syrjala KL, Andrykowski MA. Physical and psychological long-term and late effects of cancer. *Cancer* (2008) **112**:2577–92. doi:10.1002/cncr.23448
4. Polsky D, Doshi JA, Marcus S, Oslin D, Rothbard A, Thomas N, et al. Long-term risk for depressive symptoms after a medical diagnosis. *Arch Intern Med* (2005) **165**:1260–6. doi:10.1001/archinte.165.11.1260
5. Ganz PA. Monitoring the physical health of cancer survivors: a survivorship-focused medical history. *J Clin Oncol* (2006) **24**:5105–11. doi:10.1200/JCO.2006.06.0541
6. Hofman M, Ryan JL, Figueroa-Moseley CD, Jean-Pierre P, Morrow GR. Cancer-related fatigue: the scale of the problem. *Oncologist* (2007) **12**(Suppl 1):4–10. doi:10.1634/theoncologist.12-S1-4
7. Koch L, Jansen L, Brenner H, Arndt V. Fear of recurrence and disease progression in long-term (>/= 5 years) cancer survivors – a systematic review of quantitative studies. *Psychooncology* (2013) **22**:1–11. doi:10.1002/pon.3022
8. Burnham TR, Wilcox A. Effects of exercise on physiological and psychological variables in cancer survivors. *Med Sci Sports Exerc* (2002) **34**:1863–7. doi:10.1097/00005768-200212000-00001
9. Daley AJ, Crank H, Saxton JM, Mutrie N, Coleman R, Roalfe A. Randomized trial of exercise therapy in women treated for breast cancer. *J Clin Oncol* (2007) **25**:1713–21. doi:10.1200/JCO.2006.09.5083
10. Alfano CM, Smith AW, Irwin ML, Bowen DJ, Sorensen B, Reeve BB, et al. Physical activity, long-term symptoms, and physical health-related quality of life among breast cancer survivors: a prospective analysis. *J Cancer Surviv* (2007) **1**:116–28. doi:10.1007/s11764-007-0014-1
11. Peddle CJ, Au HJ, Courneya KS. Associations between exercise, quality of life, and fatigue in colorectal cancer survivors. *Dis Colon Rectum* (2008) **51**:1242–8. doi:10.1007/s10350-008-9324-2
12. Haas BK, Kimmel G, Hermanns M, Deal B. Community-based FitSTEPS for life exercise program for persons with cancer: 5-year evaluation. *J Oncol Pract* (2012) **8**:320–4. doi:10.1200/JOP.2012.000555
13. Schmitz KH, Courneya KS, Matthews C, Demark-Wahnefried W, Galvão DA, Pinto BM, et al. American college of sports medicine roundtable on exercise guidelines for cancer survivors. *Med Sci Sports Exerc* (2010) **42**:1409–26. doi:10.1249/MSS.0b013e3181e0c112
14. *2008 Physical Activity Guidelines for Americans.* U.S. Department of Health and Human Services (2008). Available from: http://www.health.gov/paguidelines/pdf/paguide.pdf
15. Holmes MD, Chen WY, Feskanich D, Kroenke CH, Colditz GA. Physical activity and survival after breast cancer diagnosis. *JAMA* (2005) **293**:2479–86. doi:10.1001/jama.293.20.2479
16. Meyerhardt JA, Giovannucci EL, Holmes MD, Chan AT, Chan JA, Colditz GA, et al. Physical activity and survival after colorectal cancer diagnosis. *J Clin Oncol* (2006) **24**:3527–34. doi:10.1200/JCO.2006.06.0855
17. Holick CN, Newcomb PA, Trentham-Dietz A, Titus-Ernstoff L, Bersch AJ, Stampfer MJ, et al. Physical activity and survival after diagnosis of invasive breast cancer. *Cancer Epidemiol Biomarkers Prev* (2008) **17**:379–86. doi:10.1158/1055-9965.EPI-07-0771
18. Meyerhardt JA, Giovannucci EL, Ogino S, Kirkner GJ, Chan AT, Willett W, et al. Physical activity and male colorectal cancer survival. *Arch Intern Med* (2009) **169**:2102–8. doi:10.1001/archinternmed.2009.412
19. Je Y, Jeon JY, Giovannucci EL, Meyerhardt JA. Association between physical activity and mortality in colorectal cancer: a meta-analysis of prospective cohort studies. *Int J Cancer* (2013) **133**:1905–13. doi:10.1002/ijc.28208
20. Courneya KS, Vallance JK, McNeely ML, Karvinen KH, Peddle CJ, Mackey JR. Exercise issues in older cancer survivors. *Crit Rev Oncol Hematol* (2004) **51**:249–61. doi:10.1016/j.critrevonc.2004.05.001
21. Pekmezi DW, Demark-Wahnefried W. Updated evidence in support of diet and exercise interventions in cancer survivors. *Acta Oncol* (2011) **50**:167–78. doi:10.3109/0284186X.2010.529822
22. Hughes SL, Seymour RB, Campbell R, Pollak N, Huber G, Sharma L. Impact of the fit and strong intervention on older adults with osteoarthritis. *Gerontologist* (2004) **44**:217–28. doi:10.1093/geront/44.2.217
23. Hughes SL, Seymour RB, Campbell RT, Huber G, Pollak N, Sharma L, et al. Long-term impact of fit and strong! on older adults with osteoarthritis. *Gerontologist* (2006) **46**:801–14. doi:10.1093/geront/46.6.801
24. Hughes SL, Seymour RB, Campbell RT, Desai P, Huber G, Chang HJ. Fit and Strong!: bolstering maintenance of physical activity among older adults with lower-extremity osteoarthritis. *Am J Health Behav* (2010) **34**:750–63. doi:10.5993/AJHB.34.6.10
25. *Facing Forward: Life After Cancer Treatment.* National Cancer Institute (2014). Available from: http://www.cancer.gov/cancertopics/coping/life-after-treatment.pdf
26. *Eating Hints: Before, During, and After Cancer Treatment.* National Cancer Institute (2014). Available from: http://www.cancer.gov/cancertopics/coping/eatinghints.pdf
27. *Facing Forward: Making a Difference in Cancer.* National Cancer Institute (2014). Available from: http://www.cancer.gov/cancertopics/facing-forward.pdf
28. *Facing Forward: When Someone You Love Have Completed Cancer Treatment.* National Cancer Institute (2014). Available from: http://www.cancer.gov/cancertopics/coping/someone-you-love-completed-cancer-treatment.pdf
29. *Follow-up Care After Cancer Treatment.* National Cancer Institute (2014). Available from: http://www.cancer.gov/cancertopics/factsheet/Therapy/followup
30. Lorig K, Stewart A, Ritter P, Gonzalez V, Laurent D, Lynch J. Chapter 2. *Construction of Measures of Behaviors, Self-Efficacy, and Outcomes, Outcome Measures for*

Health Education and Other Health Care Interventions. Thousand Oaks, CA: Sage Publications, Inc (1996). p. 10–45.

31. Avis NE, Smith KW, McGraw S, Smith RG, Petronis VM, Carver CS. Assessing quality of life in adult cancer survivors (QLACS). *Qual Life Res* (2005) **14**:1007–23. doi:10.1007/s11136-004-2147-2
32. Morey MC, Snyder DC, Sloane R, Cohen HJ, Peterson B, Hartman TJ, et al. Effects of home-based diet and exercise on functional outcomes among older, overweight long-term cancer survivors: renew: a randomized controlled trial. *JAMA* (2009) **301**:1883–91. doi:10.1001/jama.2009.643

29

Adoption of evidence-based health promotion programs: Perspectives of early adopters of Enhance® Fitness in YMCA-affiliated sites

Basia Belza[1,2]*, Miruna Petrescu-Prahova[1], Marlana Kohn[1], Christina E. Miyawaki[1,3], Laura Farren[1], Grace Kline[1] and Ann-Hilary Heston[4]

[1] Health Promotion Research Center, University of Washington, Seattle, WA, USA
[2] School of Nursing, University of Washington, Seattle, WA, USA
[3] School of Social Work, University of Washington, Seattle, WA, USA
[4] Healthy Living Department, YMCA of the USA, Chicago, IL, USA

Edited by:
Matthew Lee Smith, The University of Georgia, USA

Reviewed by:
Mary Odum, Texas A&M University, USA
Elisa Beth Hutson McNeill, Texas A&M University, USA

***Correspondence:**
Basia Belza, Health Promotion Research Center, University of Washington, 1107 NE 45th Street, Suite 200, Seattle, WA 98195, USA
e-mail: basiab@uw.edu

Purpose: To identify facilitators and barriers among early adopters of Enhance®Fitness (EF), in Young Men's Christian Association-affiliated (Y-affiliated) sites from the perspective of program staff. EF is an evidence-based group exercise program for seniors.

Methods: This qualitative study used semi-structured phone interviews with 15 staff members representing 14 Y-affiliated sites. Interviews were digitally recorded, transcribed, and analyzed using qualitative content analysis informed by the RE-AIM framework.

Findings: Staff were, on average, 48.7 years old (SD 13.5) and had been involved with EF for 5.2 years (SD 3.1). Key themes related to facilitating adoption of EF were: match with the Y mission, support from different organizational levels, match between the target population need and EF, initial and on-going financial support, presence of champions, novelty of EF, an invitation to partner with a community-based organization to offer EF, and program-specific characteristics of EF. Key themes related to barriers interfering with EF adoption included competing organizational programs and space limitations, limited resources and expertise, and costs of offering the program.

Implications: Our findings identify the types of organizational support needed for adoption of evidence-based health promotion programs like EF. Recommendations for practice, research, and policy based on the findings, including assessing organizational readiness, researching late adopters, and developing revenue streams, may help facilitate program adoption. Packaging and sharing these practical recommendations could help community-based agencies and nationally networked organizations facilitate adoption of EF and other evidence-based programs.

Keywords: older adults, RE-AIM, physical activity, dissemination, adoption, evidence-based programs, community intervention, dissemination framework

INTRODUCTION

Since the development of evidence-based medicine (EBM) over two decades ago (1), the Centers for Disease Control and Prevention (CDC) has promoted healthy aging with an emphasis on reliable, efficient, and cost-effective care models with measurable outcomes (2). The goal of evidence-based programs is to create healthier communities and prevent chronic diseases (3). Translating evidence-based programs from research studies to community practice and sustaining them is a top priority for public health researchers and practitioners.

Evidence-based health promotion programs for older adults have been adopted and implemented by organizations in communities throughout the United States (4, 5). Enhance®Fitness (EF) is an evidence-based group exercise program for frail and active older adults (6–8). The one hour classes meet three-times a week and include exercises for cardiovascular endurance, balance, flexibility, and strength. Research has demonstrated that EF improves upper and lower body muscle strength and flexibility (9, 10). EF participants report improved over-all health (9). Participation in EF has been associated with healthcare costs saving. The average increase in annual total healthcare costs was less among EF participants compared to non-participating controls in a managed health care plan ($642 vs. 1175) (6). Among Medicare beneficiaries, enrollment in EF was associated with per person medical savings of $945/year after enrollment (8). Since 2001, there have been a total of 42,560 EF participants (unduplicated) served at a total of 689 sites in 33 states and Washington DC (Susan Snyder, personal communication, Senior Services, 2014 April 14).

Senior Services (Seattle, WA, USA) licenses and disseminates EF to multipurpose social service agencies, faith-based organizations, retirement communities, and recreational organizations. With more than 10,000 community locations, Young Men's Christian Association (Y) is a leading non-profit committed to improving the nation's health and well-being by offering programs that nurture the mind, body, and spirit. From 2005 to 2012, 116 Y-affiliated community sites adopted EF. These included both classes on-site at Y brick-and-mortar buildings, and classes licensed by Ys but offered in community settings such as churches or retirement communities. These sites represent a first stage in the adoption of EF by a nationally networked organization; as such, their experience is likely to inform efforts to scale-up adoption of EF and other evidence-based programs. In this paper, we refer to these sites as early adopters (11).

Various models have been used to evaluate evidence-based health promotion programs. One of these program planning and evaluation models is RE-AIM. RE-AIM, an acronym for Reach, Effectiveness, Adoption, Implementation, and Maintenance, is a systematic process that researchers, practitioners, and policy makers use to evaluate the dissemination of health promotion programs (12). Within the RE-AIM framework, adoption refers to the "proportion and representativeness of settings willing to initiate a given program" (13). Understanding how adoption of interventions plays out in different organizational settings is critical to the current and potential impact of an intervention (14).

Previous research has identified a number of motivating factors for program adoption: participant interest and/or demand, proven safety and effectiveness for older adults, cost, and a well-rounded program structure that attracts multiple groups (13). Additionally, the availability of resources is important for program adoption (15). Facilitating factors for program adoption identified in previous studies include having a curriculum, availability of training, space, and equipment (12), awareness of the importance of promoting physical activity in the community and internal support for physical activity interventions (15), sufficient funds, leadership support, capable staff, and successful partnerships and collaborations (16). Barriers include scheduling issues, lack of space, and insufficient participant recruitment efforts (13), program cost (16, 17), and lack of leadership, and time and training (16). These findings reinforce the idea that adoption can be improved by developing organizational support and capacity to deliver a program (18).

The research question for this study was: what are the facilitators and barriers among early adopters of EF in Y-affiliated sites from the perspective of program staff. Based on our findings, we provide practice, research, and policy recommendations that may help inform the adoption of other evidence-based programs in community settings. Increasing the number of community organizations that adopt evidence-based health promotion programs for older adults will contribute to the goal of creating healthier communities and preventing chronic disease.

MATERIALS AND METHODS

DESIGN

This qualitative study used semi-structured individual phone interviews with 15 staff from 14 Y-affiliated sites that had responsibility for the oversight of EF.

MEASURE

We developed a structured interview guide for staff with questions that were informed by the RE-AIM framework (**Table 1**). We piloted our guide, which adds rigor to our data collection process (19). The interview guide contained a total of 39 questions and probes about benefits of EF, fitness checks, facilitators and barriers/challenges to offering EF, staff responsibilities, support from the Y management for offering EF, and strategies to recruit EF participants and instructors. Seven of the 39 questions included skip patterns (#5, 9, 12, 15, 16, 30, and 39). For example, item #9 asked: were you involved in the original adoption of EF? If the staff answered in the affirmative, then the follow on question was asked: if yes, how did your YMCA come about offering EF? If the staff answered not in the affirmative the interviewer immediately went onto the next question. Ten of the 39 items were close-ended or demographic items requiring short responses (#1, 2, 3, 7, 8, 17, 20, 36, 37, and 38). Additionally, we asked staff their age, duration of time involved with EF, educational level, and title of their position.

PROCEDURES

Our study was determined to be exempt by the University of Washington Institutional Review Board. We obtained administrative program records from Senior Services of all Y-affiliated program sites that had offered EF between January 2005 and June 2012. Inclusion criteria for this study were EF program management staff listed in the administrative program records from 2005 to 2012 in 116 Y-affiliated sites and who had complete contact information. Exclusion criteria were: (1) staff on this list without complete contact information, and (2) staff during the pre-enrollment screening call were determined that they did not have experience with EF. The list included 94 names of EF program management staff; of which 75 has complete contact information. Recruiting letters were sent to those 75 staff. Additionally, a Y-USA staff member (AHH) sent emails to the staff employed by Ys inviting them to participate in our study. Two reminder recruiting postcards were sent to staff who had not responded to the initial recruiting letter; reminders were sent at 2 and 4 weeks after the initial mailing. Interested staff called a study phone line or sent an email to the study email account. Twenty-five out of 75 (33%) responded to the recruiting letter, and 8 were determined ineligible for the study. Two staff were placed on a wait list. The study recruiting coordinator (LF) tracked and responded to all phone and email messages, determined eligibility, and scheduled interviews. At the beginning of each phone interview, verbal informed consent was obtained. Interviews were conducted by two members of the research team (BB and MPP). Each study participant received a gift card for $20. Interviews ranged from 30 to 71 min (average duration was 47 min) and were digitally recorded. In 2008, Gill et al. (20) note that when conducting interviews the length varies depending on the topic, researcher and participant. However, on average, the duration of interviews about health care topics is 20–60 min (20). The average length of our interview is within this range.

The interviews were transcribed by a professional transcriptionist using a "lightly edited verbatim" style for readability with an emphasis on sentence structure. This is a more frequently used style over "strictly verbatim" since it is executed without compromising the actual content or altering the intended expression (21).

Table 1 | Interview guide for Y administrative staff.

INFORMATION ABOUT THE INTERVIEWEE AND ENHANCE® FITNESS OVERSIGHT
1. What is your title with the YMCA? How long have you held this position?
2. Approximately what year did your YMCA first become involved with EF?
3. Approximately what year did you become involved with EF?
4. What are your responsibilities related to EF?
5. Are you responsible for the oversight of EF with your YMCA? a. If not, what is the title of the person responsible for oversight?
6. What are the responsibilities related to oversight of the operations of EF with your YMCA?
7. Is your YMCA still offering EF classes? Yes No
8. What, if any, other exercise classes and/or programs does/did your YMCA offer specifically for seniors (defined as older than 62 years) besides EF?
ENHANCE® FITNESS READINESS AND ADOPTION
9. *Were you involved in the original adoption of EF? a. If yes, how did your YMCA come about offering EF?
10. *What was the primary motivation for your YMCA getting involved in EF?
11. *What were some of the other motivations for your YMCA getting involved in EF?
12. *Does/did your YMCA receive funding to provide EF classes? a. If yes, what kind of funding? b. Source of funding? c. Use of funds? (Probe: staff support, participant fee offset, marketing, etc.)
13. Do you think your YMCA has/had the right and adequate number of ... to support EF classes? a. Staff b. Instructors c. Class materials (chairs, weights, etc.) d. Space/room
14. Are there any resources you wish you had, or had more of, to support EF classes at your YMCA?
15. *Is there someone at your YMCA that is a champion for EF? (A champion can be paid staff or a volunteer who helps keep classes going, recruits new participants, or works to expand the program, for example) a. If YES: can you describe some of the things this person does to champion EF?
16. Are there paid and/or volunteer staff that manage or oversee EF operations with your YMCA? (This would include scheduling classes, managing instructors, and/or answering EF questions for current or potential participants.) a. If YES: how was staff recruited or selected to manage EF with your YMCA?
17. Is the management of EF: a. Centralized and occurs at the association-level, or b. De-centralized and managed at the branch level?
18. What are/were the methods used to recruit EF instructors to teach classes with your YMCA?
19. What are/were the methods used to recruit participants to EF classes with your YMCA?
20. Location of EF classes: a. Are EF classes held at: a) your YMCA, b) off-site locations, or c) both? b. If off-site, what type of locations? If more than one site, list all sites and be specific as to type of site. (churches, senior centers, community centers, Parks and Recreation facilities, schools, and retirement communities)?
21. What is/was the primary motivation for you personally getting involved in EF? (Probe: part of my job, personal interest, etc.)
22. What are/were some of your other motivations for you getting personally involved in EF? (Probe: saw the benefits, have aging family members that had benefited from this or similar programs.)

(Continued)

Table 1 | Continued

EXPERIENCE WITH ENHANCE®FITNESS

23. What benefits do you think your YMCA gets/got from participating in EF? (Probe: member engagement, community outreach, and serving a need).
    a. Is/was your YMCA reimbursed in any way for offering EF classes?
        i. If yes, by whom?
    b. Do/did your participants pay a fee to participate in EF classes?
        i. If yes, how much?
        ii. If the fee changed over time, provide a range but note the current amount
        iii. Does your Y ever offer EF:
            1. On a sliding scale?
            2. For reduced cost?
        iv. How reasonable do you think this fee is?
        v. How does this fee compare to other like classes or programs? (Probe: More, same, less than?)
    c. Are EF classes through your YMCA available to both Y members and non-members?
        i. Does your Y track conversion rates of non-member program participants to members? (e.g., For 10 non-member participants, 1 becomes a member.)
            1. If YES: what is the conversion rate?
    d. Do you know if any of your EF participants are/were reimbursed for participating in EF, such as through health insurance?
        i. If yes, by what plan or program?
24. What do/did you like most about EF? (Probe: full classes, positive reports from participants, outcomes tracking)
25. What do/did you like least about EF? (Probe: time of the day the class is offered, instructor, room the class was held, conducting the fitness checks)
26. What are/were characteristics of EF classes that you think make them successful? (Probes: instructor ownership of the class, size of class, well-ventilated room, good time of day, room easily accessible, and class offered immediately before or after another event like a meal program)
27. What are/were characteristics of EF classes that you think are barriers to success (probe: too small of a room, mismatch between instructor and participant characteristics, high fees, time of day)?
28. <u>If the class is no longer offered:</u> why do you think EF is not/no longer offered at your YMCA? (Probe: cost of running EF, no instructor, instructor not a good match with participants, not enough participants, not large enough space, and other concurrent exercise classes)
29. What are/have been your challenges with offering EF? (Probe: finding instructors, frailty of participants, and for the participant transportation to and from class)
30. Are/were there particular issues you have faced in offering EF?
    a. If YES: can you describe these issues, and how you have handled them?
31. What does/did your YMCA do that you think makes EF appealing to: (Probes: advertising, offering at prime time, and offer it at no or low cost)
    a. Participants and members at your YMCA?
    b. The greater community that your YMCA serves?
    c. If your Y receives funding to offer EF classes (separate from member due or class fees), who are the other funders (probe: specific organization and individual)?
32. What does/did your YMCA do that you think makes EF not appealing?
33. What are the reasons you believe your YMCA has/not been able to implement/maintain EF classes?
34. Do you have any recommendations for changes to EF based on your experiences?
35. How was your experience with EF been similar to or different from other classes at the YMCA, particularly fitness classes or classes for seniors?
36. Regarding your Y members:
    a. About how many members does your YMCA serve?
    b. About what percent of your members are 65 and older?
    c. About what percent of your members are in the 50–64-year-old age range?

DEMOGRAPHIC ITEMS

37. What is your age?
38. In what education category do you fall: less than college degree, some college or college degree, and more than college degree?

CLOSING

39. Is there anything else you would like us to know about your experience with EF with your YMCA?

Items with high relevance to the findings presented in this paper are noted with an asterisk.

"Lightly edited" is simply used to refer to the reduction of superfluous words such as "hmm, ah, mm, you know, well, yeah, uh-huh." Transcripts are still considered full and complete and do not in any way deviate from representing the full intent and thoughts as expressed by each individual respondent. Transcripts were then entered and analyzed in ATLAS.ti version 7.

DATA ANALYSIS

Our research team had content expertise in dissemination and implementation science, administrative management, community-based participatory research, gerontology, public health, and healthy aging. All members of our team that were involved in the analysis had previous experience in conducting qualitative analysis. Our study used qualitative content analysis (22) to identify facilitators and barriers to the adoption of EF. A codebook was developed using a combination of *a priori* themes addressed in the interview guide and additional themes identified through the initial review of interview transcripts. The team met weekly for 3 months to discuss and come to agreement on coding rules. A dyad (BB and GK) double-coded a subset of five transcripts until agreement reached 85%. Remaining transcripts were divided between both team members (BB and GK) and coded independently. After the initial coding, we used a deductive approach (23) to review the coded text within the RE-AIM framework component of adoption (24). Descriptive statistics were calculated for demographic items including staff age, duration of involvement with EF, and education level.

RESULTS

Study participants were, on average, 48.7 years old (SD 13.5) and had been involved with EF for 5.2 years (SD 3.1). Three staff (20%) had some college education, seven (47%) had a college degree, and five (33%) had more than a college degree. Ten staff members (67%) were employed by a Y while the remaining five staff (33%) were employed by other organizations (faith-based organization, senior center, social service organization, and residential facility). Titles and levels of responsibility varied: five were Health and Wellness staff, four had roles specific to older adults, six were at the program coordinator/instructor level, and eight were at the program manager/director level or above.

Staff interviewed represented 10 different YMCA associations in six states. Fourteen out of 15 staff worked in locations where classes were conducted; one staff worked in an administrative office. Ten sites currently offered EF classes; the remaining five had previously offered EF but did not have active classes at the time of the interview.

In the remainder of this paper, we summarize our findings regarding facilitators for adoption of EF and barriers that interfered with adoption of EF, with representative quotes presented in **Tables 2** and **3**, respectively.

FACILITATORS FOR ADOPTION OF EF

Key facilitators identified by staff, which contributed to EF adoption, were match with the Y mission, support from different organizational levels, match between the target population need and EF, initial and on-going financial support, presence of champions, novelty of EF, an invitation to partner with a community-based organization to offer EF, and program-specific characteristics of EF, such as being evidence-based and having a recognizable name.

Match with the Y mission

The Y mission is to put Christian principles into practice through programs that build a healthy spirit, mind, and body for all (25). Staff employed by Ys and community organizations with whom the Y partners noted that EF's evidence-based curriculum was a good match with the Y mission since it is proven to improve older adults' physical health in a fun and engaging atmosphere that promotes social interaction. Staff expressed strong commitment to the Y mission and to addressing unmet demographic needs: "Adopting an evidence-based program fit well with the Y goals and standards and was congruent with the Y mission." The staff saw it as their responsibility to keep seniors socially and mentally involved so they were not isolated at home. Another staff member mentioned, "Our strategic initiatives and our strategies roadmap for our association states very clearly that we will have a growing focus on expanding our senior membership and increasing our programing to meet the needs of the aging population." The staff were committed to providing programs that seniors enjoyed and needed. The Ys' values promote inclusiveness, which is operationalized by staff providing programing to improve the health and well-being of older adults.

Organizational support

Support from different organizational levels of the Y also served to facilitate adoption. For example, staff were consulted when EF marketing materials were developed. This helped the staff feel like they had a say in how and to whom the program was being promoted. Staff also felt that adoption of EF was facilitated with support from junior management, Wellness Directors, Executive Directors, and CEOs.

Match with the target population

Enhance®Fitness was more easily adopted when the staff perceived there was a good fit between the needs of the target population (older adults) and the program itself (EF). Older adults were considered to be in an age bracket that had previously been underserved by the Y. A perceived gap in programing led staff to look for exercise programs like EF because it was a valuable addition for the senior community. Because EF exercises can be adapted to suit participant abilities, the staff felt it was a very inclusive program in which older adults at varying levels of function could participate. In addition, some of the EF classes were offered off-site in settings that catered to older adults and with which the Y branch had been partnering. One such setting was a retirement community. One staff commented: "the residents [in assisted living] were good candidates because they were at a point where they had not been exercising. We could start at the beginning and see where their progress was which would not have been if we brought it into our Y and tried to offer it to our regular seniors".

Financial support

Initial financial support was an important factor in the adoption of EF. Several staff members reported receiving funding through grants at the time of EF adoption to cover EF training

Table 2 | Facilitator themes for adoption of Enhance®Fitness (EF): perceptions of Y staff.

	Theme	Transcripts represented	Exemplar quotations
1	EF matches well with Y mission	8 of 15 (53%)	Adopting an evidence-based program fit well with the Y goals and standards and was congruent with the Y mission. The Y mission includes providing programing that helps to improve the health and fitness of older adults (Age 30, 11 years with the Y). It's back to the spirit of mind and body of what the YMCA does (Age 33, 11 years with the Y). We knew it was an evidence-based program, one that fit well with the Y goals and standards (Age 30, 11 years with the Y). I think it falls into our focus areas i.e., healthy living for seniors and social responsibility as well. We're being responsible when we provide those types of exercise programs (Age 29, 5 years with the Y).
2	Organizational support	5 of 15 (33%)	The association office asked us if we would be interested. Because of the clientele we have, we have lots of seniors, of course I stepped up to the plate and said: "Yes, definitely let's try this for our seniors." That's how we got involved (Age 41, 14 years with the Y). I think having a focus and support from junior management is important (Age 38, 8 years with the Y). I think you need to have an Executive Director or CEO really understanding what it means to deliver evidence-based programs (Age 38, 8 years with the Y). I think it's always good thing to bring something new in. It was driven by the Y of the USA. And then also I was asked to do this by our Health and Wellness director of the main branch (Age 51, 15 years with the Y).
3	Match with the target population	10 of 15 (67%)	We had been looking for an older adult program because we have a large aging population in our community. It has been an age bracket that had been underserved at our Y (Age 30, 11 years with the Y). We are known for the fact that we offer programing that is valuable to the community and to the seniors in the community. EF is one of those programs (Age 63, 2 years with Y-affiliated site). We are in close proximity to (low income housing) and so this is a very easy place for them to come. It's convenient for them. If we're talking about people that are low income and don't have money for public transportation, it makes it very easy for them to do something to take care of their healthy living (Age 63, 2 years with Y-affiliated site). It is completely appropriate for many health seekers and people who struggle with becoming more active or staying active (Age 38, 8 years with the Y).
4	Financial support	5 of 15 (33%)	When we started it, we started with the [state department of health]. . . . they gave us a grant basically along with other YMCAs in [the state] with all of those being downstate. They basically paid for my staff's training and they sent us. I think that they also paid for all of our equipment. They were a huge, huge partner in this and for us being able to start EF when we did (Age 33, 11 years with the Y). The [state] contacted us and we've been working with them for some other programs. They offered to help with the initial training, and that's where we learned about the program (Age 30, 11 years with the Y). We offer financial assistance. Based upon income I can give participants a certain percentage off the price of the class. And then based upon some of the grants that we have been given, I can give them even a higher percentage off. We do the best that we can to really make it happen for them. I don't like saying no to anybody (Age 29, 5 years with the Y).
5	Champions	10 of 15 (67%)	I am a go-getter and if I hear something, I go after it because it is beneficial to our residents (Age 65, 6 years with the Y-affiliated site). For me, personally, it was something else for me to offer to the seniors. I absolutely love working with the active older adults (Age 41, 14 years with the Y). The more and more I learned about it, the more I loved it. I didn't really know of any other like evidence-based programs for older adults. I really liked the pre and post-tests that they did. It just seemed like a great program (Age 33, 11 years with the Y). I told my boss about it and how I thought it would be beneficial. I told our members about it because I wanted to get them on board and get them excited. I did anything I could when the (grant sponsor) people came over. I did everything I could to promote our space (Age 60, 7 years with Y-affiliated site).

(Continued)

Table 2 | Continued

	Theme	Transcripts represented	Exemplar quotations
6	Novelty of EF	5 of 15 (33%)	I thought it would be something different, you know? I thought it would be more different and something that we could offer to our seniors (Age 41, 14 years with the Y). It was just something new and exciting, evidence-based. It was everything we wanted (Age 51, 11 years with the Y). I think it's always good thing to bring something new in (Age 51, 16 years with the Y). I just wanted to have a varied program offering, and I thought this would fit...I wanted to keep the people who come here happy with our center. I want to give them a variety of things, and so I don't want anything to be stagnant (Age 60, 7 years with Y-affiliated site).
7	Invitation to partner with another organization to offer EF	8 of 15 (53%)	I think that I thought it looked like a great program. Our partnership at the [state department of health] was so strong. They really wanted to help the YMCAs start it (Age 33, 11 years with the Y). Sometimes the senior centers request us to do a program. That is kind of how it happened. It was just really good timing when we started EF because they were requesting that we come and do some different things. We thought it would be perfect and so it just kind of fell into place (Age 33, 11 years with the Y). I was working with a grant writer at [a university]. I was looking for something that we could get through a grant. This is the something she came up with (Age 60, 7 years with Y-affiliated site). Someone [YMCA staff member] called [my manager] and said: "We have this EF class and would you want to be our pilot program?" And she said "Absolutely, yes! That's how it all started" (Age 51, 11 years with the Y).
8	Program-specific characteristics of EF such as being evidence-based and with name recognition	10 of 15 (67%)	It is evidence-based and has got solid backing. It has a proven track record and can meet the needs that are out there (Age 30, 11 years with the Y). I won't touch anything that does not have data or an evidence-based curriculum, especially as related to chronic disease management (Age 38, 8 years with the Y). It is an incentive to bring people in when they know that you have a program that is known throughout the country. It's a recognizable name. You are branded already (Age 63, 2 years with Y-affiliated site).

Table 3 | Barrier themes to adoption of Enhance®Fitness (EF): perceptions by Y staff.

	Theme	Transcripts represented	Supporting quotations
1	Competing programing	5 of 15 (33%)	For group classes we have dance, water aerobics, step aerobics, spinning, and the range of movement class from [another exercise program]. We have additional programs that are available at a cost, and those include our nutritional services; the EF classes; swimming lessons; different sports programs, and then small group training types of classes (Age 30, 11 years with the Y). We acknowledge that space is an issue ... They [wellness directors] see it as oh we already have [another program], our program for active older adults. Why would we want to do this one? (Age 38, 8 years with the Y). ... We [offer EF] off-site. We are not in our own building anymore. It was to save on rent ... The big room is often taken up with children's camps and things like that (Age 60, 7 years with Y-affiliated site).
2	Limited resources and expertise	7 of 15 (47%)	The staff did not see the benefit or the value to their people (Age 45, 10 years). ... And getting our health and wellness directors to understand and not condemn it, like "What's in it for us?" (Age 38, 8 years with the Y). ... Where are we going to put it; who is the instructor going to be; who's going to pay for this, or where are the funds coming from (Age 51, 16 years with the Y). I know the whole issue is that people don't have time. There is a lack of staff. We have it here, too, and so I know some of the issues (Age 65, 6 years with Y-affiliated site).

for their instructors, weights and other equipment, licensing fees, and/or instructor salaries. These funds also allowed Ys to offer the program at no charge to participants in some sites.

Champions

Champions for both EF and older adult programing facilitated adoption of EF. When asked to identify champions for EF, staff identified both paid staff and volunteers who fully embraced EF, and passionately and frequently promoted the program both within and outside the Y. Staff champions advocated for and secured resources to launch the EF program. Champions described themselves as "go-getters," extolled the virtues of EF, and communicated often with managers, staff, and site members about the benefits of EF. One staff champion expressed adopting the "we will make it work" attitude when it came to rolling out EF for the first time. Volunteer champions welcomed new comers, brought guests to class, and took on other tasks such as setting up fitness check areas. "[Champions] just do it on their own. Nobody asked them to do that (in reference to setting up fitness check areas). They just love the community that EF provides and obviously the physical benefits. They want to capture anybody that comes into class and really helps them feel that same way."

Novelty

Staff were looking for new and exciting programs to offer older adults. They viewed adopting EF as an opportunity to keep their programing fresh, and valued being an early adopter when the program was just getting started: "Back then [when EF was adopted] EF was kind of an experiment. There were only a few sites in the country offering it, I believe, and so I thought that it would be nice to be part of that group."

Invitation to partner

The initial adoption of EF by Y-affiliated sites was often triggered by an invitation from an established community partner, providing motivation to adopt EF. The Y has close links with community partners and values their suggestions. Being part of an active community-based network that also provides services to older adults positions the Y to be on the cutting-edge of learning when new programs are launched. Established relationships with state departments of health and affiliations with academic and philanthropic organizations were often key to adoption. These relationships afforded access to financial resources that provided initial start-up and on-going funding for EF. One staff member noted: "the opportunity to work with and partner with an outside agency to help address another portion of our population definitely interested me." There were also examples of invitations to partner with new organizations, such as assisted living communities that had never had a program like EF. An invitation from a new partner "opened doors."

Program-specific facilitators

There were program-specific facilitators that helped with adoption. Staff described EF as being unlike other programs they had offered. Most frequently mentioned was EF being evidence-based, branded, and having name recognition. Staff reported that EF was, "... an easy sale as it was proven to improve things," and "it has solid backing."

BARRIERS TO THE ADOPTION OF ENHANCE® FITNESS

A number of factors that interfered with the adoption of EF were noted such as competing senior programs and space limitations, limited staff resources, and costs of the program.

Competing programing and space limitations

Staff noted one of the barriers to offering EF was that the Y Association was already offering a number of other programs for active older adults, and the health and wellness staff did not see the need or benefit to offering another one. Additionally, in some Y sites staff reported there was a "space crunch" with rooms that would be appropriate for offering EF being allocated to other programs such as camps for children. One staff member said: "we no longer had the luxury of having two senior programs running because of space limitations." One staff that was trained to offer EF but never did said: "we were having a time and space crunch. It wasn't anything wrong with the program *per se* but we're not going to take away our already very strong programs and try something new." Off-site locations like retirement communities also had issues with finding adequate space.

Limited resources, expertise, and program costs

Another factor that interfered with the adoption of EF was the lack of staff resources, both in terms of time availability and the need to find instructors with appropriate skills for working with older adults. Staff noted that costs of the program were a potential barrier to adoption: rent, materials, and instructor costs, on the one hand, and affordability for participants, on the other, were taken into account before deciding to adopt EF.

DISCUSSION

In this study, we examined the facilitators and barriers to the adoption on EF in early adopter Y-affiliated sites. The Health Promotion Research Center (HPRC) dissemination framework provides a context for interpreting the findings from this study and informs the translation of our findings to other community-delivered, evidence-based programs (26). The HPRC dissemination framework incorporates the terminology of the RE-AIM framework such that the definition of adoption is consistent between the two frameworks.

The HPRC dissemination framework (**Figure 1**) identifies three main actors involved in the dissemination of an evidence-based program: researchers, disseminating organizations, and user organizations. Researchers and disseminating organizations partner to develop a dissemination approach that is suitable for the targeted user organizations. The approach is built on learnings about the user organization's characteristics and readiness for adoption and implementation, and is continually refined through the collaboration of the three main actors. At the same time, all actors operate within a broader context that includes both modifiable and unmodifiable components, such as funding and partnerships, and economic conditions, respectively.

Study participants identified several facilitators and barriers related to the characteristics of Y-affiliated sites, the user organizations in this study. Ys have made major strides in recent years to become leaders in community-based health promotion programs. It was readily apparent that there was a strong fit between EF and the Y mission to offer older adults an environment that promotes physical and emotional health, and the availability of resources to ensure adequate programing. This rich environment also included champions for both EF and older

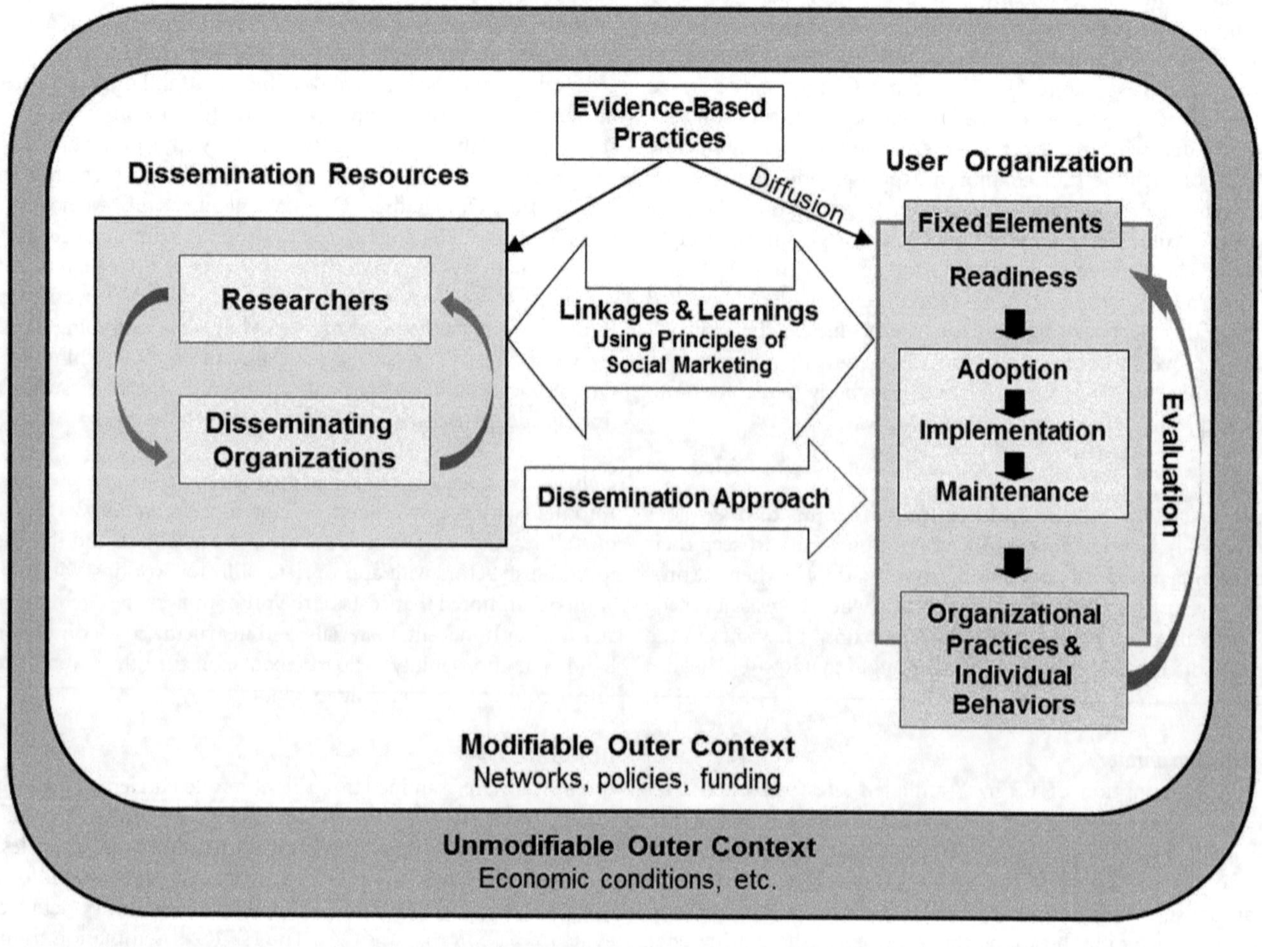

FIGURE 1 | The HPRC dissemination framework [taken from Harris et al. (26)].

adult programs. Programs with this type of fit have an enhanced ability to sustain themselves. On the other hand, our findings suggest a need for improved evaluation of organizational readiness prior to the adoption of any evidence-based program. Structured and rigorous determination of organizational readiness would help organizations avoid known barriers to successful implementation, such as competing programs, and limited space and resources. Organizational readiness for change is an important precursor to the successful implementation of health promotion programs (27).

Our study also identified facilitators related to the modifiable context in which user organizations operate. Staff noted the significant role grant funding played in the initial adoption of the program, as well as the importance of building partnerships at the local and state level.

Finally, we would like to highlight the role of the disseminating organization, Y-USA, the national office of the Y. Between 2007 and 2011, Y-USA significantly increased its national effort, Activate America®, to engage Ys in organizational and community change focused on supporting health seekers, those who struggle to adopt and maintain a healthy lifestyle. Nearly two-thirds of Y Associations committed to Activate America and built their capacity to better align their programs, practices, and policies with the needs of health seekers. This was the Y climate when EF was being brought into the organization by early adopters. The organization was primed for embracing evidence-based health promotion programs and working with a community of adults with chronic conditions. At this time, chronic disease prevention programs were introduced as well, including LIVE**STRONG** at the YMCA, a cancer survivorship program, and the YMCA's Diabetes Prevention Program (DPP).

Ackermann and colleagues tested offering DPP at Y sites (11, 28–30). Ys were able to increase the number of participants and offer DPP at a lower cost compared to other community settings, making Ys an ideal community partner. They noted a variety of factors contributing to the success of DPP offered at Ys: the Y is a nationwide, community-based organization reaching diverse U.S. communities; it has a successful history of adopting and implementing health promotion program for all age groups; it takes a group-delivery approach, which uses minimal over-all personnel cost; and it has a national policy to accept all participants regardless of their ability to pay the membership fee. Y-USA and its associations and branches nationwide are well-positioned to successfully adopt new evidence-based programs, and more broadly disseminate existing programs based on the program experience noted above, and the organizational infrastructure already in place.

There were several limitations in this study. First, we used a convenience sample. Convenience samples can introduce response bias, with those having positive experiences being more likely to participate than those with less favorable experience. However, staff who volunteered to participate in this study shared a range of experiences, both positive and negative, related to the adoption of EF. Second, our sample size of 15 may have limited our ability to reach conceptual saturation with regard to the research questions. After completing 15 interviews, the research team determined that additional interviews were unlikely to return substantively new information, and that we had reached conceptual saturation. Third, inherent in qualitative methodologies is the potential issue of transferability. To minimize issues with transferability and assure our findings would have applicability in other contexts, a partner from the Y (AHH) was actively involved in all phases of our study and another Y staff member served on our Project Advisory Group. Fourth, some of the staff had started overseeing EF up to 8 years prior to the phone interviews, resulting in potential recall bias with respect to the initial decisions and process of adopting EF. Last, Y staff who were the target of our interviews were in positions in which they had responsibilities for program management and also could adopt new initiatives like EF. When further exploring the concept of adoption, it would be valuable to also include senior leadership who are likely to be key decision makers and have an influence in whether a new program would be considered, paid for and/or adopted.

Based on the findings in this study, we propose practice, research, and policy recommendations for the adoption of evidence-based health promotion programs by community organizations. They are summarized in **Table 4**, which also includes the facilitator/barrier themes they address.

Our practice recommendations focus on organizational readiness for adopting new programs. Assessing organizational readiness, formally or informally, identifying gaps in readiness, and addressing any gaps may improve adoption (11). Organizational readiness can be evaluated through the following activities: assessing fit of the program with organizational mission; assessing overlap with other programing, and physical space and time constraints; identifying potential partners and funding/revenue models; identifying capable instructors and securing training and technical assistance for staff and potential instructors; and assessing cultural and demographic needs of the target population. Addressing these aspects of readiness may provide opportunities to open dialog with partners and stakeholders, or develop supporting resources like a business plan to support successful adoption.

The practice recommendations outlined above are based on the experience of early adopters. However, the adoption experience of majority adopters and late adopters/laggards may face different facilitators and barriers (11). Future research is needed to better understand the spectrum of adoption in all phases, and how early adopters' experience may influence later adopters. In addition, successful adoption should lead to program implementation and, ultimately, maintenance. Additional research on how adoption strategies influence subsequent implementation and maintenance of evidenced-based health promotion programs could contribute to development of best practices for the translation of research into practice.

Table 4 | Recommendations for practice, research, and policy in the adoption of evidence-based health promotion programs.

	Facilitators addressed	Barriers addressed
Recommendations for practice		
Assess fit with the organizational mission	Match with mission	
Assess fit with other programing	Novelty, match with target population	Competing programing
Identify existing community partners and new potential partners	Invitation to partner, financial support	Limited resources and expertise
Identify capable staff and instructors	Champions	Limited resources and expertise
Identify training and technical assistance for staff and potential instructors		Limited resources and expertise
Assess cultural and demographic needs of the target population	Match with target population, match with mission	
Assess physical space and time constraints		Limited resources and expertise
Assess start-up and on-going costs and offsetting funding/revenue	Financial support	Limited resources and expertise
Recommendations for research		
Explore adoption among majority and laggard adopters, and compare to early adopters		
Explore influence of adoption on implementation and maintenance		
Recommendations for policy		
Explore policy approaches to revenue development	Financial support	Limited resources and expertise

Finally, broad policy support for evidence-based programs may create an environment more primed for successful adoption. Policy support may include establishing a revenue stream to offset program costs, an approach that has been seen in other programs (30, 31). Policy approaches to developing revenue streams may be fruitful among evidence-based programs demonstrating health improvements and reductions in health care costs (6, 8).

CONCLUSION

While these recommendations are based on our study of the experience of early adopters of EF at Y-affiliated sites, they are likely applicable to other evidence-based programs conducted in community settings. Facilitators and barriers to adoption apply across programs and settings (8). Furthermore, facilitators, barriers, and recommendations address modifiable aspects of adoption that may improve success, including support of the organizational mission, available resources, and options for offsetting costs. Y-USA has successfully adopted a variety of evidence-based programs, and can serve as a model for other regionally and nationally networked community organizations. Organizations looking to adopt new programs may increase their likelihood of success by applying the recommendations appropriate to their organization and program.

ACKNOWLEDGMENTS

The authors wish to thank Susan Snyder and Meghan Thompson at Senior Services, Seattle, WA. This study was funded in part by the Centers for Disease Control and Prevention (CDC), Prevention Research Centers Program, through the University of Washington Health Promotion Research Centers Cooperative Agreement U48DP001911. The contents of this work are solely the responsibility of the authors and do not necessarily represent the official views of the CDC.

REFERENCES

1. Guyatt G, Cairns J, Churchill D, Cook D, Haynes B, Hirsh J, et al. Evidence-based medicine: a new approach to teaching the practice of medicine. *JAMA* (1992) **268**(17):2420–5. doi:10.1001/jama.1992.03490170092032
2. Pope ND, Rollins L, Chaumba J, Risler E. Evidence-based practice knowledge and utilization among social workers. *J Evid Based Soc Work* (2011) **8**(4):349–68. doi:10.1080/15433710903269149
3. *United States Senate Democrats, Democratic Policy Committee.* The patient protection and affordable care act detailed summary. Washington, DC (2010) [cited 2014 April 15]. Available from: http://www.dpc.senate.gov/healthreformbill/healthbill04.pdf.
4. National Council on Aging. *Using the Evidence Base to Promote Healthy Aging [Issue Brief].* Washington, DC (2006) [cited 2014 April 15]. Available from: http://www.ncoa.org/news-ncoa-publications/publications/issuebrief_1-r_usingeb.pdf.
5. National Council on Aging. *Evidence-Based Health Promotion Programs for Older Adults: Key Factors and Strategies Contributing to Program Sustainability [Issue Brief].* Washington, DC (2012) [cited 2014 April 15]. Available from: http://www.ncoa.org/improve-health/NCOA-Health-Promo-Issue-Brief.pdf.
6. Ackermann RT, Williams B, Nguyen HQ, Berke EM, Maciejewski ML, LoGerfo JP. Healthcare cost differences with participation in a community-based group physical activity benefit for medicare managed care health plan members. *J Am Geriatr Soc* (2008) **56**(8):1459–65. doi:10.1111/j.1532-5415.2008.01804.x
7. Belza B, Shumway-Cook A, Phelan E, Williams B, Snyder S, LoGerfo J. The effects of a community-based exercise program on function and health in older adults: the EnhanceFitness program. *J Appl Gerontol* (2006) **25**(4):291–306. doi:10.1177/0733464806290934
8. Centers for Medicare and Medicaid Services. *Report to Congress: The Centers for Medicare & Medicaid Services' Evaluation of Community-based Wellness and Prevention Programs under Section 4202 (b) of the Affordable Care Act.* Washington, DC (2013). Available from: http://innovation.cms.gov/Files/reports/CommunityWellnessRTC.pdf
9. Belza B, Snyder S, Thompson M, LoGerfo J. From research to practice: EnhanceFitness, an innovative community-based senior exercise program. *Top Geriatr Rehabil* (2010) **26**(4):299–309. doi:10.1097/TGR.0b013e3181fee69e
10. Wallace J, Buchner D, Grothaus L, Leveille S, LaCroix A, Wagner E. Implementation and effectiveness of a community-based health promotion program for older adults. *J Gerontol A Biol Sci Med Sci* (1998) **53a**(4):M301–6.
11. Rogers EM. *Diffusion of Innovations.* 5th ed. New York: Simon and Schuster (2003).
12. Glasgow RE, Klesges LM, Dzewaltowski DA, Bull SS, Estabrooks P. The future of health behavior change research: what is needed to improve translation of research into health promotion practice? *Ann Behav Med* (2004) **27**(1):3–12. doi:10.1207/s15324796abm2701_2
13. Deranaian CA, Desai P, Smith-Ray R, Seymour RB, Hughes SL. Perceived versus actual factors associated with adoption and maintenance of an evidence-based physical activity program. *Transl Behav Med* (2012) **2**(2):209–17. doi:10.1007/s13142-012-0131-x
14. Virginia Tech. *RE-AIM: A Model for the Planning, Evaluation, Reporting and Review of Translational Research and Practice.* [Internet]. Blacksburg, VA (2014) [cited 2014 April 14]. Available from: http://re-aim.org/.
15. Brownson RC, Ballew P, Dieffenderfer B, Haire-Joshu D, Heath GW, Kreuter MW, et al. Evidence-based interventions to promote physical activity: what contributes to dissemination by state health departments. *Am J Prev Med* (2007) **33**(1 Suppl):S66–73. doi:10.1016/j.amepre.2007.03.011
16. Ballew P, Brownson RC, Haire-Joshu D, Heath GW, Kreuter MW. Dissemination of effective physical activity interventions: are we applying the evidence? *Health Educ Res* (2010) **25**(2):185–98. doi:10.1093/her/cyq003
17. Pagoto SL, Kantor L, Bodenlos JS, Gitkind M, Ma Y. Translating the diabetes prevention program into a hospital-based weight loss program. *Health Psychol* (2008) **27**(1 Suppl):S91–8. doi:10.1037/0278-6133.27.1.S91
18. Gale BVP, Schaffer MA. Organizational readiness for evidence-based practice. *J Nurs Adm* (2009) **39**(2):91–7. doi:10.1097/NNA.0b013e318195a48d
19. Kohlbacher F. The use of qualitative content analysis in case study research. *Forum Qual Soc Res* (2006) **7**(1):Art.21. Available from: http://nbn-resolving.de/urn:nbn:de:0114-fqs0601211
20. Gill P, Stewart K, Treasure E, Chadwick B. Methods of data collection in qualitative research: interviews and focus groups. *Br Dent J* (2008) **204**(6):291–5. doi:10.1038/bdj.2008.192
21. Powers WR. *Transcription Techniques for the Spoken Word.* Lanham, MD: Altamira Press (2005).
22. Graneheim UH, Lundman B. Qualitative content analysis in nursing research: concepts, procedures and measures to achieve trustworthiness. *Nurse Educ Today* (2004) **24**(2):105–12. doi:10.1016/j.nedt.2003.10.001
23. Hsieh HF, Shannon SE. Three approaches to qualitative content analysis. *Qual Health Res* (2005) **15**(9):1277–88. doi:10.1177/1049732305276687
24. Glasgow RE, Vogt TM, Boles SM. Evaluating the public health impact of health promotion interventions: the RE-AIM framework. *Am J Public Health* (1999) **89**(9):1322–7. doi:10.2105/AJPH.89.9.1322
25. The YMCA. *About Us. [Internet].* Chicago, IL: YMCA of the USA (2014) [cited 2014 April 14]. Available from: http://www.ymca.net/about-us.
26. Harris JR, Cheadle A, Hannon M, Forehand M, Lichiello P, Mahoney E, et al. A framework for disseminating evidence-based health promotion practices. *Prev Chronic Dis* (2012) **9**:110081. doi:10.5888/pcd9.110081
27. Weiner B. A theory of organizational readiness for change. *Implement Sci* (2009) **4**(67):1–9. doi:10.1186/1748-5908-4-67
28. Ackermann RT. Working with the YMCA to implement the diabetes prevention program. *Am J Prev Med* (2013) **44**(4 Suppl 4):S352–6. doi:10.1016/j.amepre.2012.12.010
29. Ackermann RT, Finch EA, Caffrey HM, Lipscomb ER, Hays LM, Saha C. Long-term effects of a community-based lifestyle intervention to prevent type 2 diabetes: the DEPLOY extension pilot study. *Chronic Illn* (2011) **7**(4):279–90. doi:10.1177/1742395311407532

30. Ackermann RT, Marrero DG. Adapting the diabetes prevention program lifestyle intervention for delivery in the community: the YMCA model. *Diabetes Educ* (2007) **33**(1):69. doi:10.1177/0145721706297743
31. Nguyen HQ, Ackermann RT, Maciejewski M, Berke E, Patrick M, Williams B, et al. Managed-medicare health club benefit and reduced health care costs among older adults. *Prev Chronic Dis* (2008) **5**(1):A14.

30

Effect of physical activity, social support, and skills training on late-life emotional health

Mark B. Snowden[1], Lesley E. Steinman[2]*, Whitney L. Carlson[1], Kara N. Mochan[3,4], Ana F. Abraido-Lanza[5], Lucinda L. Bryant[6], Michael Duffy[7], Bob G. Knight[8], Dilip V. Jeste[9], Katherine H. Leith[10], Eric J. Lenze[11], Rebecca G. Logsdon[12], William A. Satariano[13], Damita J. Zweiback[14,15] and Lynda A. Anderson[16,17]

[1] Department of Psychiatry and Behavioral Sciences, University of Washington School of Medicine, Seattle, WA, USA
[2] Health Promotion Research Center, University of Washington, Seattle, WA, USA
[3] University of Washington School of Nursing with Environmental Health Focus, Seattle, WA, USA
[4] Adolescent Medicine, Seattle Children's, Seattle, WA, USA
[5] Department of Sociomedical Sciences, Columbia University Mailman School of Public Health, New York, NY, USA
[6] Department of Community and Behavioral Health, Colorado School of Public Health, University of Colorado Denver, Aurora, CO, USA
[7] Department of Educational Psychology, Counseling Psychology Program, Texas A&M University, College Station, TX, USA
[8] Davis School of Gerontology and Department of Psychology, University of Southern California, Los Angeles, CA, USA
[9] Sam and Rose Stein Institute for Research on Aging and Department of Psychiatry, University of California San Diego, San Diego, CA, USA
[10] College of Social Work, University of South Carolina, Columbia, SC, USA
[11] Department of Psychiatry, Washington University School of Medicine, St Louis, MO, USA
[12] Department of Psychosocial and Community Health, University of Washington School of Nursing, Seattle, WA, USA
[13] School of Public Health, University of California Berkeley, Berkeley, CA, USA
[14] Division of Chronic Disease and Injury Prevention, Michigan Department of Community Health, Lansing, MI, USA
[15] Healthy Aging Council and Health Equity Council, National Association of Chronic Disease Directors, Atlanta, GA, USA
[16] National Center for Chronic Disease Prevention and Health Promotion, Centers for Disease Control and Prevention, Atlanta, GA, USA
[17] Rollins School of Public Health, Emory University, Atlanta, GA, USA

Edited by:
Matthew Lee Smith, The University of Georgia, USA

Reviewed by:
Eli Carmeli, Haifa University, Israel
Brittany Rosen, University of Cincinnati, USA

****Correspondence:***
Lesley E. Steinman, MSW, MPH, Health Promotion Research Center, University of Washington, Seattle, WA. 1107 NE 45th Street, Suite 200, Seattle, WA 98105, USA
e-mail: lesles@uw.edu

Purpose: Given that emotional health is a critical component of healthy aging, we undertook a systematic literature review to assess whether current interventions can positively affect older adults' emotional health.

Methods: A national panel of health services and mental health researchers guided the review. Eligibility criteria included community-dwelling older adult (aged ≥ 50 years) samples, reproducible interventions, and emotional health outcomes, which included multiple domains and both positive (well-being) and illness-related (anxiety) dimensions. This review focused on three types of interventions – physical activity, social support, and skills training – given their public health significance and large number of studies identified. Panel members evaluated the strength of evidence (quality and effectiveness).

Results: In all, 292 articles met inclusion criteria. These included 83 exercise/physical activity, 25 social support, and 40 skills training interventions. For evidence rating, these 148 interventions were categorized into 64 pairings by intervention type and emotional health outcome, e.g., strength training targeting loneliness or social support to address mood. 83% of these pairings were rated at least fair quality. Expert panelists found sufficient evidence of effectiveness only for skills training interventions with health outcomes of decreasing anxiety and improving quality of life and self-efficacy. Due to limitations in reviewed studies, many intervention–outcome pairings yielded insufficient evidence.

Conclusion: Skills training interventions improved several aspects of emotional health in community-dwelling older adults, while the effects for other outcomes and interventions lacked clear evidence. We discuss the implications and challenges in moving forward in this important area.

Keywords: mental health, aged, health promotion, review

INTRODUCTION

Emotional health is increasingly viewed as a multidimensional construct that includes both positive and illness-related dimensions. Hendrie et al. (1) characterized emotional health as self-efficacy, depression, hostility and anger, anxiety, psychological stress, optimism, self-esteem, quality of life, and other domains assessed by multidimensional measures. A report (2) using data from the Behavioral Risk Factor Surveillance System (BRFSS) (3) identified six indicators reflecting positive and illness-related emotional health outcomes in older adults: social and emotional support; life satisfaction; frequent mental distress; current depression; lifetime diagnosis of depression; and lifetime diagnosis of anxiety disorders.

Mental health is increasingly viewed as part of public health's mission, as important as physical health in contributing to overall health and well being (2). Epidemiologic data links a range of health outcomes, particularly mortality and cardiovascular disease, to emotions (1). Despite the public health importance, little is currently known about the effectiveness of interventions to promote emotional health in community-dwelling older adults. One of the few available reports (4) reviews studies from UK, finding some evidence to support significant small-to-moderate improvements in emotional health from select exercise programs including mixed exercise programs, strength and resistance, aerobic, walking, and individually targeted health promotion interventions. However, it also indicated a clear shortage of robust evidence for effective programs to improve late-life emotional health.

Although this review (4) addressed several important questions, a more rigorous review of the scientific literature is warranted. The primary objective of this systematic literature review was to identify interventions to promote emotional health of older adults aged 50 years and older. We sought to expand Windle and colleagues work by encompassing a wider range of community-based interventions, including more than UK-based studies, examining multiple domains of emotional health incorporating both positive and illness-related dimensions, and addressing community-dwelling older adults.

MATERIALS AND METHODS

DATA SOURCES

Conceptual framework and definition of emotional health

This review used the NIH's Cognitive and Emotional Health Project (1, 5) to guide the development of our conceptual framework and definition of emotional health (**Figure 1**). Interventions to promote emotional health can influence various determinants of emotional health. These determinants include substance use and other behaviors, cognitive factors, psychosocial factors, emotional factors, and chronic conditions. Risk and protective factors for emotional health also included less modifiable biological and genetic factors and demographics. For the purpose of this review, we focused on interventions aimed at modifiable determinants.

Borrowing from Hendrie and colleagues, we defined emotional health comprehensively as including both emotion regulation concepts (e.g., the ability to control/regulate emotions) and emotion intelligence (e.g., the ability to recognize and use emotions constructively). Most importantly, emotional health is multidimensional, involving positive mental health constructs, such as life satisfaction as well as illness-related domains such as anxiety. We used Hendrie and colleagues' emotional health domains (1) and added "general well being" and "social support," given research describing the relevance of these constructs to emotional health (6–8). The emotional health constructs used in this review are provided in the first row of **Table 1**. Finally, based on the literature, the conceptual model included longer term health outcomes associated with emotional health, including reductions in mortality and improvements in functional ability, morbidity of chronic conditions, and overall quality of life (entailing both physical and emotional well being).

Expert panel and review methods

This review was guided by an eight-member expert panel of health services and mental health researchers from around the United States representing psychology, psychiatry, geriatrics, public health, and social work. The systematic review methods were derived from the *Guide to Community Preventive Services* ("The *Guide*") (9, 10) and the systematic literature review of strategies to address late-life depression (11), using a formal process to identify relevant studies, assess their quality, and summarize the evidence. We searched the peer-reviewed literature through

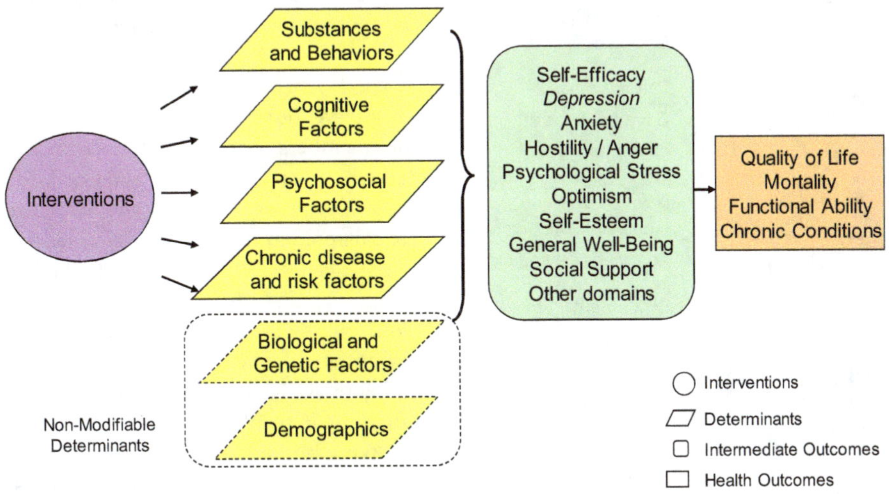

FIGURE 1 | Conceptual framework.

Table 1 | Search terms used in electronic searches.

Construct	Search terms	
Emotional health	Emotional health	*Interpersonal trust*
	Self-efficacy	*Positive Energy*
	Locus of control	Happiness
	Personal control	*Contentment*
	Personal mastery	*Hardiness*
	Powerlessness	*Resilience*
	Sense of coherence	Emotional vitality
	Depression	*Shame*
	Hopelessness	*Guilt*
	Hostility	*Regret*
	Anger	*Emotion regulation*
	Type A behavior	*Emotional control*
	Anxiety	Well being
	Environmental demands	*Altruism*
	Life events	*Sadness*
	Stress	Fear
	Mood states	*Neuroticism*
	Positive affect	*Boredom*
	Negative affect	*Capacity to care*
	Optimism	Life satisfaction
	Self-esteem	Spirituality
	Quality of life	Caregiver burden
	Loneliness	Acculturation
	Social support	Discrimination
Intervention	Intervention	Reminiscence therapy
	Treatment	Assertiveness training
	Prevention	Strengths-based
	Exercise	Positive psychology
	Physical activity	Social support
	CBT	Spirituality
	Psychotherapy	Complementary and alternative medicine
	Life review	Integrated medicine stress management
	Meditation	Anger management
	Mindfulness	Coping skills
Community based	Community	Primary care
	Home	Community health center
	Neighborhood	
Older adults	Older adults	Middle-Aged
	Aged	Limits of 40 and older (to include 50 and older)
	Elderly	
Study design	Clinical trial	Experimental replication
	Multicenter study	Follow-up study
	Randomized controlled trial	Field study
	Randomized clinical trial	Non-clinical case study
	Evaluation studies	Qualitative study
	Clinical case study	Quantitative study
	Empirical study	

Note: We did not find any physical activity, social support, or skills training intervention studies that targeted the emotional health outcomes in italics.

June 2008 and updated the search in June 2012 using PubMed (www.ncbi.nlm.nih.gov), CINAHL (http://www.ebscohost.com/academic/cinahl-plus-with-full-text/), and PsycINFO (www.apa.org/pubs/databases/psycinfo/index.aspx) databases. Subject headings and text words reflected our study aims, including key concepts of "emotional health," "older adults," "community based," and "intervention"; specific terms are provided in **Table 1**. References to meta-analyses and review papers were also examined, and expert panelists reviewed the citations of included articles.

STUDY SELECTION

Study inclusion criteria were (1) published data on populations aged 50 years and older, (2) community-based sample and setting, (3) clearly described intervention; and (4) "emotional health" operationalized using the list of constructs determined by the expert panel (see **Table 1**). There were no restrictions on sample size or study design. Articles were excluded if they: were not available in English; reported only a review of the literature, meta-analysis, or commentary; focused exclusively on inpatient or institutionalized persons. We included articles from any country as long as they were published in English. We excluded interventions that targeted depression given the overlap with a previously conducted review focusing on late-life depression (11). The emotional component of quality of life measures was included [e.g., the role emotional subscale of the SF-36 (12)]; however, physical subscales were excluded. For studies aimed at addressing outcomes not strictly emotional in nature (e.g., spirituality, caregiver burden), we required the inclusion of at least one other emotional health outcome from the list of constructs.

We used a two-step screening process evaluating abstracts and where necessary full text to assess whether articles met inclusion criteria. A standardized form was used to systematically collect key data from each article, including study design, sample size, intervention setting, outcome measures, results, and indicators of study quality. Data were compiled in summary tables that the expert panel used for the evidence rating. As employed in our prior review (11), we grouped articles into intervention type-emotional health outcome pairings to categorically rate the evidence. For example, skills training interventions aimed at reducing anxiety were paired together.

Expert panel members rated the quality and effectiveness of each intervention–outcome pairing (**Table 2**). For quality rating, panel members independently rated the set of studies for each intervention–outcome pairing as *Good, Fair,* or *Limited.* Because few pairings received a vote of "good," the good and fair categories were collapsed into a single category labeled "at least fair" quality. For effectiveness ratings, the panel members independently rated each intervention–outcome pairing as *Strong, Sufficient,* or *Insufficient.* For any pairing rated as insufficient, panel members were asked to record whether the rating was due to (1) an insufficient number of available studies or (2) a sufficient number of available studies but an insufficient amount of data to determine effectiveness. As established at the start of the review process, final determination of quality and effectiveness was based on 80% agreement among panel members. The panel met to discuss areas of disagreement and panel members were allowed to change their votes after the discussion; however, they were not required to reach consensus.

RESULTS

A total of 3,926 articles were identified in the initial search (1,250 from PubMed, 1,025 from PsycINFO, 1,631 from CINAHL, and 20 from reference lists of review articles or meta-analyses). 553 articles were duplicates and were eliminated (**Figure 2**). Two hundred ninety-two articles were eligible for inclusion, with the majority of the ineligible being excluded due to having too young of a sample size, not being an intervention study, or not having an emotional health outcome. Of the 292 eligible articles, the expert panel focused on three types of interventions relevant to public health practice and with ample studies for rating the evidence. These comprised a total of 148 of the 292 found articles: physical activity and/or exercise ($n = 83$), skills training ($n = 40$), and social support ($n = 25$) (**Table 3**). More than half of the studies (57%) were from the US or Canada, 19% were from European studies, 12% were from Australia or New Zealand, and 11% were from Asia. Thirty-nine percent of the articles specified that a theoretical framework that was used to inform the development of the intervention – one-third of the studies that evaluate an exercise or a social support intervention used a theoretical framework, while two-thirds of skills training interventions used a theoretical framework. Across interventions, the most common frameworks used across interventions were social cognitive theory, self-efficacy, and social learning theory. Other theories include the progressively lowered stress threshold model, the self-care deficit nursing theory of Orem, mindfulness meditation, self-management model of illness behavior, stress and coping theoretical framework, stress process models of caregiving, the transtheoretical model of behavior change, stages of change, negotiated adherence model, motivational interviewing, transforming hope theory, and Yalom group theory.

The physical activity and/or exercise interventions included aerobic activity, strength training, balance and flexibility interventions, motivational strategies, and a combination of exercise types. The skills training group included self-management [e.g., Chronic Disease Self-Management Program (CDSMP)], psycho-education, anger management, and stress management interventions. The social support group included interventions targeting direct or indirect provision of social support (e.g., interventions designed to improve ability to obtain support).

The 148 studies were subsequently grouped into 64 intervention type–outcome pairings, or categories, for rating the evidence, such as social support interventions aimed at elevating mood

Table 2 | Indicators of quality and effectiveness for rating the evidence.

Quality indicators	Effectiveness indicators
Well-described study population and intervention	Study quality
Sampling	Study design
Inclusion/exclusion criteria	Number of studies
Data analysis	Consistency across studies
Interpretation of results	Statistical results

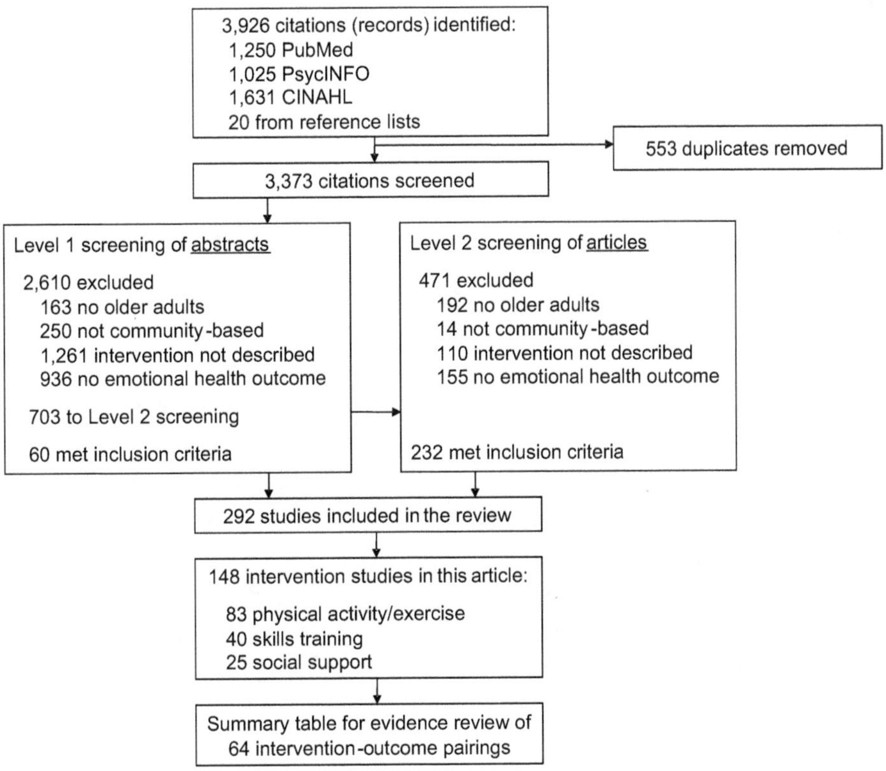

FIGURE 2 | Literature review flow chart.

Table 3 | Intervention–outcome pairings for skills training, social support + skills training, and physical activity interventions.

Intervention	Emotional health outcome	# Of studies (*n*)[a]	Quality rating	Effectiveness rating
Skills training	Anger	3 (258) (13–15)	At least fair	Insufficient (no consensus)
Skills training	Anxiety	11 (1,346) (13, 16–25)	At least fair	Sufficient
Skills training	Mood	5 (988) (13, 18, 26, 27, 76)	At least fair	Insufficient (no consensus)
Skills training	Other positive outcomes	2 (99) (29, 145)	At least fair	Insufficient (not enough studies)
Skills training	Psychological well being/distress	4 (1,449) (31, 32, 124, 142)	At least fair	Insufficient (multiple studies, inconclusive data)
Skills training	Quality of life	11 (1,417) (17, 22, 29, 31, 35–41)	At least fair	Sufficient
Skills training	Self-efficacy	16[b] (3,735) (14, 15, 18, 20, 24, 26, 27, 30, 35, 39, 41–46, 175)	At least fair	Sufficient
Skills training	Spirituality	3[b] (283) (23, 27, 65, 148)	Limited	Insufficient (not enough studies)
Skills training	Stress	4[b] (500) (39, 45, 46, 98, 142)	At least fair	Insufficient (multiple studies, inconclusive data)
Social support	Anxiety	3[b] (502) (34, 93, 135, 138)	At least fair	Insufficient (no consensus)
Social support	Loneliness	2 (313) (72, 108)	Limited	Insufficient (not enough studies)
Social support	Mood	2[b] (144) (72, 109, 113)	Limited	Insufficient (not enough studies)
Social support	Other positive outcomes	1 (39) (83)	Limited	Insufficient (not enough studies)
Social support	Psychological well being/distress	5[b] (704) (31, 34, 89, 128, 135, 139)	At least fair	Insufficient (multiple studies, inconclusive data)
Social support	Quality of life	3[b] (450) (31, 34, 135, 138)	At least fair	Insufficient (no consensus)
Social support	Self-efficacy/locus of control	1 (39) (83)	Limited	Insufficient (not enough studies)
Social support + skills training	Anxiety	5 (580) (54, 63, 70, 100, 143)	At least fair	Insufficient (multiple studies, inconclusive data)
Social support + skills training	Mood	1 (144) (70)	At least fair	Insufficient (not enough studies)
Social support + skills training	Other negative outcomes	2 (415) (47, 82)	At least fair	Insufficient (not enough studies)
Social support + skills training	Other positive outcomes	3[c] (58) (33, 66)	At least fair	Insufficient (no consensus)
Social support + skills training	Psychological well being/distress	6 (1,041) (14, 47, 70, 82, 144, 174)	Limited	Insufficient (multiple studies, inconclusive data)
Social support + skills training	Quality of life	3[b,c] (393) (66, 109, 113, 121)	At least fair	Insufficient (no consensus)
Social support + skills training	Self-efficacy/locus of control	3 (408) (65, 70, 121)	At least fair	Insufficient (no consensus)
Motivation/counseling	Mood	1 (86) (103)	At least fair	Insufficient (not enough studies)
Motivation/counseling	Other positive outcomes	2 (969) (71, 79)	At least fair	Insufficient (No consensus)
Motivation/counseling	Quality of life	4 (850) (52, 64, 71, 120)	At least fair	Insufficient (Multiple studies, inconclusive data)
Motivation/counseling	Self-efficacy/mastery	5 (567) (71, 79, 92, 112, 176)	At least fair	Insufficient (multiple studies, inconclusive data)

(Continued)

Table 3 | Continued

Intervention	Emotional health outcome	# Of studies (*n*)[a]	Quality rating	Effectiveness rating
Motivation/counseling	Stress	2 (1,712) (79, 118)	At least fair	Insufficient (no consensus)
Aerobic: walking	Anxiety	3 (507) (59, 102, 146)	At least fair	No Consensus (btw sufficient and insufficient, multiple studies)
Aerobic: other aerobic activities	Anxiety	4 (361) (57, 73, 114, 136)	At least fair	Insufficient (multiple studies, inconclusive data)
Aerobic: walking	Caregiver burden	1[b] (100) (60, 102)	At least fair	Insufficient (not enough studies)
Aerobic: walking	Mood	2 (170) (107, 147)	At least fair	Insufficient (no consensus)
Aerobic: walking	Other positive outcomes	1 (582) (101)	At least fair	Insufficient (not enough studies)
Aerobic: other aerobic activities	Other positive outcomes	2 (150) (57, 114)	At least fair	Insufficient (not enough studies)
Aerobic: walking	Quality of life	6 (1,273) (56, 101, 104, 123, 130, 147)	At least fair	Insufficient (multiple studies, inconclusive data)
Aerobic: other aerobic activities	Quality of life	6 (823) (51, 57, 117, 134, 151, 179)	At least fair	Insufficient (multiple studies, inconclusive data)
Aerobic: walking	Psychological distress and well-being	91 (28)	At least fair	Insufficient (not enough studies)
Aerobic: other aerobic activities	Psychological distress and well being	101 (136)	At last fair	Insufficient (not enough studies)
Aerobic: walking	Self-efficacy/mastery/locus of control	1 (32) (62)	NC	Insufficient (not enough studies)
Aerobic: Other aerobic activities	Self-efficacy/mastery/locus of control	3 (231) (56, 106, 114)	NC	Insufficient (no consensus)
Aerobic: walking	Stress	2[b] (457) (59, 60, 102)	At least fair	No consensus (btw sufficient and insufficient, not enough studies)
Strength/resistance	Anxiety	1 (42) (129)	At least fair	Insufficient (not enough studies)
Strength/resistance	Fear of falling	2 (94) (48, 150)	At least fair	Insufficient (no consensus)
Strength/resistance	Loneliness	1[b] (32) (84, 129)	At least fair	Insufficient (not enough studies)
Strength/resistance	Mood	2 (144) (69, 153)	At least fair	Insufficient (no consensus)
Strength/resistance	Psychological well being/distress	2 (124) (134, 153)	At least fair	Insufficient (not enough studies)
Strength/resistance	Quality of life	13[b] (1,000) (28, 68, 75, 84, 115, 119, 122, 126, 132–134, 137, 153, 177)	At least fair	Insufficient (multiple studies, inconclusive data)
Strength/resistance	Self-efficacy/locus of control	7[b] (442) (75, 115, 126, 129, 132, 137, 153, 177)	At least fair	Insufficient (multiple studies, inconclusive data)
Stretch/flexibility/ balance/agility	Anxiety	1 (88) (96)	NC	Insufficient (not enough studies)
Stretch/flexibility /balance/agility	Fear of falling	2[b] (422) (53, 90, 181)	At least fair	No consensus (btw sufficient and insufficient)
Stretch/flexibility/ balance/agility	Mood	5 (307) (49, 87, 95, 116, 147)	At least fair	Insufficient (no consensus)
Stretch/flexibility/ balance/agility	Other positive outcomes	1[b] (200) (53, 182)	At least fair	Insufficient (not enough studies)

(Continued)

Table 3 | Continued

Intervention	Emotional health outcome	# Of studies (*n*)[a]	Quality rating	Effectiveness rating
Stretch/flexibility/balance/agility	Psychological well being/distress	1[b] (200) (53, 182)	At least fair	Insufficient (not enough studies)
Stretch/flexibility/balance/agility	Quality of life	8[b] (853) (48, 51, 53, 87, 94, 96, 132, 147, 181)	At least fair	Insufficient (multiple studies, inconclusive data)
Stretch/flexibility/balance/agility	Self-efficacy/mastery/locus of control	5 (465) (48, 90, 94, 95, 132)	At least fair	No consensus (btw strong, sufficient, insufficient)
Stretch/flexibility/balance/agility	Stress	1 (39) (95)	NC	Insufficient (not enough studies)
Combination	Anxiety	3 (485) (91, 180, 182)	At least fair	Insufficient (no consensus)
Combination	Fear of falling	2 (200) (85, 88)	At least fair	Insufficient (no consensus)
Combination	Mood	3 (257) (81, 97, 173)	At least fair	Insufficient (no consensus)
Combination	Other positive outcomes	3 (459) (91, 131, 178)	At least fair	Insufficient (multiple studies, inconclusive data)
Combination	Psychological well being/distress	6 (748) (97, 131, 133, 180, 182, 184)	At least fair	Insufficient (multiple studies, inconclusive data)
Combination	Quality of life	16 (7,492) (55, 61, 78, 80, 81, 85, 86, 88, 97, 99, 110, 111, 149, 152, 182, 183)	At least fair	Insufficient (multiple studies, inconclusive data)
Combination	Self-efficacy/mastery/locus of control	5[b] (654) (77, 92, 105, 125, 127, 183)	At least fair	Insufficient (multiple studies, inconclusive data)
Combination	Stress	1 (187) (180)	NC	Insufficient (not enough studies)

NC, no consensus.

[a]Article citations for each intervention–outcome pairing are provided in this column. Some of the 148 studies are listed in more than one intervention–outcome pairing.

[b]Several studies are reported in more than one article (e.g., article #40 and article #41 describe the same study using different analyses).

[c]Article #62 reported on two different positive outcomes, self-esteem and life satisfaction.

(**Table 3**). For quality, 53 (83%) of the intervention–outcome pairings were rated as having "at least fair" quality; only 11% of these had good quality. For effectiveness, a majority of pairings (89%) were deemed to have insufficient evidence, due to lack of studies (two or fewer) or inconclusive evidence (mixed results within or across studies). Herein, we will report findings for the three intervention–outcome pairings for which sufficient evidence was found. For further information about categories not presented or on detailed summary data tables, please contact the corresponding author.

INTERVENTION–OUTCOME PAIRINGS WITH SUFFICIENT EVIDENCE

Skills training

Sufficient evidence was found for effectiveness of skills training interventions to reduce anxiety and to promote quality of life and self-efficacy (from a total of 38 studies). These studies were rated as having "at least fair" quality. Of these studies, 11 were aimed at reducing anxiety, of which four involved randomized controlled trials (RCT). They involved 1,346 participants and represented a diverse subject population (e.g., caregivers and people with breast cancer, heart disease, or arthritis). Only three studies reported dropout rates, and in two of these, that rate was below 20%. Study duration varied from 2 to 12 months, although generally the active phase ranged from 6 to 8 weeks.

The report by López et al. (16) focused on caregivers in which the majority of care was provided to persons living with dementia (80%).They found a 38% decrease in mean anxiety score in the Hospital Anxiety and Depression Scale (HADS) (154) for traditional format skills training (60 min weekly over a period of 8 weeks) involving cognitive behavioral approaches, assertiveness training, self-esteem building exercises, and problem-solving skills training. The other studies using the HADS found a 10–20% decrease in anxiety scores after intervention (17, 18). The Williams (19) study of 71 women with breast cancer found no effect for a 20-min audiotape to teach skills for decreasing sleep, anxiety, and fatigue problems encountered during chemotherapy. Two non-randomized, controlled trials did not show a significant effect. One focused on asthma self-management and another focused on Chinese older adults with history of depression or anxiety, although there was a non-significant trend toward effectiveness ($p < 0.10$) (20, 21). Five single-group studies revealed mixed results (13, 22–25).

Eleven additional skills training studies aimed at emotional health as measured by the subscales of a quality of life measure such as the SF-36. There were eight RCTs, two quasi-experimental studies, and one single-group study. A total of 1,417 participants were included in these studies, with sample sizes ranging from 35 to 320, averaging between 75 and 100 participants. The duration of the interventions ranged from 1 week to 8 months, averaging between 6 and 8 weeks. Interventions included both group and individual-level activities. Dropout rates of less than 20% were reported for all but two studies. Seven studies [five RCTs (17, 35–39) and one non-RCT (40)] reported statistically significant improvements in at least one emotional health subscale of the SF-36 Quality of Life measure. Specifically, statistically significant improvements were reported for the *vitality and role limitations emotional* SF-36 subscales for Barnason et al.'s (35) phone-based home communication intervention for older adults with ischemic heart failure ($p < 0.01$). Similarly, Grant et al.'s (36) social problem-solving phone partnership for adult caregivers of stroke survivors improved quality of life subdomains ($p = 0.013$). McHugh et al.'s (17) share care health education and motivational interviewing program for adults waiting for elective CABG ($p = 0.000$), and Wallace et al.'s (37) nurse visit to develop a customized health plan for older adults exercising at a local senior center were found to be effective ($p = 0.02$). No significant improvements in *vitality* were found for Markle-Reid et al.'s (26, 38) individual-level program to bolster personal and environmental resources of frail, older home care clients although this study did find improvement using the *role limitation emotional* subscale. In addition to Grant et al. (36), Markle-Reid et al. (38), McHugh et al. (17), and Wallace et al. (37) studies, Hughes et al. (39) study of a workshop intervention for women with self-reported disabilities all reported significant improvements in the SF-36 *mental health* subscale. Furthermore, two studies (38, 40) found significant improvements in the *mental health composite* SF-36 measure (including vitality, mental health, and role limitation emotional). Significant improvements were demonstrated in two studies using emotional health subscales of quality of life-specific measures for older adults with heart failure (13, 22–25, 31, 35–38). The remaining two studies (29, 41) did not find improvements in emotional health subscales of different quality of life measures.

Sixteen skills training intervention studies were directed at improving self-efficacy. These studies included 11 RCTs, two observational studies, and three single-group studies. Seven of the studies were of interventions using the CDSMP. A total of 3,735 participants received skills training interventions, with sample sizes ranging from 33 to 728. Study duration averaged 6 to 8 weeks. Dropout rates, reported in half the studies, were less than 20%. The frequency of the skills training interventions was rarely reported. When reported, adherence to the intervention was typically less than 80%. The interventions were delivered most often in a group format and the control groups were generally usual care and wait-list control conditions. Eight of the 11 RCTs (14, 15, 26, 27, 35, 42–46) reported significant improvements in self-efficacy; three of the significant studies used CDSMP (15, 42, 45). Four of the five non-RCT studies (15, 20, 24, 32) also demonstrated significant improvements in self-efficacy. All but Smith et al. (20) study were single-group designs with 20–32% dropout rates.

Exercise and social support

The expert panel did not find sufficient evidence for either exercise or social support interventions to improve emotional health.

OTHER INTERVENTION–OUTCOME PAIRINGS

Skills training

The expert panel found insufficient evidence for 20 other skills training interventions that focused on other emotional health outcomes such as mood and stress. Most of these pairings were of at least fair quality. In addition, 82 studies were found that reported on the effects of physical activity and/or exercise on emotional health outcomes, and 25 studies looked at social support interventions. There was insufficient evidence of effectiveness for most of these intervention–outcome pairings and the panel rated most of the pairings as at least fair quality.

Exercise and physical activity

The expert panel did not reach consensus for several physical activity and exercise intervention–outcome pairings. First, the panel was split between ratings of sufficient and insufficient for stretching, flexibility, balance, or agility interventions to decrease fear of falling. Second, panel members did not agree on whether there was sufficient evidence that stretching, flexibility, balance or agility interventions improved self-efficacy, mastery, or locus of control. Panel members raised concerns about limited numbers of studies for any single outcome and about mixed results observed across the study outcomes. Finally, the expert panelists were split between evidence ratings of sufficient and insufficient for walking interventions that targeted anxiety or stress. Insufficient evidence was found for all other exercise and physical activity interventions.

Social support

The expert panel found insufficient evidence that the reviewed social support interventions improved emotional health.

DISCUSSION

This review examined three broad types of interventions designed to promote emotional health: physical activity and/or exercise, skills training, and social support. Among the interventions rated as having at least fair quality and sufficient evidence, we found that skills training interventions reduced anxiety; enhanced self-efficacy; and improved vitality, role functioning related to emotional limitations, and emotional health as measured in quality of life subscales. Skills training interventions are theorized to promote positive domains of emotional health through cognitive reframing, strengthening coping resources, and increasing the amount of support (or quality of support). We acknowledge that skills training may improve emotional health through improved self-efficacy, though the panel chose to view self-efficacy as its own emotional health domain. These interventions are designed for older adults with chronic conditions (e.g., arthritis, heart disease, physical disabilities) or informal caregivers (e.g., spouses, adult children) of older adults coping with dementia, stroke survivors, or mental illness making them quite generalizable. These populations were targeted by these interventions because chronic conditions or caregiving responsibilities increase the need for skills training, support, information, and resources.

The CDSMP was used as an intervention in seven of the skills training studies that showed sufficient evidence for improving quality of life or self-efficacy or decreasing anxiety. CDSMP has been shown to enhance stress management techniques, improve communication with physicians, increase confidence in ability to manage the condition, and improve role function (32, 42, 155–159). Improving self-management skills has been shown to impact other aspects of participants' lives, such as their ability to manage their emotions, choose healthy foods and exercise activities, and activate their social network (158). This review is limited by its end date of June 2008. While it is beyond the scope of this project to conduct an updated systematic literature review, we recently searched for other review papers on skills training, exercise and/or physical activity, and social support interventions to promote emotional health. We found two review papers (160, 161) that reported similar findings as we report above, namely, sufficient evidence for skills training interventions impact on self-efficacy and quality of life and insufficient evidence for other emotional health outcomes. We also searched for intervention studies for those areas where sufficient evidence was found. Our search yielded 10 recently published articles (162–171), none of which reported different findings than reported above.

We defined "insufficient evidence of effectiveness" in two ways: either there were not enough studies of at least fair quality, or there were multiple studies with inconclusive data. Insufficient evidence did not mean that interventions were clearly ineffective. Very few intervention–outcome pairings were rated as at least fair quality. The expert panel identified the following common quality limitations: lack of descriptive information about the interventions, limited information about the statistical methods and analyses, and small sample sizes or underpowered studies. Additionally, features of some of the study designs made it difficult to detect changes in emotional health. For example, many studies included emotional health outcome measures that may not be responsive to small changes from programs of limited intensity and duration, and sampling "emotionally healthy" subjects that created ceiling effects. In fact, many of the reviewed aerobic physical activity interventions did not meet current national guidelines (140) for 150 min per week of moderate-intensity activity (though all reviewed strength/resistance interventions did meet existing criteria of 2 days per week).

Our review included a wide range of emotional health constructs. Some outcomes were entirely emotional (e.g., anxiety), whereas others included a mix of cognitive, emotional, and behavioral domains (e.g., self-efficacy). In addition, some studies included emotional health outcomes as their primary outcomes, whereas others included emotional health as intermediate outcomes or mediators of other health outcomes. Finally, there was a dearth of intervention studies on certain emotional health constructs, such as hopelessness, shame, guilt, regret, fear, neuroticism, boredom, positive energy, contentment, hardiness, resilience, emotional stability, emotional regulation/control, altruism, capacity to care, and happiness. In particular, positive constructs were underrepresented in the available literature. We were not surprised that there was limited evidence on interventions to promote emotional health, and particularly any studies lacking in positive emotional health constructs given the tendency (up until recently) to focus on disease prevention over health promotion. We anticipate that more research will include emotional health outcomes as models such as the socio-ecological model (67, 172) and guidelines such as the Public Health Action Plan to Integrate Mental Health Promotion and Mental Illness Prevention with Chronic Disease Prevention, 2011–2015 (74) emphasize the importance of emotional health in the larger public health goals.

Future research needs to address these quality concerns by attending to limitations with both internal and external validity. One way to do so is to use the RE-AIM framework, a conceptual approach for evaluating the translation of research into practice in "real-world" settings (141). RE-AIM stands for reach, effectiveness, adoption, implementation fidelity, and maintenance – five areas, which, if addressed, ensure that essential program goals are retained during the implementation process, resulting in greater external validity. More research is also needed to investigate the longer term, maintenance effects of interventions to promote positive emotional health, and address illness-related domains in older adults as most of the studies here were of short-term effectiveness. The prominence of theories such as social cognitive theory, social learning theory, and self-efficacy theory in those interventions with sufficient evidence may also be helpful to consider in future intervention design and development as they may have contributed to the optimization of participants' quality of life and self-efficacy and minimization of anxiety symptoms.

Despite the gaps in the current research, our systematic review provides important information about interventions that can promote emotional health outcomes in community-dwelling older adults. Specifically, we found that skills training interventions resulted in improvements in both illness-related (anxiety) and positive (quality of life and self-efficacy) domains of emotional health. Given that more than one in four Americans lives with two or more concurrent chronic conditions, the challenges of managing multiple chronic conditions among the growing numbers of older persons are significant (50). One of the overarching goals of the U.S. Department of Health and Human Services' Strategic Framework (58), *Optimum Health and Quality of Life for Individuals with Multiple Chronic Conditions*, is to "maximize the use of proven self-care management and other services by individuals with multiple chronic conditions." As shown in this review, skills training interventions can offer important benefits in the realm of promoting emotional health in older adults. Given the expanding proportion of older adults in the US and globally, we hope this review will help in addressing some of challenges identified in this important area of study.

ACKNOWLEDGMENTS

This research was made possible through a contract with the National Association of Chronic Disease Directors (NACDD) to the University of Washington Health Promotion Research Center and funded by the CDC Healthy Aging Program's Healthy Brain Initiative (U48-DP000050). The findings and conclusions in this article are those of the authors and do not necessarily represent the official position of the Centers for Disease Control and Prevention.

REFERENCES

1. Hendrie HC, Albert MS, Butters MA, Gao S, Knopman DS, Launer LJ, et al. The NIH cognitive and emotional health project: report of the critical evaluation study committee. *Alzheimers Dement* (2006) **2**:12–32. doi:10.1016/j.jalz.2005.11.004
2. Centers for Disease Control and Prevention (CDC) and National Association of Chronic Disease Directors (NACDD). *The State of Mental Health and Aging in America Issue Brief 1: What Do the Data Tell Us?*. National Association of Chronic Disease Directors (2008). Available from: http://www.cdc.gov/aging/pdf/mental_health.pdf
3. Centers for Disease Control and Prevention (CDC). *Behavioral Risk Factor Surveillance System Survey Data*. Atlanta, GA: U.S. Department of Health and Human Services, Centers for Disease Control and Prevention (2006).
4. Windle G, Linck P, Morgan R, Hughes D, Burholt V, Reeves C, et al. *Public Health Interventions to Promote Mental Well-Being in People Aged 65 and Over: Systematic Review of Effectiveness and Costs-Effectiveness*. (2008). Available from: http://www.nice.org.uk/guidance/index.jsp?action=folder&o=36395
5. National Institutes of Health (NIH). *Cognitive and Emotional Health Project: The Healthy Brain*. (2001). Available from: http://trans.nih.gov/cehp/HBPemot.htm
6. Stevens A, Coon D, Wisniewski S, Vance D, Arguelles S, Belle S, et al. Measurement of leisure time satisfaction in family caregivers. *Aging Ment Health* (2004) **8**:450–9. doi:10.1080/13607860410001709737
7. Dickinson P, Neilson G, Agee M. The sustainability of mentally healthy schools initiatives: insights from the experiences of a co-educational secondary school in Aotearoa/New Zealand. *Int J Ment Health Promot* (2004) **6**(2):34–9. doi:10.1080/14623730.2004.9721929
8. Haley W, Roth D, Coleton M, Ford G, West C, Collins R, et al. Appraisal, coping, and social support as mediators of well-being in black and white family caregivers of patients with Alzheimer's disease. *J Consult Clin Psychol* (1996) **64**:121–9. doi:10.1037/0022-006X.64.1.121
9. Briss P, Zaza S, Pappaioanou M, Fielding J, Wright-De Agüero L, Truman BI, et al. Developing an evidence-based guide to community preventive services-methods. *Am J Prev Med* (2000) **18**(1S):35–43. doi:10.1016/S0749-3797(99)00119-1
10. Norris S, Nichols PJ, Caspersen CJ, Glasgow RE, Engelgau MM, Jack L, et al. The effectiveness of disease and case management for people with diabetes: a systematic review. *Am J Prev Med* (2002) **22**(4S):15–38. doi:10.1016/S0749-3797(02)00423-3
11. Frederick JT, Steinman LE, Prohaska T, Satariano WA, Bruce M, Bryant L, et al. Community-based treatment of late life depression—an expert panel informed literature review. *Am J Prev Med* (2007) **33**(3):222–49. doi:10.1016/j.amepre.2007.04.035
12. Ware JE, Sherbourne CD. The MOS 36-item short form health survey (SF-36). I. Conceptual framework and item selection. *Med Care* (1992) **30**:473–83. doi:10.1097/00005650-199206000-00002
13. Mizuno E, Hosak T, Ogihara R, Higano H, Mano Y. Effectiveness of a stress management program for family caregivers of the elderly at home. *J Med Dent Sci* (1999) **46**(4):145–53.
14. Coon DW, Thompson L, Steffen A, Sorocco K, Gallagher-Thompson D. Anger and depression management: psychoeducational skill training interventions for women caregivers of a relative with dementia. *Gerontologist* (2003) **43**(5):678–89. doi:10.1093/geront/43.5.678
15. Steffen AM. Anger management for dementia caregivers: a preliminary study using video and telephone interventions. *Behav Ther* (2000) **31**(2):281–99. doi:10.1080/13607860903420989
16. López J, Crespo M, Zarit SH. Assessment of the efficacy of a stress management program for informal caregivers of dependent older adults. *Gerontologist* (2007) **47**(2):205–14. doi:10.1093/geront/47.2.205
17. McHugh F, Lindsay GM, Hanlon P, Hutton I, Brown MR, Morrison C, et al. Nurse led shared care for patients on the waiting list for coronary artery bypass surgery: a randomised controlled trial. *Heart* (2001) **86**(3):317–23. doi:10.1136/heart.86.3.317
18. Barlow JH, Turner AP, Wright CC. A randomized controlled study of the arthritis self-management programme in the UK. *Health Educ Res* (2000) **15**(6):665–80. doi:10.1093/her/15.6.665
19. Williams SA, Schreier AM. The role of education in managing fatigue, anxiety, and sleep disorders in women undergoing chemotherapy for breast cancer. *Appl Nurs Res* (2005) **18**(3):138–47. doi:10.1016/j.apnr.2004.08.005
20. Smith C, Hancock H, Blake-Mortimer J, Eckert K. A randomised comparative trial of yoga and relaxation to reduce stress and anxiety. *Complement Ther Med* (2007) **15**(2):77–83. doi:10.1016/j.ctim.2006.05.001
21. Dai Y, Zhang S, Yamamoto J, Ao M, Belin TR, Cheung F, et al. Cognitive behavioral therapy of minor depressive symptoms in elderly Chinese Americans: a pilot study. *Community Ment Health J* (1999) **35**(6):537–42. doi:10.1023/A:1018763302198
22. Hui E, Lee PS, Woo J. Management of urinary incontinence in older women using videoconferencing versus conventional management: a randomized controlled trial. *J Telemed Telecare* (2006) **12**(7):343–7. doi:10.1258/135763306778682413
23. Kretzer K, Davis J, Easa D, Johnson J, Harrigan R. Self identity through Ho'oponopono as adjunctive therapy for hypertension management. *Ethn Dis* (2007) **17**(4):624–8.
24. Wright CC, Barlow JH, Turner AP, Bancroft GV. Self-management training for people with chronic disease: an exploratory study. *Br J Health Psychol* (2003) **8**(Pt 4):465–76. doi:10.1348/135910703770238310
25. Ishizaki J, Meguro K, Ohe K, Kimura E, Tsuchiya E, Ishii H, et al. Therapeutic psychosocial intervention for elderly subjects with very mild Alzheimer disease in a community: the tajiri project. *Alzheimer Dis Assoc Disord* (2002) **16**(4):261–9. doi:10.1097/00002093-200210000-00008
26. Brody BL, Roch-Levecq AC, Gamst AC, Maclean K, Kaplan RM, Brown SI. Self-management of age-related macular degeneration and quality of life: a randomized controlled trial. *Arch Ophthalmol* (2002) **120**(11):1477–83. doi:10.1001/archopht.120.11.1477
27. Cunningham AJ. Integrating spirituality into a group psychological therapy program for cancer patients. *Integr Cancer Ther* (2005) **4**(2):178–86. doi:10.1177/1534735405275648
28. Evcik D, Sonel B. Effectiveness of a home-based exercise therapy and walking program on osteoarthritis of the knee. *Rheumatol Int* (2002) **22**(3):103–6. doi:10.1007/s00296-002-0198-7
29. Duggleby WD, Degner L, Williams A, Wright K, Cooper D, Popkin D, et al. Living with hope: initial evaluation of a psychosocial hope intervention for older palliative home care patients. *J Pain Symptom Manage* (2007) **33**(3):247–57. doi:10.1016/j.jpainsymman.2006.09.013
30. Kline KS, Scott LD, Britton AS. The use of supportive-educative and mutual goal-setting strategies to improve self-management for patients with heart failure. *Home Healthc Nurse* (2007) **25**(8):502–10. doi:10.1097/01.NHH.0000289104.60043.7d
31. Scott LD, Setter-Kline K, Britton AS. The effects of nursing interventions to enhance mental health and quality of life among individuals with heart failure. *Appl Nurs Res* (2004) **17**(4):248–56. doi:10.1016/j.apnr.2004.09.004
32. Lorig KR, Sobel DS, Stewart AL, Brown BW Jr, Bandura A, Ritter P, et al. Evidence suggesting that a chronic disease self-management program can improve health status while reducing hospitalization: a randomized trial. *Med Care* (1999) **37**(1):5–14. doi:10.1097/00005650-199901000-00003
33. Davis LL. Telephone-based interventions with family caregivers: a feasibility study. *J Fam Nurs* (1998) **4**(3):255–70. doi:10.1177/107484079800400303
34. Mant J, Winner S, Roche J, Wade DT. Family support for stroke: one year follow up of a randomised controlled trial. *J Neurol Neurosurg Psychiatry* (2005) **76**(7):1006–8. doi:10.1136/jnnp.2004.048991
35. Barnason SL, Zimmerman L, Nieveen J, Schmaderer M, Carranza B, Reilly S. Impact of a home communication intervention for coronary artery bypass graft patients with ischemic heart failure on self-efficacy, coronary disease risk factor modification, and functioning. *Heart Lung* (2003) **32**(3):147–58. doi:10.1016/S0147-9563(03)00036-0
36. Grant JS, Elliott TR, Weaver M, Bartolucci AA, Giger JN. Telephone intervention with family caregivers of stroke survivors after rehabilitation. *Stroke* (2002) **33**(8):2060–5. doi:10.1161/01.STR.0000020711.38824.E3
37. Wallace JI, Buchner DM, Grothaus L, Leveille S, Tyll L, LaCroix AZ, et al. Implementation and effectiveness of a community-based health promotion program for older adults. *J Gerontol A Biol Sci Med Sci* (1998) **53**(4):M301–6. doi:10.1093/gerona/53A.4.M301
38. Markle-Reid M, Weir R, Browne G, Roberts J, Gafni A, Henderson S. Health promotion for frail older home care clients. *J Adv Nurs* (2006) **54**(3):381–95. doi:10.1111/j.1365-2648.2006.03817.x
39. Hughes RB, Robinson-Whelen S, Taylor HB, Hall JW. Stress self-management: an intervention for women with physical disabilities. *Womens Health Issues* (2006) **16**(6):389–99. doi:10.1016/j.whi.2006.08.003

40. Pischke CR, Weidner G, Elliott-Eller M, Ornish D. Lifestyle changes and clinical profile in coronary heart disease patients with an ejection fraction of <or=40% or >40% in the multicenter lifestyle demonstration project. *Eur J Heart Fail* (2007) **9**(9):928–34. doi:10.1016/j.ejheart.2007.05.009
41. Kocken PL, Voorham AJJ. Effects of a peer-led senior health education program. *Patient Educ Couns* (1998) **34**(1):15–23. doi:10.1016/S0738-3991(98)00038-X
42. Swerissen H, Belfrage J, Weeks A, Jordan L, Walker C, Furler J, et al. A randomised control trial of a self-management program for people with a chronic illness from Vietnamese, Chinese, Italian and Greek backgrounds. *Patient Educ Couns* (2006) **64**(1–3):360–8. doi:10.1016/j.pec.2006.04.003
43. Barlow JH, Williams B, Wright CC. Instilling the strength to fight the pain and get on with life': learning to become an arthritis self-manager through an adult education programme. *Health Educ Res* (1999) **14**(4):533–44. doi:10.1093/her/14.4.533
44. Lorig K, Gonzalez VM, Ritter P. Community-based Spanish language arthritis education program: a randomized trial. *Med Care* (1999) **37**(9):957–63. doi:10.1097/00005650-199909000-00011
45. Solomon P, Draine J, Mannion E, Meisel M. Impact of brief family psychoeducation on self-efficacy. *Schizophr Bull* (1996) **22**(1):41–50. doi:10.1093/schbul/22.1.41
46. Solomon P, Draine J, Mannion E, Meisel M. Effectiveness of two models of brief family education: retention of gains by family members of adults with serious mental illness. *Am J Orthopsychiatry* (1997) **67**(2):177–86. doi:10.1037/h0080221
47. Forster A, Young J. Specialist nurse support for patients with stroke in the community: a randomised controlled trial. *BMJ* (1996) **312**(7047):1642–6. doi:10.1136/bmj.312.7047.1642
48. Liu-Ambrose T, Khan KM, Eng JJ, Lord SR, McKay HA. Balance confidence improves with resistance or agility training. *Gerontology* (2004) **50**(6):373–82. doi:10.1159/000080175
49. Ross MC, Bohannon AS, Davis DC, Gurchiek L. The effects of a short-term exercise program on movement, pain, and mood in the elderly: results of a pilot study. *J Holist Nurs* (1999) **17**(2):139–47. doi:10.1177/089801019901700203
50. Anderson G. *Chronic Care: Making the Case for Ongoing Care.* Robert Wood Johnson Foundation: (2010). Available from: http://www.rwjf.org/content/dam/farm/reports/reports/2010/rwjf54583
51. Daley AJ, Crank H, Saxton JM, Mutrie N, Coleman R, Roalfe A. Randomized trial of exercise therapy in women treated for breast cancer. *J Clin Oncol* (2007) **25**(13):1713–21. doi:10.1200/JCO.2006.09.5083
52. Kolt GS, Schofield GM, Kerse N, Garrett N, Oliver M. Effect of telephone counseling on physical activity for low-active older people in primary care: a randomized, controlled trial. *J Am Geriatr Soc* (2007) **55**(7):986–92. doi:10.1111/j.1532-5415.2007.01203.x
53. Kutner NG, Barnhart H, Wolf SL, McNeely E, Xu T. Self-report benefits of Tai Chi practice by older adults. *J Gerontol B Psychol Sci Soc Sci* (1997) **52**(5):242–6. doi:10.1093/geronb/52B.5.P242
54. Hartford K, Wong C, Zakaria D. Randomized controlled trial of a telephone intervention by nurses to provide information and support to patients and their partners after elective coronary artery bypass graft surgery: effects of anxiety. *Heart Lung* (2002) **31**(3):199–206. doi:10.1067/mhl.2002.122942
55. Smart N, Haluska B, Jeffriess L, Marwick TH. Predictors of a sustained response to exercise training in patients with chronic heart failure: a telemonitoring study. *Am Heart J* (2005) **150**(6):1240–7. doi:10.1016/j.ahj.2005.01.035
56. Clark DO, Stump TE, Damush TM. Outcomes of an exercise program for older women recruited through primary care. *J Aging Health* (2003) **15**(3):567–85. doi:10.1177/0898264303253772
57. Courneya KS, Friedenreich CM, Quinney HA, Fields AL, Jones LW, Fairey AS. A randomized trial of exercise and quality of life in colorectal cancer survivors. *Eur J Cancer Care* (2003) **12**(4):347–57. doi:10.1046/j.1365-2354.2003.00437.x
58. U.S. Department of Health and Human Services. *Multiple Chronic Conditions—A Strategic Framework: Optimum Health and Quality of Life for Individuals with Multiple Chronic Conditions.* Washington, DC: (2010). Available from: http://www.hhs.gov/ash/initiatives/mcc/mcc_framework.pdf
59. King AC, Taylor CB, Haskell WL. Effects of differing intensities and formats of 12 months of exercise training on psychological outcomes in older adults. *Health Psychol* (1993) **12**(4):292–300. doi:10.1037/0278-6133.12.5.405
60. King AC, Baumann K, O'Sullivan P, Wilcox S, Castro C. Effects of moderate-intensity exercise on physiological, behavioral, and emotional responses to family caregiving: a randomized controlled trial. *J Gerontol A Biol Sci Med Sci* (2002) **57**(1):M26–36. doi:10.1093/gerona/57.1.M26
61. Focht BC, Brawley LR, Rejeski WJ, Ambrosius WT. Group-mediated activity counseling and traditional exercise therapy programs: effects on health-related quality of life among older adults in cardiac rehabilitation. *Ann Behav Med* (2004) **28**(1):52–61. doi:10.1207/s15324796abm2801_7
62. Gary R. Exercise self-efficacy in older women with diastolic heart failure: results of a walking program and education intervention. *J Gerontol Nurs* (2006) **32**(7):31–9.
63. Gendron CE, Poitras LR, Engels ML, Dastoor DP, Sirota SE, Barza SL, et al. Skills training with supporters of the demented. *J Am Geriatr Soc* (1986) **34**(12):875–80.
64. Halbert JA, Silagy CA, Finucane PM, Withers RT, Hamdorf PA. Physical activity and cardiovascular risk factors: effect of advice from an exercise specialist in Australian general practice. *Med J Aust* (2000) **173**(2):84–7.
65. Slivinske LR, Fitch VL. The effect of control enhancing interventions on the well-being of elderly individuals living in retirement communities. *Gerontologist* (1987) **27**(2):176–81. doi:10.1093/geront/27.2.176
66. Acorn S. Assisting families of head-injured survivors through a family support programme. *J Adv Nurs* (1995) **21**(5):872–7. doi:10.1046/j.1365-2648.1995.21050872.x
67. *Promoting Positive Mental Health Through A Socio-Ecological Approach.* Centers for Addictions Research of BC (2011). Available from: http://www.heretohelp.bc.ca/sites/default/files/CARBC-campusdoc1.pdf
68. Chien MY, Yang RS, Tsauo JY. Home-based trunk-strengthening exercise for osteoporotic and osteopenic postmenopausal women without fracture – a pilot study. *Clin Rehabil* (2005) **19**(1):28–36. doi:10.1191/0269215505cr844oa
69. Etkin CD, Prohaska TR, Harris BA, Latham N, Jette A. Feasibility of implementing the strong for life program in community settings. *Gerontologist* (2006) **46**(2):284–92. doi:10.1093/geront/46.2.284
70. Hébert R, Lévesque L, Vézina J, Lavoie JP, Ducharme F, Gendron C, et al. Efficacy of a psychoeducative group program for caregivers of demented persons living at home: a randomized controlled trial. *J Gerontol B Psychol Sci Soc Sci* (2003) **58B**(1):S58–67. doi:10.1093/geronb/58.1.S58
71. Stewart AL, Mills KM, Sepsis PG, King AC, McLellan BY, Roitz K, et al. Evaluation of CHAMPS, a physical activity promotion program for older adults. *Ann Behav Med* (1997) **19**(4):353–61. doi:10.1007/BF02895154
72. Stewart M, Craig D, MacPherson K, Alexander S. Promoting positive affect and diminishing loneliness of widowed seniors through a support intervention. *Public Health Nurs* (2001) **18**(1):54–63. doi:10.1046/j.1525-1446.2001.00054.x
73. Molloy GJ, Johnston DW, Gao C, Witham MD, Gray JM, Argo IS. Effects of an exercise intervention for older heart failure patients on caregiver burden and emotional distress. *Eur J Cardiovasc Prev Rehabil* (2006) **13**(3):381–7. doi:10.1097/01.hjr.0000198916.60363.85
74. Centers for Disease Control and Prevention. *Public Health Action Plan to Integrate Mental Health Promotion and Mental Illness Prevention with Chronic Disease Prevention, 2011–2015.* Atlanta: U.S. Department of Health and Human Services (2011).
75. Singh NA, Clements KM, Singh MA. The efficacy of exercise as a long-term antidepressant in elderly subjects: a randomized, controlled trial. *J Gerontol A Biol Sci Med Sci* (2001) **56**(8):M497–504. doi:10.1093/gerona/56.8.M497
76. Garand L, Buckwalter KC, Lubaroff D, Tripp-Reimer T, Frantz RA, Ansley TN. A pilot study of immune and mood outcomes of a community-based intervention for dementia caregivers: the PLST intervention. *Arch Psychiatr Nurs* (2002) **16**(4):156–67. doi:10.1053/apnu.2002.34392
77. Inokuchi S, Matsusaka N, Hayashi T, Shindo H. Feasibility and effectiveness of a nurse-led community exercise programme for prevention of falls among frail elderly people: a multi-centre controlled trial. *J Rehabil Med* (2007) **39**(6):479–85. doi:10.2340/16501977-0080
78. Losito J, Murphy S, Thomas M. The effects of group exercise on fatigue and quality of life during cancer treatment. *Oncol Nurs Forum* (2006) **33**(4):821–5. doi:10.1188/06.ONF.821-825
79. Anderson RT, King A, Stewart AL, Camacho F, Rejeski WJ. Physical activity counseling in primary care and patient well-being: do patients benefit? *Ann Behav Med* (2005) **30**(2):146–54. doi:10.1207/s15324796abm3002_7

80. Munro JF, Nicholl JP, Brazier JE, Davey R, Cochrane T. Cost effectiveness of a community based exercise programme in over 65 year olds: cluster randomised trial. *J Epidemiol Community Health* (2004) **58**(12):1004–10. doi:10.1136/jech.2003.014225
81. Mutrie N, Campbell AM, Whyte F, McConnachie A, Emslie C, Lee L, et al. Benefits of supervised group exercise programme for women being treated for early stage breast cancer: pragmatic randomised controlled trial. *BMJ* (2007) **334**(7592):517. doi:10.1136/bmj.39094.648553.AE
82. Toseland RW, Rossiter CM, Peak T, Smith GC. Comparative effectiveness of individual and group interventions to support family caregivers. *Soc Work* (1990) **35**(3):209–17.
83. Bogat G, Jason LA. An evaluation of two visiting programs for elderly community residents. *Int J Aging Hum Dev* (1983) **17**(4):267–80. doi:10.2190/6AQX-1TDM-DEL4-3T6L
84. Jette AM, Harris BA, Sleeper L, Lachman ME, Heislein D, Giorgetti M, et al. A home-based exercise program for nondisabled older adults. *J Amer Geriatr Soc* (1996) **44**(6):644–9.
85. Lin MR, Wolf SL, Hwang HF, Gong SY, Chen CY. A randomized, controlled trial of fall prevention programs and quality of life in older fallers. *J Am Geriatr Soc* (2007) **55**(4):499–506. doi:10.1111/j.1532-5415.2007.01146.x
86. Austin EN, Johnston YA, Morgan LL. Community gardening in a senior center: a therapeutic intervention to improve the health of older adults. *Ther Recreation J* (2006) **40**(1):48–56.
87. Chen KM, Snyder M, Kirchbaum K. Tai chi and well-being of Taiwanese community-dwelling elders. *Clin Gerontol* (2001) **24**(3–4):137–56. doi:10.1300/J018v24n03_12
88. Devereux K, Robertson D, Briffa NK. Effects of a water-based program on women 65 years and over: a randomised controlled trial. *Aust J Physiother* (2005) **51**(2):102–8. doi:10.1016/S0004-9514(05)70038-6
89. Logiudice D, Waltrowicz W, Brown K, Burrows C, Ames D, Flicker L. Do memory clinics improve the quality of life of carers? A randomized pilot trial. *Int J Geriatr Psychiatry* (1999) **14**(8):626–32. doi:10.1002/(SICI)1099-1166(199908)14:8<626::AID-GPS990>3.0.CO;2-5
90. Li F, Fisher KJ, Harmer P, McAuley E. Falls self-efficacy as a mediator of fear of falling in an exercise intervention for older adults. *J Gerontol B Psychol Sci Soc Sci* (2005) **60**(1):34–40. doi:10.1093/geronb/60.1.P34
91. Means KM, O'Sullivan PS, Rodell DE. Psychosocial effects of an exercise program in older persons who fall. *J Rehabil Res Dev* (2003) **40**(1):49–58. doi:10.1682/JRRD.2003.01.0049
92. Resnick B, Orwig D, Yu-Yahiro J, Hawkes W, Shardell M, Hebel JR, et al. Testing the effectiveness of the exercise plus program in older women post-hip fracture. *Ann Behav Med* (2007) **34**(1):67–76. doi:10.1007/BF02879922
93. Drummond MF, Mohide EA, Tew M, Streiner DL, Pringle DM, Gilbert JR. Economic evaluation of a support program for caregivers of demented elderly. *Int J Technol Assess Health Care* (1991) **7**(2):209–19. doi:10.1017/S0266462300005109
94. Hartman CA, Manos TM, Winter C, Hartman DM, Li B, Smith JC. Effects of T'ai Chi training on function and quality of life indicators in older adults with osteoarthritis. *J Am Geriatr Soc* (2000) **48**(12):1553–9.
95. Taylor-Piliae RE, Haskell WL, Waters CM, Froelicher ES. Change in perceived psychosocial status following a 12-week Tai Chi exercise programme. *J Adv Nurs* (2006) **54**(3):313–29. doi:10.1111/j.1365-2648.2006.03809.x
96. Cheung BM, Lo JL, Fong DY, Chan MY, Wong SH, Wong VC, et al. Randomised controlled trial of qigong in the treatment of mild essential hypertension. *J Hum Hypertens* (2005) **19**(9):697–704. doi:10.1038/sj.jhh.1001884
97. Christopher KA, Morrow LL. Evaluating a community-based exercise program for women cancer survivors. *Appl Nurs Res* (2004) **17**(2):100–8. doi:10.1016/S0897-1897(04)00024-2
98. Gross CR, Kreitzer MJ, Russas V, Treesak C, Frazier PA, Hertz MI. Mindfulness meditation to reduce symptoms after organ transplant: a pilot study. *Adv Mind Body Med* (2004) **20**(2):20–9.
99. Papaioannou A, Adachi JD, Winegard K, Ferko N, Parkinson W, Cook RJ, et al. Efficacy of home-based exercise for improving quality of life among elderly women with symptomatic osteoporosis-related vertebral fractures. *Osteoporos Int* (2003) **14**(8):677–82. doi:10.1007/s00198-003-1423-2
100. Smith TL, Toseland RW. The effectiveness of a telephone support program for caregivers of frail older adults. *Gerontologist* (2006) **46**(5):620–9. doi:10.1093/geront/46.5.620
101. Fisher K, Li FA. Community-based walking trial to improve neighborhood quality of life in older adults: a multilevel analysis. *Ann Behav Med* (2004) **28**(3):186–94. doi:10.1207/s15324796abm2803_7
102. Castro CM, Wilcox S, O'Sullivan P, Baumann K, King AC. An exercise program for women who are caring for relatives with dementia. *Psychosom Med* (2002) **64**(3):458–68. doi:10.1097/00006842-200205000-00010
103. Pinto BM, Frierson GM, Rabin C, Trunzo JJ, Marcus BH. Home-based physical activity intervention for breast cancer patients. *J Clin Oncol* (2005) **23**(15):3577–87. doi:10.1200/JCO.2005.03.080
104. Stewart AL, King AC, Haskell WL. Endurance exercise and health-related quality of life in 50-65 year-old adults. *Gerontologist* (1993) **33**(6):782–9. doi:10.1093/geront/33.6.782
105. Hughes SL, Seymour RB, Campbell RT, Huber G, Pollak N, Sharma L, et al. Long-term impact of fit and strong! on older adults with osteoarthritis. *Gerontologist* (2006) **46**(6):801–14. doi:10.1093/geront/46.6.801
106. Senuzun F, Fadiloglu C, Burke LE, Payzin S. Effects of home-based cardiac exercise program on the exercise tolerance, serum lipid values and self-efficacy of coronary patients. *Eur J Cardiovasc Prev Rehabil* (2006) **13**(4):640–5. doi:10.1097/01.hjr.0000198445.41860.ec
107. Shin Y. The effects of a walking exercise program on physical function and emotional state of elderly Korean women. *Public Health Nurs* (1999) **16**(2):146–54. doi:10.1046/j.1525-1446.1999.00146.x
108. Heller K, Thompson MG, Trueba PE, Hogg JR, Vlachos-Weber I. Peer support telephone dyads for elderly women: was this the wrong intervention? *Am J Community Psychol* (1991) **19**(1):53–74. doi:10.1007/BF00942253
109. Dröes RM, Breebaart E, Ettema TP, van Tilburg W, Mellenbergh GJ. Effect of integrated family support versus day care only on behavior and mood of patients with dementia. *Int Psychogeriatr* (2000) **12**(1):99–115. doi:10.1017/S1041610200006232
110. Ruhland JL, Shields RK. The effects of a home exercise program on impairment and health-related quality of life in persons with chronic peripheral neuropathies. *Phys Ther* (1997) **77**(10):1026–39.
111. Alexander MJL, Butcher JE, MacDonald PB. Effect of a water exercise program on walking gait, flexibility, strength, self-reported disability and other psycho-social measures of older individuals with arthritis. *Physiother Can* (2001) **53**(3):203–11.
112. Bennett JA, Young HM, Nail LM, Winters-Stone K, Hanson G. A telephone-only motivational intervention to increase physical activity in rural adults: a randomized controlled trial. *Nurs Res* (2008) **57**(1):24–32. doi:10.1097/01.NNR.0000280661.34502.c1
113. Dröes RM, Meiland F, Schmitz M, van Tilburg W. Effect of combined support for people with dementia and carers versus regular day care on behaviour and mood of persons with dementia: results from a multi-centre implementation study. *Int J Geriatr Psychiatry* (2004) **19**(7):673–84. doi:10.1002/gps.1142
114. Emery CF, Gatz M. Psychological and cognitive effects of an exercise program for community-residing older adults. *Gerontologist* (1990) **30**(2):184–8. doi:10.1093/geront/30.2.184
115. Foley A, Halbert J, Hewitt T, Crotty M. Does hydrotherapy improve strength and physical function in patients with osteoarthritis – a randomised controlled trial comparing a gym based and a hydrotherapy based strengthening programme. *Ann Rheum Dis* (2003) **62**(12):1162–7. doi:10.1136/ard.2002.005272
116. Jeong S, Kim MT. Effects of a theory-driven music and movement program for stroke survivors in a community setting. *Appl Nurs Res* (2007) **20**(3):125–31. doi:10.1016/j.apnr.2007.04.005
117. Savage P, Ricci MA, Lynn M, Gardner A, Knight S, Brochu M, et al. Effects of home versus supervised exercise for patients with intermittent claudication. *J Cardiopulm Rehabil* (2001) **21**(3):152–7. doi:10.1097/00008483-200105000-00006
118. Wilcox S, Dowda M, Griffin SF, Rheaume C, Ory MG, Leviton L, et al. Results of the first year of active for life: translation of 2 evidence-based physical activity programs for older adults into community settings. *Am J Health* (2006) **96**(7):1201–9. doi:10.2105/AJPH.2005.074690
119. Beaupre LA, Lier D, Davies DM, Johnston DB. The effect of a preoperative exercise and education program on functional recovery, health related quality of life, and health service utilization following primary total knee arthroplasty. *J Rheumatol* (2004) **31**(6):1166–73.
120. Kerse N, Elley C, Robinson E, Arroll B. Is physical activity counseling effective for older people? A cluster randomized, controlled trial in primary care. *J Am Geriatr Soc* (2005) **53**(11):1951–6. doi:10.1111/j.1532-5415.2005.00466.x

121. van den Heuvel ET, Witte LP, Stewart RE, Schure LM, Sanderman R, Meyboom-de Jong B. Long-term effects of a group support program and an individual support program for informal caregivers of stroke patients: which caregivers benefit the most? *Patient Educ Couns* (2002) **47**(4):291–9. doi:10.1016/S0738-3991(01)00230-0
122. Barrett CJ, Smerdely P. A comparison of community-based resistance exercise and flexibility exercise for seniors. *Aust J Physiother* (2002) **48**(3):215–9. doi:10.1016/S0004-9514(14)60226-9
123. Hernández MT, Rubio TM, Ruiz FO, Riera HS, Gil RS, Gómez JC. Results of a home-based training program for patients with COPD. *Chest* (2000) **118**(1):106–14. doi:10.1378/chest.118.1.106
124. Murray J, Manela M, Shuttleworth A, Livingston G. An intervention study with husband and wife carers of older people with a psychiatric illness. *J Affect Disord* (1997) **46**(3):279–84. doi:10.1016/S0165-0327(97)00098-0
125. Stenstrom CH. Home exercise in rheumatoid arthritis functional class II: goal setting versus pain attention. *J Rheumatol* (1994) **21**(4):627–34.
126. Greendale GA, Salem GJ, Young JT, Damesyn M, Marion M, Wang MY, et al. A randomized trial of weighted vest use in ambulatory older adults: strength, performance, and quality of life outcomes. *J Am Geriatr Soc* (2000) **48**(3): 305–11.
127. Hughes SL, Seymour RB, Campbell R, Pollak N, Huber G, Sharma L. Impact of the fit and strong intervention on older adults with osteoarthritis. *Gerontologist* (2004) **44**(2):217–28. doi:10.1093/geront/44.2.217
128. Larson J, Franzén-Dahlin A, Billing E, Arbin M, Murray V, Wredling R. The impact of a nurse-led support and education programme for spouses of stroke patients: a randomized controlled trial. *J Clin Nurs* (2005) **14**(8):995–1003. doi:10.1111/j.1365-2702.2005.01206.x
129. Tsutsumi T, Don BM, Zaichkowsky LD, Delizonna LL. Physical fitness and psychological benefits of strength training in community dwelling older adults. *Appl Human Sci* (1997) **16**(6):257–66. doi:10.2114/jpa.16.257
130. van Uffelen JG, Chin A, Paw MJ, Hopman-Rock M, van Mechelen W. The effect of walking and vitamin B supplementation on quality of life in community-dwelling adults with mild cognitive impairment: a randomized, controlled trial. *Qual Life Res* (2007) **16**(7):1137–46. doi:10.1007/s11136-007-9219-z
131. Chin A, Paw MJ, de Jong N, Schouten EG, van Staveren WA, Kok FJ. Physical exercise or micronutrient supplementation for the wellbeing of the frail elderly? A randomised controlled trial. *Br J Sports Med* (2002) **36**(2):126–31. doi:10.1136/bjsm.36.2.126
132. King AC, Pruitt LA, Phillips W, Oka R, Rodenburg A, Haskell WL. Comparative effects of two physical activity programs on measured and perceived physical functioning and other health-related quality of life outcomes in older adults. *J Gerontol A Biol Sci Med Sci* (2000) **55**(2):M74–83. doi:10.1093/gerona/55.2.M74
133. Bravo G, Gauthier P, Roy PM, Payette H, Gaulin P. A weight-bearing, water-based exercise program for osteopenic women: its impact on bone, functional fitness, and well-being. *Arch Phys Med Rehabil* (1997) **78**(12):1375–80. doi:10.1016/S0003-9993(97)90313-0
134. de Vreede PL, van Meeteren NL, Samson MM, Wittink HM, Duursma SA, Verhaar HJ. The effect of functional tasks exercise and resistance exercise on health-related quality of life and physical activity. A randomised controlled trial. *Gerontology* (2007) **53**(1):12–20. doi:10.1159/000095387
135. Mant J, Carter J, Wade DT, Winner S. Family support for stroke: a randomised controlled trial. *Lancet* (2000) **356**(9232):808–13. doi:10.1016/S0140-6736(05)67276-5
136. Blumenthal JA, Emery CF, Madden DJ, Schniebolk S, Walsh-Riddle M, George LK. Long-term effects of exercise on psychological functioning in older men and women. *J Gerontol* (1991) **46**(6):352–61. doi:10.1093/geronj/46.6.P352
137. Singh NA, Stavrinos TM, Scarbek Y, Galambos G, Liber C, Fiatarone Singh MA. A randomized controlled trial of high versus low intensity weight training versus general practitioner care for clinical depression in older adults. *J Gerontol A Biol Sci Med Sci* (2005) **60**(6):768–76. doi:10.1093/gerona/60.6.768
138. Barker C. The value of home support for cancer patients: a study. *Nurs Stand* (1997) **11**(32):34–7. doi:10.7748/ns1997.04.11.32.34.c2453
139. Walsh K, Jones L, Tookman A, Mason C, McLoughlin J, Blizard R, et al. Reducing emotional distress in people caring for patients receiving specialist palliative care. Randomised trial. *Br J Psychiatry* (2007) **190**:142–7. doi:10.1192/bjp.bp.106.023960
140. Centers for Disease Control and Prevention. *Physical Activity Guidelines for Older Adults.* Division of Nutrition, Physical Activity, and Obesity, National Center for Chronic Disease Prevention and Health Promotion (2011). Available from: http://www.cdc.gov/physicalactivity/everyone/guidelines/olderadults.html
141. Glasgow RE, McKay HG, Piette JD, Reynolds KD. The re-aim framework for evaluating interventions: what can it tell us about approaches to chronic illness management? *Patient Educ Couns* (2001) **44**:119–27. doi:10.1016/S0738-3991(00)00186-5
142. Ducharme F, Trudeau D. Qualitative evaluation of a stress management intervention for elderly caregivers at home: a constructivist approach. *Issues Ment Health Nurs* (2002) **23**(7):691–713. doi:10.1080/01612840290052820
143. Harding R, Higginson IJ, Leam C, Donaldson N, Pearce A, George R, et al. Evaluation of a short-term group intervention for informal carers of patients attending a home palliative care service. *J Pain Symptom Manage* (2004) **27**(5):396–408. doi:10.1016/j.jpainsymman.2003.09.012
144. Hunkeler EM, Meresman JF, Hargreaves WA, Fireman B, Berman WH, Kirsch AJ, et al. Efficacy of nurse telehealth care and peer support in augmenting treatment of depression in primary care. *Arch Fam Med* (2000) **9**(8):700–8. doi:10.1001/archfami.9.8.700
145. Malde S. Guided autobiography: a counseling tool for older adults. *J Couns Dev* (1988) **66**(6):290–3. doi:10.1002/j.1556-6676.1988.tb00872.x
146. Mock V, Dow KH, Meares CJ, Grimm PM, Dienemann JA, Haisfield-Wolfe ME, et al. Effects of exercise on fatigue, physical functioning, and emotional distress during radiation therapy for breast cancer. *Oncol Nurs Forum* (1997) **24**(6):991–1000.
147. Oken BS, Zajdel D, Kishiyama S, Flegal K, Dehen C, Haas M, et al. Randomized, controlled, six-month trial of yoga in healthy seniors: effects on cognition and quality of life. *Altern Ther Health Med* (2006) **12**(1):40–7.
148. Slivinske LR, Kosberg JI. Assessing the effect of a personal health management system within retirement communities: a preliminary investigation. *Gerontologist* (1984) **24**(3):280–5. doi:10.1093/geront/24.3.280
149. Villaverde-Gutiérrez C, Araújo E, Cruz F, Roa JM, Barbosa W, Ruíz-Villaverde G. Quality of life of rural menopausal women in response to a customized exercise programme. *J Adv Nurs* (2006) **54**(1):11–9. doi:10.1111/j.1365-2648.2006.03784.x
150. Hauer K, Specht N, Schuler M, Bärtsch P, Oster P. Intensive physical training in geriatric patients after severe falls and hip surgery. *Age Ageing* (2002) **31**(1):49–57. doi:10.1093/ageing/31.1.49
151. Headley JA, Ownby KK, John LD. The effect of seated exercise on fatigue and quality of life in women with advanced breast cancer. *Oncol Nurs Forum* (2004) **31**(5):977–83. doi:10.1188/04.ONF.977-983
152. Helbostad JL, Sletvold O, Moe-Nilssen R. Home training with and without additional group training in physically frail old people living at home: effect on health-related quality of life and ambulation. *Clin Rehabil* (2004) **18**(5):498–508. doi:10.1191/0269215504cr761oa
153. Sims J, Hill K, Davidson S, Gunn J, Huang N. Exploring the feasibility of a community-based strength training program for older people with depressive symptoms and its impact on depressive symptoms. *BMC Geriatr* (2006) **6**:18. doi:10.1186/1471-2318-6-18
154. Zigmond AS, Snaith RP. The hospital anxiety and depression scale. *Acta Psychiatr Scand* (1983) **67**:361–70. doi:10.1111/j.1600-0447.1983.tb09716.x
155. Kennedy A, Reeves D, Bower P, Middleton E, Richardson G, Gardner C, et al. The effectiveness and cost effectiveness of a national lay-led self care support programme for patients with long-term conditions: a pragmatic randomised controlled trial. *J Epidemiol Community Health* (2007) **61**(3):254–61. doi:10.1136/jech.2006.053538
156. Lorig KR, Ritter PL, Gonzalez VM. Hispanic chronic disease self-management: a randomized community-based outcome trial. *Nurs Res* (2003) **52**(6):361–9. doi:10.1097/00006199-200311000-00003
157. Dongbo F, Fu H, McGowan P, Yi-E S, Lizhen Z, Huiqin Y, et al. Implementation and quantitative evaluation of chronic disease self-management programme in Shanghai, China: randomized controlled trial. *Bull World Health Organ* (2003) **81**(3):174–82.
158. Lorig KR, Ritter PL, Laurent DD, Plant K. Internet-based chronic disease self-management: a randomized trial. *Med Care* (2006) **44**(11):964–71. doi:10.1097/01.mlr.0000233678.80203.c1

159. Griffiths C, Motlib J, Azad A, Ramsay J, Eldridge S, Feder G, et al. Randomised controlled trial of a lay-led self-management programme for Bangladeshi patients with chronic disease. *Br J Gen Pract* (2005) **55**(52O):831–7.
160. Berkman ND, Sheridan SL, Donahue KE, Halpern DJ, Viera A, Crotty K, et al. Health literacy interventions and outcomes: an updated systematic review. *Evid Rep Technol Assess* (*Full Rep*) (2011) **1999**:1–941.
161. Coberley C, Rula EY, Pope JE. Effectiveness of health and wellness initiatives for seniors. *Popul Health Manag* (2011) **14**(Suppl 1):S45–50. doi:10.1089/pop.2010.0072
162. Gitlin LN, Chernett NL, Fields Harris L, Palmer D, Hopkins P, Dennis MP. Harvest health: translation of the chronic disease self-management program for older African Americans in a senior setting. *Gerontologist* (2008) **48**:698–705. doi:10.1093/geront/48.5.698
163. Hochhaltera AK, Song J, Rush J, Sklar L, Stevens A. Making the most of your healthcare intervention for older adults with multiple chronic illnesses. *Patient Educ Couns* (2010) **81**:207–13. doi:10.1016/j.pec.2010.01.018
164. Jerant A, Moore-Hill M, Franks P. Home-based, peer-led chronic illness self-management training: findings from a 1-year randomized controlled trial. *Ann Fam Med* (2009) **7**:319–27. doi:10.1370/afm.996
165. Jonker AAGC, Comijs HC, Knipscheer KCPM, Deeg DJH. Promotion of self-management in vulnerable older people: a narrative literature review of outcomes of the chronic disease self-management program (CDSMP). *Eur J Ageing* (2009) **6**:303–14. doi:10.1007/s10433-009-0131-y
166. Ritter PL, Lee J, Lorig K. Moderators of chronic disease self-management programs: who benefits? *Chronic Illn* (2011) **7**:162–72. doi:10.1177/1742395311399127
167. Rose MA, Arenson C, Harrod P, Salkey R, Santana A, Diamond J. Evaluation of the chronic disease self-management program with low-income, Urban, African American older adults. *J Community Health Nurs* (2008) **25**(4):193–202. doi:10.1080/07370010802421178
168. Smeulders ESTF, van Haastregt JCM, Janssen-Boyne JJJ, Stoffers HEJH, van Eijk JTM, Kempen GIJM. Feasibility of a group-based self-management program among congestive heart failure patients. *Heart Lung* (2009) **38**:499–512. doi:10.1016/j.hrtlng.2009.01.007
169. Smeulders ESTF, van Haastregt JCM, Ambergen T, Stoffers HEJH, Janssen-Boyne JJJ, Uszko-Lencer NHKM, et al. Heart failure patients with a lower educational level and better cognitive status benefit most from a self-management group programme. *Patient Educ Couns* (2010) **81**:214–21. doi:10.1016/j.pec.2010.01.003
170. Tomioka M, Braun KL, Compton M, Tanoue L. Adapting Stanford's chronic disease self-management program to Hawaii's multicultural population. *Gerontologist* (2012) **52**(1):121–32. doi:10.1093/geront/gnr054
171. Frosch DL, Rincon D, Ochoa S, Mangione CM. Activating seniors to improve chronic disease care: results from a pilot intervention study. *J Am Geriatr Soc* (2010) **58**(8):1496–503. doi:10.1111/j.1532-5415.2010.02980.x
172. McLeroy KR, Bibeau D, Steckler A, Glanz K. An ecological perspective on health promotion programs. *Health Educ Q* (1988) **15**(4):351–77. doi:10.1177/109019818801500401
173. Engels HJ, Drouin J, Zhu W, Kazmierski JF. Effects of low-impact, moderate-intensity exercise training with and without wrist weights on functional capacities and mood states in older adults. *Gerontology* (1998) **44**(4):239–44. doi:10.1159/000022018
174. Friedland JF, McColl M. Social support intervention after stroke: results of a randomized trial. *Arch Phys Med Rehabil* (1992) **73**(6):573–81.
175. Groessl EJ, Cronan TA. A cost analysis of self-management programs for people with chronic illness. *Am J Community Psychol* (2000) **28**(4):455–80. doi:10.1023/A:1005184414241
176. Richeson NE, Croteau KA, Jones DA, Farmer BC. Effects of a pedometer-based intervention on the physical performance and mobility-related self-efficacy of community-dwelling older adults: an interdisciplinary preventive health care intervention. *Ther Recreation J* (2006) **40**(1):18–32.
177. Singh NA, Clements KM, Fiatarone MA. A randomized controlled trial of progressive resistance training in depressed elders. *J Gerontol A Biol Sci Med Sci* (1997) **52**(1):M27–35. doi:10.1093/gerona/52A.1.M27
178. Stevenson JS, Topp R. Effects of moderate and low intensity long-term exercise by older adults. *Res Nurs Health* (1990) **13**(4):209–18. doi:10.1002/nur.4770130403
179. Stiggelbout M, Popkema DY, Hopman-Rock M, de Greef M, van Mechelen W. Once a week is not enough: effects of a widely implemented group based exercise programme for older adults: a randomised controlled trial. *J Epidemiol Community Health* (2004) **58**(2):83–8. doi:10.1136/jech.58.2.83
180. Williams P, Lord SR. Effects of group exercise on cognitive functioning and mood in older women. *Aust N Z J Public Health* (1997) **21**(1):45–52. doi:10.1111/j.1467-842X.1997.tb01653.x
181. Wolf SL, Barnhart HX, Kutner NG, McNeely E, Coogler C, Xu T, et al. Selected as the best paper in the 1990s: reducing frailty and falls in older persons: an investigation of tai chi and computerized balance training. *J Am Geriatr Soc* (2003) **51**(12):1794–803. doi:10.1046/j.1532-5415.2003.51566.x
182. Yu DS, Lee DT, Woo J, Hui E. Non-pharmacological interventions in older people with heart failure: effects of exercise training and relaxation therapy. *Gerontology* (2007) **53**(2):74–81. doi:10.1159/000096427
183. Greendale GA, Hirsch SH, Hahn TJ. The effect of a weighted vest on perceived health status and bone density in older persons. *Qual Life Res* (1993) **2**(2):141–52. doi:10.1007/BF00435733
184. Bravo G, Gauthier P, Roy PM, Payette H, Gaulin P, Harvey M, et al. Impact of a 12-month exercise program on the physical and psychological health of osteopenic women. *J Am Geriatr Soc* (1996) **44**(7):756–62.

31

Healthcare providers' perceptions and self-reported fall prevention practices: Findings from a large New York health system

Matthew Lee Smith[1]*, Judy A. Stevens[2], Heidi Ehrenreich[2], Ashley D. Wilson[3], Richard J. Schuster[4], Colleen O'Brien Cherry[4] and Marcia G. Ory[3]

[1] Department of Health Promotion and Behavior, College of Public Health, The University of Georgia, Athens, GA, USA
[2] National Center for Injury Prevention and Control, Centers for Disease Control and Prevention, Atlanta, GA, USA
[3] Department of Health Promotion and Community Health Sciences, Texas A&M Health Science Center School of Public Health, College Station, TX, USA
[4] Center for Global Health, College of Public Health, The University of Georgia, Athens, GA, USA

Edited by:
Michal Grivna, United Arab Emirates University, United Arab Emirates

Reviewed by:
Laura Rudkin, University of Texas Medical Branch, USA
Koustuv Dalal, Örebro University, Sweden

***Correspondence:**
Matthew Lee Smith, Department of Health Promotion and Behavior, College of Public Health, The University of Georgia, #345E Wright Hall, Health Science Campus, Athens, GA 30602, USA
e-mail: health@uga.edu

Among older adults, falls are the leading cause of injury-related deaths and emergency department visits, and the incidence of falls in the United States is rising as the number of older Americans increases. Research has shown that falls can be reduced by modifying fall-risk factors using multifactorial interventions implemented in clinical settings. However, the literature indicates that many providers feel that they do not know how to conduct fall-risk assessments or do not have adequate knowledge about fall prevention. To help healthcare providers incorporate older adult fall prevention (i.e., falls risk assessment and treatment) into their clinical practice, the Centers for Disease Control and Prevention's (CDC) Injury Center has developed the Stopping Elderly Accidents, Deaths, and Injuries (STEADI) tool kit. This study was conducted to identify the practice characteristics and providers' beliefs, knowledge, and fall-related activities before they received training on how to use the STEADI tool kit. Data were collected as part of a larger State Fall Prevention Project funded by CDC's Injury Center. Completed questionnaires were returned by 38 medical providers from 11 healthcare practices within a large New York health system. Healthcare providers ranked falls as the lowest priority of five conditions, after diabetes, cardiovascular disease, mental health, and musculoskeletal conditions. Less than 40% of the providers asked most or all of their older patients if they had fallen during the past 12 months. Less than a quarter referred their older patients to physical therapists for balance or gait training, and <20% referred older patients to community-based fall prevention programs. Less than 16% reported they conducted standardized functional assessments with their older patients at least once a year. These results suggest that implementing the STEADI tool kit in clinical settings could address knowledge gaps and provide the necessary tools to help providers incorporate fall-risk assessment and treatment into clinical practice.

Keywords: clinical practice, fall prevention, fall screening, intervention science

INTRODUCTION

Falls are the leading cause of death and emergency department visits for injury among older adults (1), and the direct medical costs for these injuries are estimated to be more than $30 billion dollars annually (2). Falls are caused by a number of risk factors usually classified as either intrinsic (e.g., age, sex, chronic diseases, medication side effects, gait and/or balance problems, muscle weakness) or extrinsic (e.g., environmental factors such as uneven surfaces, poor lighting, and lack of railings and/or grab bars) (3–7). It is expected that the incidence of falls and associated injuries will continue to rise as the nation's population of older adults increases. However, fall risk can be reduced through multifactorial interventions that are implemented in clinical settings (8, 9).

The American and British Geriatrics Societies (AGS/BGS) have published a clinical practice guideline to reduce falls (10). However, primary care physicians have been slow to put the AGS/BGS guideline into clinical practice because many feel that they do not know how to conduct fall-risk assessments or do not have adequate knowledge about fall prevention (11, 12). To help healthcare providers incorporate older adult fall prevention into their clinical practice, experts at Centers for Disease Control and Prevention's (CDC) Injury Center developed the Stopping Elderly Accidents, Deaths, and Injuries (STEADI) tool kit. The tool kit is based on the AGS/BGS clinical practice guideline (10), applies concepts from Wagner's Chronic Care Model (CCM) (13) to fall risk, and includes input from healthcare providers (14). It contains basic information about falls, standardized gait and balance assessment tests, case studies, and conversation starters. In addition, there are educational handouts about fall prevention specifically designed for older patients and their friends and family.

The contents of the STEADI tool kit and supplemental resources are available online (15).

Data for this study were collected as part of a larger 5-year project begun in 2011. This project funded three state health departments (Colorado, New York, Oregon) to integrate clinical and evidence-based community fall prevention programs in selected communities. This study describes the beliefs, knowledge, and fall-related activities of 38 healthcare providers from 11 healthcare practices within a large New York health system, prior to receiving training about implementing the STEADI tool kit. This community case study describes the current attributes, perceptions, and self-reported practices of healthcare providers. The results underscore the need to enhance providers' knowledge about fall prevention and for clinical resources to support falls screening, assessment, and treatment.

MATERIALS AND METHODS

At part of a cooperative agreement with the CDC, the STEADI evaluation and implementation teams (led by the Texas A&M Health Science Center and The University of Georgia, respectively) developed a provider training based on academic detailing called the Clinical Engagement and Education (CEE) session (16). These teams trained the state grantees to conduct CEE sessions and developed, tested, and refined the evaluation materials and processes.

The purpose of the CEE session was to help clinicians find innovative ways to incorporate STEADI into their clinical practice (16). The 1-h session was led by a physician fall prevention "Champion" who had been identified and trained by the state grantee, and was open to all clinicians and office personnel in the practice. These interactive sessions were designed to bring healthcare providers and office staff together to discuss the burden of older adult falls and to foster collective decisions about fall prevention activities that they could implement during clinical visits with older adult patients (16).

DATA COLLECTION

Clinical Engagement and Education session data about the characteristics of the practice, provider characteristics, and provider beliefs, knowledge, and fall-related activities were collected from two sources. First, office personnel completed a registration form after the practice agreed to participate in the CEE session. This form provided general information about the healthcare group (e.g., number of years the practice has been in business, the number of employees, size of the patient base).

Second, each CEE session participant was asked to complete a two-page questionnaire at the beginning of the CEE Session. The 35-item questionnaire took approximately 15 min to complete and asked for the participant's characteristics (i.e., job title, gender), opinions about fall-risk factors, practice priorities, and activities conducted during clinical visits with older patients. Responses consisted of Likert scales and closed-response formats. Institutional Review Board approval was obtained from Texas A&M University to conduct descriptive analyses using de-identified data.

MEASURES

Providers were asked to rate each of five health conditions from 1 (low) to 10 (high) in response to the question, "When thinking about your older patients, please rate the level of priority given to conditions in your practice." Then, given a list of eight fall-risk factors, providers were asked to, "Rate the extent to which you believe the following items are fall-risk factors for your older patients." Each factor was rated from 1 (low) to 10 (high). Finally, they were asked, "In the past month, approximately what percent of your older patients have you referred to attend community fall prevention programs?"

Given a list of 10 intervention activities, providers were asked to report the proportion of older patients who received specific fall interventions at least once a year. Examples of intervention activities included discussing prescription medications, discussing mobility aids, assessing visual acuity, and performing standardized physical functioning assessments. Responses were measured using five-point Likert scales but, based on the frequency distribution, these were collapsed into three categories: none, a few or some, and most or all.

Other items asked of providers, but not presented in tables, included the average amount of time (in minutes) they spent with an older patient during a typical visit and the average amount of time (in minutes) they spent assessing fall risk during a typical visit with an older patient. Providers were also asked their level of agreement with statements including, "My older patients are reluctant to tell me they have fallen;" "It is important to perform a standardized fall-risk assessment with older adults;" "Gait and balance tests are easy to perform;" and "I have adequate time during a clinical visit to assess fall risk among my older patients." Responses were measured using four-point Likert scales but, based on the frequency distribution, these were collapsed into two categories: agree and disagree.

STATISTICAL ANALYSES

Given the limited number of participants in this study, data are described but no tests for statistical significance were performed. Some data are presented in tabular form and others are described in the text.

RESULTS

PRACTICE CHARACTERISTICS

Between September 2012 and June 2013, 11 New York based practices within United Healthcare, a managed healthcare company, hosted 11 CEE sessions. These practices had existed for an average of 20 years (range: 5–30 years). Each practice served an average of 6,365 patients (range: 320–12,000 patients) and, on average, 43% of these patients (range: 20–70%) were aged 65 years or older. Each practice employed an average of 15 medical personnel (range: 4–30 employees) that included between one and six physicians.

PROVIDER CHARACTERISTICS

Forty-nine persons attended the CEE sessions. For this study, office personnel ($n = 5$) and those with missing socio-demographic data ($n = 6$) were excluded. Therefore, data are presented for 38 medical providers. Of these, 34% were nurses, 26% physicians, 18% nurse practitioners, 8% physician assistants, 8% medical assistants, and 3% specialty care providers. The median age was 38 years (range: 23–69 years), and 84% were female.

PROVIDER BELIEFS AND KNOWLEDGE

Table 1 shows the participants' level of priority given to specific health conditions and beliefs about fall-risk factors among older adults. Of the five health conditions, diabetes received the highest average score (8.4) while falls received the lowest (7.1). Of eight fall-risk factors, a history of falling received the highest average score (8.1). Postural hypotension received the lowest average score (6.1).

PROVIDER FALL-RELATED ACTIVITIES

Providers reported that a typical office visit with an older patient lasted on average 20.7 (±9.9) minutes (range: 0–60 min). The time spent assessing fall-risk factors averaged 3.8 (±2.5) minutes (range: 0–10 min). Approximately, 66% of respondents agreed or strongly agreed with the statement, "I have adequate time during a clinical visit to assess fall risk among my older patients."

Table 2 shows the proportion of respondents who delivered specific fall interventions to their older patients at least once a year. Over 81% of providers discussed details about prescribed medications with most or all of their older patients. About 47% conducted a cognitive screening with most or all of their older patients, and 37% asked most or all of their older patients about falls during the past 12 months.

All providers reported that it was important to perform a standardized fall-risk assessment and said gait and balance tests were easy to perform. Just over one-third of the providers routinely asked their older patients if they had fallen in the past year. Yet, about 61% of providers agreed or strongly agreed with the statement, "My older patients are reluctant to tell me they have fallen." As shown in **Table 2**, fewer than 16% reported that they conducted either the *Timed Up and Go* test, *30-s Chair Stand*, or *4-Stage Balance Test* with most or all of their older patients at least once a year.

Thirty-one providers reported that they referred on average 20% (±18.5%) of their older adult patients to community fall prevention programs (range: 10–100%). Similarly, 32 providers reported that they referred on average 22% (±18.8%) of their older patients to physical therapy for gait and/or balance retraining (range: 10–100%).

DISCUSSION

This study examined the beliefs, knowledge, and fall-related activities conducted among 38 healthcare providers. These data, collected at the beginning of the CEE session, showed that the providers considered all five specified health conditions were high priority. However, falls were considered a lower priority than chronic conditions such as diabetes and cardiovascular disease.

Despite clinical guidelines (10), few providers routinely asked their older patients if they had fallen in the past year. This is especially troubling since providers reported that their patients were reluctant to tell them that they had fallen. These data further indicated that few providers actually conducted standardized tests to assess gait and balance, although these tests are seen as both important and easy to perform. The low assessment rate by providers was partially counterbalanced by patient referrals to physical therapy to address gait or balance problems.

Prior research suggests that primary care providers feel that they do not know how to conduct fall-risk assessments and this study found that providers were not conducting multifactorial risk assessments on every patient (11, 12, 17). These are missed opportunities for prevention that are likely to result in higher fall rates. An important next step is to make fall prevention a routine part of clinical care. This requires educating providers about how to conduct fall-risk assessments and providing them with the necessary tools to streamline the process. Promising approaches include educating providers about the STEADI tool

Table 1 | Healthcare providers' priorities and beliefs about the importance of issues facing older adult patients.

	N	Median	Mean	SD	Range	
					Minimum	Maximum
Priority given to health conditions[a]						
Diabetes	37	9	8.35	1.69	3	10
Cardiovascular disease, including stroke	37	8	8.08	1.99	3	10
Mental health, including depression	34	8	7.44	2.22	3	10
Musculoskeletal conditions	37	8	7.35	1.93	3	10
Falls	37	7	7.05	2.15	3	10
Beliefs about fall-risk factors for older patients[a]						
History of falling	38	9	8.11	2.35	3	10
Balance issues	38	9	7.95	2.27	3	10
Gait issues	37	9	7.68	2.46	2	10
Environmental issues within the home	38	8	7.16	2.09	3	10
Medication issues	38	8	7.13	2.47	2	10
Neurological issues	38	7	6.68	2.35	2	10
Vision issues	35	7	6.66	2.35	2	10
Postural hypotension	36	6	6.11	2.51	2	10

[a] *All items measured on a scale from 1 = low to 10 = high.*

Table 2 | Proportion of older patients for whom activities are performed at least once a year.

	N	None (%)	A few/ some (%)	Most/ all (%)
Discuss details about their prescribed medications (e.g., number, type, dose, side effects)	37	0.0	18.9	81.1
Conduct a cognitive screening	34	11.8	41.2	47.1
Discuss their use of mobility aids	37	5.4	56.8	37.8
Collect fall history over the past 12 months	38	18.4	44.7	36.8
Educate about their specific fall-risk factors	36	16.7	52.8	30.6
Follow-up with patients who are at risk for falling within 30 days of their clinical visit	36	16.7	55.6	27.8
Assess their visual acuity	35	5.7	77.1	17.1
Conduct the *Timed Up and Go* test	32	53.1	31.3	15.6
Conduct the *30-s Chair Stand* test	34	58.8	32.4	8.8
Conduct the *4-Stage Balance* test	35	65.7	25.7	8.6

kit as well as providing them with additional resources such as online provider education and clinical decision support modules that are integrated into the provider's electronic health records (EHR) system.

LIMITATIONS

A limitation of this study is that provider data were available for only 38 healthcare providers from one healthcare organization in one state, so findings must be considered preliminary. While study data were obtained from a diverse set of healthcare providers, the small number of respondents made it impossible to examine how the knowledge, beliefs, and activities differed by provider or practice type. Further investigation is warranted to assess such differences. Additionally, these data were collected pre-intervention, before the healthcare providers were introduced to the tool kit. Because insufficient follow-up data were collected post-intervention, changes in healthcare providers' beliefs and behaviors could not be assessed. Further investigation is warranted to examine the impact of the STEADI tool kit on healthcare providers' perceptions and clinical practice.

The approach used for recruiting healthcare practices to receive training in using the STEADI tool kit may have limited participation; it may have selected those participants who were especially interested in fall prevention. This would suggest that the frequency of fall-risk assessments (e.g., collecting fall history, conducting standardized gait, and balance tests) actually might be lower among healthcare providers.

Another limitation was associated with hosting CEE sessions in healthcare practices. State health department grantees were required to first identify and then train a highly motivated provider Champion. This was a difficult and labor-intensive process because the grantees had to first establish new partnerships with healthcare provider groups. Future efforts will include developing an online training for STEADI with continuing education (CE) credits, and creating a software module to integrate STEADI's fall prevention processes into EHR.

Lastly, the study relied on self-reported estimates of fall prevention activities that could not be confirmed by objective measures such as medical chart reviews. These estimates may not accurately reflect the true frequencies of these activities in primary care settings.

CONCLUSION

This study found that most healthcare providers did not consider falls as high a priority as other chronic conditions among older patients, and did not routinely assess and address these patients' fall-risk factors. The STEADI tool kit may be a valuable resource to help providers incorporate fall-risk assessment, treatment, and/or referral into clinical practice. However, providers must first be convinced that falls are a priority issue among their older patients, and devote as much, or more, time to assessing falls risks and educating patients about appropriate programs to reduce fall risks. Future studies will focus on educating providers about the STEADI tool kit, their adoption of STEADI, and STEADI's impact on fall-risk screening, assessment, and treatment.

ACKNOWLEDGMENTS

The authors would like to thank Margaret Kaniewski, MPH, Public Health Advisor at the CDC, and the staff at the New York State Department of Health, Bureau of Occupational Health and Injury Prevention, for their significant contributions to this work. We thank Dr. Frank Floyd, and UHS Physician Practices for collecting the study data. Additional thanks are given to Natalie Martin for her contribution to the STEADI implementation and training process. This research was supported by the CDC, National Center for Injury Prevention and Control, under Cooperative Agreement Number 1U48 DP001924 with the Texas A&M Health Science Center School of Rural Public Health Center for Community Health Development, and by an appointment to the Research Participation Program at the CDC, administered by the Oak Ridge Institute for Science and Education, through an interagency agreement between the U.S. Department of Energy and CDC. *Disclaimer:* The findings and conclusions in this report are those of the authors and do not necessarily represent the official position of the Centers for Disease Control and Prevention.

REFERENCES

1. *Web-Based Injury Statistics Query and Reporting System (WISQARS) [Database on the Internet]*. National Center for Injury Prevention and Control (2012). Available from: http://www.cdc.gov/injury/wisqars/index.html
2. Stevens JA, Corso PS, Finkelstein EA, Miller TR. The costs of fatal and non-fatal falls among older adults. *Inj Prev* (2006) **12**(5):290–5. doi:10.1136/ip.2005.011015
3. Tinetti ME, Speechley M, Ginter SF. Risk factors for falls among elderly persons living in the community. *N Engl J Med* (1988) **319**(26):1701–7.
4. Tinetti M, Doucette J, Claus E, Marottoli R. Risk factors for serious injury during falls by older persons in the community. *J Am Geriatr Soc* (1995) **43**(11):1214–21.
5. Tinetti ME, McAvay G, Claus E. Does multiple risk factor reduction explain the reduction in fall rate in the Yale FICSIT trial? *Am J Epidemiol* (1996) **144**(4):389–99. doi:10.1093/oxfordjournals.aje.a008940
6. Kannus P, Sievänen H, Palvanen M, Järvinen T, Parkkari J. Prevention of falls and consequent injuries in elderly people. *Lancet* (2005) **366**:1885–93. doi:10.1016/S0140-6736(05)67604-0

7. Stevens M, Holman CAJ, Bennett N. Preventing falls in older people: impact of an intervention to reduce environmental hazards in the home. *J Am Geriatr Soc* (2001) **49**(11):1442–7. doi:10.1046/j.1532-5415.2001.4911235.x
8. Haines TP, Bennell KL, Osborne RH, Hill KD. Effectiveness of targeted falls prevention programme in subacute hospital setting: randomised controlled trial. *BMJ* (2004) **328**(7441):676. doi:10.1136/bmj.328.7441.676
9. Cameron ID, Murray GR, Gillespie LD, Robertson MC, Hill KD, Cumming RG, et al. Interventions for preventing falls in older people in nursing care facilities and hospitals. *Cochrane Database Syst Rev* (2010) **1**(1):CD005465. doi:10.1002/14651858.CD005465.pub2
10. American Geriatrics Society, British Geriatrics Society. *AGS/BGS Clinical Practice Guideline: Prevention of Falls in Older Persons.* New York, NY: American Geriatrics Society (2010).
11. Chou WC, Tinetti ME, King MB, Irwin K, Fortinsky RH. Perceptions of physicians on the barriers and facilitators to integrating fall risk evaluation and management into practice. *J Gen Intern Med* (2006) **21**(2):117–22. doi:10.1007/s11606-006-0244-3
12. Fortinsky RH, Iannuzzi-Sucich M, Baker DI, Gottschalk M, King MB, Brown CJ, et al. Fall-risk assessment and management in clinical practice: views from healthcare providers. *J Am Geriatr Soc* (2004) **52**(9):1522–6. doi:10.1111/j.1532-5415.2004.52416.x
13. Wagner EH. Chronic disease management: what will it take to improve care for chronic illness? *Eff Clin Pract* (1998) **1**:2–4.
14. Stevens JA, Phelan EA. Development of STEADI: a fall prevention resource for health care providers. *Health Promot Pract* (2012) **14**(5):706–14. doi:10.1177/1524839912463576
15. Centers for Disease Control and Prevention (CDC). *STEADI (Stopping Elderly Accidents, Deaths & Injuries) Tool Kit for Health Care Providers.* Atlanta, GA (2013) [Cited 2014 July 14]. Available from: http://www.cdc.gov/homeandrecreationalsafety/Falls/steadi/index.html?s_cid=tw_injdir154
16. Schuster RJ, Cherry COB, Smith ML. The clinician engagement and education session modernizing "academic detailing. *Am J Med Qual* (2013) **28**(6):533–5. doi:10.1177/1062860613491976
17. Rubenstein LZ, Solomon DH, Roth CP, Young RT, Shekelle PG, Chang JT, et al. Detection and management of falls and instability in vulnerable elders by community physicians. *J Am Geriatr Soc* (2004) **52**(9):1527–31. doi:10.1111/j.1532-5415.2004.52417.x

Permissions

 Every chapter published in this book has been scrutinized by our experts. Their significance has been extensively debated. The topics covered herein carry significant findings which will fuel the growth of the discipline. They may even be implemented as practical applications or may be referred to as a beginning point for another development.

The contributors of this book come from diverse backgrounds, making this book a truly international effort. This book will bring forth new frontiers with its revolutionizing research information and detailed analysis of the nascent developments around the world.

We would like to thank all the contributing authors for lending their expertise to make the book truly unique. They have played a crucial role in the development of this book. Without their invaluable contributions this book wouldn't have been possible. They have made vital efforts to compile up to date information on the varied aspects of this subject to make this book a valuable addition to the collection of many professionals and students.

This book was conceptualized with the vision of imparting up-to-date information and advanced data in this field. To ensure the same, a matchless editorial board was set up. Every individual on the board went through rigorous rounds of assessment to prove their worth. After which they invested a large part of their time researching and compiling the most relevant data for our readers.

The editorial board has been involved in producing this book since its inception. They have spent rigorous hours researching and exploring the diverse topics which have resulted in the successful publishing of this book. They have passed on their knowledge of decades through this book. To expedite this challenging task, the publisher supported the team at every step. A small team of assistant editors was also appointed to further simplify the editing procedure and attain best results for the readers.

Apart from the editorial board, the designing team has also invested a significant amount of their time in understanding the subject and creating the most relevant covers. They scrutinized every image to scout for the most suitable representation of the subject and create an appropriate cover for the book.

The publishing team has been an ardent support to the editorial, designing and production team. Their endless efforts to recruit the best for this project, has resulted in the accomplishment of this book. They are a veteran in the field of academics and their pool of knowledge is as vast as their experience in printing. Their expertise and guidance has proved useful at every step. Their uncompromising quality standards have made this book an exceptional effort. Their encouragement from time to time has been an inspiration for everyone.

The publisher and the editorial board hope that this book will prove to be a valuable piece of knowledge for researchers, students, practitioners and scholars across the globe.

List of Contributors

Chivon A. Mingo
Gerontology Institute, College of Arts and Sciences, Georgia State University, Atlanta, GA, USA

Matthew Lee Smith
Department of Health Promotion and Behavior, College of Public Health, The University of Georgia, Athens, GA, USA

SangNam Ahn
Division of Health Systems Management and Policy, School of Public Health, The University of Memphis, Memphis, TN, USA
Department of Health Promotion and Community Health Sciences, School of Public Health, Texas A&M Health Science Center, College Station, TX, USA

Luohua Jiang
Department of Epidemiology and Biostatistics, School of Public Health, Texas A&M Health Science Center, College Station, TX, USA

Jinmyoung Cho
Department of Health Promotion and Community Health Sciences, School of Public Health, Texas A&M Health Science Center, College Station, TX, USA
Baylor Scott & White Health, Center for Applied Health Research, Temple, TX, USA

Samuel D.Towne Jr. and Marcia G. Ory
Department of Health Promotion and Community Health Sciences, School of Public Health, Texas A&M Health Science Center, College Station, TX, USA

Luohua Jiang
Department of Epidemiology and Biostatistics, School of Public Health, Texas A&M Health Science Center, College Station, TX, USA

Matthew Lee Smith
Department of Health Promotion and Behavior, College of Public Health, The University of Georgia, Athens, GA, USA

Shuai Chen
Department of Statistics, Texas A&M University, College Station, TX, USA

SangNam Ahn
Division of Health Systems Management and Policy, School of Public Health, The University of Memphis, Memphis, TN, USA
Department of Health Promotion and Community Health Sciences, School of Public Health, Texas A&M Health Science Center, College Station, TX, USA

Kristie P. Kulinski
National Council on Aging,Washington, DC, USA

Kate Lorig
Stanford Patient Education Research Center, Department of Medicine, Stanford School of Medicine, Palo Alto, CA, USA

Marcia G. Ory
Department of Health Promotion and Community Health Sciences, School of Public Health, Texas A&M Health Science Center, College Station, TX, USA

Samuel D.Towne Jr. and Marcia G. Ory
Department of Health Promotion and Community Health Sciences, Texas A&M Health Science Center, School of Public Health, College Station, TX, USA

Matthew Lee Smith
Department of Health Promotion and Behavior, College of Public Health, University of Georgia, Athens, GA, USA

SangNam Ahn
Department of Health Promotion and Community Health Sciences, Texas A&M Health Science Center, School of Public Health, College Station, TX, USA
Division of Health Systems Management and Policy, School of Public Health, The University of Memphis, Memphis, TN, USA

Matthew Lee Smith
Department of Health Promotion and Behavior, College of Public Health, The University of Georgia, Athens, GA, USA

SangNam Ahn
Division of Health Systems Management and Policy, School of Public Health, The University of Memphis, Memphis, TN, USA
Department of Health Promotion and Community Health Sciences, Texas A&M Health Science Center, School of Public Health, College Station, TX, USA

Luohua Jiang
Department of Epidemiology and Biostatistics, Texas A&M Health Science Center, School of Public Health, College Station, TX, USA

Kristie P. Kulinski
National Council on Aging,Washington, DC, USA

Marcia G. Ory
Department of Health Promotion and Community Health Sciences, Texas A&M Health Science Center, School of Public Health, College Station, TX, USA

Kristie P. Kulinski
National Council on Aging,Washington, DC, USA

Michele Boutaugh
Administration on Aging, Administration for Community Living, Atlanta, GA, USA

Matthew Lee Smith
Department of Health Promotion and Behavior, College of Public Health, The University of Georgia, Athens, GA, USA

Marcia G. Ory 4
Department of Health Promotion and Community Health Sciences, School of Public Health, Texas A&M Health Science Center, College Station, TX, USA

Kate Lorig
Stanford Patient Education Research Center, Department of Medicine, Stanford School of Medicine, Palo Alto, CA, USA

Matthew Lee Smith
Department of Health Promotion and Behavior, College of Public Health, The University of Georgia, Athens, GA, USA

Marcia G. Ory and Scott Horel
Department of Health Promotion and Community Health Sciences, Texas A&M Health Science Center, School of Public Health, College Station, TX, USA

SangNam Ahn
Department of Health Promotion and Community Health Sciences, Texas A&M Health Science Center, School of Public Health, College Station, TX, USA
Division of Health Systems Management and Policy, School of Public Health, The University of Memphis, Memphis, TN, USA

Kristie P. Kulinski
National Council on Aging,Washington, DC, USA

Luohua Jiang
Department of Epidemiology and Biostatistics, Texas A&M Health Science Center, School of Public Health, College Station, TX, USA

Deborah Paone
Paone & Associates, LLC, Minneapolis, MN, USA

Shuo Liu
Department of Social Medicine and Management, School of Public Health, Peking University, Beijing, China

Kate Lorig
Department of Medicine, Stanford Patient Education Research Center, Stanford School of Medicine, Palo Alto, CA, USA

SangNam Ahn
Division of Health Systems Management and Policy, School of Public Health, The University of Memphis, Memphis, TN, USA
Department of Health Promotion and Community Health Sciences, Texas A&M Health Science Center, School of Public Health, College Station, TX, USA

Matthew Lee Smith
Department of Health Promotion and Behavior, College of Public Health, The University of Georgia, Athens, GA, USA

Mary Altpeter
Center for Health Promotion and Disease Prevention, The University of North Carolina at Chapel Hill, Chapel Hill, NC, USA

Basia Belza
School of Nursing, Biobehavioral Nursing and Health Systems, The University ofWashington, Seattle,WA, USA

Lindsey Post
Division of Health Systems Management and Policy, School of Public Health, The University of Memphis, Memphis, TN, USA

Marcia G. Ory
Department of Health Promotion and Community Health Sciences, Texas A&M Health Science Center, School of Public Health, College Station, TX, USA

Ellen C. Schneider
Center for Health Promotion and Disease Prevention, University of North Carolina at Chapel Hill, Chapel Hill, NC, USA

(Bonita) Lynn Beattie
Falls Free® Initiative, National Council on Aging,Washington, DC, USA

Matthew Lee Smith
Department of Health Promotion and Behavior, College of Public Health, The University of Georgia, Athens, GA, USA

Kristie P. Kulinski
National Council on Aging,Washington, DC, USA

Marcia G. Ory
Department of Health Promotion and Community Health Sciences, Texas A&M Health Science Center School of Public Health, College Station, TX, USA

Luohua Jiang
Department of Epidemiology, School of Medicine, University of California Irvine, Irvine, CA, USA

Kate Lorig
Stanford Patient Education Research Center, Department of Medicine, Stanford University School of Medicine, Palo Alto, CA, USA

SangNam Ahn
Department of Health Promotion and Community Health Sciences, Texas A&M Health Science Center School of Public Health, College Station, TX, USA
Division of Health Systems Management and Policy, School of Public Health, The University of Memphis, Memphis, TN, USA

SangNam Ahn
Division of Health Systems Management and Policy, School of Public Health, The University of Memphis, Memphis, TN, USA
Department of Health Promotion and Community Health Sciences, School of Public Health, Texas A&M Health Science Center, College Station, TX, USA

Matthew Lee Smith
Department of Health Promotion and Behavior, College of Public Health, The University of Georgia, Athens, GA, USA

Jinmyoung Cho
Department of Health Promotion and Community Health Sciences, School of Public Health, Texas A&M Health Science Center, College Station, TX, USA
Center for Applied Health Research, Baylor Scott & White Healthcare, Temple, TX, USA

Luohua Jiang
Department of Epidemiology, School of Medicine, University of California Irvine, Irvine, CA, USA

Lindsey Post
Division of Health Systems Management and Policy, School of Public Health, The University of Memphis, Memphis, TN, USA

Marcia G. Ory
Department of Health Promotion and Community Health Sciences, School of Public Health, Texas A&M Health Science Center, College Station, TX, USA

Colette Joy Browning
Royal District Nursing Service Institute, St Kilda, VIC, Australia
School of Primary Health Care, Monash University
School of Primary Health Care, Monash University, Melbourne, VIC, Australia

HuiYang
School of Primary Health Care, Monash University
School of Primary Health Care, Monash University, Melbourne, VIC, Australia

Tuohong Zhang
Research Center for Ageing and Health Services, Department of Global Health, Peking University, Beijing, China

Anna Chapman and Joanne Enticott
School of Primary Health Care, Monash University
School of Primary Health Care, Monash University, Melbourne, VIC, Australia

Shane Andrew Thomas
School of Primary Health Care, Monash University
School of Primary Health Care, Monash University, Melbourne, VIC, Australia
The University of Adelaide, Adelaide, SA, Australia

Rashmita Basu and Angela K. Hochhalter
Baylor Scott & White Health, Temple, TX, USA

Marcia G. Ory and Samuel D.Towne Jr.
Department of Health Promotion and Community Health Sciences, School of Public Health, Texas A&M Health Science Center, College Station, TX, USA

Matthew Lee Smith
Department of Health Promotion and Behavior, College of Public Health, The University of Georgia, Athens, GA, USA

SangNam Ahn
Division of Health Systems Management and Policy, School of Public Health, The University of Memphis, Memphis, TN, USA

Marcia G. Ory and Ashley D. Wilson
Department of Health Promotion and Community Health Sciences, Texas A&M Health Science Center School of Public Health, College Station, TX, USA

Matthew Lee Smith
Department of Health Promotion and Behavior, The University of Georgia College of Public Health, Athens, GA, USA

Erin M. Parker, Judy A. Stevens, Heidi Ehrenreich and Robin Lee
National Center for Injury Prevention and Control, Centers for Disease Control and Prevention, Atlanta, GA, USA

Luohua Jiang
Department of Epidemiology and Biostatistics, Texas A&M Health Science Center School of Public Health, College Station, TX, USA

Shuai Chen
Department of Statistics, Texas A&M University, College Station, TX, USA

Philip Lloyd Ritter, Audrey Alonis, Diana D. Laurent and Kate Lorig
Stanford Patient Education Research Center, Stanford School of Medicine, Stanford, CA, USA

Marcia G. Ory
School of Public Health, Texas A&M University, College Station, TX, USA

Matthew Lee Smith
College of Public Health, The University of Georgia, Athens, GA, USA

Luohua Jiang
Department of Epidemiology & Biostatistics, School of Public Health, Texas A&M Health Science Center, College Station, TX, USA

MichiyoTomioka and Kathryn L. Braun
Office of Public Health Studies, University of Hawai'i at M¯anoa, Honolulu, HI, USA

Betsy C. Risendal and Andrea Dwyer
Community and Behavioral Health, Colorado School of Public Health, Aurora, CO, USA

RichardW. Seidel
Carilion Clinic, Virginia Tech Carilion School of Medicine, Roanoke, VA, USA

Kate Lorig
School of Medicine, Stanford University, Stanford, CA, USA

Letoynia Coombs
Colorado Health Outcomes, University of Colorado, Aurora, CO, USA

Marcia G. Ory
Health Promotion and Community Health Sciences, Texas A&M Health Science Center School of Public Health, College Station, TX, USA

Marcia G. Ory and Ashley D. Wilson
Department of Health Promotion and Community Health Sciences, Texas A&M Health Science Center, College Station, TX, USA

Matthew Lee Smith
Department of Health Promotion and Behavior, The University of Georgia College of Public Health, Athens, GA, USA

Luohua Jiang
Department of Epidemiology, University of California, Irvine, CA, USA
Department of Statistics, Texas A&M University, College Station, TX, USA

Robin Lee4, Judy A. Stevens4 and Erin M. Parker
National Center for Injury Prevention and Control, Centers for Disease Control and Prevention, Atlanta, GA, USA

Shuai Chen
Department of Statistics, Texas A&M University, College Station, TX, USA

Matthew Lee Smith, Mark G. Wilson, David M. DeJoy, Heather Padilla and Heather Zuercher
Workplace Health Group, Department of Health Promotion and Behavior, College of Public Health, The University of Georgia, Athens, GA, USA

Phaedra Corso
Department of Health Policy and Management, College of Public Health, The University of Georgia, Athens, GA, USA

RobertVandenberg
Department of Management, Terry College of Business, The University of Georgia, Athens, GA, USA

Kate Lorig
Stanford Patient Education Research Center, Department of Medicine, Stanford School of Medicine, Palo Alto, CA, USA

Marcia G. Ory
Department of Health Promotion and Community Health Sciences, Texas A&M Health Science Center School of Public Health, College Station, TX, USA

Marcia G. Ory, Doris Howell, Alyson Zollinger and Cindy Quinn
Department of Health Promotion and Community Health Sciences, Texas A&M Health Science Center School of Public Health, College Station, TX, USA

Alan B. Stevens
Baylor Scott & White Health, Temple, TX, USA

Matthew Lee Smith
Department of Health Promotion and Behavior, College of Public Health, The University of Georgia, Athens, GA, USA

Suzanne M. Swierc
Big Brothers Big Sisters of South Texas, San Antonio, TX, USA

Julie A. St. John
Department of Public Health, Graduate School of Biomedical Sciences, Texas Tech University Health Sciences Center, Abilene, TX, USA

Tiffany E. Shubert
Division of Geriatrics, School of Medicine, University of North Carolina at Chapel Hill, Chapel Hill, NC, USA

Matthew Lee Smith
College of Public Health, The University of Georgia, Athens, GA, USA

Cherie A. Rosemond
Center for Health Promotion and Disease Prevention, University of North Carolina at Chapel Hill, Chapel Hill, NC, USA

Doris A. Howell
Program on Healthy Aging, Texas A&M Health Science Center School of Public Health, College Station, TX, USA

Christopher E. Beaudoin
Department of Communication, Texas A&M University, College Station, TX, USA

Marcia G. Ory
Department of Health Promotion and Community Health Sciences, Texas A&M Health Science Center School of Public Health, College Station, TX, USA

Tiffany E. Shubert and Cristine B. Clarke
Center for Aging and Health, University of North Carolina, School of Medicine, Chapel Hill, NC, USA

Matthew Lee Smith
College of Public Health, The University of Georgia, Athens, GA, USA

Marcia G. Ory
Department of Health Promotion and Community Health Sciences, Texas A&M School of Public Health, College Station, TX, USA

Stephanie A. Bomberger
University of North Carolina Center for Health Promotion and Disease Prevention, Chapel Hill, NC, USA

Ellen Roberts and Jan Busby-Whitehead
Division of Geriatrics, University of North Carolina, School of Medicine, Chapel Hill, NC, USA

Jinmyoung Cho
Center for Applied Health Research, Baylor Scott & White Health, Temple, TX, USA
Department of Health Promotion and Community Health Science, Texas A&M Health Science Center, USA

Matthew Lee Smith
Department of Health Promotion and Community Health Science, Texas A&M Health Science Center School of Public Health, College Station, TX, USA
Department of Health Promotion and Behavior, The University of Georgia, Athens, GA, USA

Tiffany E. Shubert
School of Medicine, University of North Carolina, Chapel Hill, NC, USA

Luohua Jiang
Department of Epidemiology, School of Medicine, University of California, Irvine, CA, USA
Department of Epidemiology and Biostatistics, Texas A&M Health Science Center School of Public Health, College Station, TX, USA

SangNam Ahn
Department of Health Promotion and Community Health Science, Texas A&M Health Science Center School of Public Health, College Station, TX, USA
Division of Health Systems Management and Policy, The University of Memphis, Memphis, TN, USA

Marcia G. Ory
Department of Health Promotion and Community Health Science, Texas A&M Health Science Center School of Public Health, College Station, TX, USA

Marcia G. Ory, Shinduk Lee and Alyson Zollinger
Department of Health Promotion and Community Health Sciences, Texas A&M Health Science Center, School of Public Health, College Station, TX, USA

Kiran Bhurtyal
Office of Surveillance, Evaluation, and Research, Texas Department of State Health Services, Austin, TX, USA

Ann-Hilary Heston
Healthy Living Department,YMCA of the USA, Chicago, IL, USA

Luohua Jiang
Department of Epidemiology and Biostatistics, Texas A&M Health Science Center, School of Public Health, College Station, TX, USA

Matthew Lee Smith
Department of Health Promotion and Behavior, College of Public Health, The University of Georgia, Athens, GA, USA

Laura Farren1 and Lesley Steinman
Health Promotion Research Center, University ofWashington, Seattle,WA, USA

Mark Snowden
Department of Psychiatry and Behavioral Sciences, Harborview Medical Center, University ofWashington, Seattle,WA, USA

Maria Monroe-DeVita
Division of Public Behavioral Health and Justice Policy, Department of Psychiatry and Behavioral Sciences, University ofWashington, Seattle,WA, USA

Samuel D.Towne Jr. and Marcia G. Ory
Department of Health Promotion and Community Health Sciences, Texas A&M Health Science Center School of Public Health, College Station, TX, USA

Matthew Lee Smith
Department of Health Promotion and Behavior, College of Public Health, The University of Georgia, Athens, GA, USA

SangNam Ahn
Department of Health Promotion and Community Health Sciences, Texas A&M Health Science Center School of Public Health, College Station, TX, USA
Division of Health Systems Management and Policy, School of Public Health, The University of Memphis, Memphis, TN, USA

Mary Altpeter
University of North Carolina at Chapel Hill, Chapel Hill, NC, USA

Basia Belza
Biobehavioral Nursing and Health Systems, School of Nursing, University ofWashington, Seattle,WA, USA

Kristie Patton Kulinski
National Council on Aging,Washington, DC, USA

Jana Reynolds
Baylor Scott & White Health, Temple, TX, USA
Baylor Charles A. Sammons Cancer Center, Baylor University Medical Center at Dallas, Dallas, TX, USA

LorieThibodeaux
Baylor Scott & White Health, Temple, TX, USA
Seton Medical Center, Austin, TX, USA

Luohua Jiang
School of Rural Public Health, Texas A&M Health Science Center, College Station, TX, USA

Kevin Francis and Angie Hochhalter
Baylor Scott & White Health, Temple, TX, USA

Basia Belza
Health Promotion Research Center, University ofWashington, Seattle,WA, USA
School of Nursing, University ofWashington, Seattle,WA, USA

Miruna Petrescu-Prahova, Marlana Kohn, Laura Farren and Grace Kline
Health Promotion Research Center, University ofWashington, Seattle,WA, USA

Christina E. Miyawaki
Health Promotion Research Center, University ofWashington, Seattle,WA, USA
School of SocialWork, University ofWashington, Seattle,WA, USA

Mark B. Snowden and Whitney L. Carlson
Department of Psychiatry and Behavioral Sciences, University ofWashington School of Medicine, Seattle,WA, USA

Lesley E. Steinman
Health Promotion Research Center, University ofWashington, Seattle,WA, USA

Kara N. Mochan
University ofWashington School of Nursing with Environmental Health Focus, Seattle,WA, USA
Adolescent Medicine, Seattle Children's, Seattle,WA, USA

Ana F. Abraido-Lanza
Department of Sociomedical Sciences, Columbia University Mailman School of Public Health, NewYork, NY, USA

Lucinda L. Bryant
Department of Community and Behavioral Health, Colorado School of Public Health, University of Colorado Denver, Aurora, CO, USA

Michael Duffy
Department of Educational Psychology, Counseling Psychology Program, Texas A&M University, College Station, TX, USA

Bob G. Knight
Davis School of Gerontology and Department of Psychology, University of Southern California, Los Angeles, CA, USA

DilipV. Jeste
Sam and Rose Stein Institute for Research on Aging and Department of Psychiatry, University of California San Diego, San Diego, CA, USA

Katherine H. Leith
College of SocialWork, University of South Carolina, Columbia, SC, USA

Eric J. Lenze
Department of Psychiatry,Washington University School of Medicine, St Louis, MO, USA

Rebecca G. Logsdon
Department of Psychosocial and Community Health, University ofWashington School of Nursing, Seattle,WA, USA

William A. Satariano
School of Public Health, University of California Berkeley, Berkeley, CA, USA

Damita J. Zweiback
Division of Chronic Disease and Injury Prevention, Michigan Department of Community Health, Lansing, MI, USA
Healthy Aging Council and Health Equity Council, National Association of Chronic Disease Directors, Atlanta, GA, USA

Lynda A. Anderson
National Center for Chronic Disease Prevention and Health Promotion, Centers for Disease Control and Prevention, Atlanta, GA, USA
Rollins School of Public Health, Emory University, Atlanta, GA, USA

Matthew Lee Smith
Department of Health Promotion and Behavior, College of Public Health, The University of Georgia, Athens, GA, USA

Judy A. Stevens and Heidi Ehrenreich
National Center for Injury Prevention and Control, Centers for Disease Control and Prevention, Atlanta, GA, USA

Ashley D. Wilson and Marcia G. Ory
Department of Health Promotion and Community Health Sciences, Texas A&M Health Science Center School of Public Health, College Station, TX, USA

Richard J. Schuster and Colleen O'Brien Cherry
Center for Global Health, College of Public Health, The University of Georgia, Athens, GA, USA

Index